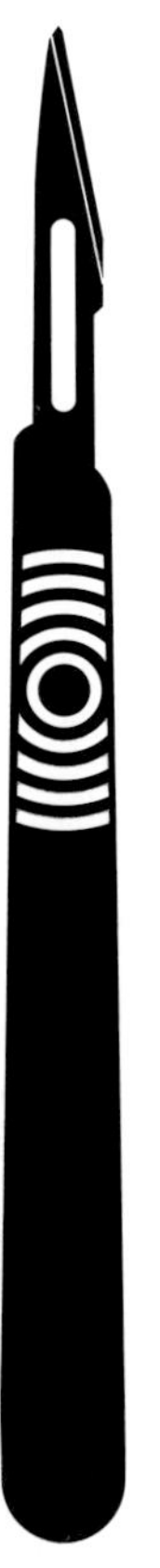

Aesthetic Surgery

ED. ANGELIKA TASCHEN

TASCHEN

KÖLN LONDON LOS ANGELES MADRID PARIS TOKYO

VII.

The World's most Famous Aesthetic Surgeons 178

Interviews by Eva Karcher, Munich and Richard Rushfield, Los Angeles

---

VIII.

Statements by the World's most Famous Aesthetic Surgeons 260

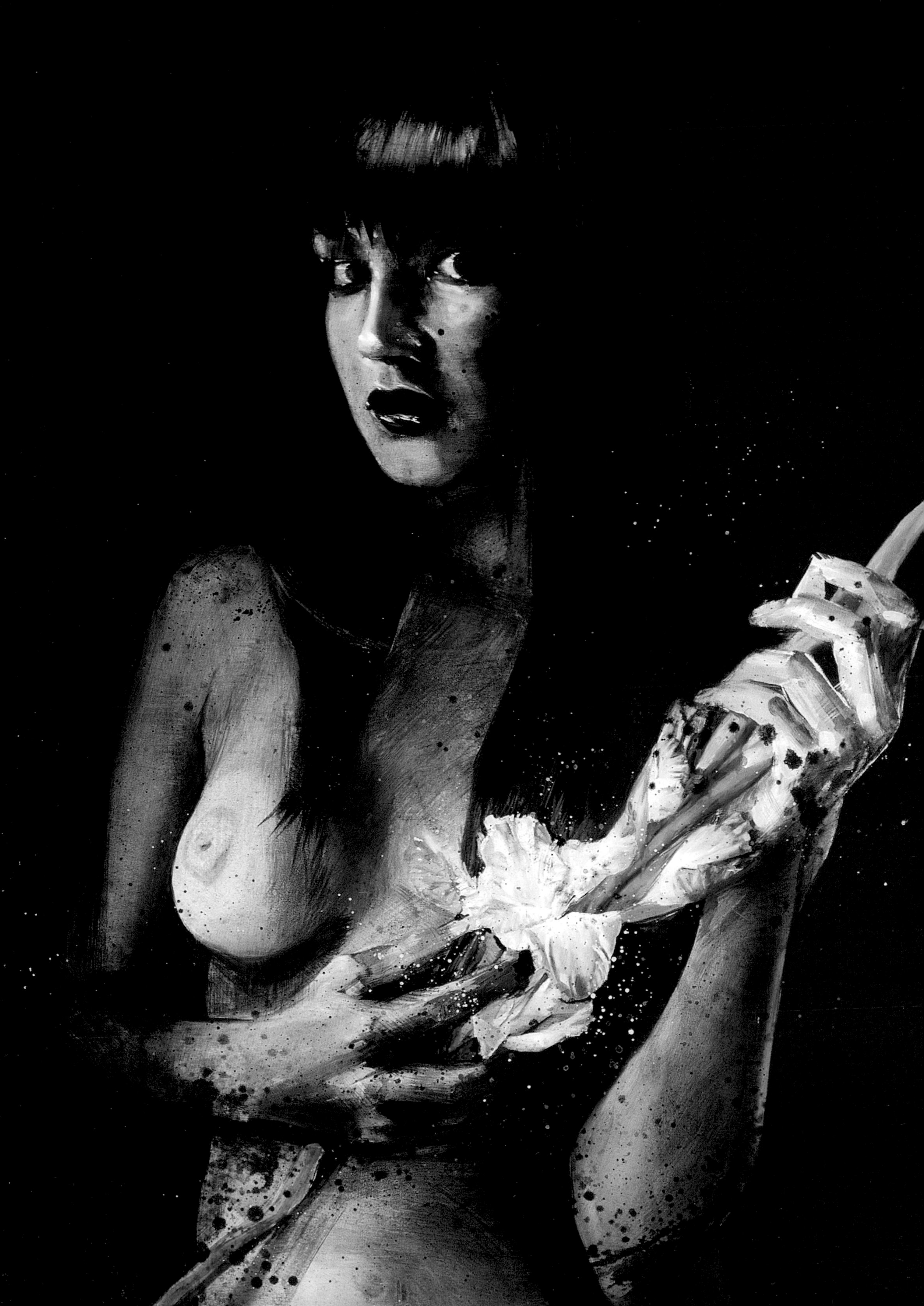

I.

BEAUTY AND BEAUTY SURGERY

Preface by
ANGELIKA TASCHEN

Beauty and Beauty Surgery

ANGELIKA TASCHEN, Berlin

Aesthetic surgery is booming. Especially in the last decade, the annual growth figure for surgical treatments has risen drastically all over the world: in the United States, for example, 2.1 million operations were performed in 1997, a figure that reached 8.8 million by 2003. With such a steep increase, the statistics undeniably reflect an explosion in popularity. Cosmetic methods and surgical techniques are becoming more sophisticated and the results are improving continually. Faster healing, lower pain levels and less visible scarring tempt more and more people to try out surgery. The age range of the patients is also widening – treatments are becoming increasingly popular with young people. Correspondingly, the technical scope of aesthetic surgery is ever broadening.

Unlike in previous decades, aesthetic surgery is no longer the prerogative of the rich. Women as well as men from all walks of life regularly have breast enlargements or reductions, liposuction, hair transplants, facelifts, blepharoplasty, Botox injections and numerous other treatments. A thriving industry has emerged, including its own tourism branch – offering scalpel safaris to South Africa and budget operations in the Near and Far East, for example in Thailand. Paralleling the overall rise in operative treatment, the share of male patients has risen considerably. In 2002, more than 15 percent of surgical patients were male, a tendency that has continued to climb since. Interestingly, almost all of the first patients in the history of aesthetic surgery – which reaches further back than most readers would be inclined to think – were men. Only at the end of the 19th century did the number of female patients begin to outweigh the number of male patients.

Humanity's search for ways to enhance physical beauty is as old as mankind itself. The beginnings of aesthetic surgery go right back to the beginnings of medicine. Accounts of rhinoplasties and scar treatment can be traced back as far as Ancient Egypt, but it was really the emergence of syphilis in 15th-century Europe that established the need for reconstructive surgery: As a result of the first epidemic in 1495, countless victims' faces were disfigured. Culturally, this was highly stigmatising. Surgical techniques were quickly developed to treat the disease's symptoms, in particular the disfigured noses. Most of the patients were men, desperate to be rid of the disgrace of being infected and culturally vilified. In this time, the concept of anaesthesia was still unheard of – sedation was only discovered in 1846 – and there was little knowledge about the existence, causes and treatment of infections. Surgery, therefore, was not only excruciatingly painful but also bore a substantial risk of postoperative death.

In 1597, a rhinoplasty – performed by the Bolognese surgeon Gaspare Tagliacozzi and documented in 22 woodcuts complete with Latin captions – took more than 20 days to be completed. The patient had to endure this time without any painkillers or anaesthetics. The pain that was experienced defies description. In the chapter "The Astonishing History of Aesthetic Surgery," you will find reproductions of most of the 22 plates from Tagliacozzi's milestone reference work, providing feasible visual descriptions of this surgical procedure. Tagliacozzi's method of reconstructing a nose was imitated right up to the beginning of the 20th century. Over the centuries, other medical practitioners similarly developed techniques that have retained their validity to the present day. The different methods of rhinoplasty, blepharoplasty and other operative corrections encountered throughout modern history are depicted here with a selection of illustrations from historical medicine manuals. Nearly every historical reference work on plastic surgery ever published is held at the Health Sciences Library of Columbia University (New York). I was permitted to research the books of the library liberally and extensively, and the reproductions presented here were photographed from these sources.

It may surprise some to learn that the history of aesthetic surgery was not written by the surgeons of the United States in the 20th century, but predominantly by German doctors who also worked in the field of plastic surgery. Carl Ferdinand von Graefe (1787–1840), Eduard Zeis (1807–1868), Hermann Eduard Fritze (1811–1866), Johann Friedrich Dieffenbach (1792–1847) and Jacques

fig. previous pages

Martin Eder "Don't Trust Violence", Oil on canvas on wood, 130 x 100 cm, 2003. Collection of Rosette Delug, courtesy of EIGEN+ART gallery, Leipzig/Berlin. Photo: © Uwe Walter

Joseph (1865–1934) are but some of the pioneers who have defined the practices of aesthetic surgery around the world. In pre-war Germany, these men performed a multitude of operations as well as publishing details of their surgical innovations. Their books disseminated the techniques in question around the entire globe.

Cosmetic surgery as we know it today had many of its roots in World War I, again largely to the credit of German surgeons. The number of war invalids and disfigured victims was so overwhelming that surgeons were forced to improvise and experiment, and in the course of their work they developed innovative new surgical techniques.

Only with the expertise gained during and after the war was it possible to turn pretty starlets into flawless beauties of the silver screen. As cinema's significance as a medium for mass entertainment and manipulation was rising, film was both defining and propagating the aesthetics of female beauty. From the silent film era to the early 1930s, the film industry flourished particularly in Germany. Under the Nazi regime, however, many filmmakers emigrated to Hollywood. To this day, Hollywood is the epicentre of the international film industry. The new cinematic icons and idols based themselves in Hollywood, and with them they brought a flock of plastic surgeons to satisfy their endless need for beautification. Soon, a significant aesthetic surgery industry emerged in Hollywood, and Los Angeles is still home to the biggest per-capita number of cosmetic surgeons.

In the 1920s, Hollywood introduced the concept of the camera close-up, an extreme zoom into the actor's face that not only engages the viewer's emotions but also mercilessly reveals any flaws in the face of the actor or actress shown. Accordingly, studio mogul Louis B. Mayer forced Greta Garbo to get her teeth fixed; Marlene Dietrich had a rhinoplasty (nose job) in 1929, and Rita Hayworth had to get her hairline shifted. Marilyn Monroe got rid of "bumps on the nose" as well as having a "small flaw around the chin" corrected with cartilage, as writer Norman Mailer reveals. There is conflicting information about her breasts – the claim that Marilyn had complained about her inflamed and suppurating breasts shortly before her death is now doubted. Apparently, she had had an injection of liquid silicone, which was later taken off the market.

To this day, Hollywood's big-budget productions define concepts of beauty for women around the world – as well as for men. Actors and actresses are turned into role models of physical aesthetics, blueprints for our perception of beauty. In the past, the higher echelons of society determined the styles and standards of beauty; people have always looked up to and striven for the next step up on the social ladder. In times of famine, voluptuous bodies were regarded as beautiful. When men and women worked the fields, a pale complexion was favoured; now that many work in offices, a tan is preferable – to show that holidays are affordable (despite the fact that the bronze skin colour usually comes from the tanning studio). In the Roaring Twenties, androgynous faces and bodies were popular, as homosexuality and bisexuality were being treated more openly; in the 1950s, the buxom pin-up girl was favoured, as women's lives were focused on finding a husband and becoming a mother. All of these female and male images are reflected and perpetuated in the movies. In order to satisfy the requirements of their character stereotypes and the revealing dimensions of the cinema screen, most actors and actresses have had to resort to cosmetic surgery to protect their careers. Today, this is truer than ever.

When the well-known German actress Hildegard Knef had a facelift in the United States in the 1980s, audiences were shocked upon her return to Germany. "Too late, too much," many of the critics concluded. This deterring "Knef" effect is deeply ingrained – hardly any celebrities or other public figures in Germany ever admit to cosmetic surgery. Currently, talkshow host Sabine Christiansen is suing a magazine that claimed she had a facelift, similarly the actress Christine Kauffmann, ex-wife of Tony Curtis. German chancellor Gerhard Schröder even sued tabloids that claimed he dyed his hair.

Aesthetic surgery is treated more candidly in the US. Many celebrities openly talk about the operations they have undergone. Phyllis Diller was the first to breach the erstwhile taboo, making headlines in 1971 when she publicly divulged details of her operations. Supposedly she once said, "the only parts left of my original body are my elbows." Cher only admitted to surgical treatments much later, and Jane Fonda initially derided "those plastic blow-up tits" – until her husband left her in 1988 and she had a breast enlargement. The actress, a former counter-culture icon, has had numerous other surgical treatments since. "Baywatch" star Pamela Anderson loves to celebrate her body and its alterations in public, informing the press of every minute change: her breasts get enlarged, reduced and enlarged again; her lips are enlarged; old tattoos are removed, new tattoos are added.

In the US, entire TV series – soap operas, documentaries and reality soaps – are being produced to deal with the phenomenon of cosmetic surgery. They have proven to be hugely successful and quickly spread around the world. ABC's "Extreme Makeover" is one of the biggest successes to date. The show's application form promises prospective candidates that, should they be selected, "we will give you a truly Cinderella-like experience by changing your looks completely in an effort to transform your life and destiny, and to make your dreams come true." In each episode, the participant is first shown in the relative squalor of her pre-"Makeover" life; next, she is chauffeured from operation to operation in a stately limousine. The made-over participant then recuperates at the luxurious "Makeover Mansion," situated in the Hollywood Hills and featuring a great panoramic view, a swimming pool, a high-tech gym and state-of-the-art entertainment technology. The highlight of the show unfolds at the end – beautiful Cinderella, operated on extensively and completely re-styled, finally gets to meet up with her friends and family. In Germany, more than 3,000 hopefuls applied to the TV channel RTL to be included in a local series based on "Extreme Makeover." After the series was produced, however, it was shelved; the German Society for Aesthetic Plastic Surgery boycotted it.

In July 2003, the soap opera "Nip/Tuck" was aired for the first time. By October 2004, 30 episodes were screened; the series was so successful that a new season has already been planned for 2005. The story is set in South Florida, presenting the lives of two surgeons working at a cosmetic surgery centre. "Nip/Tuck" deals with the darker sides of surgical beautification, presenting failed operations, infidelity, criminal plots, drugs and ruthless capitalist greed. The operations shown are bloody orgies, the setting resembling a butchery rather than a sterile surgical theatre.

In direct competition to "Extreme Makeover," Fox has produced "The Swan" – a highly successful reality show that reaches 15 million viewers per screening in the US alone. 17 female and male candidates, mostly plain-looking, shy people who can't afford cosmetic surgery, have so far received an all-round surgical renewal with countless different treatments – for free. Usually, the operations would cost up to US$ 250,000. A professional team consisting of a personal coach, a therapist, a fitness trainer, a dentist and several cosmetic surgeons is assigned to each selected participant. Over a period of three months, they work on the physical, mental and emotional transformation of their "ugly duckling." The participants do not have access to any mirrors in this time, and contact to their families is restricted to three weekly telephone calls of no more than ten minutes. The highlight of the show is the beauty pageant held at the end of the series – one of the formerly ugly ducklings is crowned the most beautiful swan. In each episode, a finalist for the pageant is selected: two participants are presented to the audience with detailed flashbacks to their three-month beautification regime, and the viewers vote on the best results. The German TV channel Pro Sieben has bought the rights to "The Swan".

Another series takes the concept one step further – MTV's "I Want A Famous Face" has been a hot topic of debate even among the most cynical of Hollywood's glamour set. The first season presented six 30-minute episodes, which have now also been aired by MTV Germany – albeit accompanied by great controversy and slotted exclusively after 11pm (similarly the German version of the "The Swan"). The Head of the German Commission for the Protection of Minors against Harmful Media Content, Wolf-Dietrich Ring, had his reasons for keeping these shows well out of primetime: "Young viewers are at a crucial stage of developing their own identity. These programmes suggest that appearance is all that matters, and that appearance can furthermore be manipulated at will. A negative influence on the formative development of minors cannot be excluded." In the MTV show, a pair of twins suddenly looked like a pair of Brad Pitts, one man was turned into Jennifer Lopez (complete with breasts), other participants were transformed into Elvis Presley, Kate Winslet, Pamela Anderson and Britney Spears. However, MTV didn't sponsor the required operations. A main consultant for this series was Dr. Randal Hayworth, one of the two plastic surgeons also featured on "Extreme Makeover." Hayworth has openly and willingly admitted that his Los Angeles practice has benefited greatly from the increased interest in cosmetic surgery generated by the series.

In stark contrast to this attitude, many surgeons – including numerous Americans – warn of the exaggerated and unrealistic expectations created by series such as these. They are concerned that people will believe everything is possible, instantly; that cosmetic surgery will degenerate into a coveted product of consumer hype, where the risks to body and soul are ignored and neglected.

The reality TV series mentioned are extremely popular, and new formats are being developed all over the world. Newspapers are also increasingly engaging in the topic of cosmetic surgery with lengthy articles and exposés. The book market offers countless reference guides that explain how to find the best surgeon, how much to pay for an operation, what happens during surgery, how long healing takes etc. Many of these publications are written by surgeons who themselves run large-scale practices and medical centres. As well as these practical guides, plenty of specialist medical literature is available. As yet, however, there hasn't been a comprehensive publication that presents and discusses the cultural, sociological, historical, spiritual and ethnic details of the topic. The book at hand traces the history and ethnic contexts of aesthetic surgery, as well as addressing some fundamental questions – why people want cosmetic surgery despite having healthy bodies, for example, or how surgeons feel about themselves, their work and their profession, and if they perceive an artistic dimension in their work. The book also traces the historical development of different surgical techniques – failures and successes alike – and takes a closer look at the pioneering surgeons and patients involved. The future of aesthetic surgery is also discussed.

An in-depth technical chapter depicts and describes all the techniques, treatments and possibilities currently offered in the field of cosmetic surgery. The before-and-after illustrations that accompany this chapter provide telling evidence of the methods described.

Foremostly, however, this book examines the relationship between age and beauty. As society itself is growing older, the cult of youth and beauty is becoming more significant than ever. Throughout the world, aging is no longer regarded as a natural process but as a condition that should be averted by any possible means – especially with the help of cosmetic surgery. In addition, the world's concerted push for globalisation is fast standardising the aesthetics of human beauty everywhere. In Brazil, the traditional ideal of female beauty stipulates small breasts and accentuated buttocks, but in keeping with today's globalised aesthetics, many Brazilian women are now getting breast enlargements instead of reductions. All over the world, a homogenised ideal of beauty is being defined by the media – predominantly in advertising and Hollywood blockbusters. Beauty is being reduced to a handful of actors, actresses and models. With the help of cosmetic surgery, these are easily imitated; liposuction, breast implants and reductions, rhinoplasties, lip injections, Botox treatments, facelifts etc. bring physical perfection within everybody's reach. Even the vagina can now be rejuvenated – hardly any part of the body, intimate or not, can still be taken to faithfully indicate the true age of a person.

In China, women get their legs extended in torturous stretching procedures that often last for several months; the fashion models of the world, advertising clothes and products in China like everywhere else, have "beautiful" long legs. In Japan and other countries of the Far East, children and teenagers get their eyelids operated on to look more Western, whereas African Americans get their noses and lips narrowed – everywhere, people are subordinating their individual identity to the so-called Caucasian ideal of beauty.

40 of the world's most prominent surgeons were interviewed for this book. They were asked what beauty and aging meant to them; if they believed beauty was based on appearance; if wrinkled old people could still be considered beautiful; if beautiful people had better sex; which living human beings and which artworks they considered beautiful; if they regarded themselves as artists; and what they thought the future holds for cosmetic surgery. All of the practitioners interviewed were given the same 19 questions. The range and depth of answers was greater than I could have imagined. Seeing that it is the basis of their livelihood, I had assumed that external appearance meant much more to plastic surgeons than their answers now suggest. At least the prolific surgeons, it turns out, have highly complex and unusual ideas about beauty, and it is precisely this refusal to conform to obvious aesthetic norms that makes a surgeon excellent.

When asked whether they believed beautiful people had better sex, the answers were very similar across the board – again a surprising result. Most surgeons agreed that beauty and the quality of sexual experience were unrelated or even had a negative effect: either the beautiful person or his/her partner could potentially experience stress caused by exaggerated sexual expectation. With beauty out of the equation, plain-looking people are perceived to have equally fulfilling sex, and sex is even perceived to improve with age.

When asked about their more well-known patients, the surgeons uniformly refused to break their professional vows of secrecy. Whereas the Hippocratic oath stipulates secrecy "for the benefit of the sick," these practitioners frequently operate on perfectly healthy people, so the relevance of the oath is debatable. It certainly would have been interesting to find out first-hand which surgeon has worked on which celebrity! In the harsh reality of the industry, on the other hand, there are cautionary examples such as Sharon Stone's current case against a cosmetic surgeon who supposedly had claimed in a magazine and on his website to have performed a facelift on Stone; in his defence, the surgeon declared that he only used Stone's face as an example for a special facelifting technique.

In fact, a chapter initially planned about celebrities and their surgical beautification treatments had to be dropped to avoid legal complications. Even Michael Jackson has claimed in television interviews that he has only had two operations on his nose and chin – after a pyrotechnics-related accident while filming a Pepsi Cola commercial, supposedly – and that his skin is only as white as it is because of a pigment cell disorder. Experts in the field disagree – Jackson's surgeon Steven Hoefflin is estimated to have performed at least 20 operations on the pop star's nose. As Stuttgart surgeon Rolf Münker reads the physical evidence: "The ridge of the singer's nose was narrowed so much that in the end, the tip simply fell off." Faced with such a challenging scenario, Hoefflin may well have used silicone injections and reconstructed the nose with cartilage from the ears – a method that frequently leaves visible "gaps" in the shape of the nose. At the end of the treatment, the nose was stabilised, but it had lost most of its natural appearance. Other stars, in contrast, are very candid about their operations. Rap star Lil' Kim makes no excuses: "I do whatever will make me feel good. I'm simply improving my external appearance."

There is a great internet site to debunk the beauty myths surrounding celebrities, describing itself as "the good, the bad and the ugly of plastic surgery" – www.awfulplasticsurgery.com. New entries and incidents are added to the website on a near-daily basis. Its archive offers illuminating before / after comparisons for stars such as Meg Ryan, Jennifer Lopez, Linda Evans, Courtney Love, Victoria Beckham, Lil' Kim, Catherine Zeta-Jones, Emanuelle Beart, Billy Bob Thornton, Burt Reynolds, Al Pacino and many more. Insightful commentaries are provided throughout.

Considering the global boom in cosmetic surgery, largely fuelled by Hollywood's lavish productions and surgically beautified actors and actresses (their faces manipulated by a few Botox or collagen injections at the very least), it is not surprising that some of the films produced engage in this topic to a greater or lesser degree. This is described in detail in the chapter under the slogan "Identity Under the Knife."

Inevitably, any discussion of the topic of aesthetic surgery leads to a much broader topic: the significance of aesthetics and beauty per se. Scientific experiments have shown that when given the choice, even three-year-olds will instinctively approach a beautiful person rather than a less attractive person. According to behavioural research, men almost invariably prefer women with full lips, slender legs, shiny hair and smooth skin, as well as statistically favouring some waist / hip proportions over others. Job interviews are also influenced by the applicant's appearance; in many cases, the better-looking person gets the job before the better-qualified one. A pretty waitress simply gets more tips. According to sociologist Bernd Guggenheimer, beauty is the high road to social success. Of course, the beauty craze is not just a recent symptom of our consumer-oriented culture, as is commonly claimed. The main difference to the past, in fact, is that today there are more opportunities of creating beauty – and of making it accessible to large parts of the population.

Throughout the history of humanity, man has searched for beauty. Antique portraits by Phidas, but also by Michelangelo or Leonardo da Vinci, demonstrate our longing for physical perfection. The aesthetics displayed by these artists are valid to this day. Most of the surgeons interviewed in this book refer to Michelangelo or to the arts of antiquity when asked which historical works of art embody beauty to them. In this respect, the history of art can also be read as a grand history of beauty! In its course, certain ideals of beauty recur over large leaps of time – yet no matter how divergent the cultural eras may be, their aesthetics are often uncannily similar.

Today, a face or a body can be surgically manipulated and enhanced, but can surgery actually make a person more beautiful? Many of the surgeons interviewed have emphasised that a pretty shell is not enough to endow a person with beauty. For somebody to be truly beautiful, non-physical qualities such as spirit, aura and charisma are essential. I sometimes ask myself if in several decades, when those old people that haven't received cosmetic surgery will be a minority – a likely scenario at least in the Western world! –, they will be regarded as particularly beautiful for not having introduced foreign substances into their bodies and having declined to manipulate their appearance?

After years of examining and researching the subject of aesthetic surgery and after seeing with my own eyes surgical results that were so convincing that anybody would agree reconstructive surgery is a blessing, I am still deeply convinced that real beauty is based on truth. Looking at beauty in a larger context, it only truly touches me when it is authentic and real, when it isn't just an external mask but emanates from within. This applies equally to people, art, music, literature or even sex. True beauty has the power and scope to be profound, to make sense.

Stendhal wrote that "beauty is a promise of happiness," while Dostoyevsky claimed that "beauty will save the world." It remains to be seen if these sublime qualities are also evident in a beauty that has been manipulated.

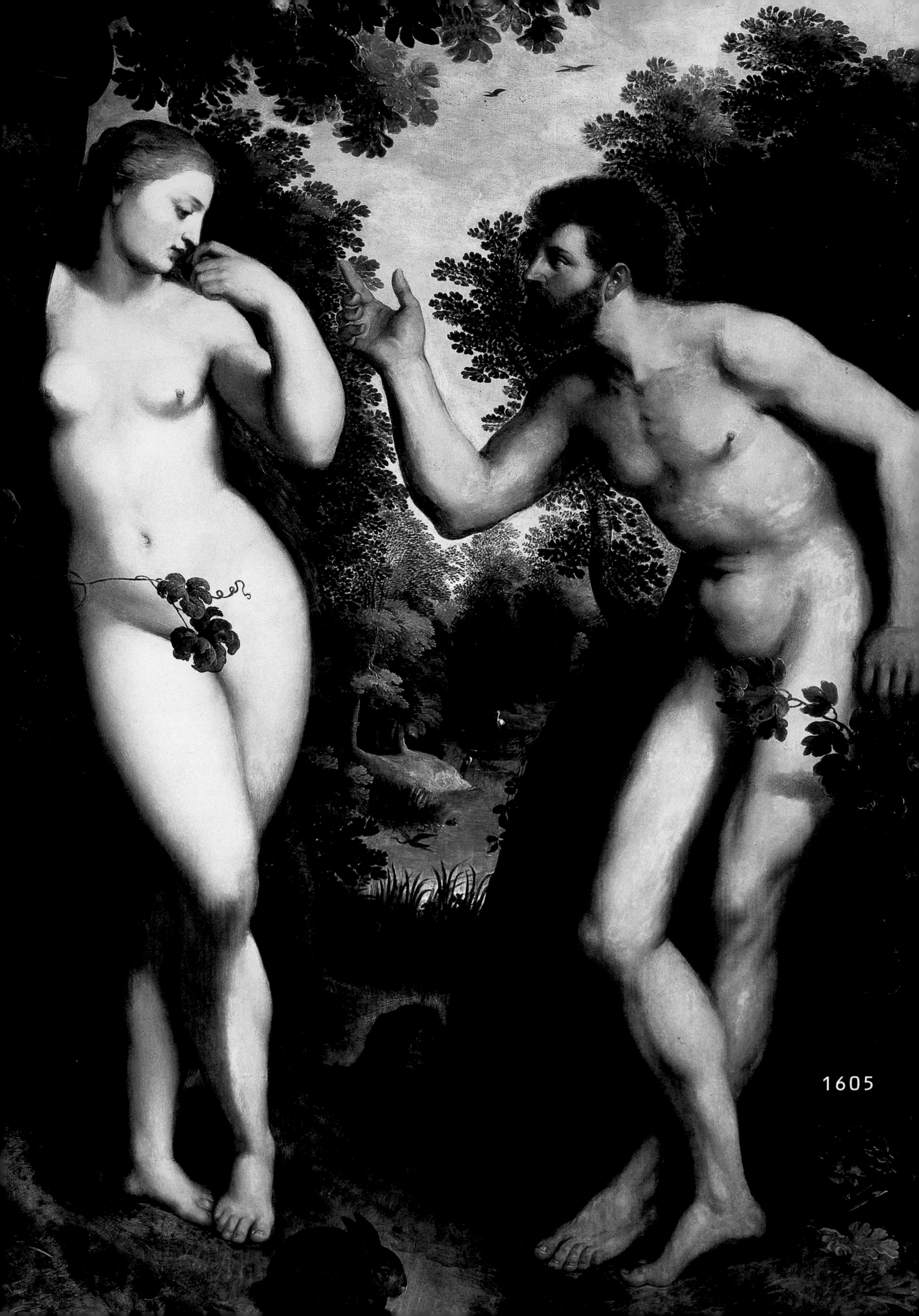
1605

II.

BEAUTY IN ART

---

compiled by

ANGELIKA TASCHEN

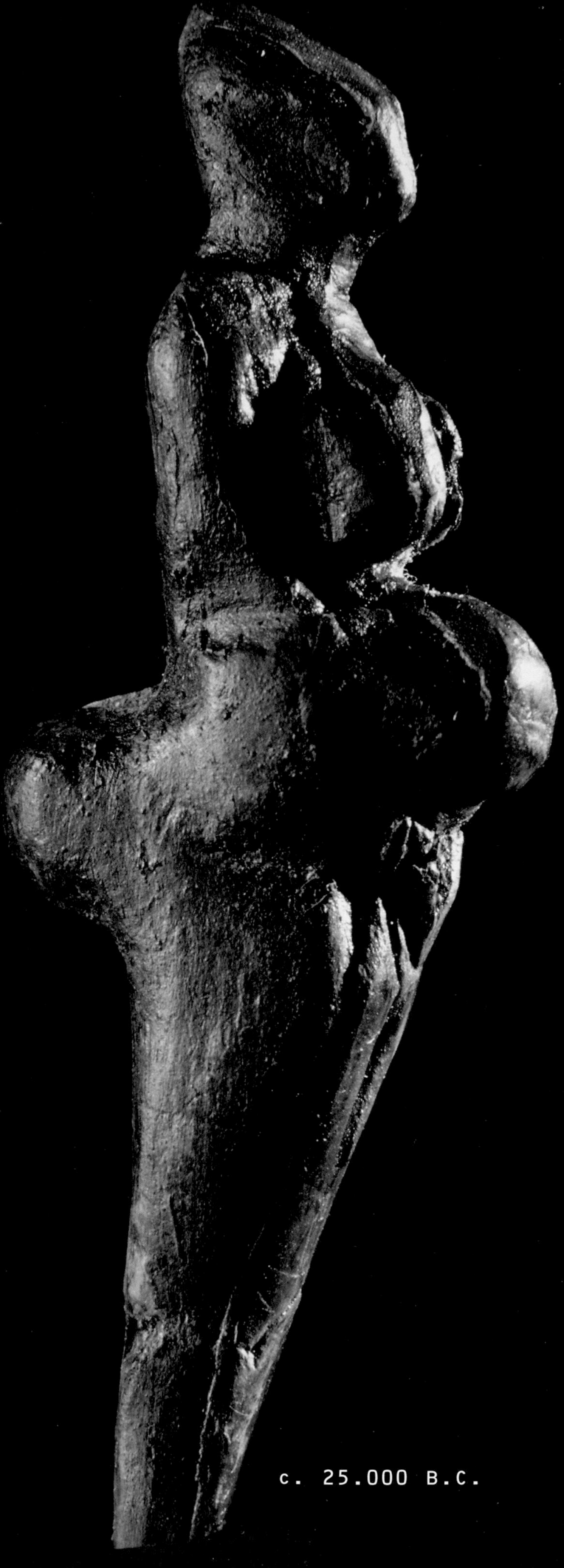

c. 25.000 B.C.

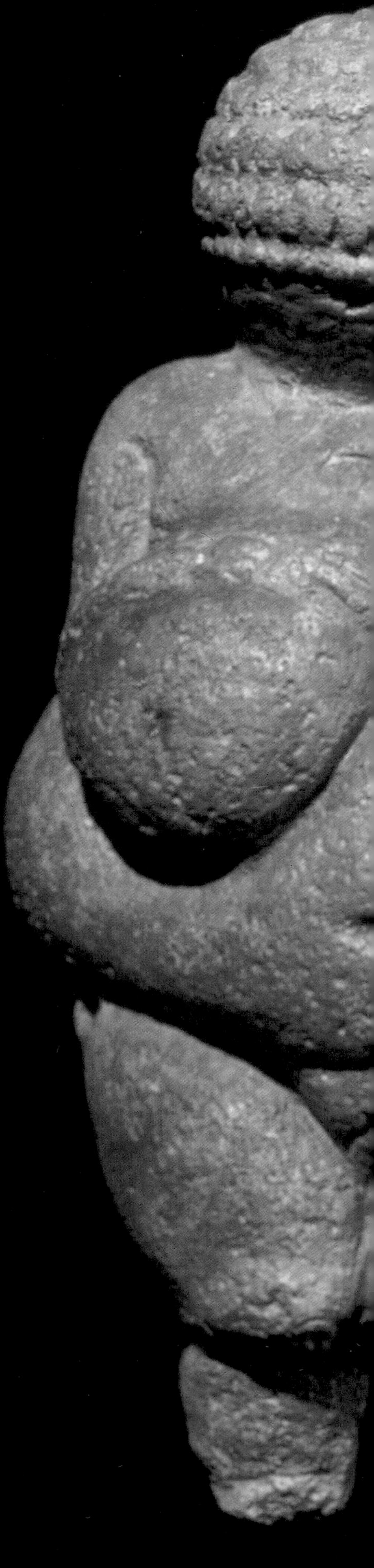

c. 25.000 B.C.

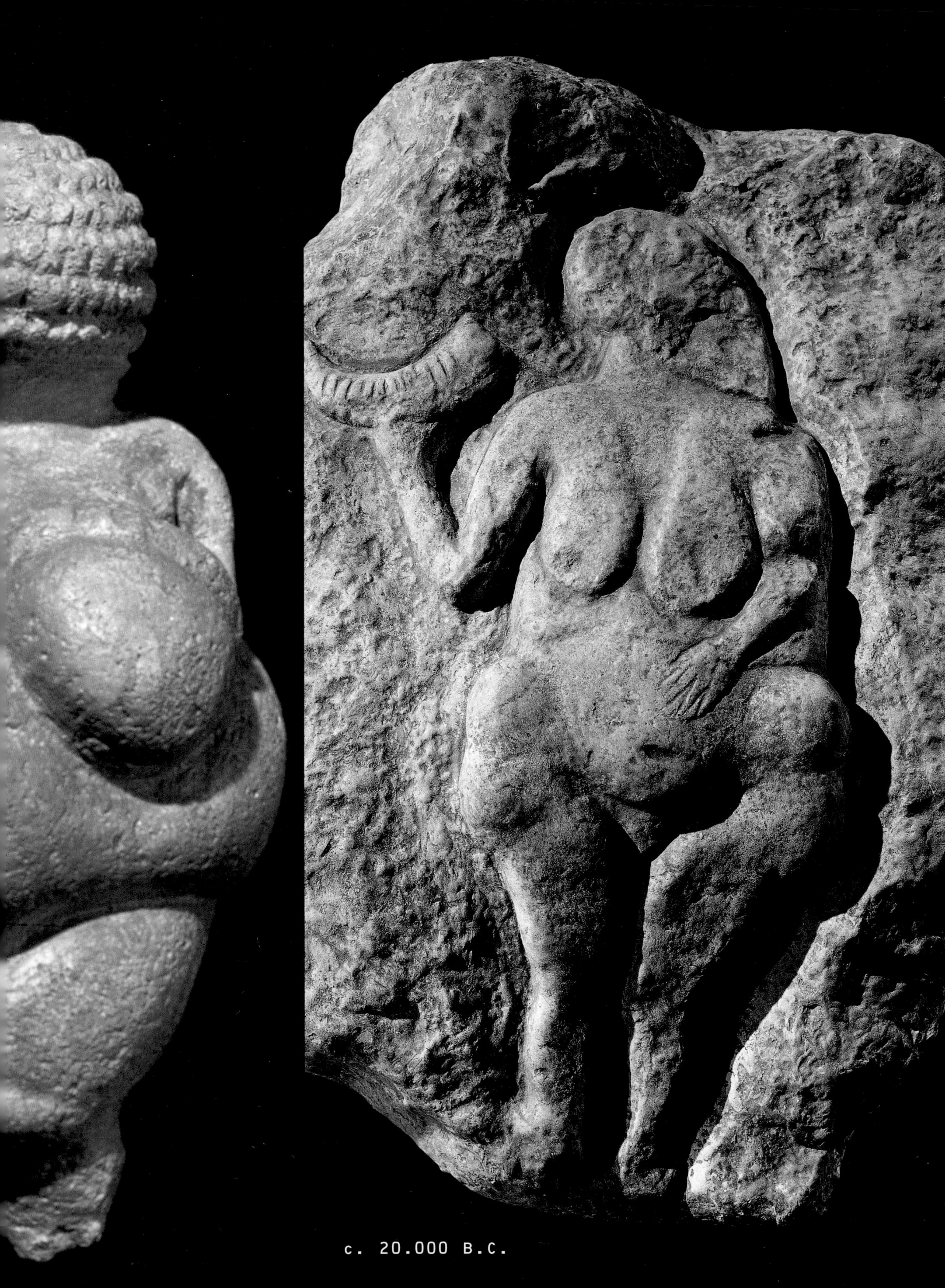

c. 20.000 B.C.

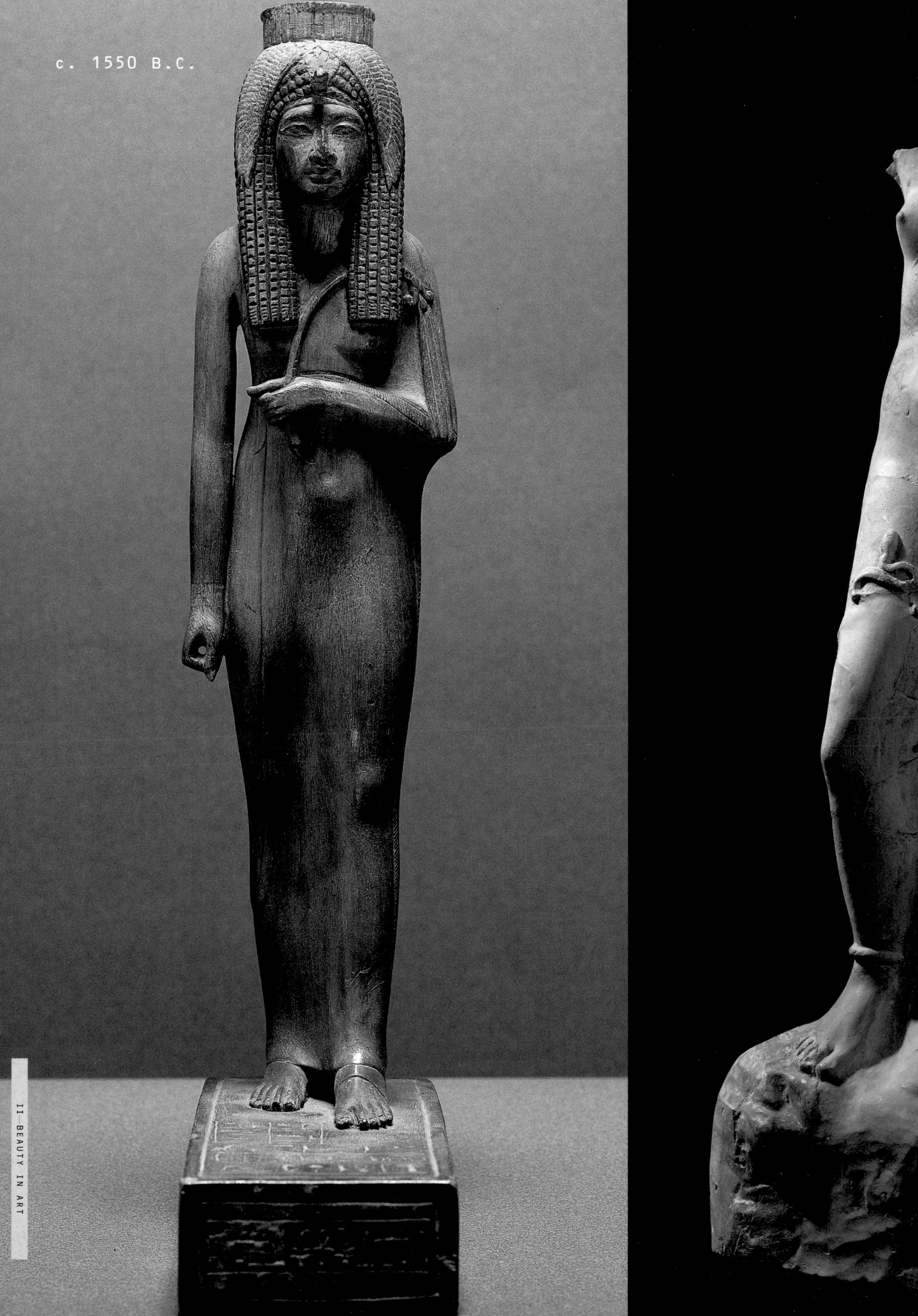
c. 1550 B.C.

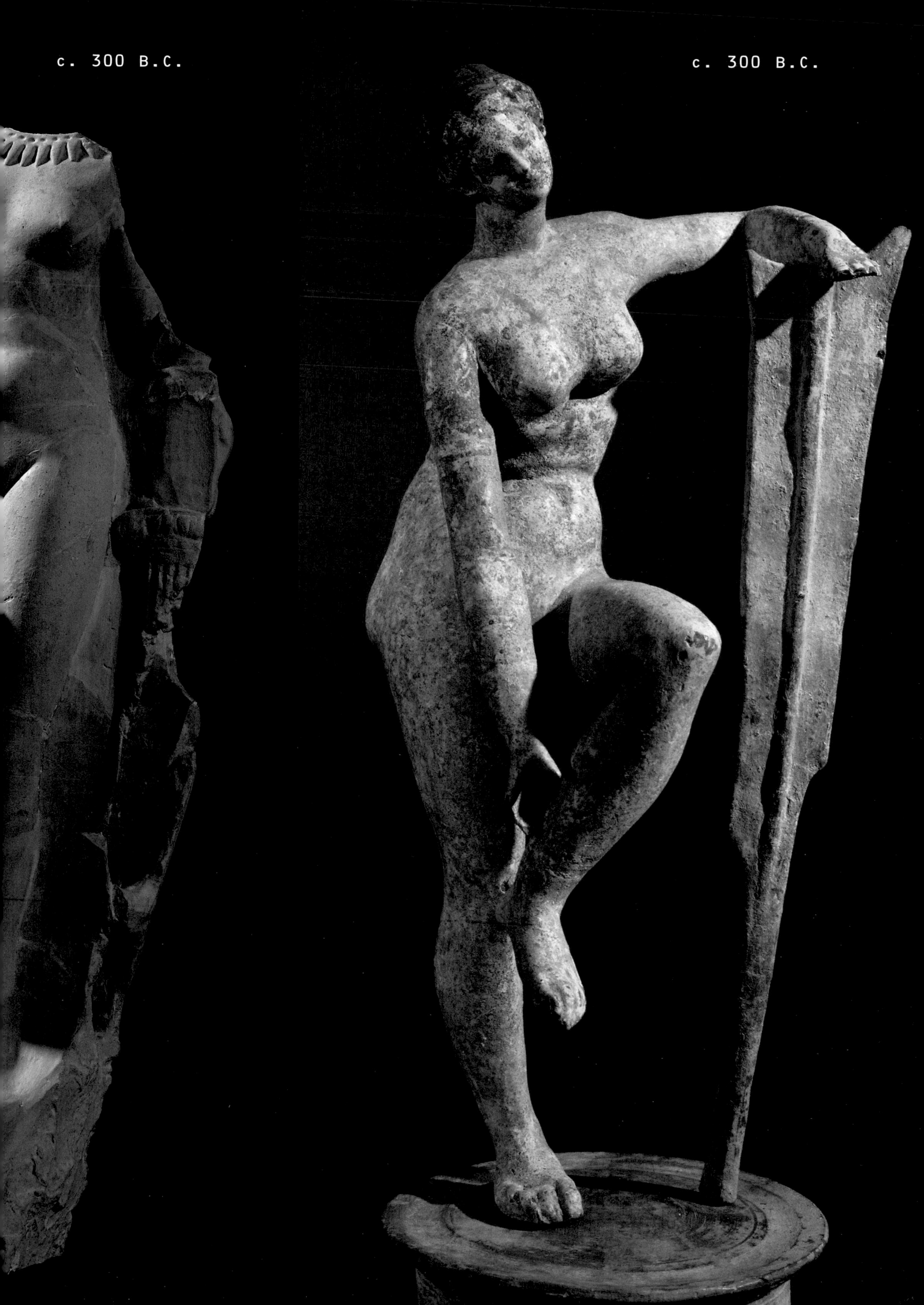
c. 300 B.C.
c. 300 B.C.

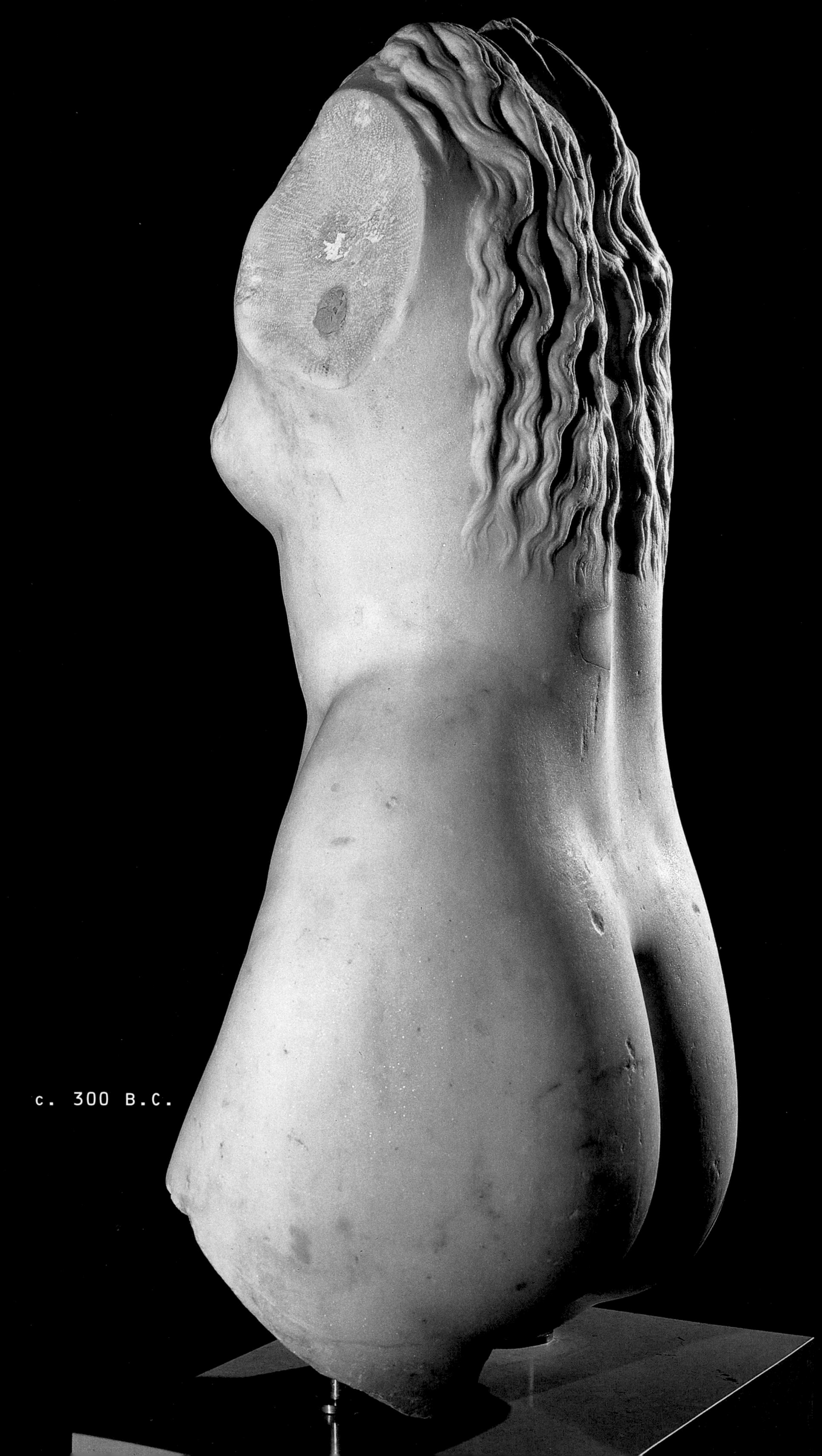

c. 300 B.C.

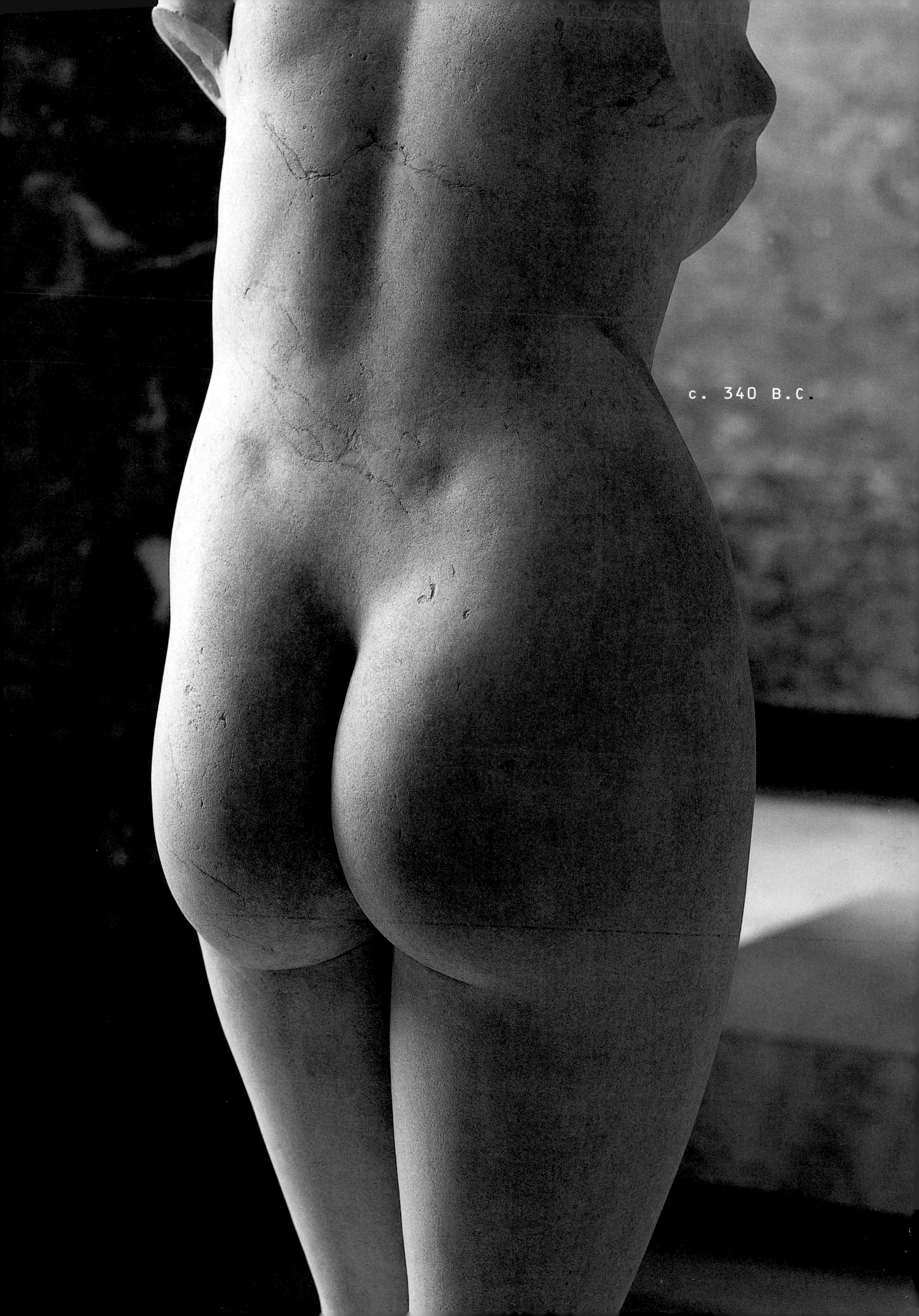
c. 340 B.C.

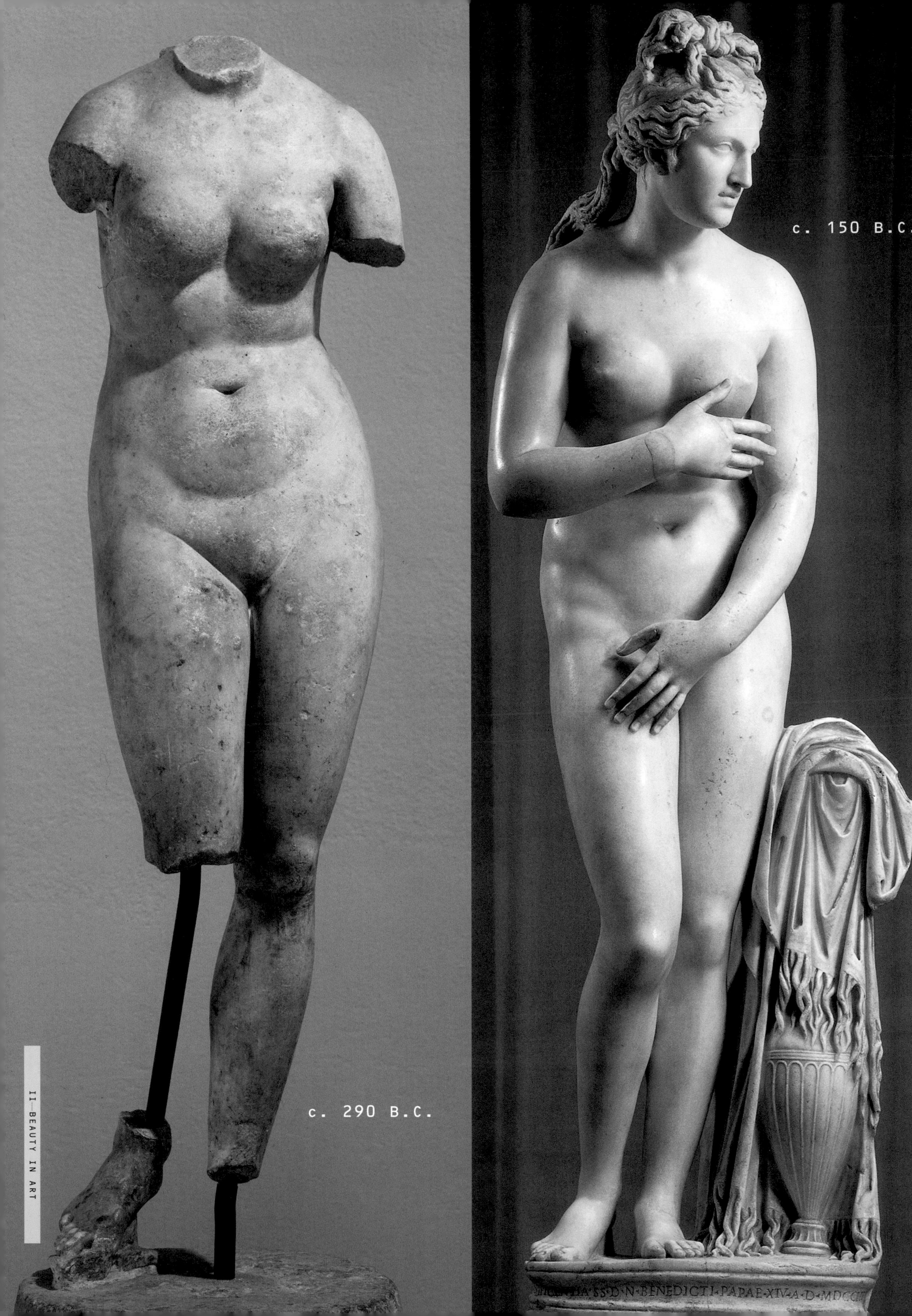

c. 290 B.C.

c. 150 B.C.

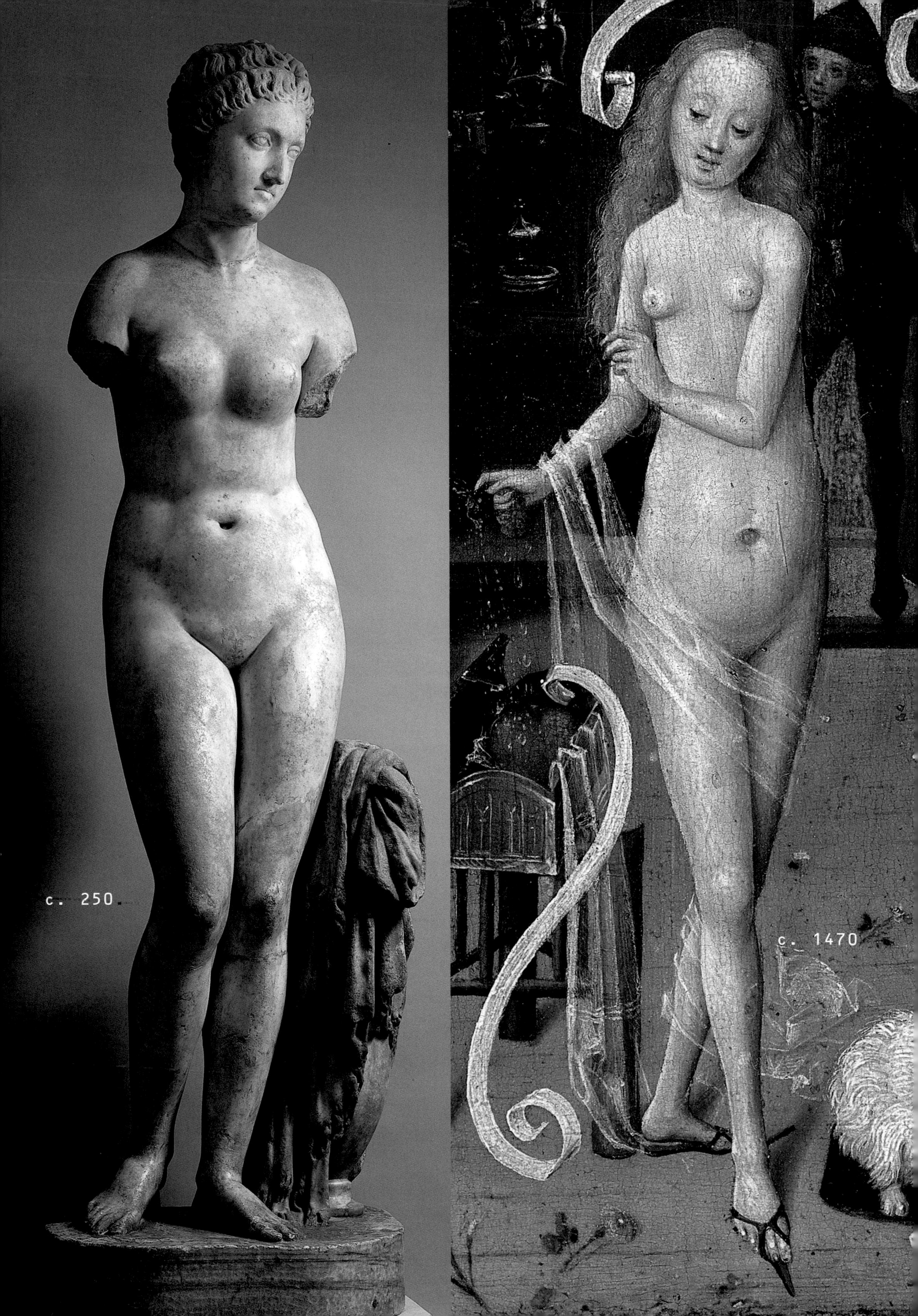
c. 250
c. 1470

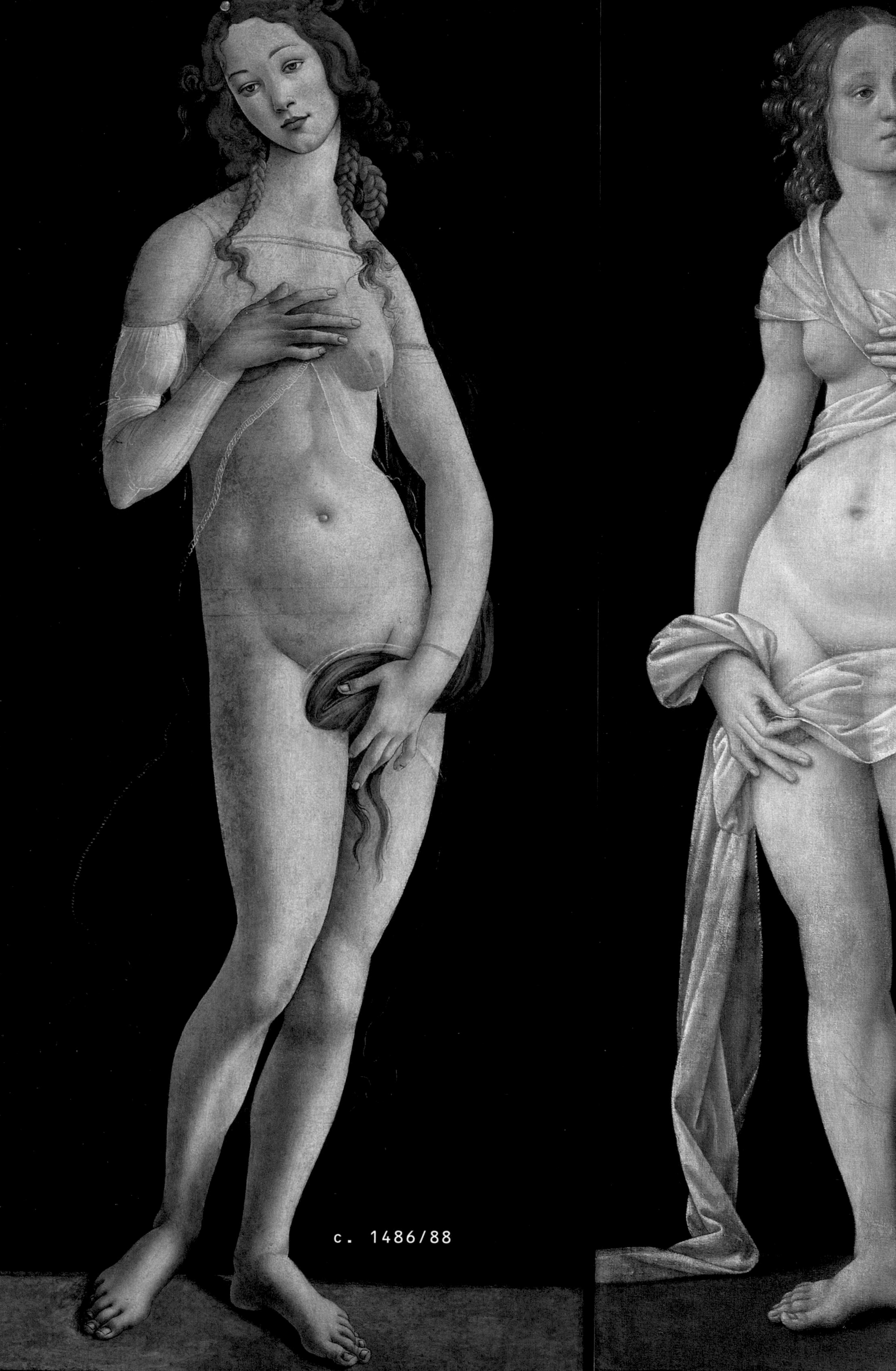

c. 1486/88

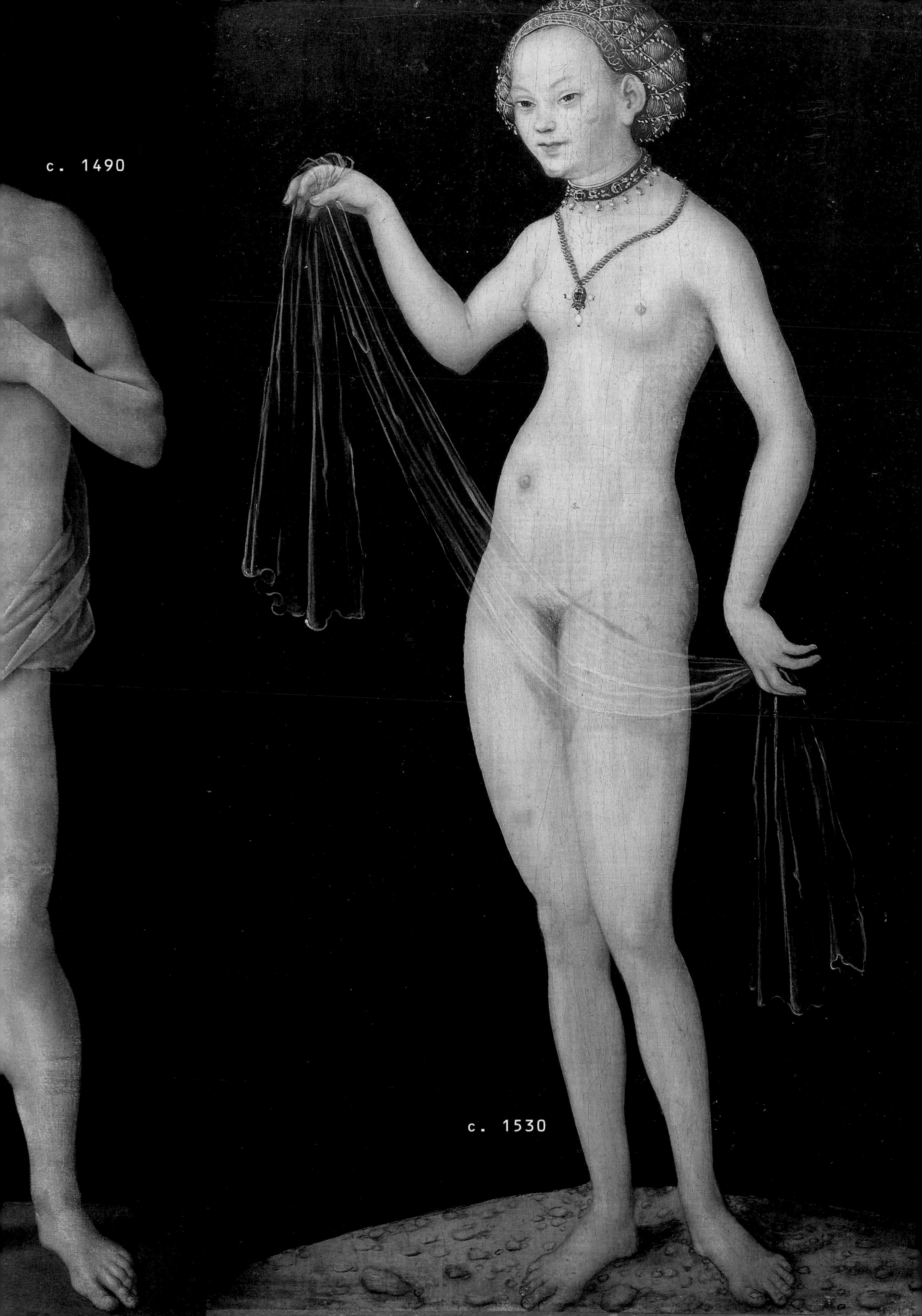
c. 1490
c. 1530

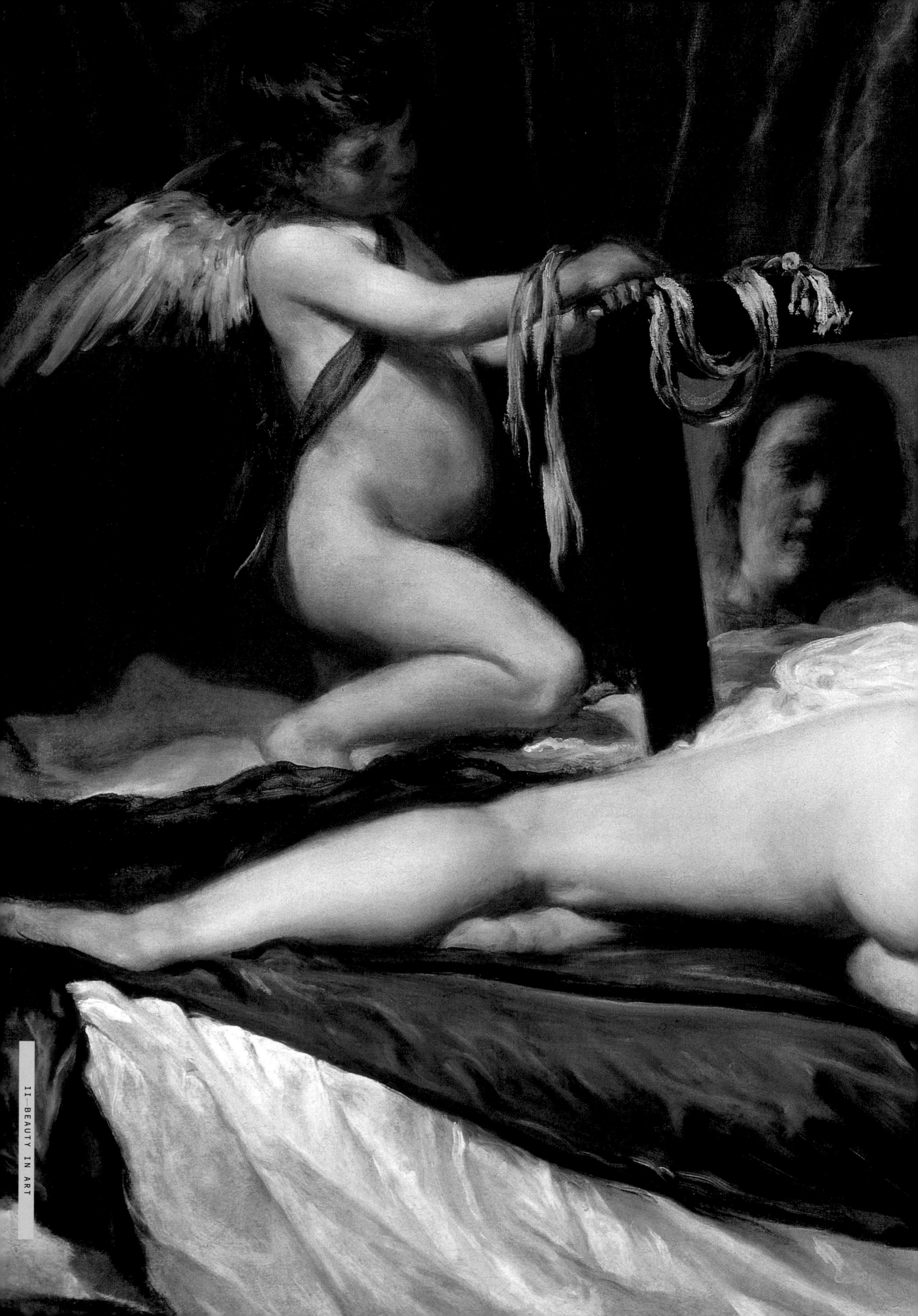

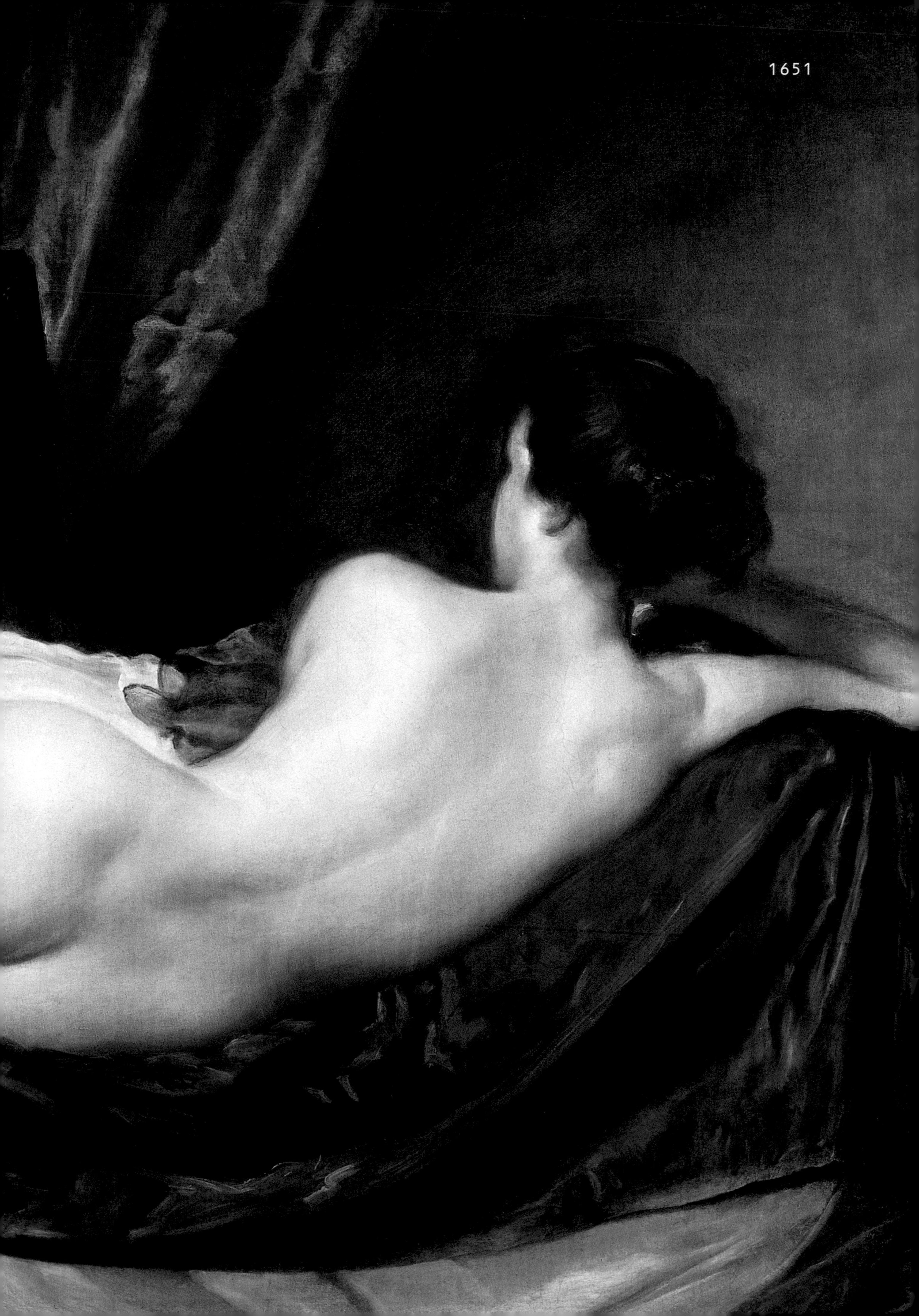

c. 1797

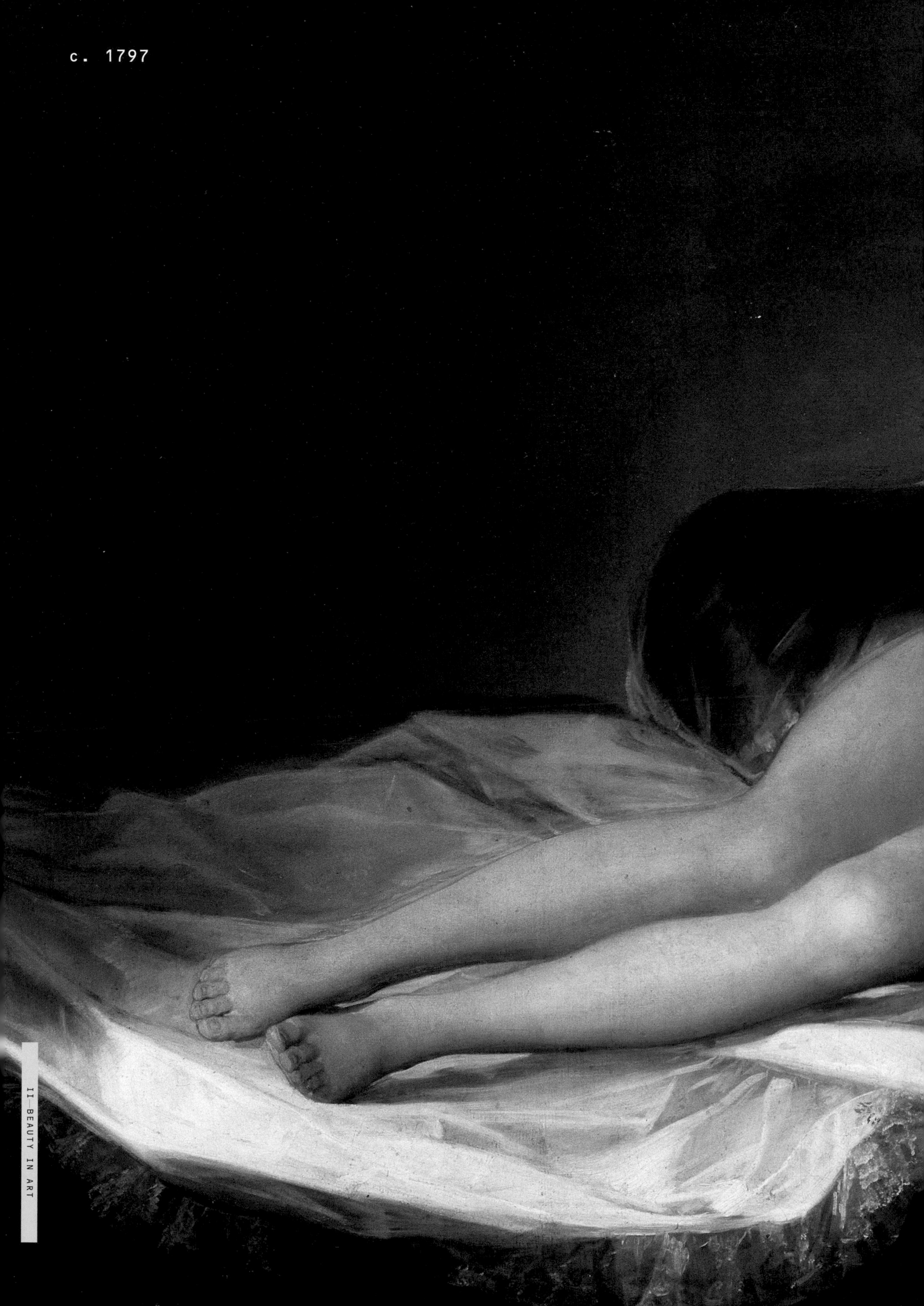

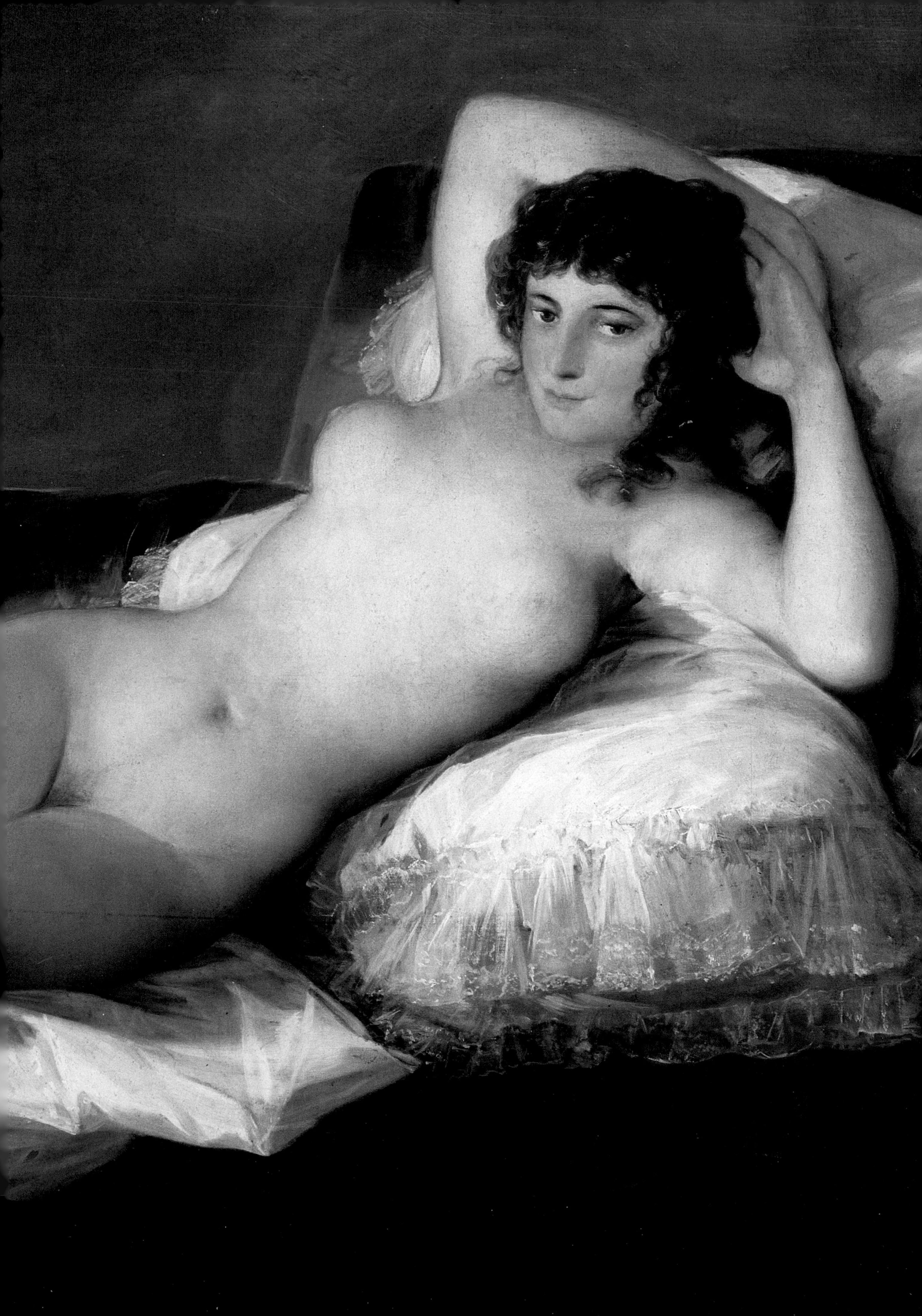

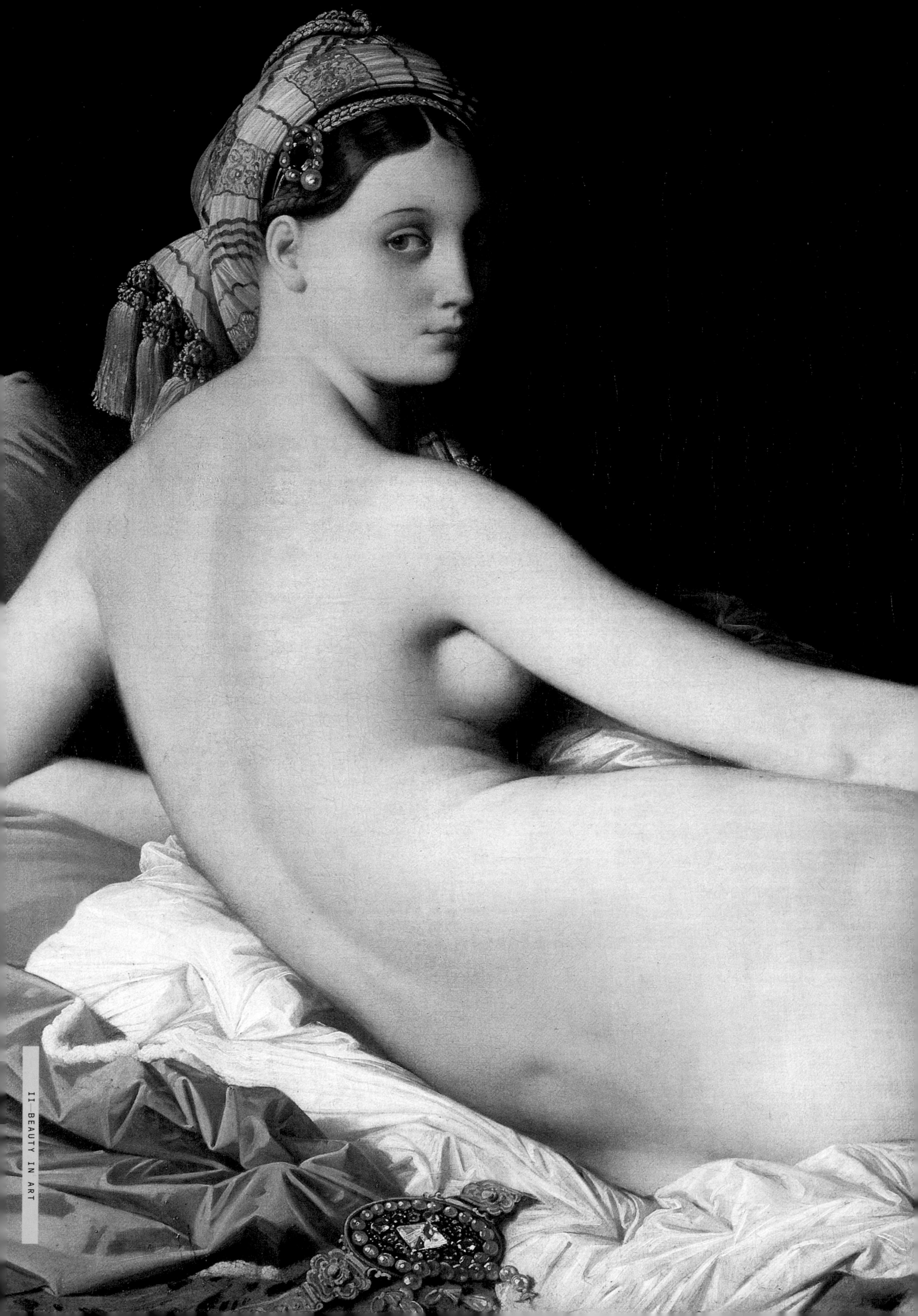

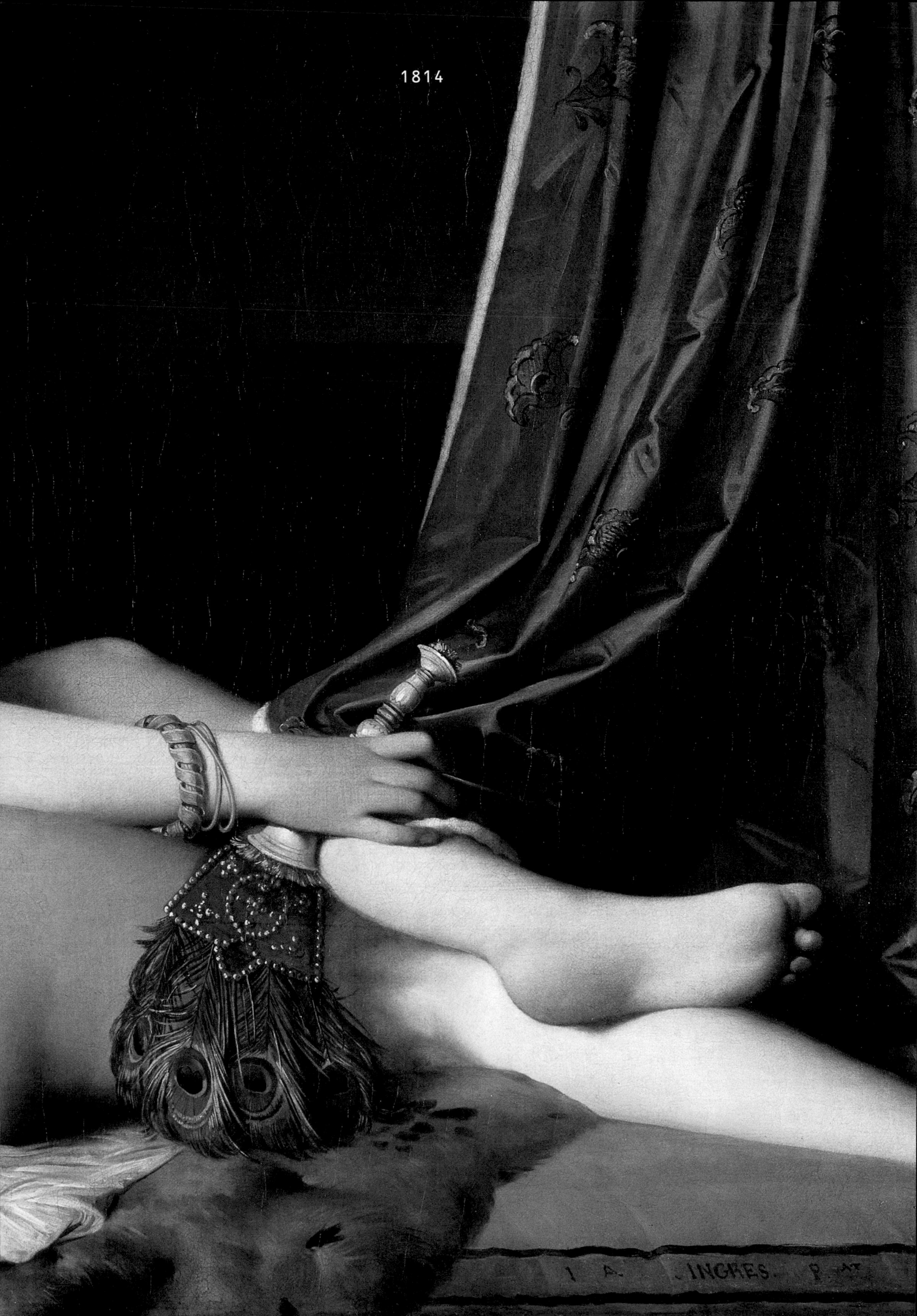

1814

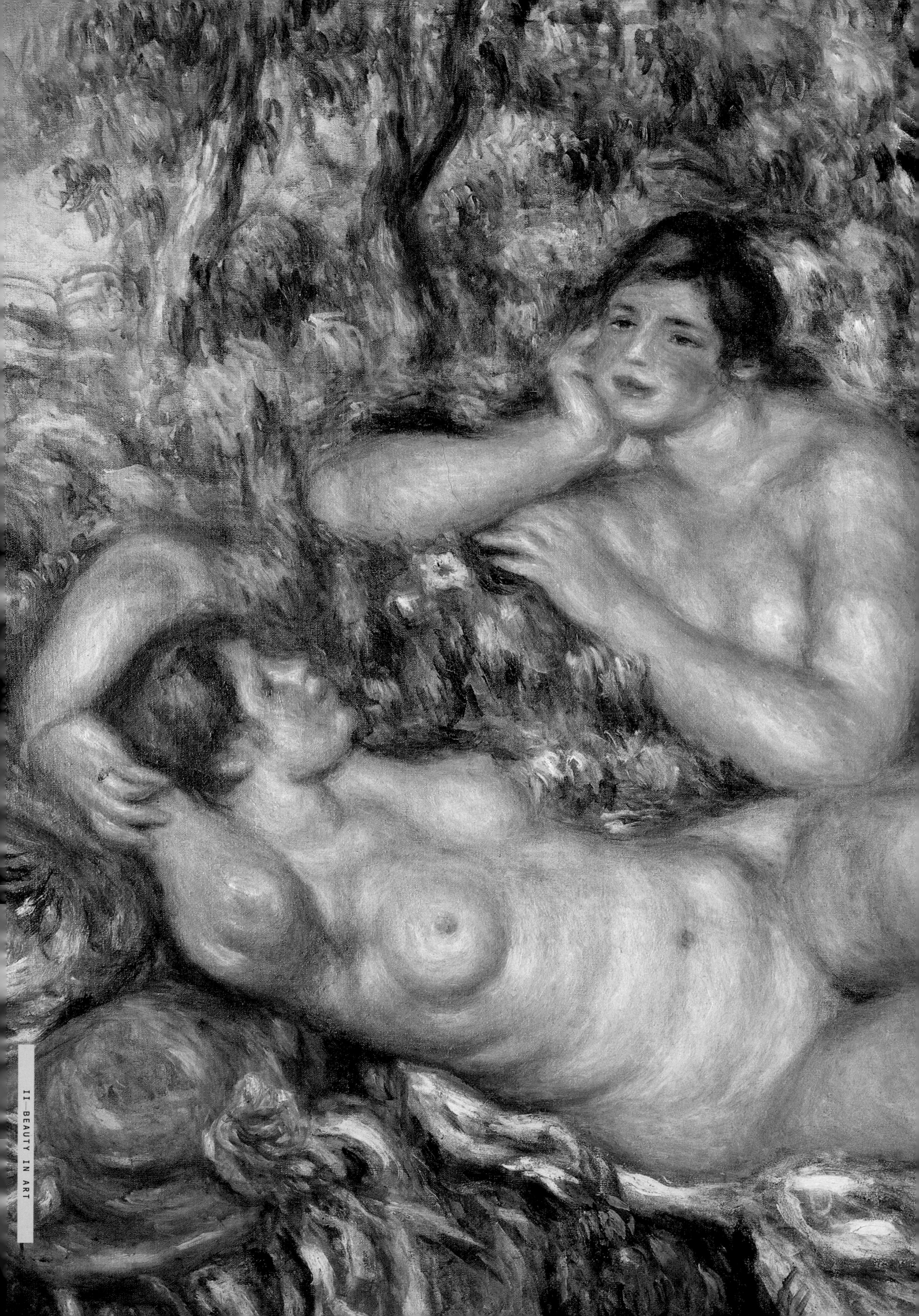

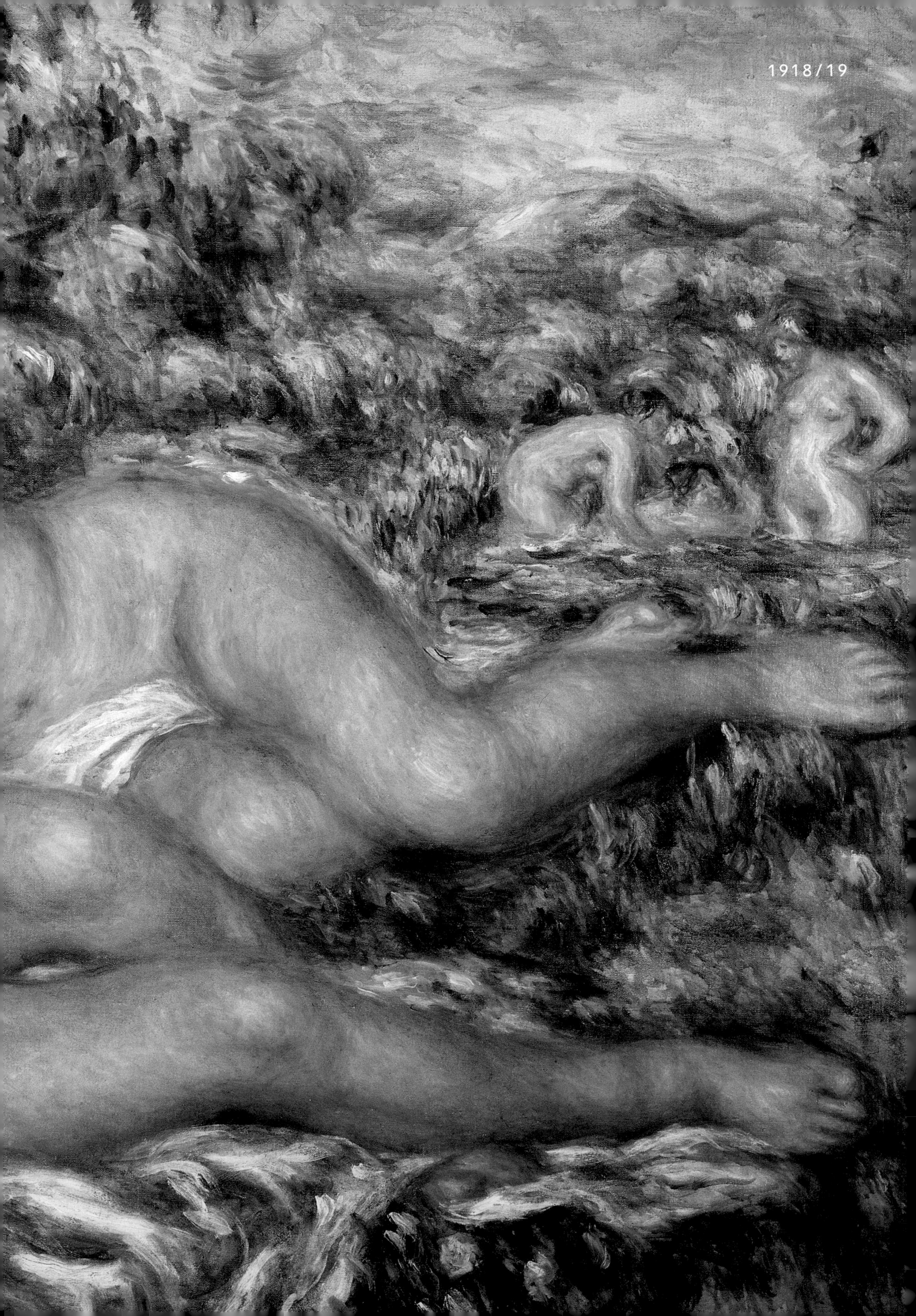

1918/19

1914

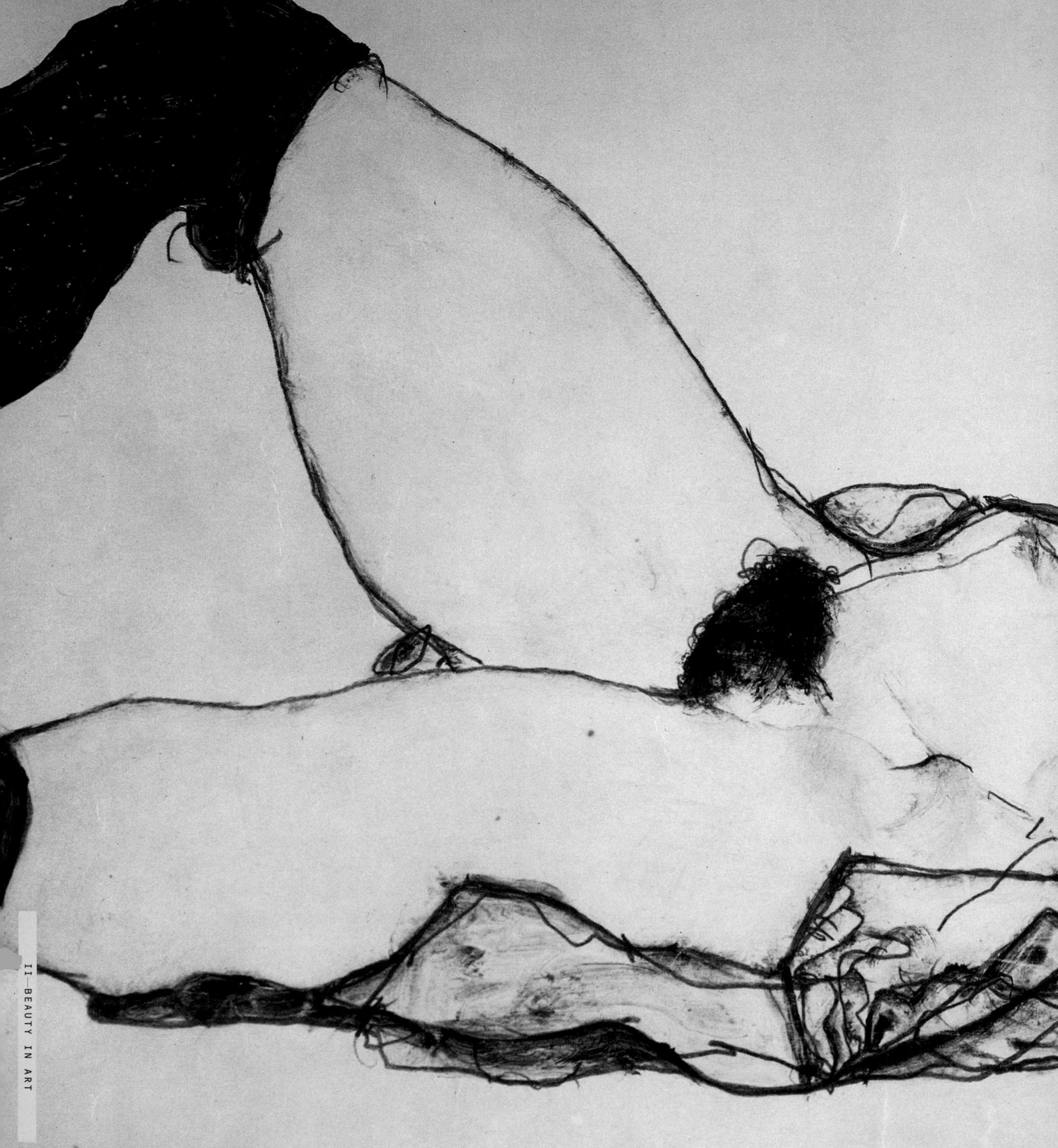

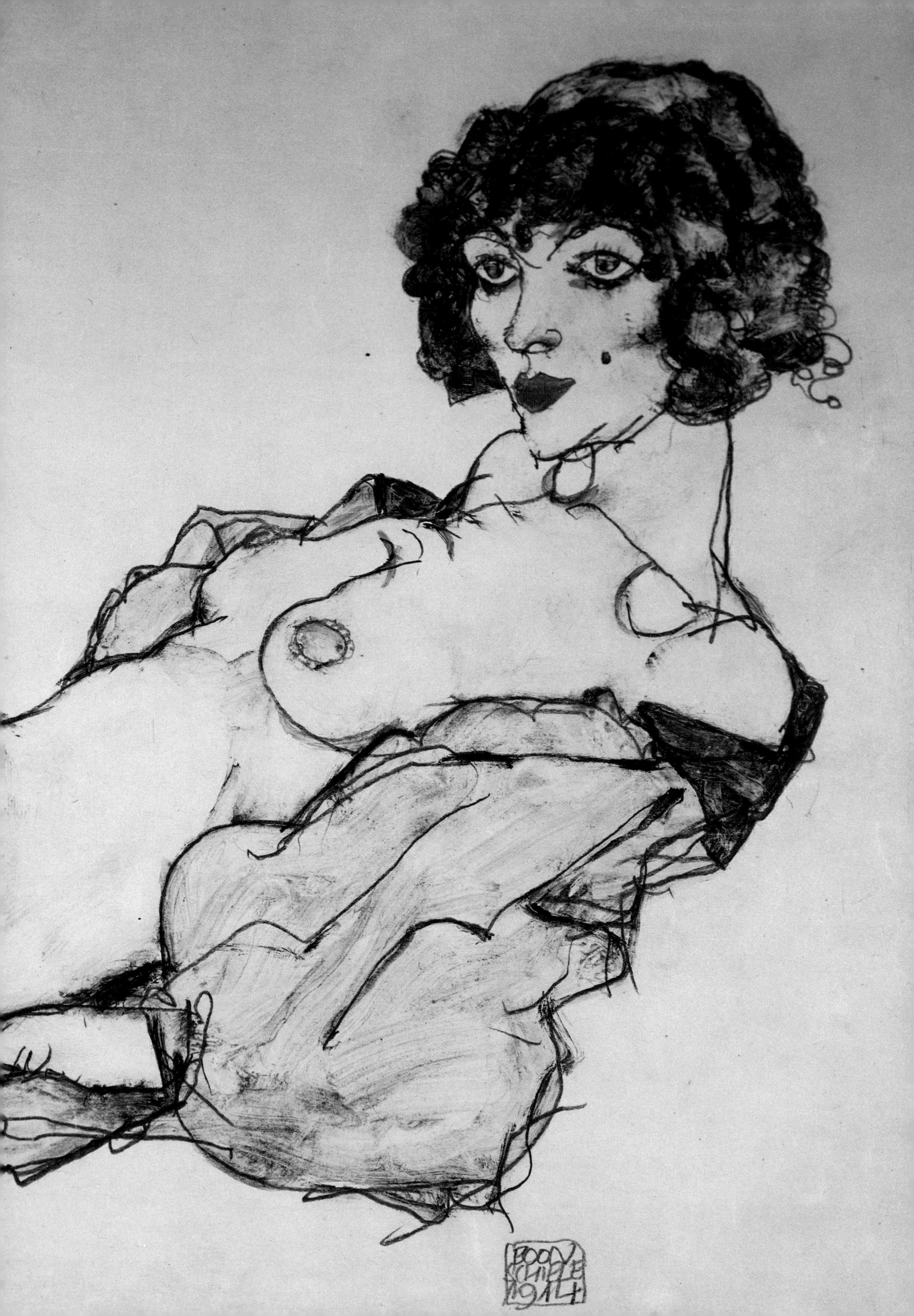
EGON
SCHIELE
1914

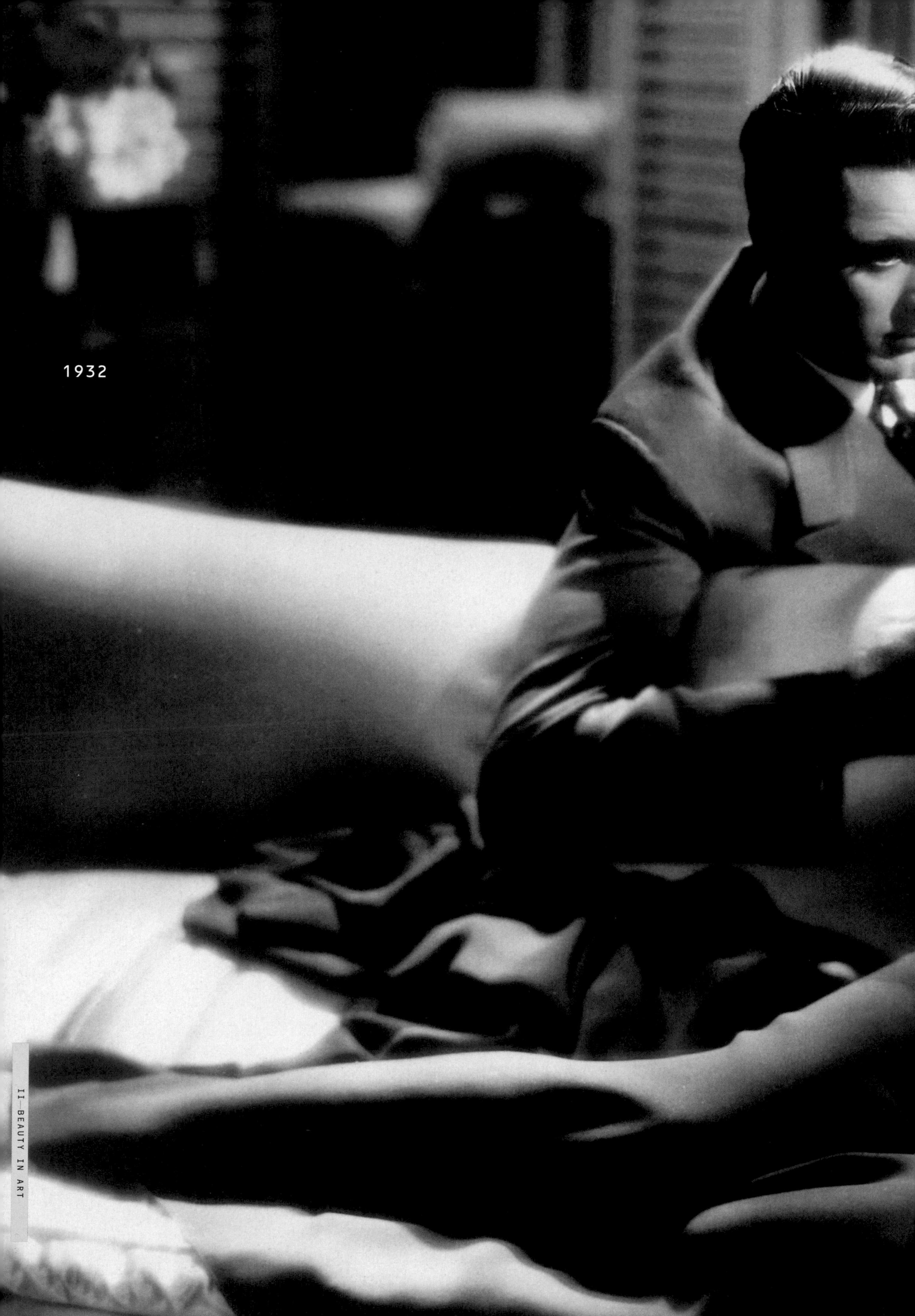

1932

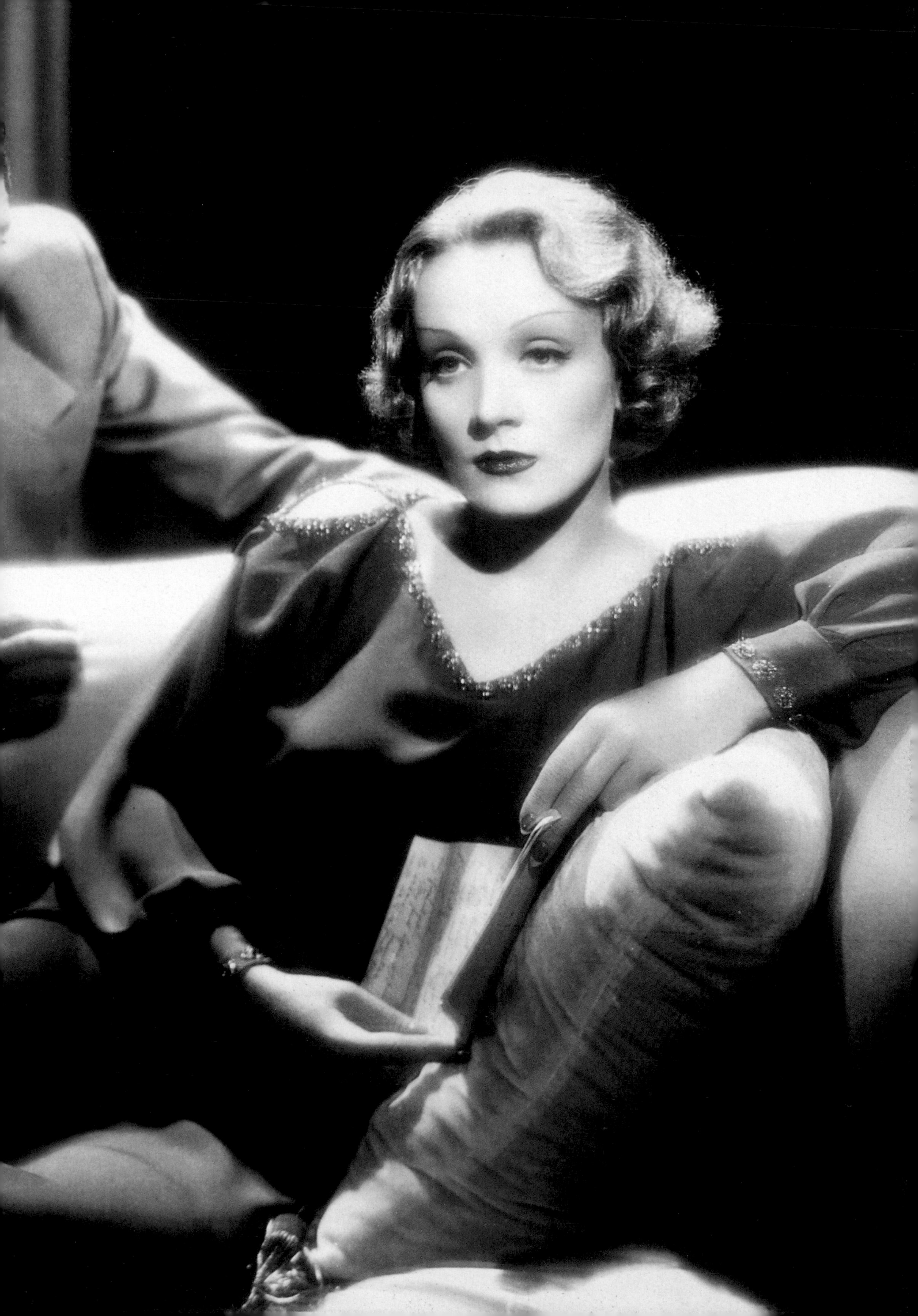

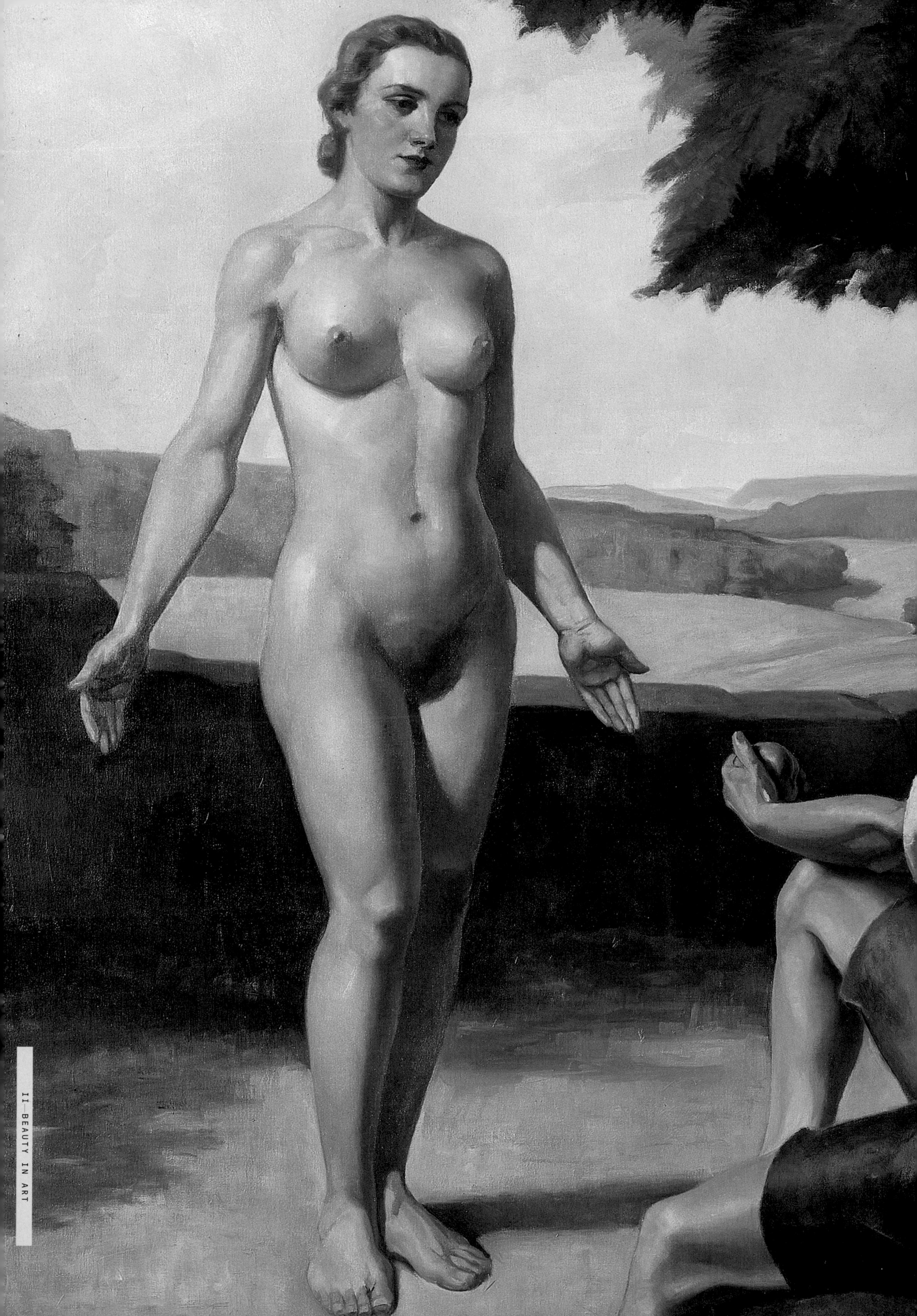

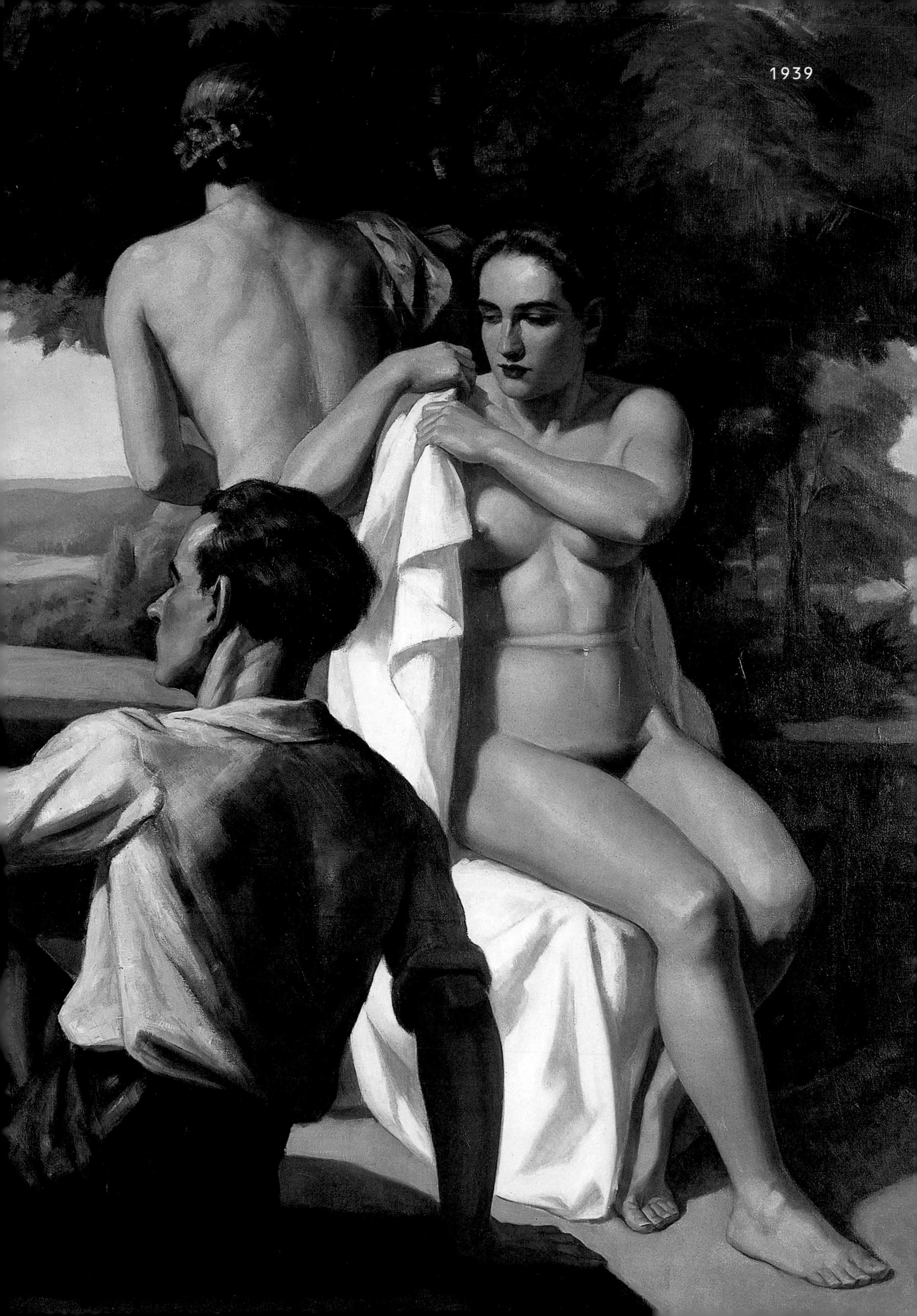

1939

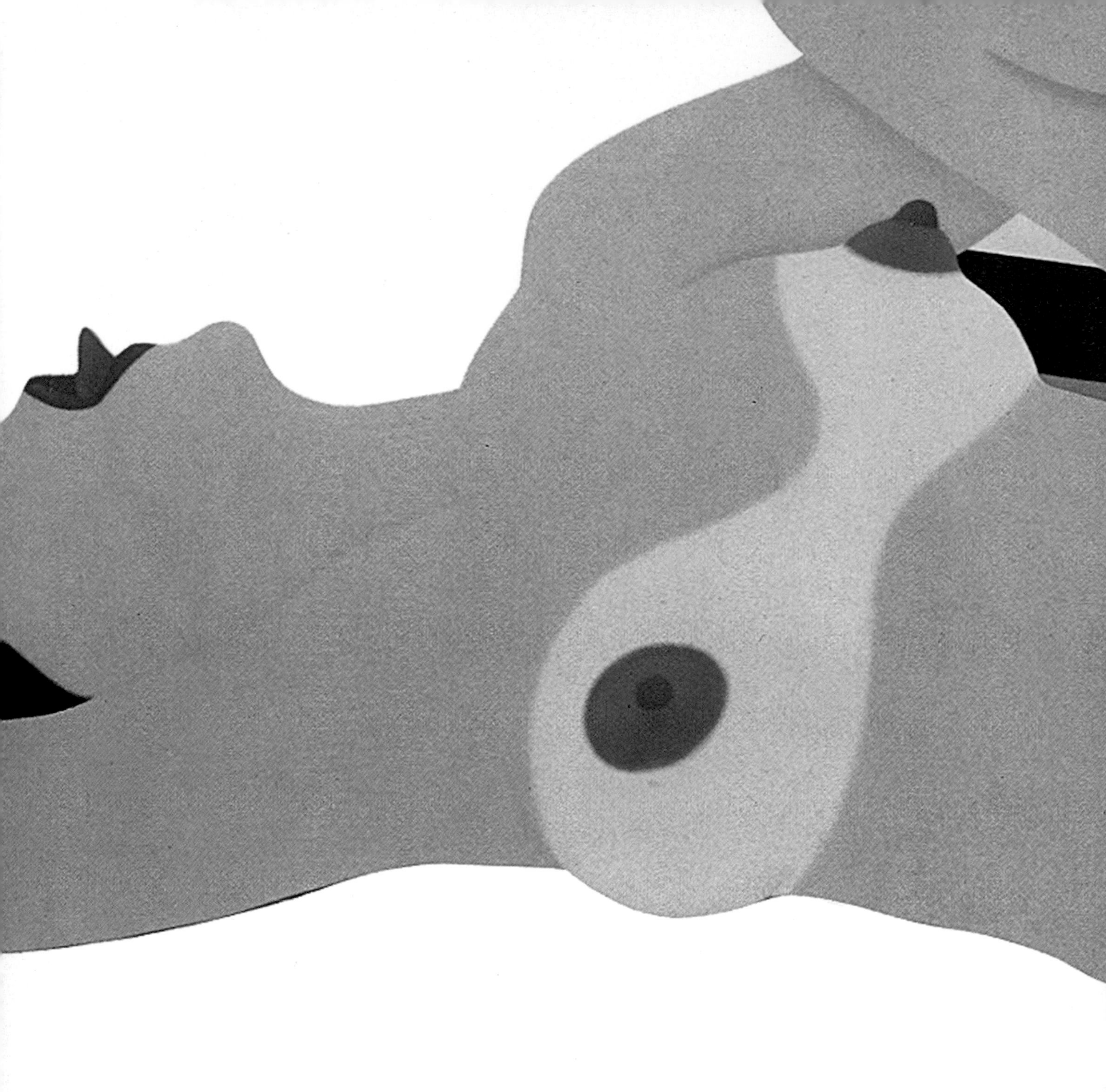

1967

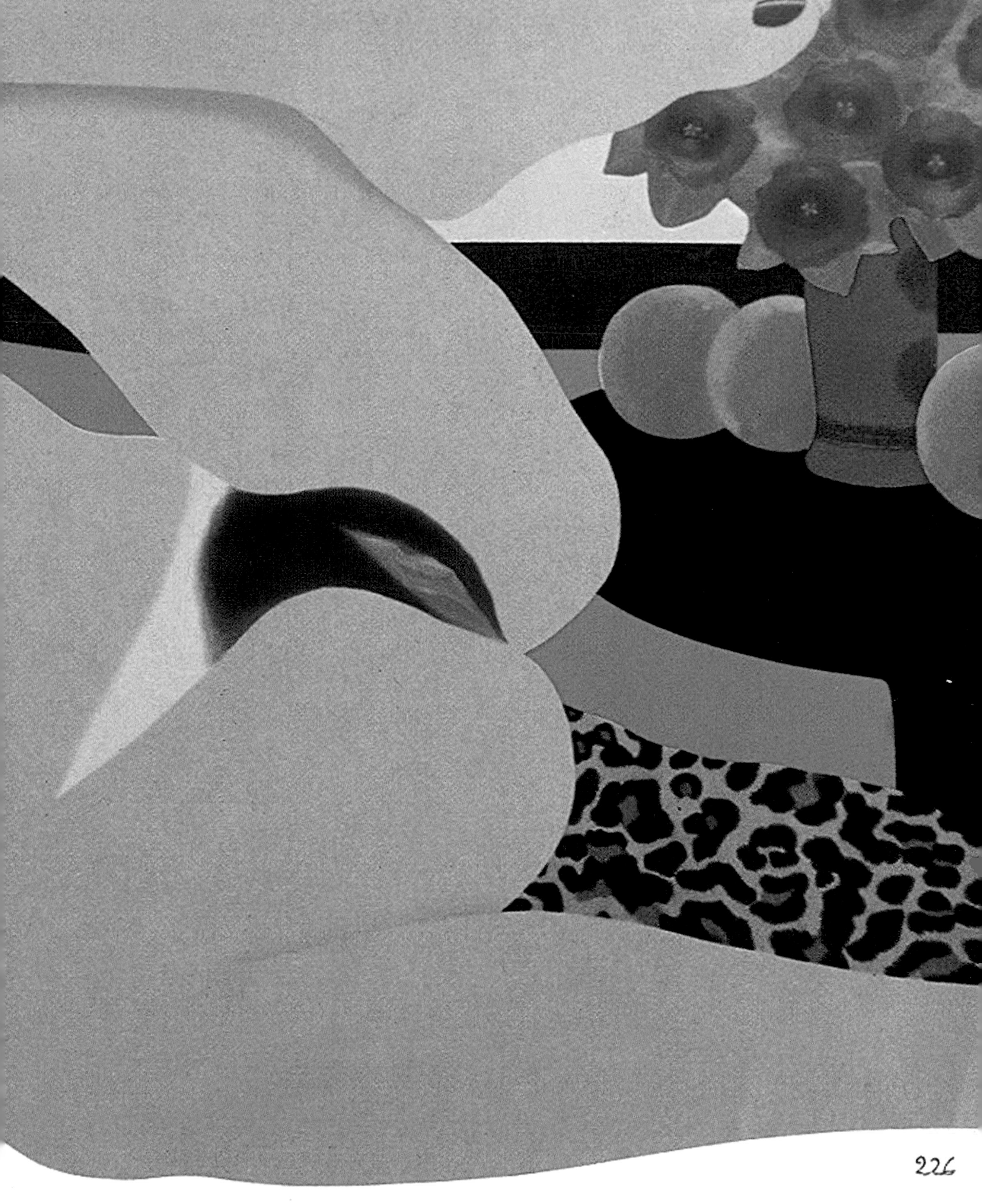

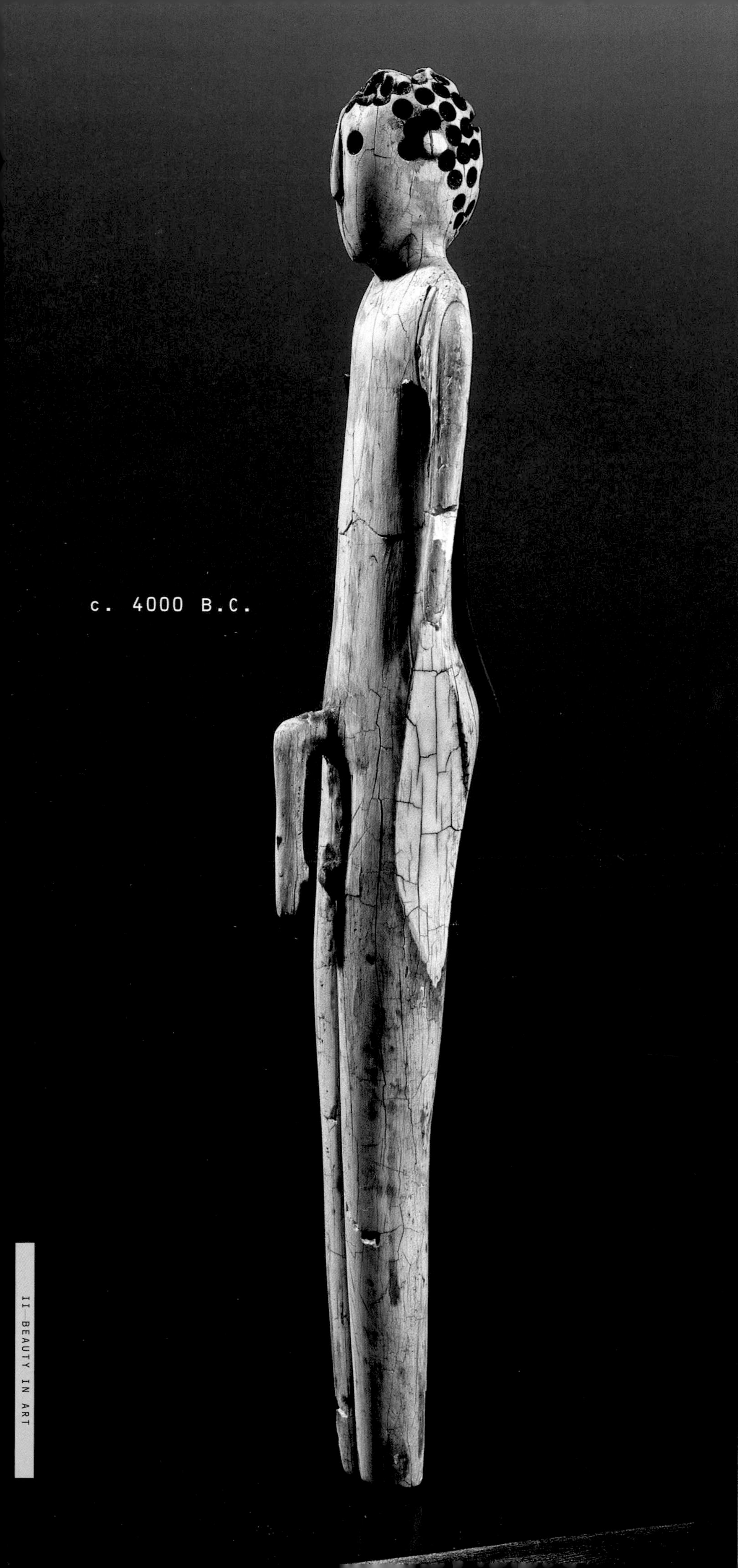

c. 530 B.C.

c. 4000 B.C.

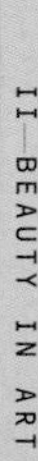

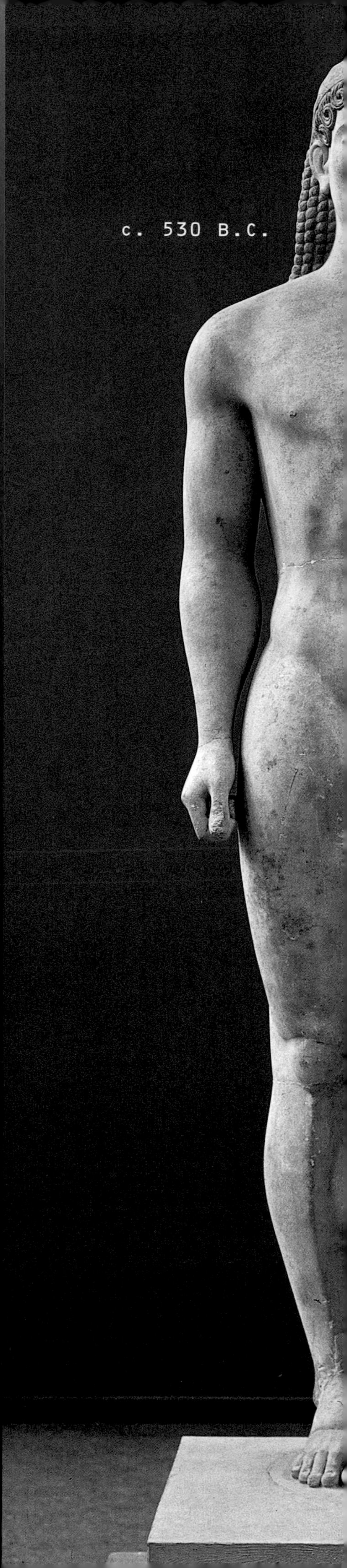

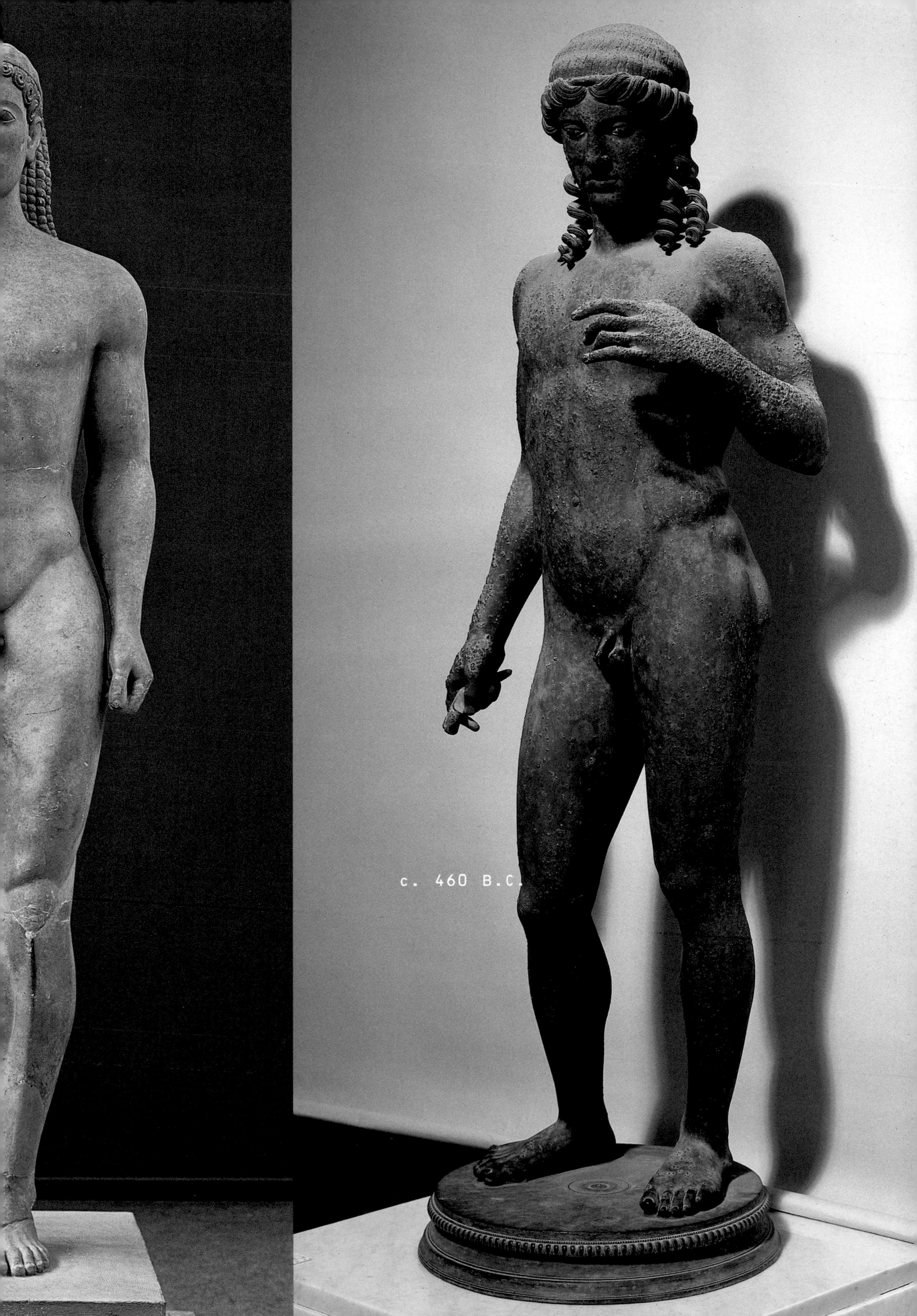

c. 460 B.C.

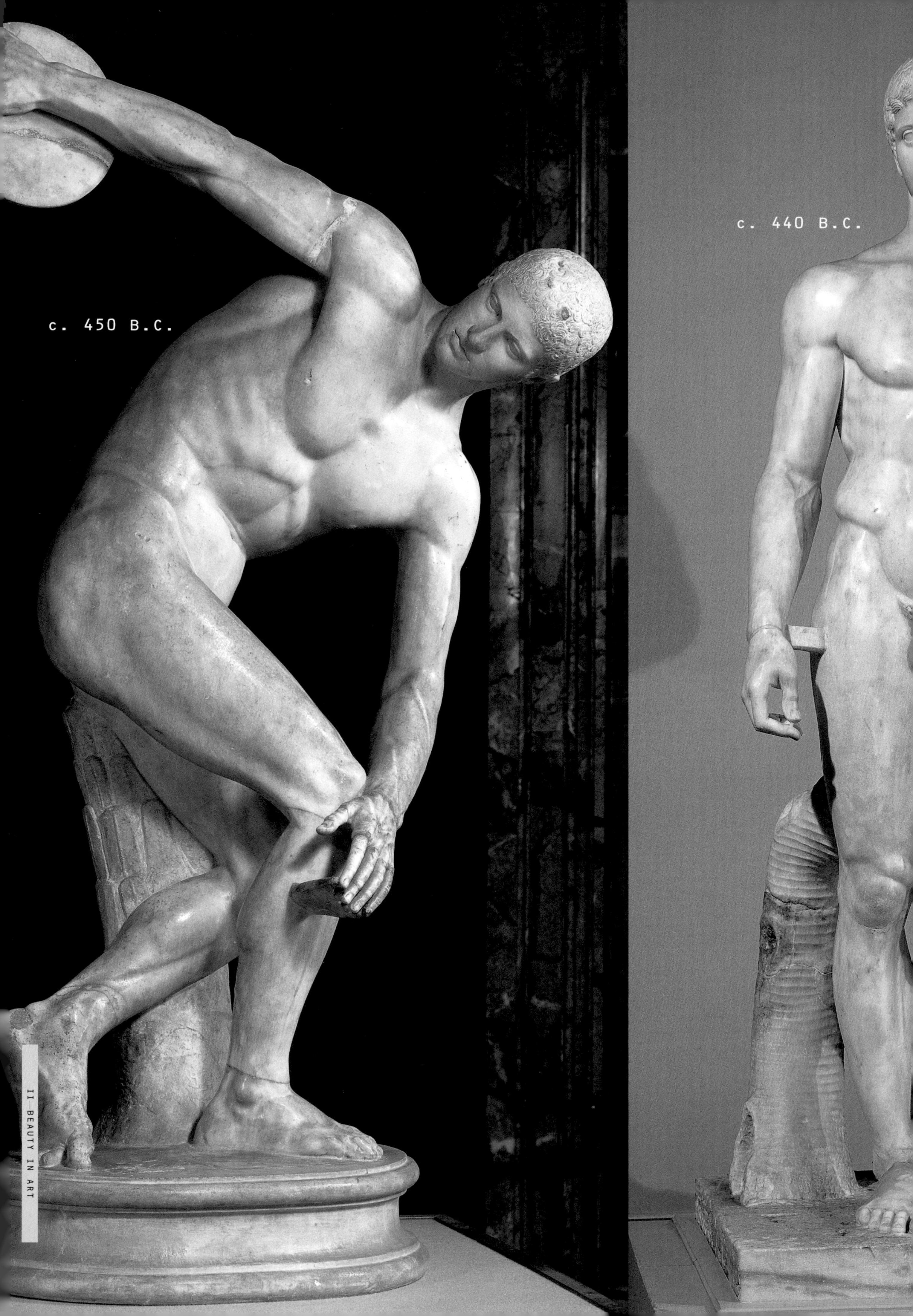
c. 450 B.C.
c. 440 B.C.

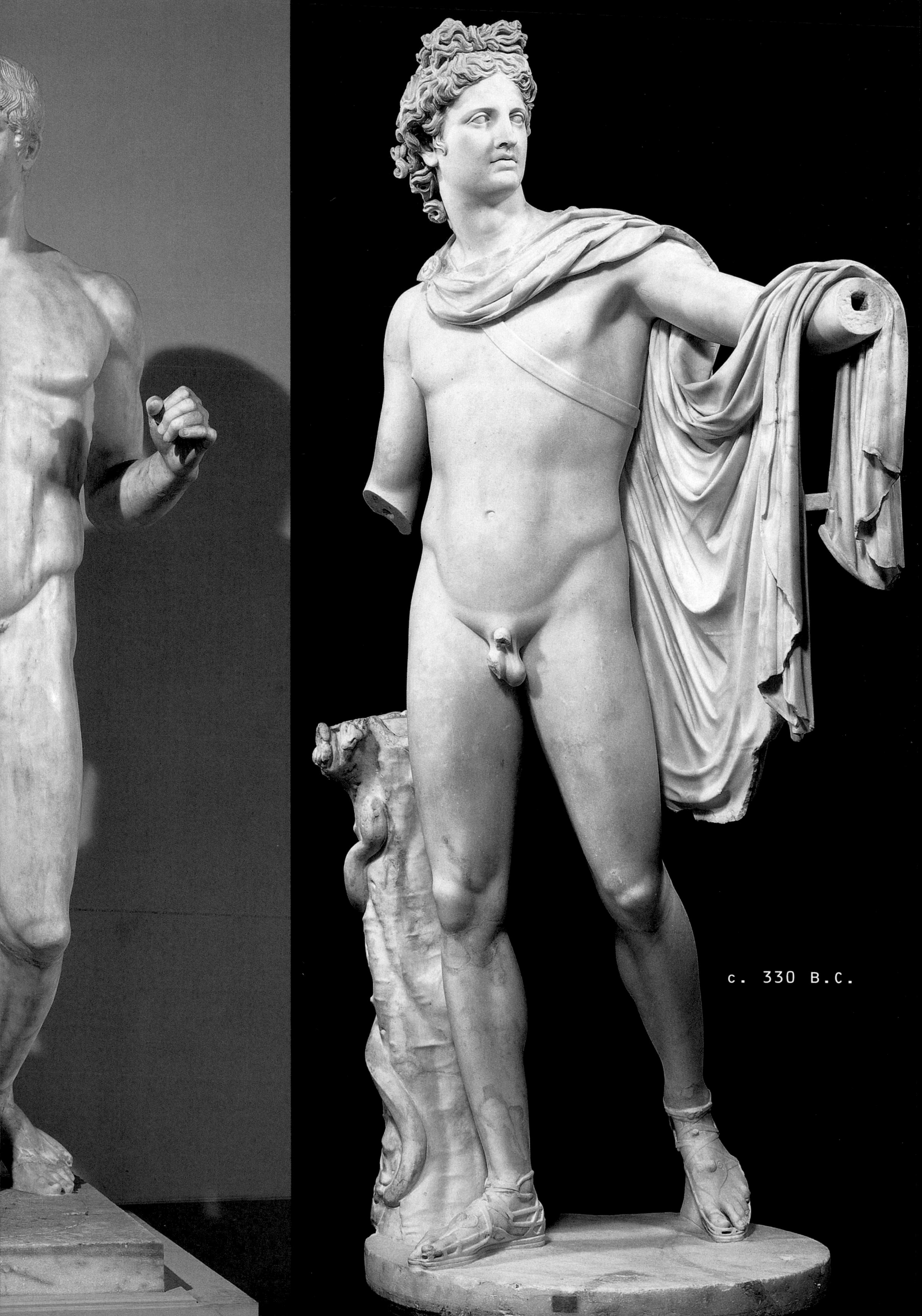

c. 330 B.C.

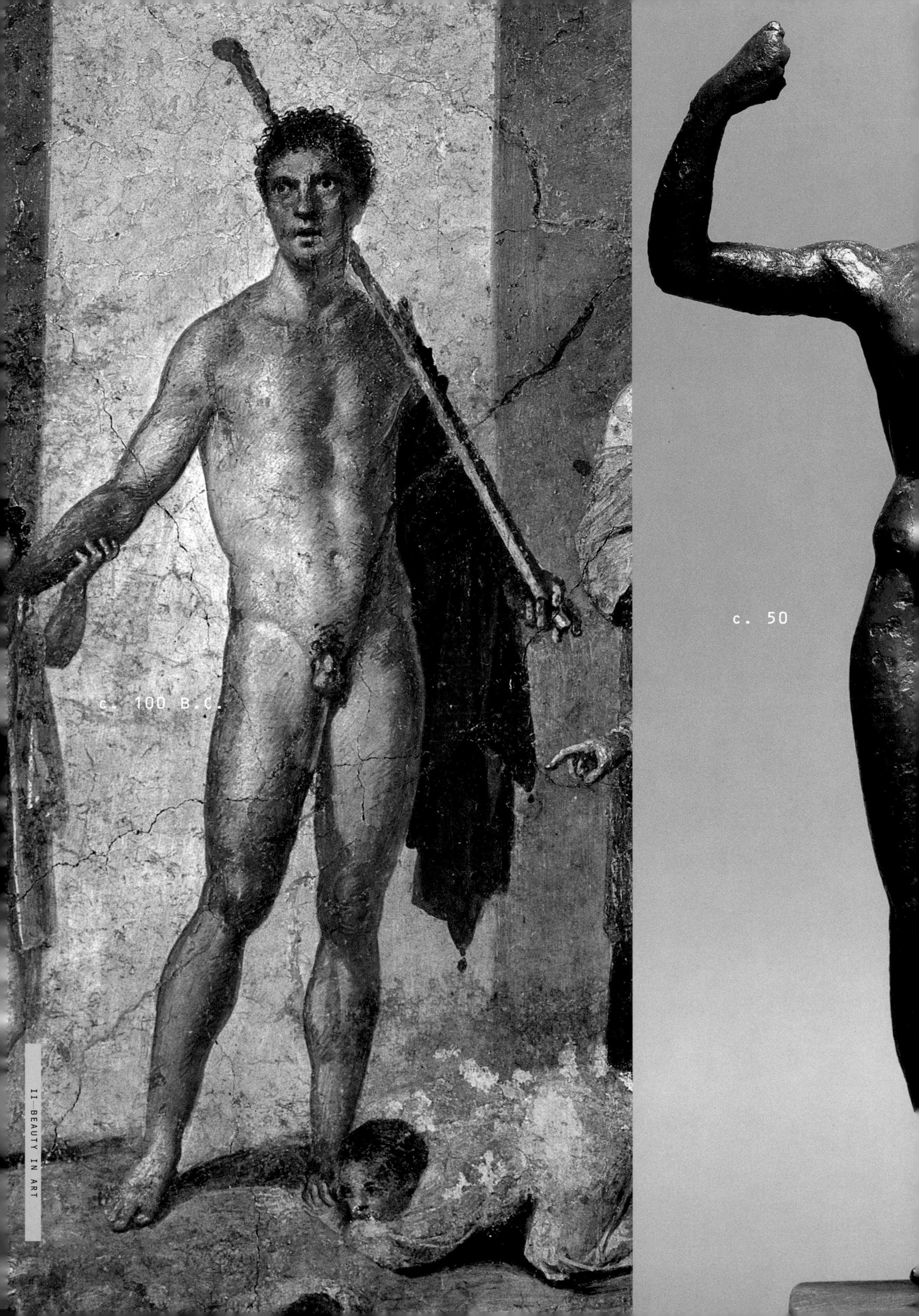
c. 100 B.C.
c. 50

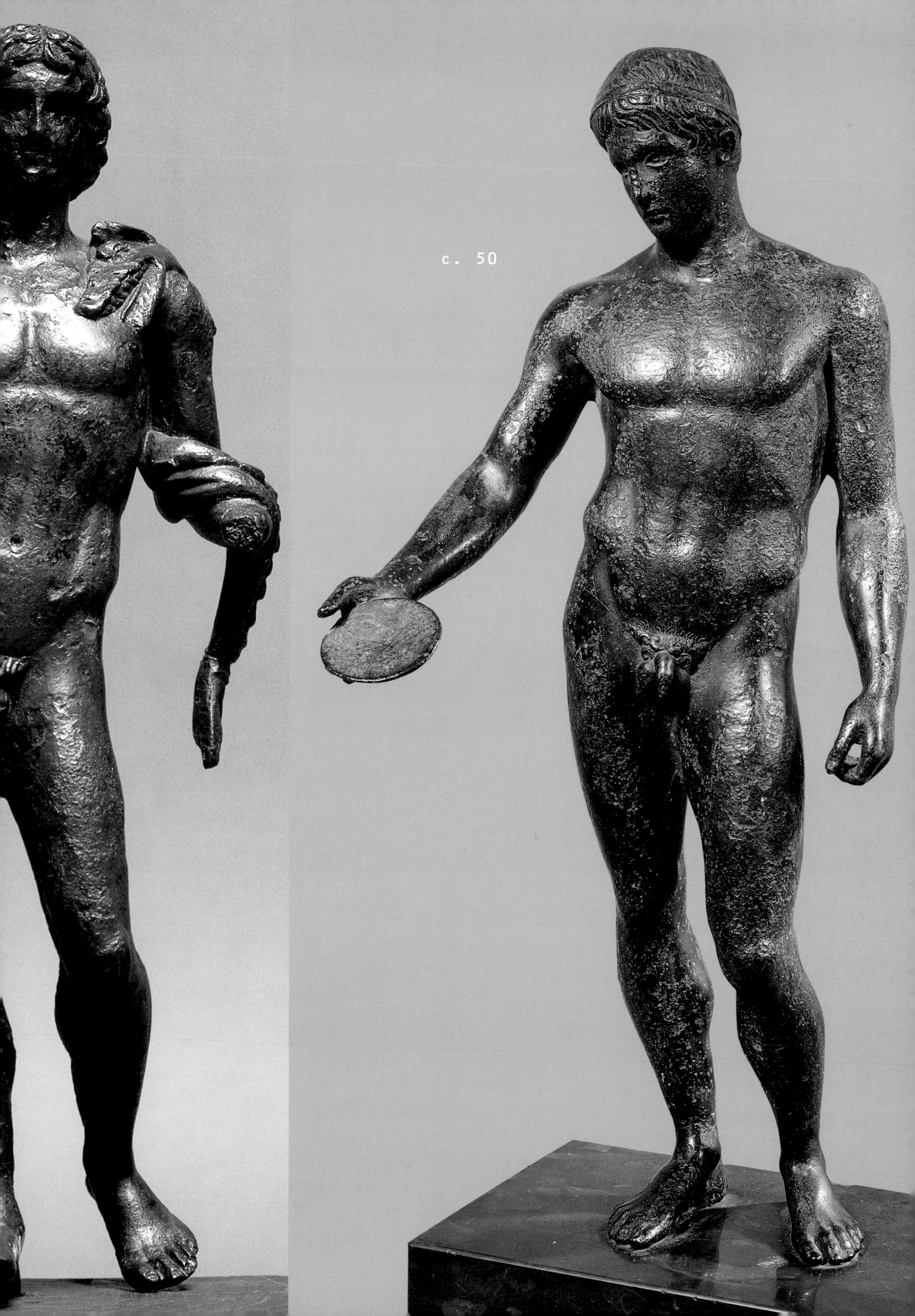
c. 50

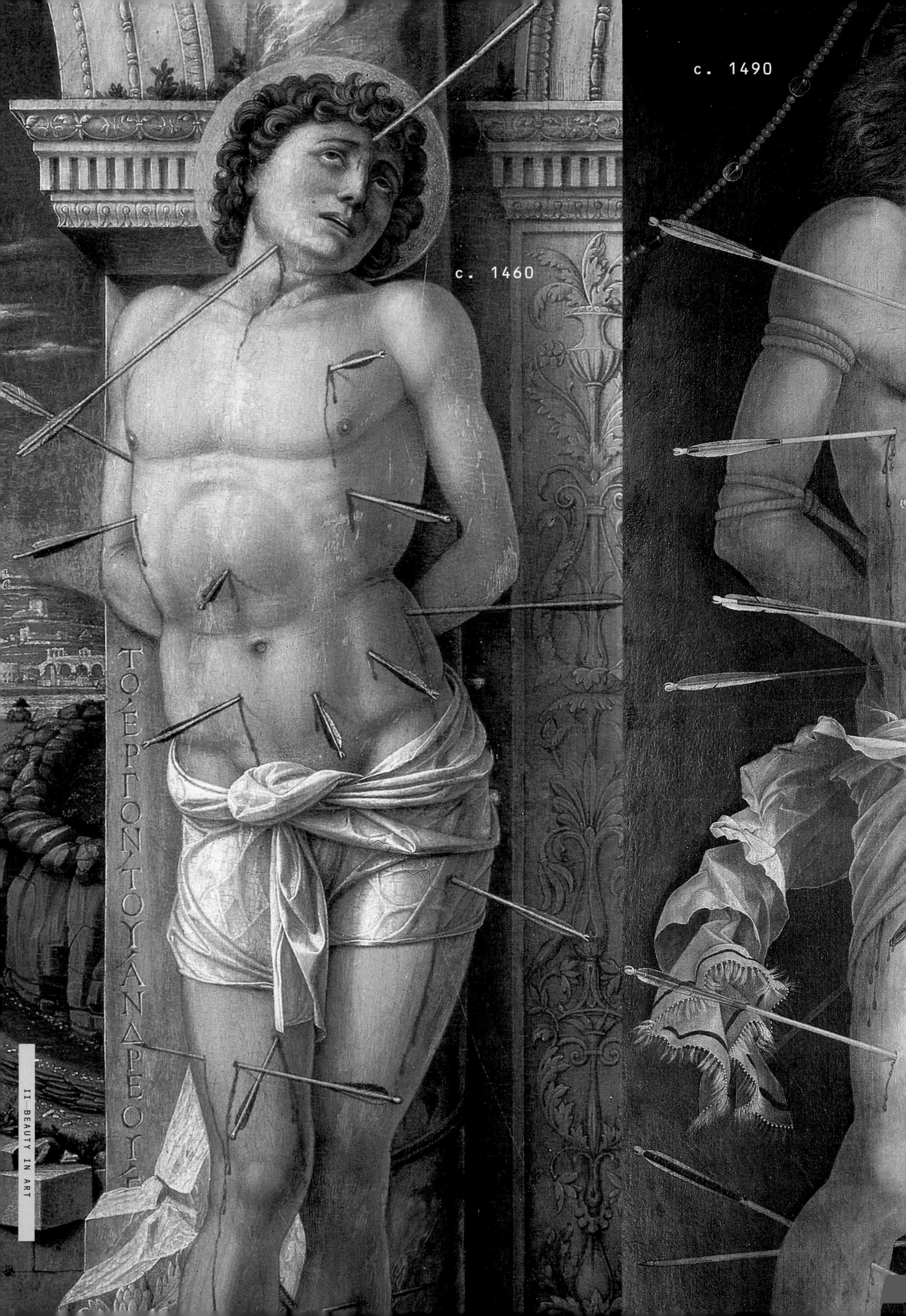

c. 1460

c. 1490

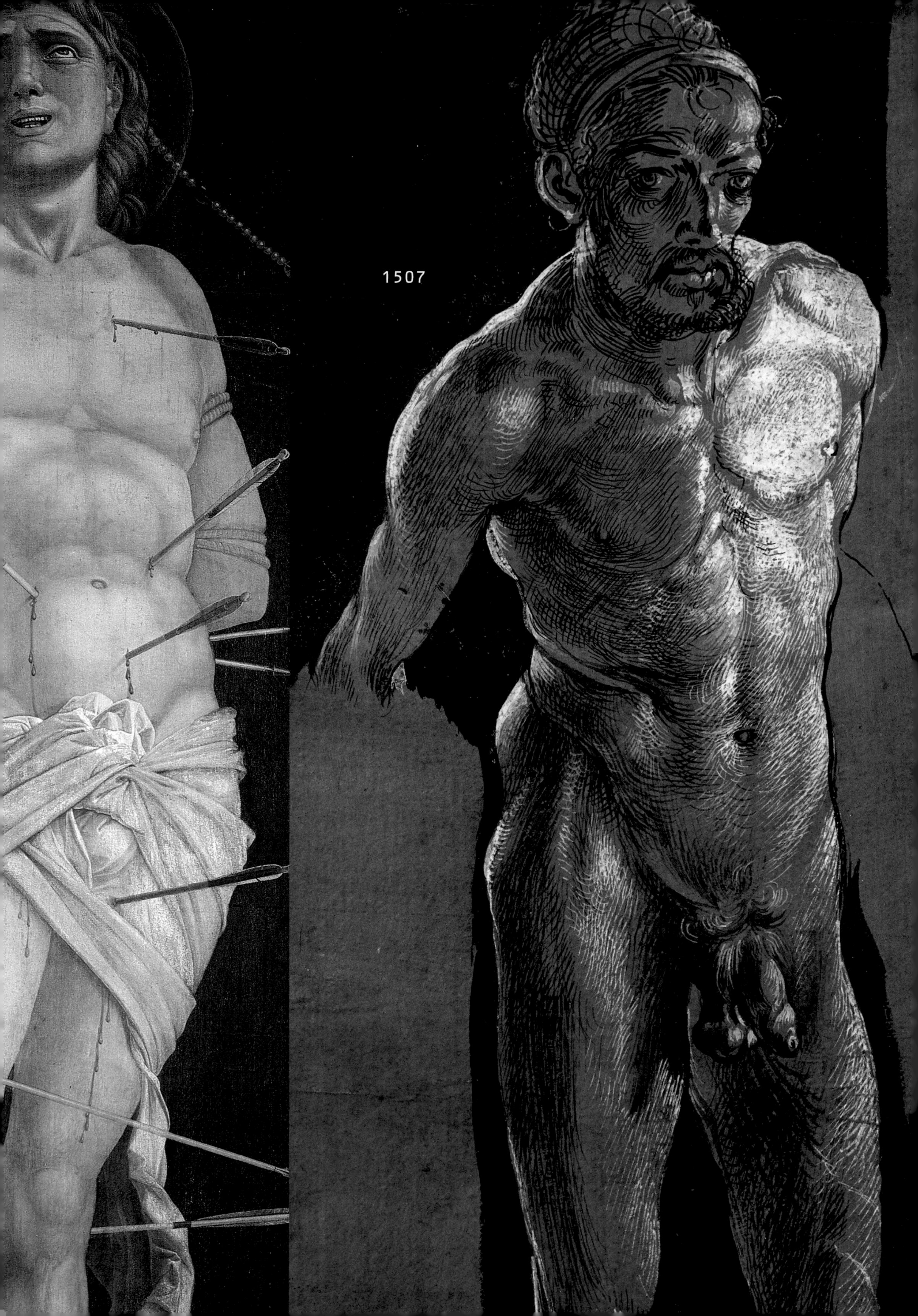

1507

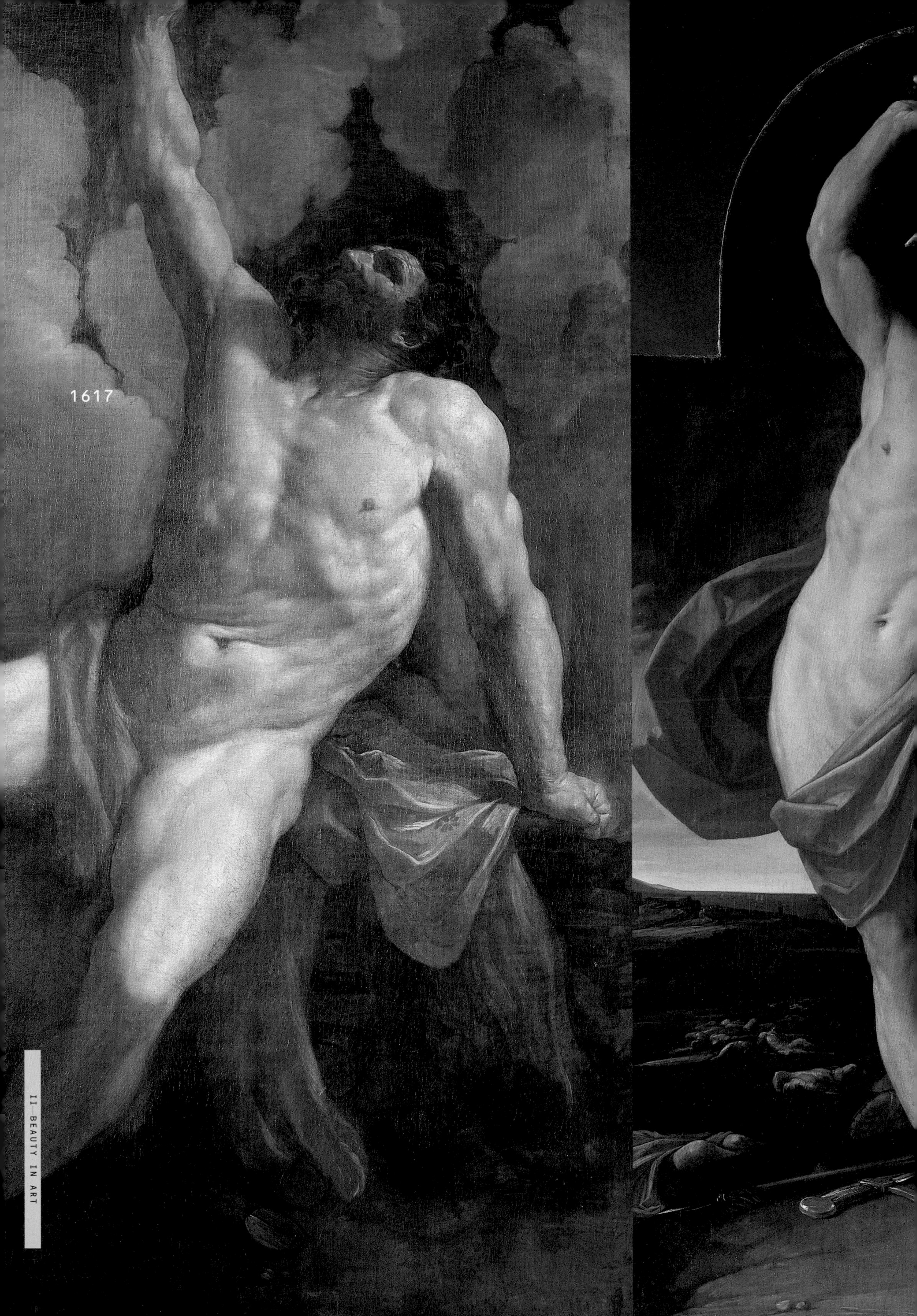
1617

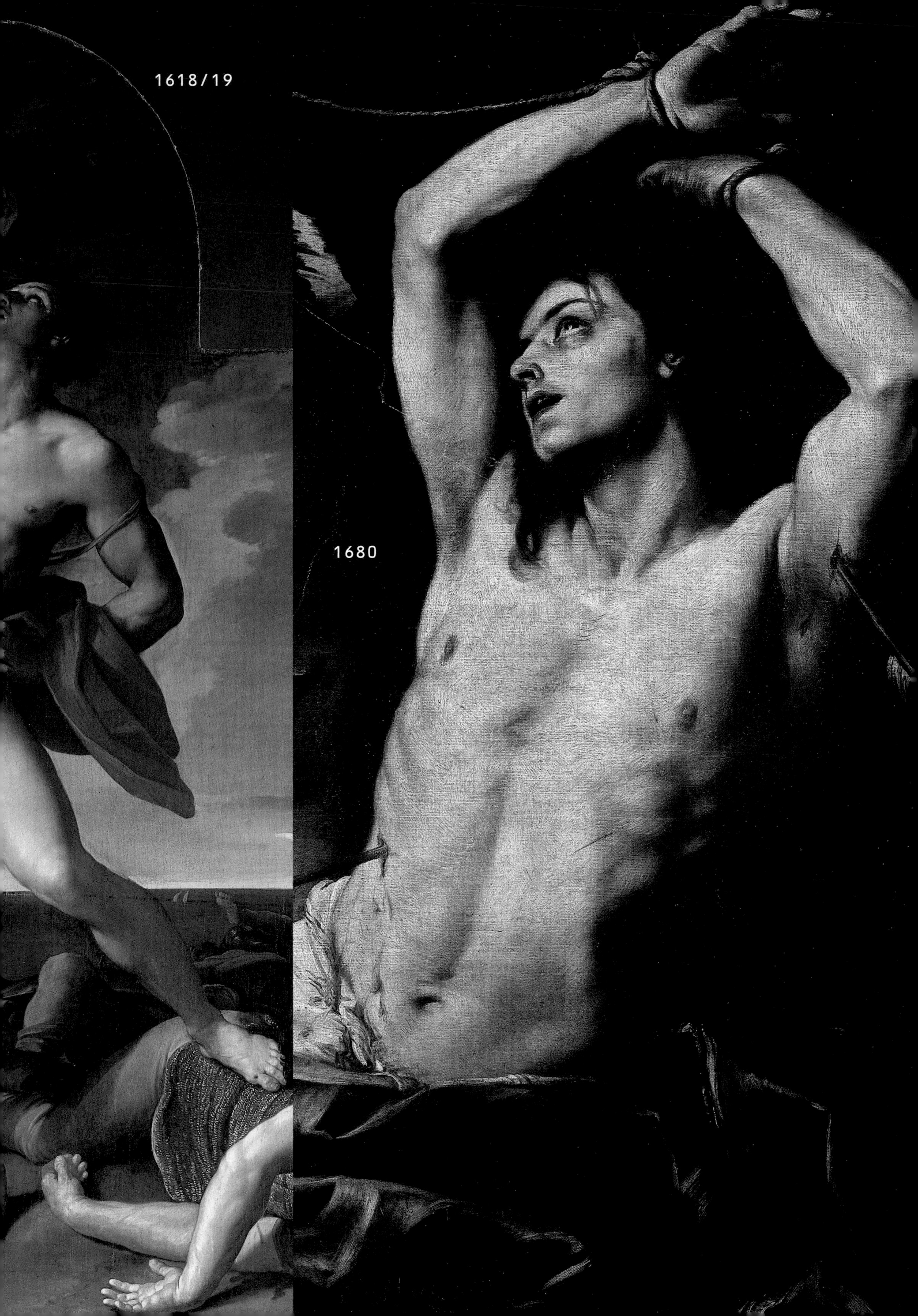
1618/19
1680

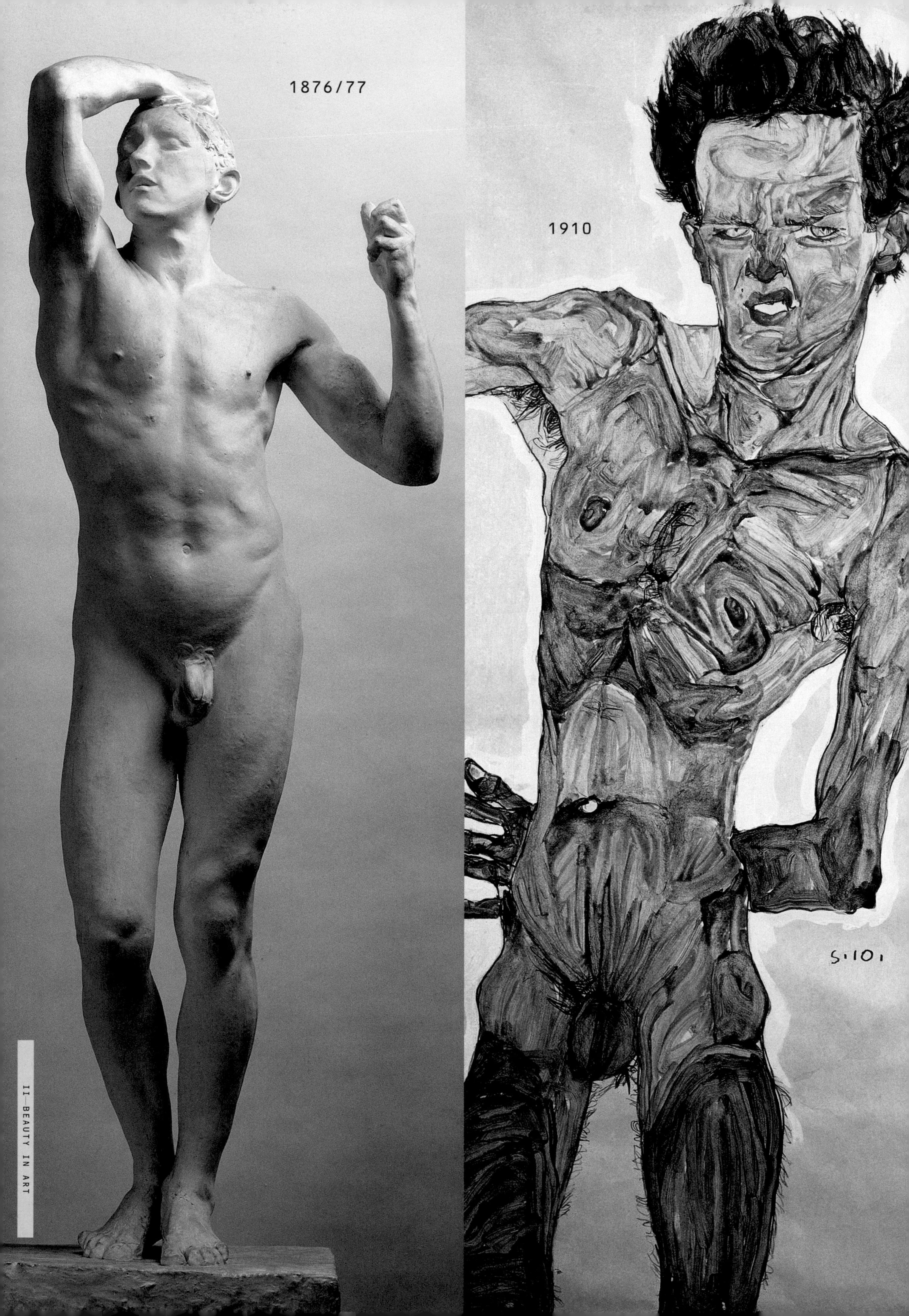

1876/77

1910

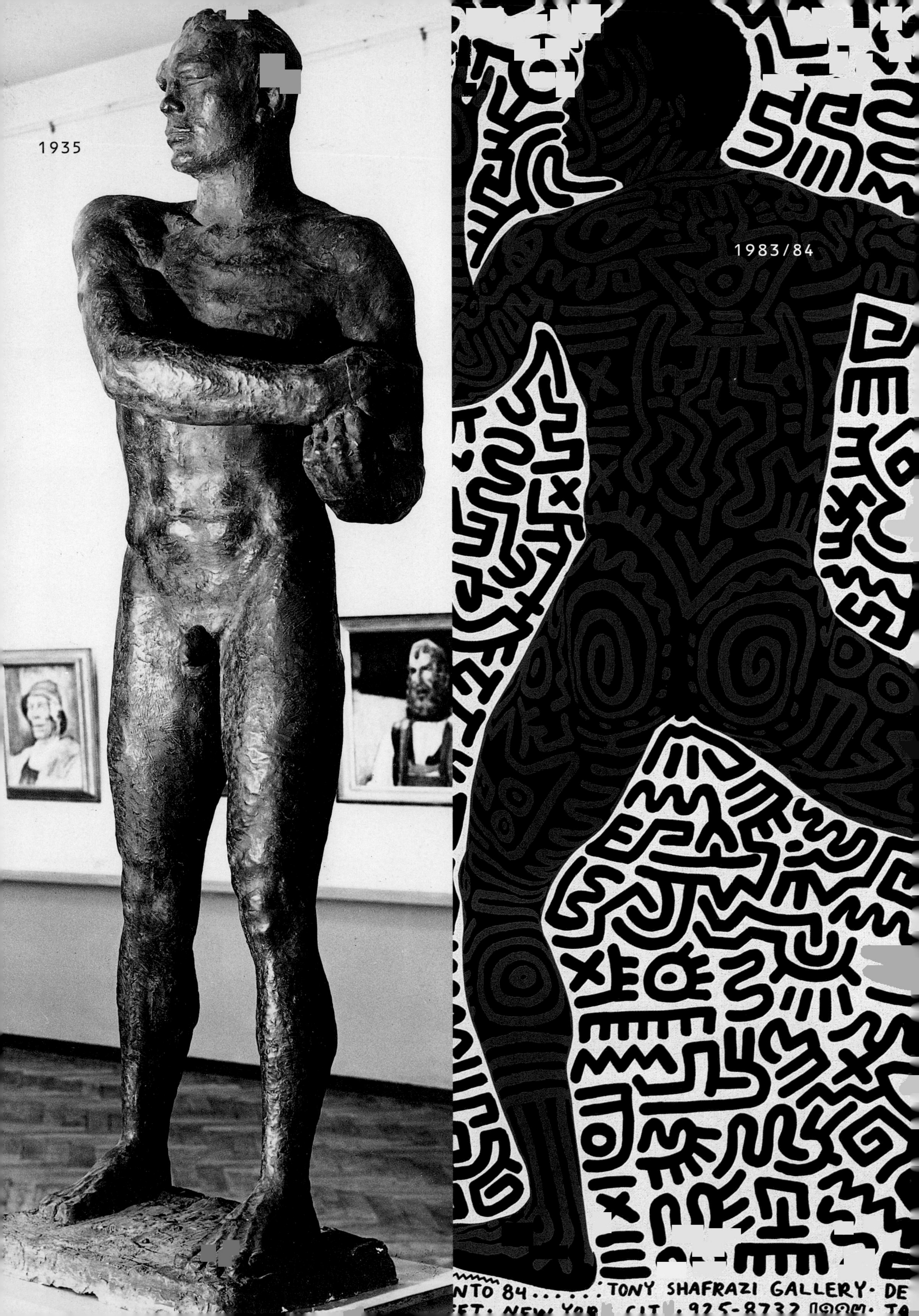

1935

1983/84

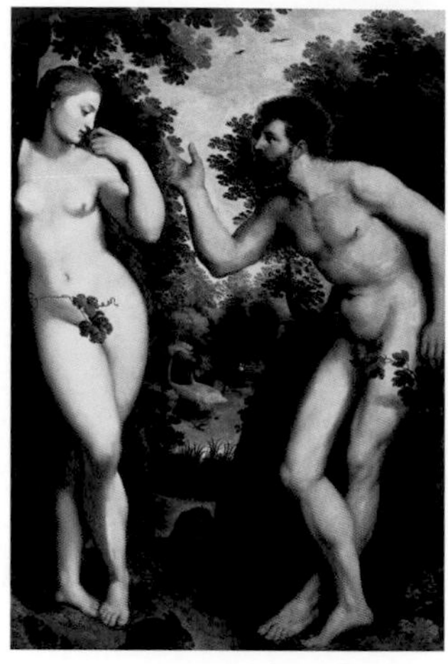

Peter Paul Rubens: Adam and Eve in Paradise, 1605. Rubenshuis, Antwerp. © akg-images

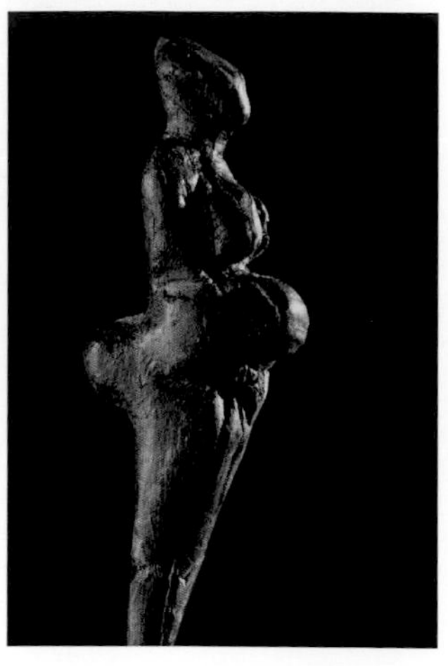

The Grimaldi Venus. Steatite figure. Palaeolithic, c. 25,000 B. C. Height: 4.5 cm. Musée des Antiquites Nationales, St-Germain-en Laye. © akg-images / Erich Lessing

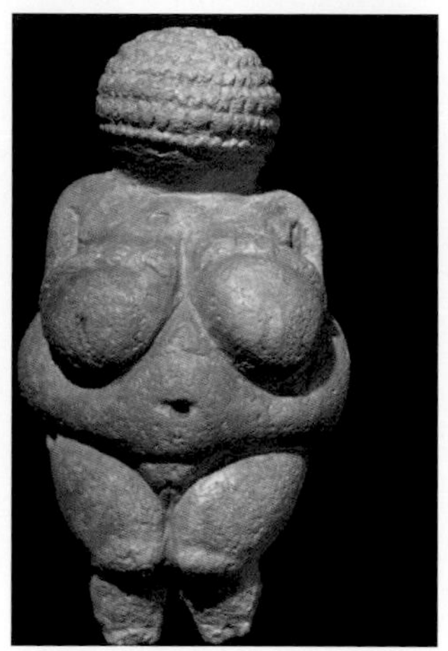

Venus of Willendorf, c. 20,000 B. C. Naturhistorisches Museum, Vienna. © bridgemanart.com

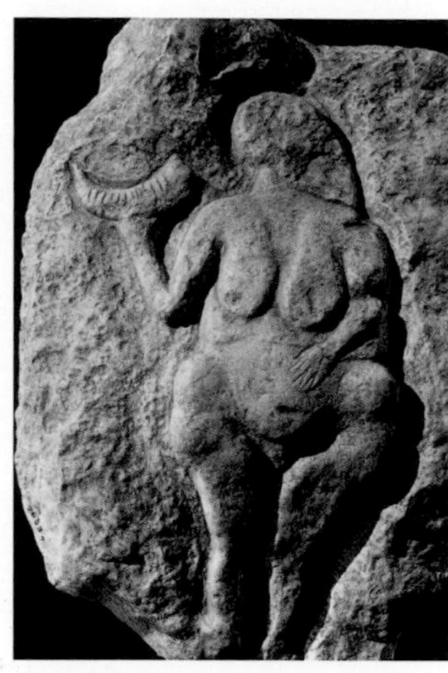

Woman With Bison Horn. Low relief on a limestone block, c. 20,000 B. C. Musée d'Aquitaine, Bordeaux. © bridgemanart.com

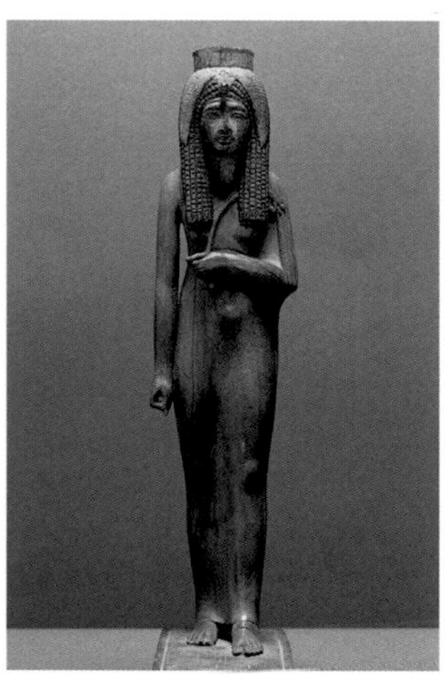

Ahmose-Nefertari. Painted wood statuette, height: 43cm, c. 1550 B. C. Found in Dayr al-Madinah. Musée du Louvre, Paris. © bridgemanart.com

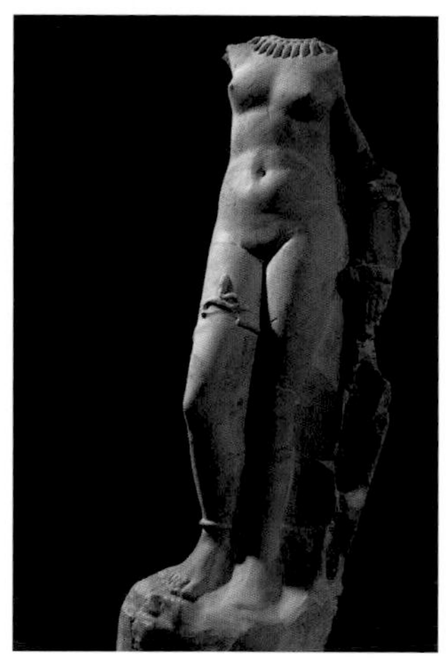

Headless Aphrodite. Clay figurine, hellenistic period, c. 300 B. C. Found in Mount Karmel. Israel Museum, Jerusalem. © akg-images / Erich Lessing

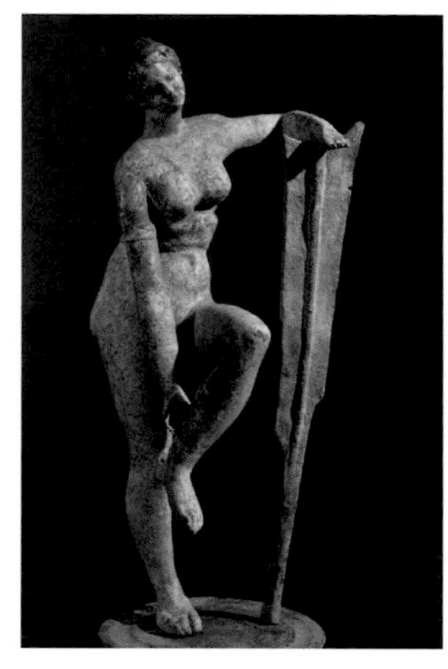

Bathing Aphrodite Leaning Against a Steering Oar. Greek terracotta figurene, hellenistic period, c. 300 B. C. National Maritime Museum, Haifa. © akg-images / Erich Lessing

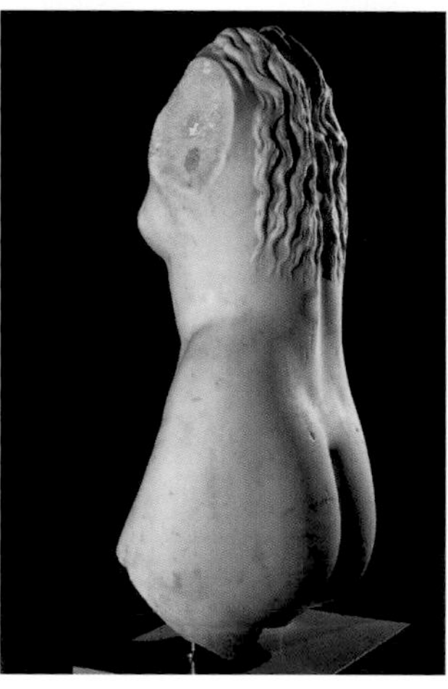

Aphrodite Anadyomene. Greek sculpture, marble, c. 300 B. C. Bibliothèque Nationale, Paris. © akg-images / Erich Lessing

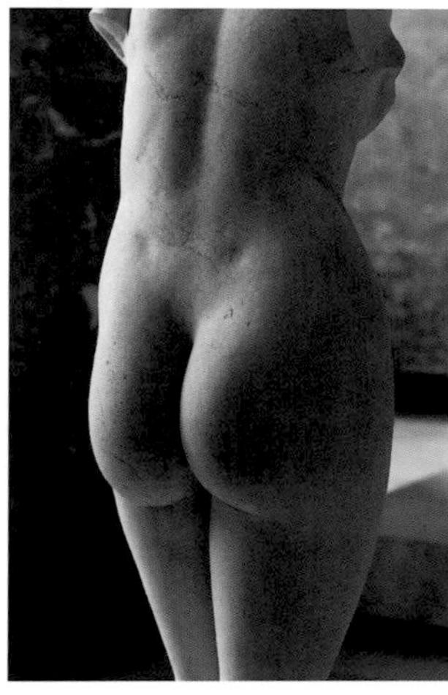

Torso of Aphrodite of Knidos. Roman copy after original by Praxiteles. Marble, c. 340 B. C. Musée du Louvre, Paris. © akg-images / Erich Lessing

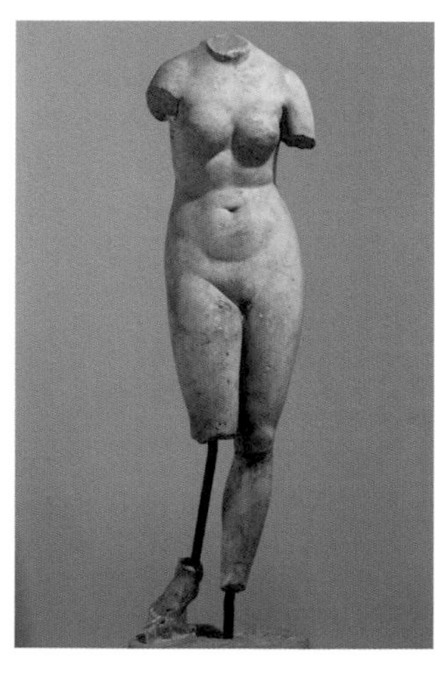

Statue of Aphrodite, with similarities to the Medici Venus. Roman copy based on Praxiteles, marble c. 300 B. C. Museo Archeologico Nazionale, Aquileia. © akg-images / Cameraphoto

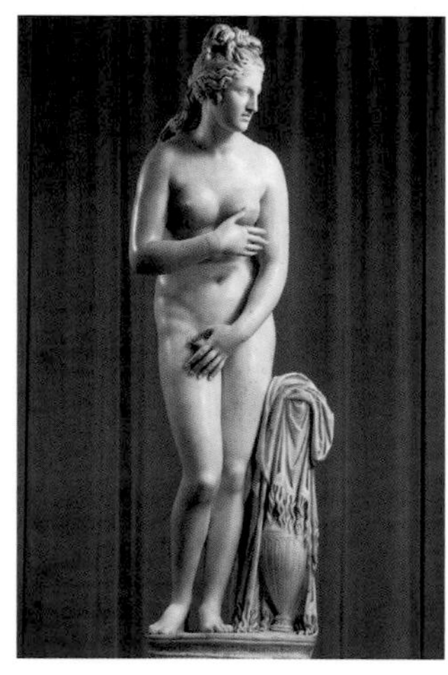

So called Capitoline Venus. Roman marble copy (c. 150 B. C.) after a hellenistic statue c. 290 B.C. Musei Capitolini, Rome. © 1990, Photo Scala, Florence

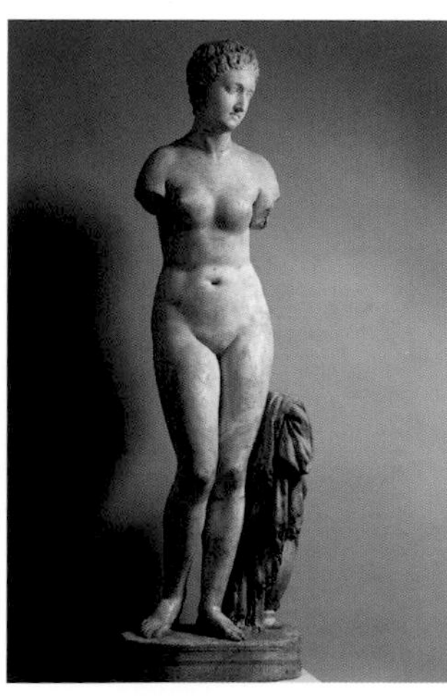

Faustina the Younger, wife of the Roman Emperor Marcus Aurelius, as Venus. Roman marble. 3rd century, Height: 180 cm. Imperial Palace, Pavlovsk. © akg-image

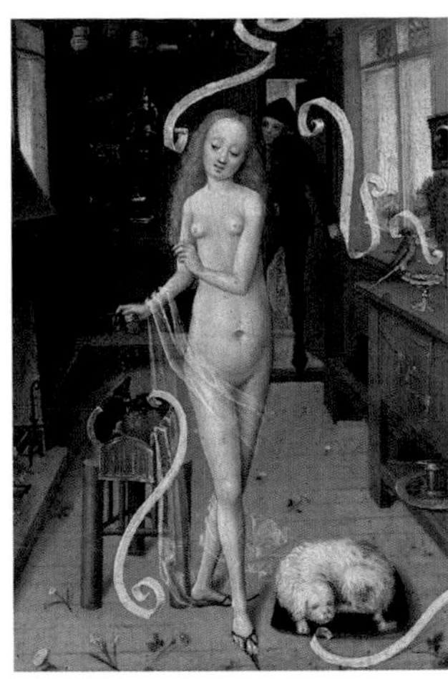

Lower Rhine Master of the 15th century: Der Liebeszauber (Love Spell), c. 1470. Oil on wood, 24 x 18 cm. Museum der Bildenden Künste, Leipzig. © Christoph Sandig – ARTOTHEK

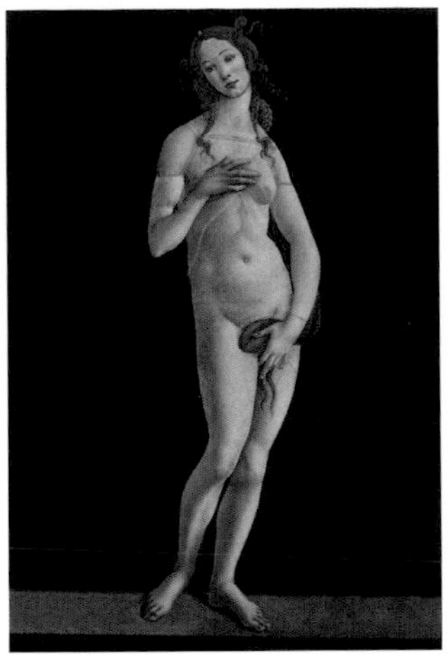

The workshop of Sandro Botticelli: Venus, c. 1486/88. Oil on canvas, 158 x 68.5 cm. Galleria Sabauda, Turin. © 1990, Photo Scala, Florence – courtesy of the Ministero Beni e Attività Culturali

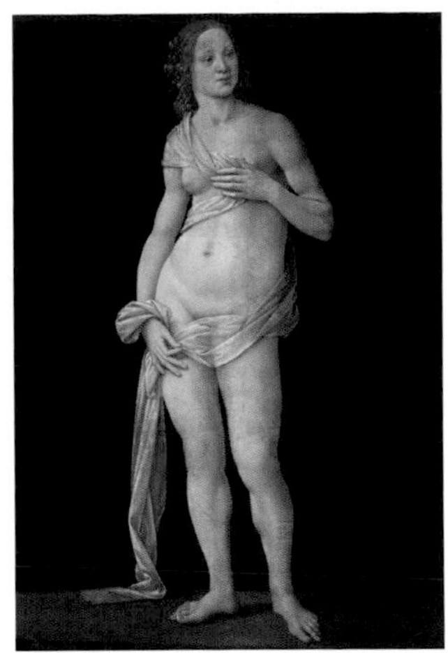

Lorenzo di Credi: Venus, c. 1490. Oil on canvas, 151 x 69 cm. Galleria degli Uffizi, Florence. © 1990, Photo Scala, Florence – courtesy of the Ministero Beni e Attività Culturali

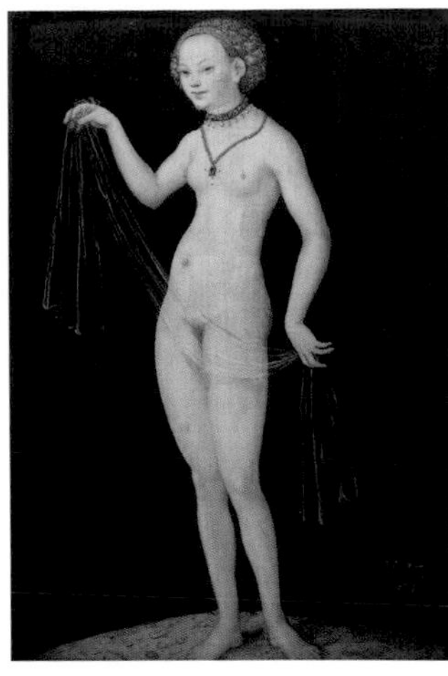

Lucas Cranach the Elder: Venus and Cupid, c. 1530. Oil on panel, 38.1 x 27 cm. National Gallery of Scotland, Edinburgh. © bridgemanart.com

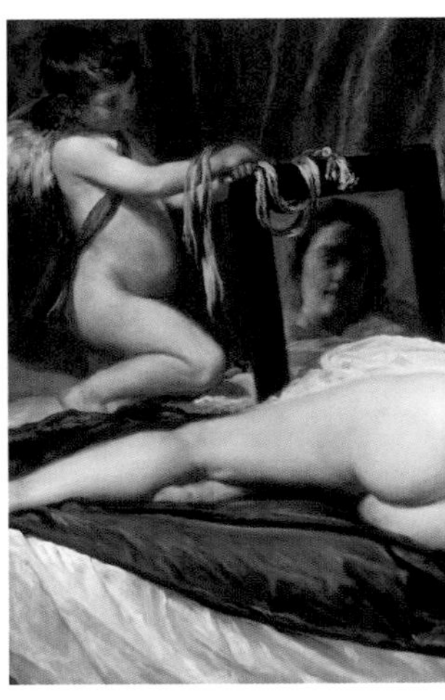

Diego Velázquez: Venus with Mirror (The Rokeby Venus), 1651. Oil on canvas, 122.5 x 177 cm. National Gallery, London. © bridgemanart.com

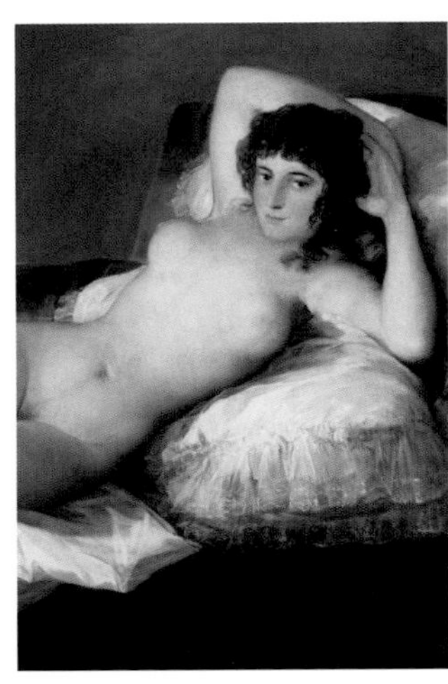

Francisco de Goya: La Maja Desnuda (The Naked Maja), c. 1797. Oil on canvas, 97 x 190 cm. Museo del Prado, Madrid. © 1990, Photo Scala, Florence

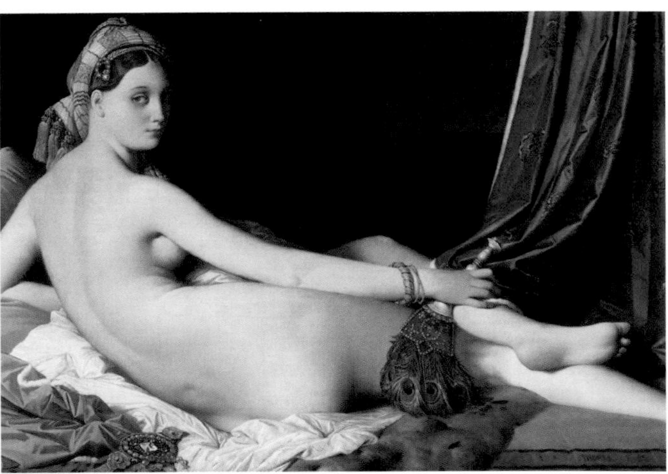

Jean Auguste Dominique Ingres: La Grande Odalisque (The Large Odalisque), 1814. Oil on canvas, 91 x 162 cm. Musée du Louvre, Paris. © 1990, Photo Scala, Florence

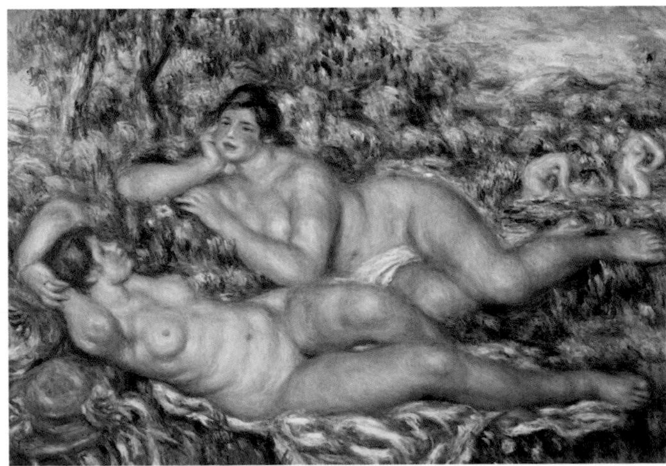

Pierre Auguste Renoir: Les Baigneuses (The Bathers), 1918/19. Oil on canvas, 110 x 160 cm. Musée d'Orsay, Paris. © 1997, Photo Scala, Florence

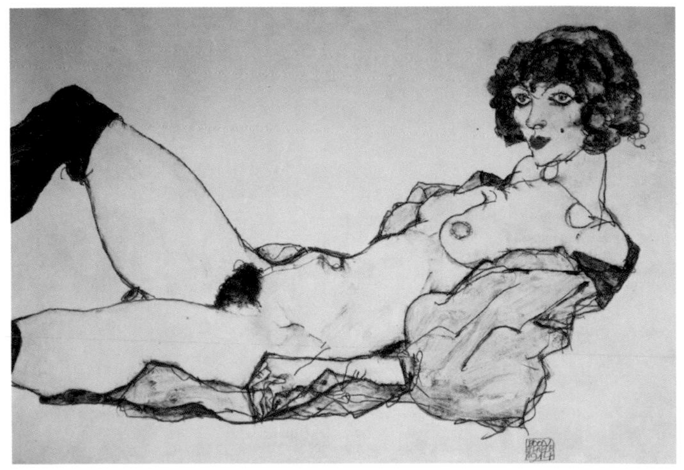

Egon Schiele: Reclining Nude with Green Stockings, 1914. Black chalk and gouache, 30.5 x 46 cm. (private collection). © Christie's – ARTOTHEK

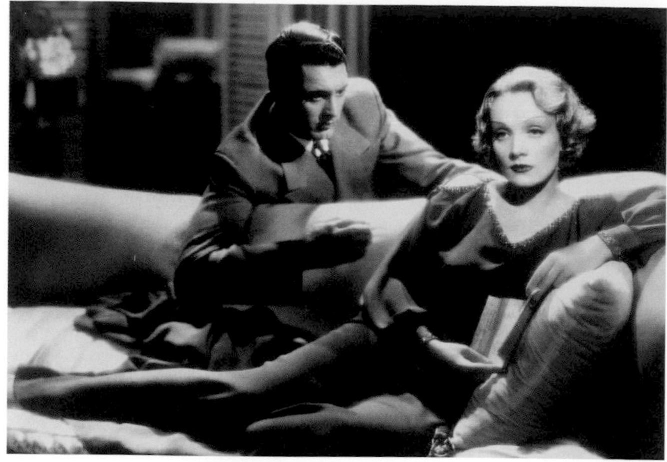

Blonde Venus (USA 1932; directed by Josef von Sternberg). Scene with Cary Grant and Marlene Dietrich. © *akg-images*

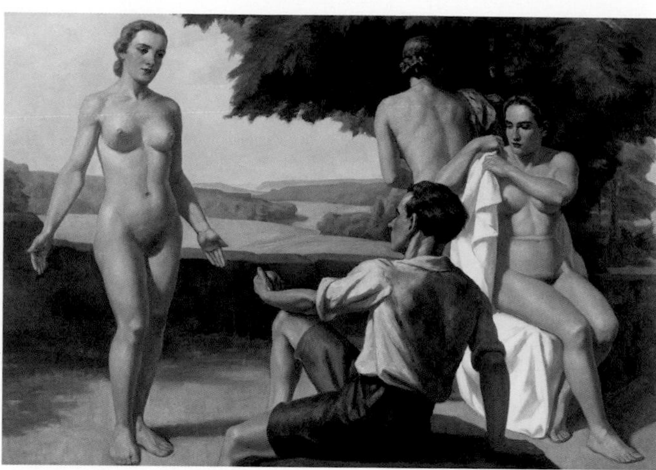

Ivo Saliger: The Judgement of Paris (Das Urteil des Paris), 1939. Oil on canvas, 160 x 200 cm. Property of the Federal Republic of Germany. © *Ernst Reinhold- ARTOTHEK*

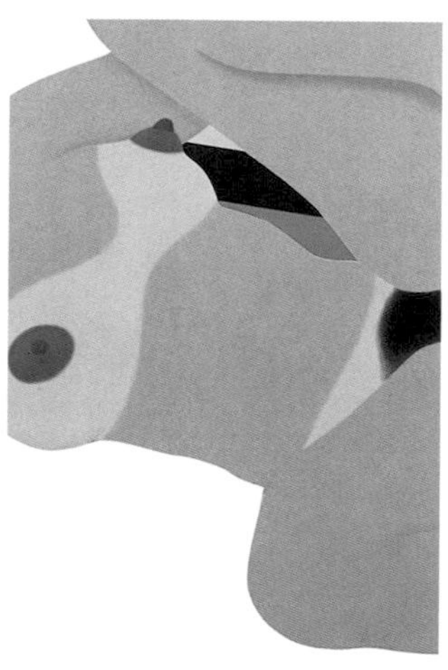

Tom Wesselmann: Great American Nude No. 91, 1967. Private collection.

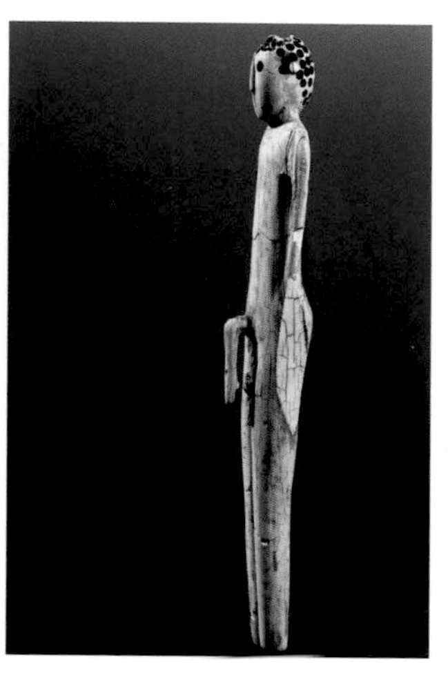

Figure of a Man. Ivory, height: 23.5 cm. Egyptian, predynastic, 1st Negade age (Negade I), c. 4000–3800 B. C. France, private collection. © *akg-images / Erich Lessing*

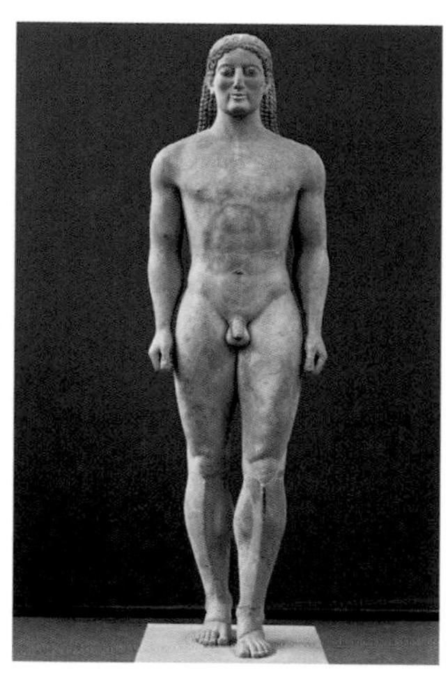

Statue of a Kouros. Ascribed to Myron. Marble, c. 600 B. C. National Archaeological Museum, Athens. © *1990, Photo Scala, Florence*

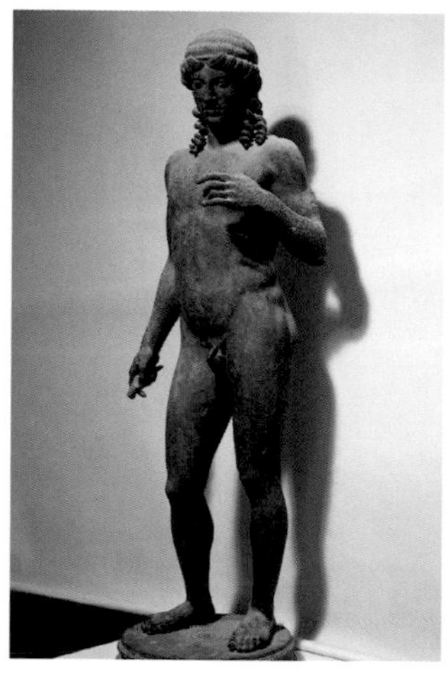

Statue of the so called warrior A from Riace. More than life-size, c. 460 B. C. Sculpture, bronze. Museo Archeologico Nazionale, Reggio. © *bridgemanart.com*

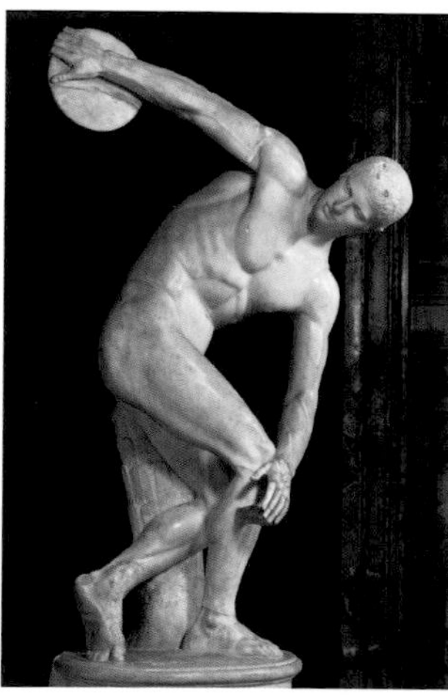

Diskobolus (Discus Thrower). Roman copy after Myron, c. 450 B. C. Marble, height: 125 cm. Museo Nazionale Romano, Rome. © *1990, Photo Scala, Florence – courtesy of the Ministero Beni e Attività Culturali*

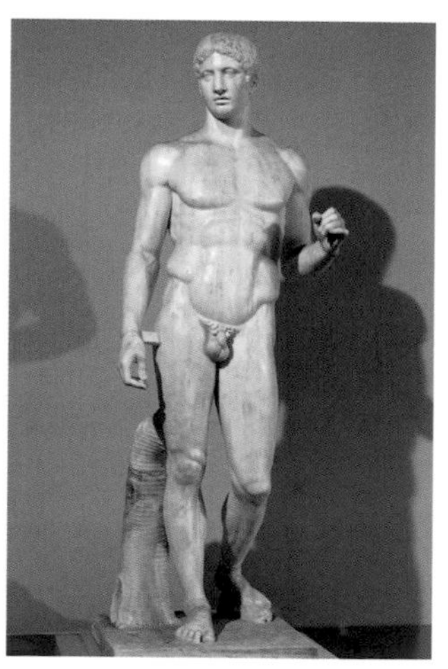

Doryphoros (Speer Carrier) by Polyklet. Copy, after a bronze original, c. 440 B. C. Marble. Museo Nazionale Archeologico, Naples. © *2003, Photo Scala, Florence – courtesy of the Ministero Beni e Attività Culturali*

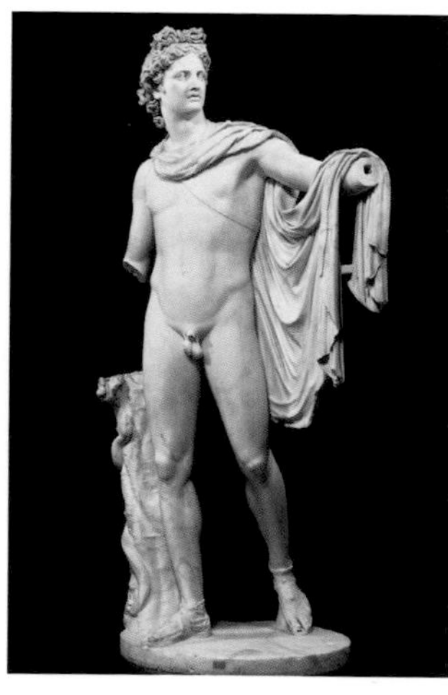

The Apollo Belvedere. Plaster cast of the Roman marble copy, after a bronze original attributed to Leochares, around 330 B. C. 225 x 113 x 82 cm. Museo Pio-Clementino, Vatican, Vatican City. © *1990, Photo Scala, Florence*

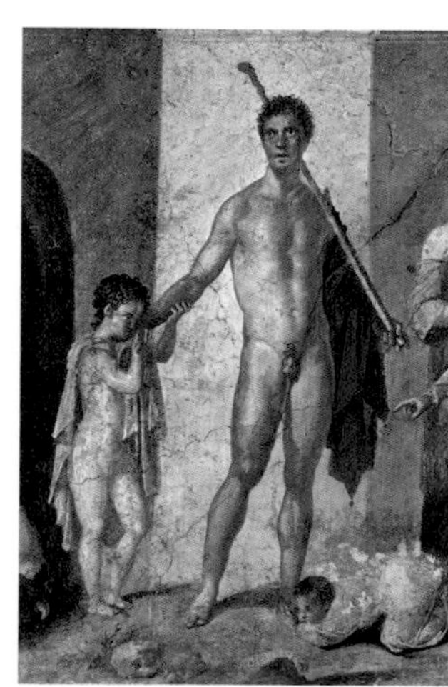

Triumph of Theseus as Victor over the Minotaur. Roman wall painting, c. 100 B. C. after an original from the 3rd century B. C. Museo Nazionale Archeologico, Naples © *2003, Photo Scala, Florence / Fotografica Foglia*

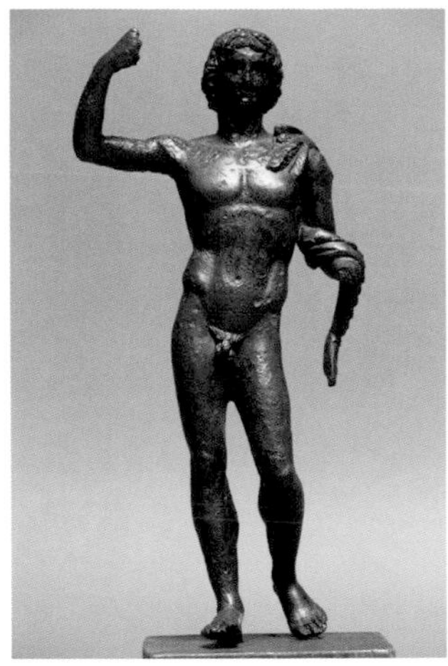

Statuette of Alexander the Great. Roman, c. 50. Bronze. Museo Civico, Trevisio. © akg-images / Cameraphoto

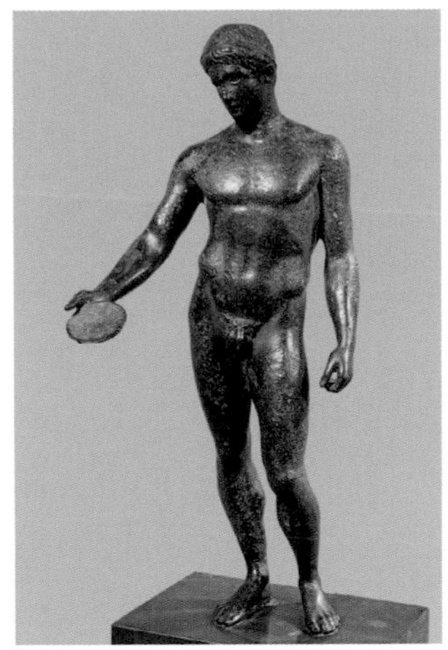

Statue of an young man. Roman, c. 50. Bronze. Museo Nazionale Archaelogico, Naples. © bridgemanart.com

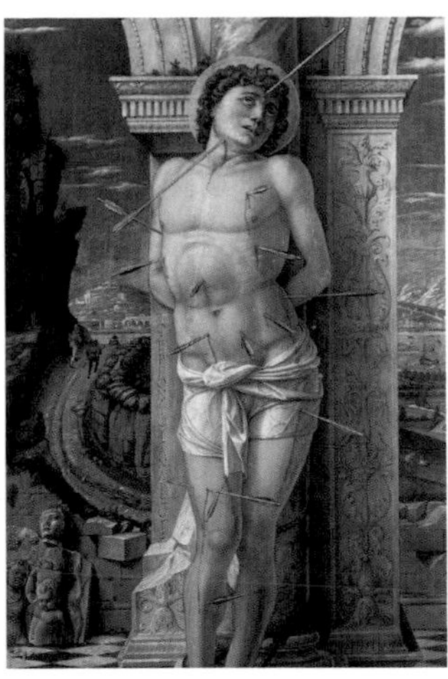

Andrea Mantegna: St. Sebastian, c. 1460. Oil on wood, 68 x 30 cm. Kunsthistorisches Museum, Vienna. © bridgemanart.com

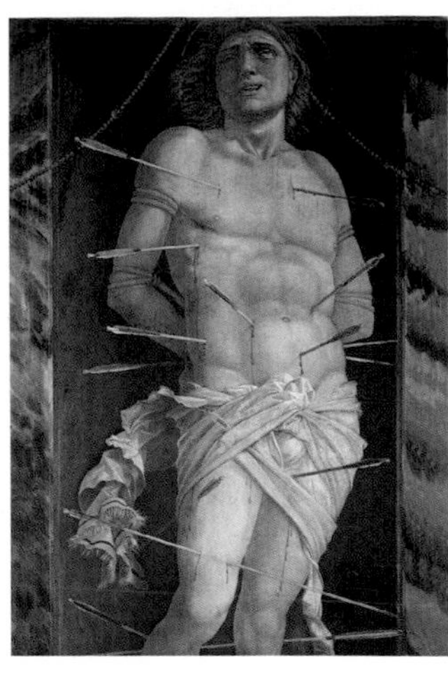

Andrea Mantegna: St. Sebastian, c. 1490. Oil on canvas, 210 x 91 cm. Ca' d'Oro, Galleria Franchetti, Venice. © 1990, Photo Scala, Florence – courtesy of the Ministero Beni e Attività Culturali

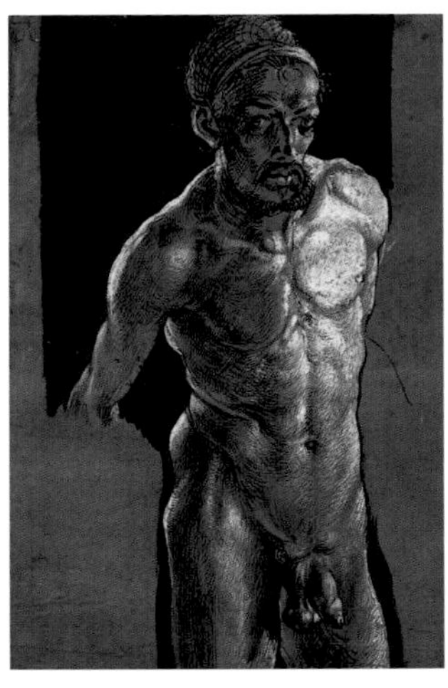

Albrecht Dürer: Nude Study (Self Portrait), 1507. Ink and wash on stained (green) paper, 29.2 x 15.4 cm. Staatliche Kunstsammlung, Schlossmuseum, Weimar. © bridgemanart.com

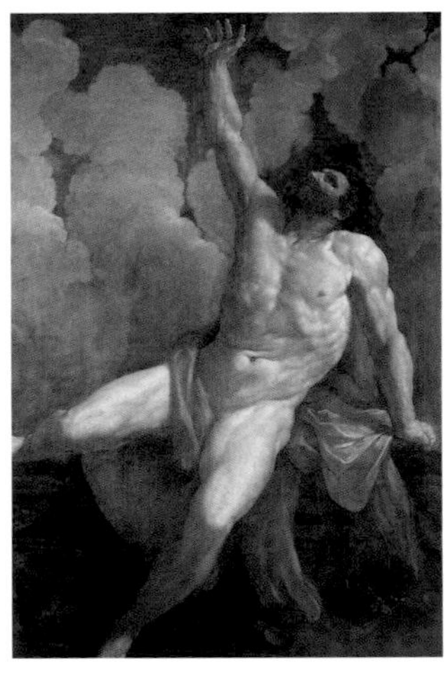

Guido Reni: Hercules on the Pyre, 1617. Oil on canvas, 260 x 192 cm. Musée du Louvre, Paris. © akg-images / Erich Lessing

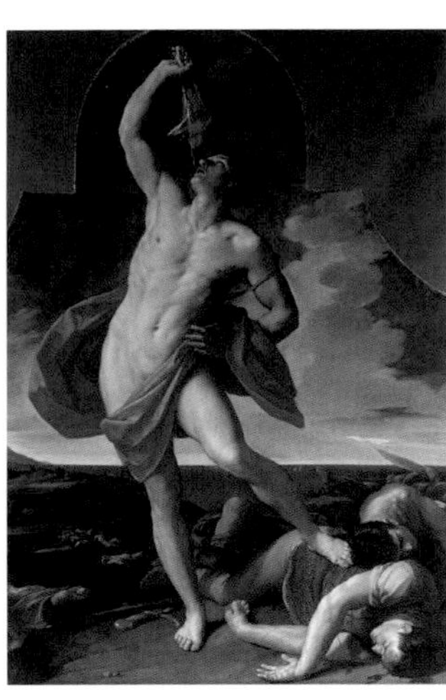

Guido Reni: Samson Victorious, 1618/19. Oil on canvas, 260 x 223 cm. Pinacoteca Nazionale, Bologna. © bridgemanart.com

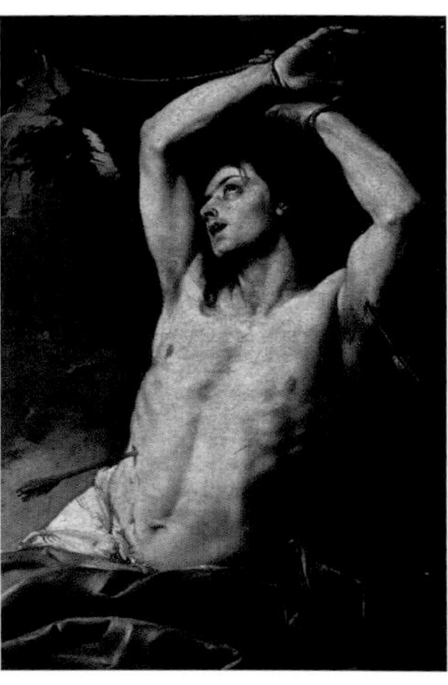

Gian Battista Beinaschi: St. Sebastian, 1680. Oil on canvas, 131 x 97 cm. © akg-images

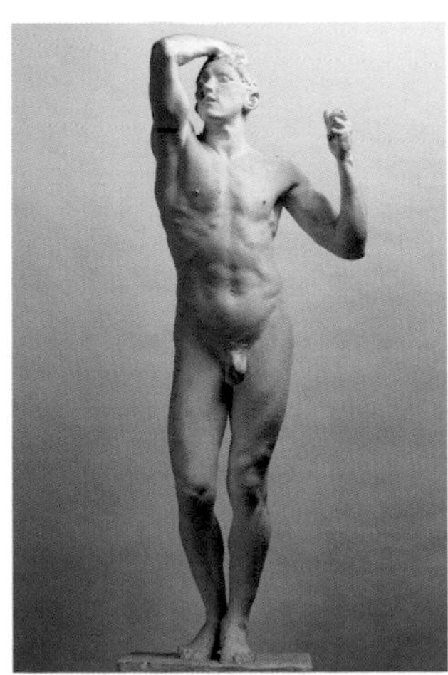

Auguste Rodin: The Age of Bronze, 1876/77. Bronze, 178 x 59 x 61.5 cm. Hermitage, Petersburg. © bridgemanart.com

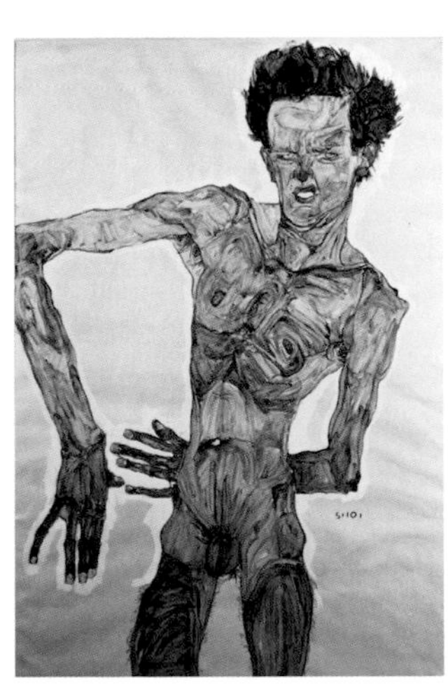

Egon Schiele: Male Nude (Self Portrait), 1910. Pencil, watercolor and opaque colours on paper, 55.7 x 36.8 cm. Graphische Sammlung Albertina, Vienna. © bridgemanart.com

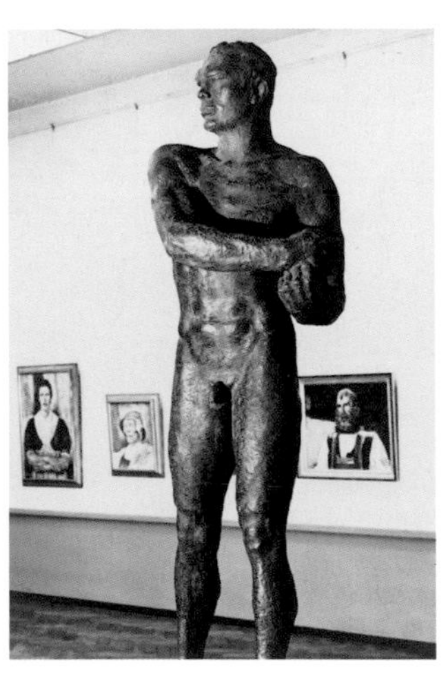

Josef Thorak: Max Schmeling, 1935. Sculpture. © akg-images

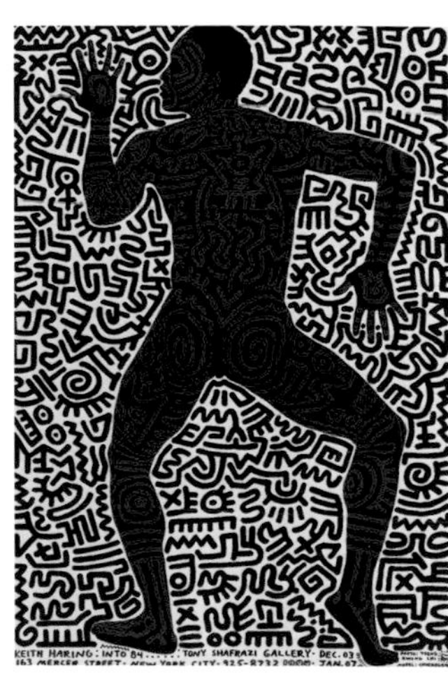

Keith Haring: The Choreographer Bill T. Jones, 1983/84. Offset poster, 89.5 x 59 cm. Private collection. © akg-images

Icon Octaua.

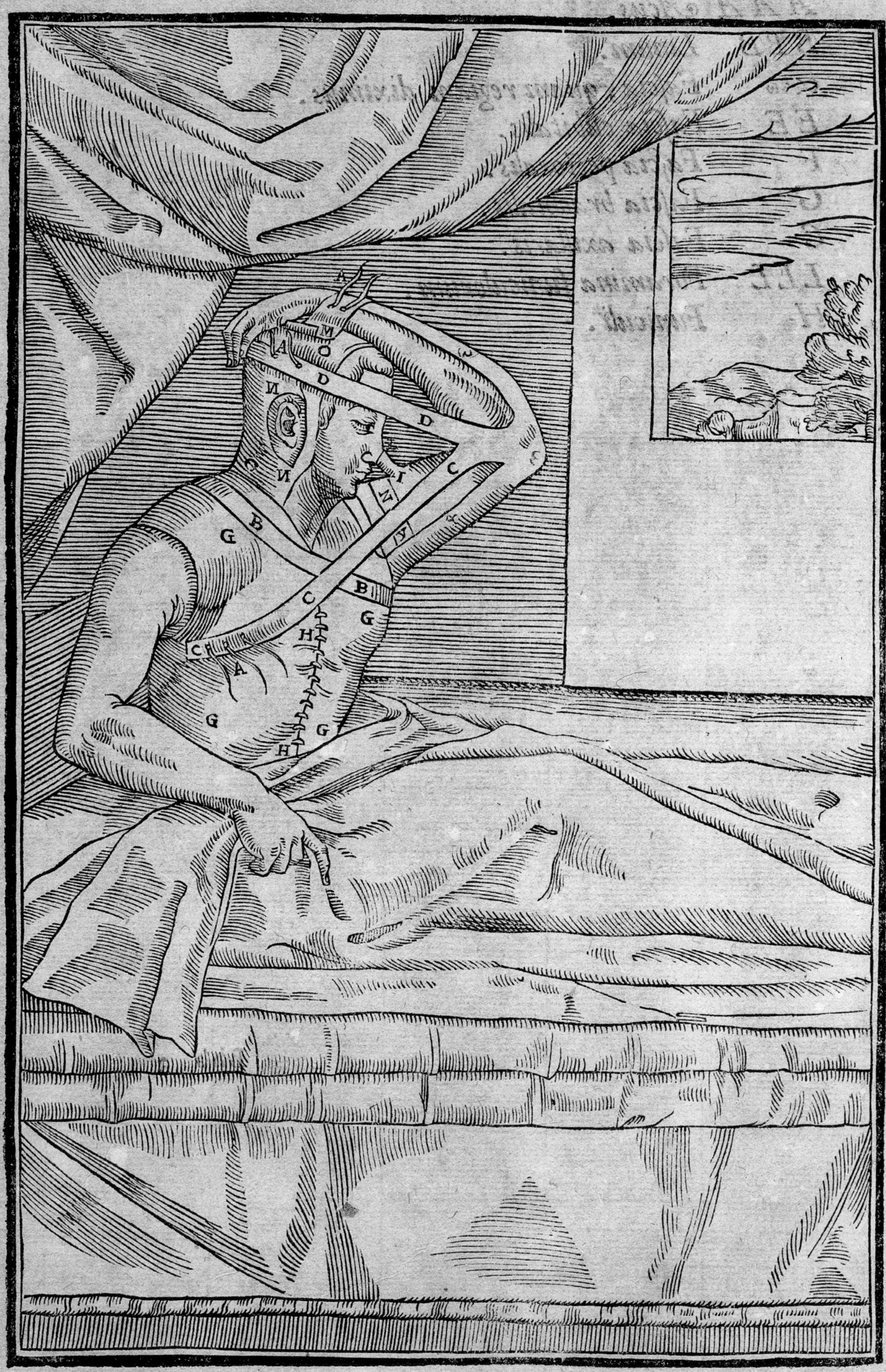

III.

THE ASTONISHING HISTORY OF AESTHETIC SURGERY

Text by

SANDER L. GILMAN

III.

The Astonishing History of Aesthetic Surgery

SANDER L. GILMAN, Chicago

The history of aesthetic surgery can be rather neatly divided into the world before the end of the 19th century and the world afterwards. It is between 1840 and 1900 that virtually all of the present procedures for the aesthetic alternation of the body are introduced. They build, of course, on earlier developments in surgery. The initial patients, with few exceptions, were men, a fact seemingly lost in the history of aesthetic surgery. But why is there an explosion of both patient interest and surgical innovation at that specific moment in time? Such surgery prior to the 19th century with the introduction of antisepsis (no infection) in 1867 and anesthesia (no pain) in 1846 was undertaken only when it was truly a functional necessity. Aesthetic surgery demanded something in addition.

THE

BOSTON MEDICAL AND SURGICAL JOURNAL.

Vol. XXXV. Wednesday, November 18, 1846. No. 16.

INSENSIBILITY DURING SURGICAL OPERATIONS PRODUCED BY INHALATION.

Read before the Boston Society of Medical Improvement, Nov. 9th, 1846, an abstract having been previously read before the American Academy of Arts and Sciences, Nov. 3d, 1846.

By Henry Jacob Bigelow, M.D., one of the Surgeons of the Massachusetts General Hospital.

[Communicated for the Boston Medical and Surgical Journal.]

It has long been an important problem in medical science to devise some method of mitigating the pain of surgical operations. An efficient agent for this purpose has at length been discovered. A patient has been rendered completely insensible during an amputation of the thigh, regaining consciousness after a short interval. Other severe operations have been performed without the knowledge of the patients. So remarkable an occurrence will, it is believed, render the following details relating to the history and character of the process, not uninteresting.

On the 16th of Oct., 1846, an operation was performed at the hospital, upon a patient who had inhaled a preparation administered by Dr. Morton, a dentist of this city, with the alleged intention of producing insensibility to pain. Dr. Morton was understood to have extracted teeth under similar circumstances, without the knowledge of the patient. The present operation was performed by Dr. Warren, and though comparatively slight, involved an incision near the lower jaw of some inches in extent. During the operation the patient muttered, as in a semi-conscious state, and afterwards stated that the pain was considerable, though mitigated; in his own words, as though the skin had been scratched with a hoe. There was, probably, in this instance, some defect in the process of inhalation, for on the following day the vapor was administered to another patient with complete success. A fatty tumor of considerable size was removed, by Dr. Hayward, from the arm of a woman near the deltoid muscle. The operation lasted four or five minutes, during which time the patient betrayed occasional marks of uneasiness; but upon subsequently regaining her consciousness, professed not only to have felt no pain, but to have been insensible to surrounding objects, to have known nothing of the operation, being only uneasy about a child left at home. No doubt, I think, existed, in the minds of those who saw this operation, that the unconsciousness was real; nor could the imagination be accused of any share in the production of these remarkable phenomena.

I subsequently undertook a number of experiments, with the view of ascertaining the nature of this new agent, and shall briefly state them,

16

fig. 1

The Introduction of Anesthesia in 1846

Anesthesia became generally accepted and central to the practice of surgery after the discovery of ether anesthesia by William Thomas Green Morton (1819—1868) in 1846. (fig. 1) The further development by the 1880s of local anesthesia, in the form of cocaine for surgery of the eye as well as spinal, the so called subarachnoid anesthesia and epidural anesthesia meant that the greater risk of dying under general anesthesia, could be avoided. Local anesthe sia has played a central part in the development of aesthetic surgery as a widely practiced specialty. It is one of the primary factors in the successful outcome of the patient, who can follow the procedure and, unlike the patient under general anesthesia, does not morbidly fantasize about the opening of the body while unconscious.[1] The patient's perception of autonomy is central to the popularity of aesthetic surgery.

The Introduction of Antisepsis in 1867

The movement toward antisepsis paralleled the development of anesthesia. In 1867 Joseph Lord Lister (1827—1912) provided a model for antisepsis, which became generally accepted by the end of the 19th century.[2] The potential

1 — Sanford Gifford, "Cosmetic Surgery and Personality Change: A Review and Some Clinical Operations," in Robert M. Goldwyn, ed., *The Unfavorable Result in Plastic Surgery: Avoidance and Treatment* (Boston: Little, Brown, and Co., 1972), p. 30.

2 — See Owen and Sarah Wangensteen, *The Rise of Surgery: from Empiric Craft to Scientific Discipline* (Minneapolis: University of Minnesota Press, 1978), pp. 275—

fig. previous pages:

Support bandage developed by Gaspare Tagliacozzi (1545—1599). Tagliacozzi taught at the University of Bologna. In 1597, he published the first book to give a detailed description of rebuilding a nose, including engravings. © Columbia University Health Sciences Library. Photo: Dwight Primiano

fig. 1

The first press article about the use of anaesthesia was published in 1846. Boston dentist William Thomas Green Morton (1819–1868) had discovered the sedative property of ether and introduced local anaesthesia in his practice. © Columbia University Health Sciences Library. Photo: Dwight Primiano

fig. 2

A Braun sedation unit from the 1920s, used predominantly for rhinoplasties. The patient was administered a precisely dosed flow of ether or chloroform via a metal mask. Source: J. Joseph, Nasenplastik und sonstige Gesichtsplastik, Leipzig 1931

fig. 3

Immanuel Kant (1724—1804) proposed a philosophy according to which every person has the right to pursue happiness and sensibly look after his or her body. Even in Kant's time, this could be interpreted as the individual's moral right to have aesthetic surgery. © Archivo Iconografico, S.A. / CORBIS

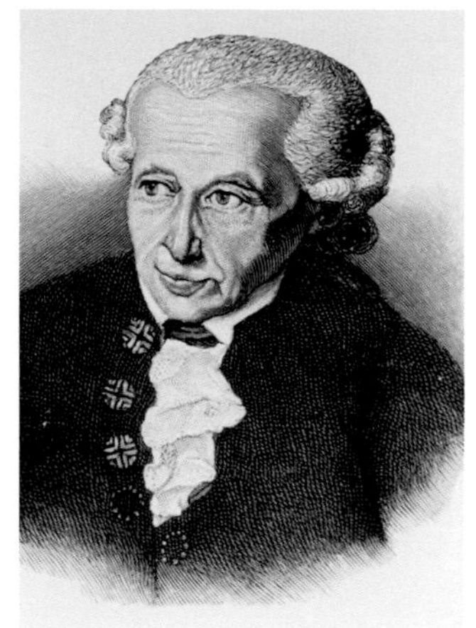

fig. 3

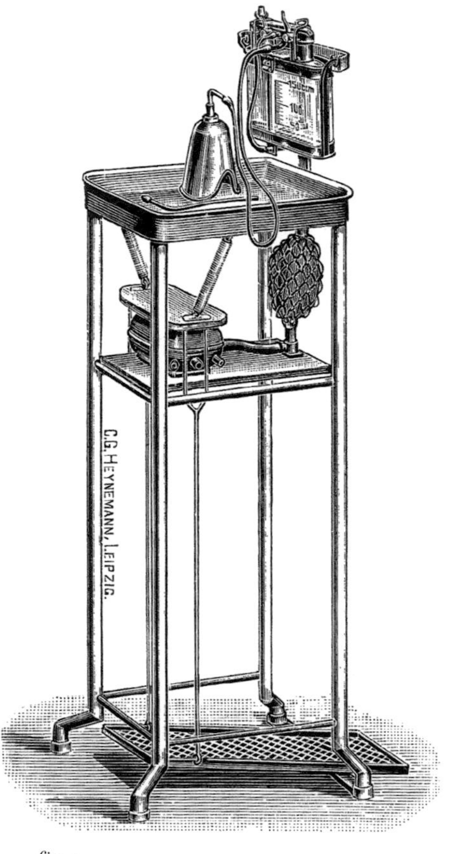

fig. 2

avoidance of infection meant that patients' anxiety about cutting the skin was lessened. The acceptance of antisepsis for all surgery was relatively slow but was strongly encouraged by aesthetic surgeons. On November 26, 1877 Robert F. Weir (1838—1927), one of the major figures in the creation of American aesthetic surgery, said in a talk before the New York Medical Association, that the British and German acceptance of this procedure had outpaced that of the United States. He urged that the smallest detail of the cleansing of patient, surgeon, instruments, and surgical theater be carried out so that the patient was not placed at needless risk.[3] Once this was done, the risks attendant on aesthetic surgery decreased sharply because of the reduction in the high incidence of infection.

The Enlightenment: Happiness as the Goal of Aesthetic Surgery

With pain and infection removed or reduced, aesthetic surgery came into its own. Yet anesthesia and antisepsis were necessary but not sufficient to mark the beginning of the modern history of aesthetic surgery. It was the Enlightenment philosophy in the 19th century that each individual could remake him or herself in the pursuit of happiness, which provided the basis for the modern culture of aesthetic surgery. Indeed it is remarkable how often aesthetic surgeons describe happiness as the goal of the surgery.[4] You can make yourself happy by being able to actively par-

326. On the historical context of general surgery as it applies to the history of aesthetic surgery see Christopher Lawrence, ed., *Medical Theory, Surgical Practice* **(London: Routledge, 1992); P. B. Adamson, "Surgery in Ancient Mesopotamia,"** *Medical History* **35 (1991): 428—35; Ulrich Trohler, "To Operate or not to Operate?: Scientific and Extraneous Factors in Therapeutical Controversies within the Swiss Society of Surgery 1913—1988,"** *Clio Medica* **22 (1991): 89—113; Martin Duke,** *The Development of Medical Techniques and Treatments: From Leeches to Heart Surgery Madison* **(Madison, Conn.: International Universities Press, 1991); Marie-Christine Pouchelle,** *The Body and Surgery in the Middle Ages*, **trans. Rosemary Morris (New Brunswick, N. J.: Rutgers Univ. Press, 1990); J. Thompson Rowling, "The Rise and Decline of Surgery in Dynastic Egypt,"** *Antiquity* **63 (1989): 312—19; Daniel de Moulin,** *A History of Surgery, with Emphasis on the Netherlands* **(Dordrecht: Nijhoff, 1988); Mark Ravitch,** *A Century of Surgery: The History of the American Surgical Association* **(Philadelphia: Lippincott, 1981); Ben Barker-Benfield, "Sexual Surgery in Late 19th-Century America,"** *International Journal of Health Services* **5 (1975): 279—98; Scott Earle, ed.,** *Surgery in America: From the Colonial Era to the 20th Century*, **second edition, (New York: Praeger, 1983); Noble S. R. Maluf, "Use of Veins in Surgery: A History,"** *Sudhoffs Archiv für Geschichte der Medizin und der Naturwissenschaften* **67 (1983): 50—73; A. L. Wyman, "The Surgeoness: The Female Practitioner of Surgery, 1400—1800,"** *Medical History* **28 (1984): 22—41; Gert H. Brieger, "Medicine and Surgery in 1909,"** *Transactions and Studies of the College of Physicians of Philadelphia* **7 (1985): 17—25.**

3 — Excerpted in Gert H. Brieger, ed., *Medical America in the Nineteenth Century: Readings from the Literature* **(Baltimore: The Johns Hopkins University Press, 1972), pp. 198—200.**

4 — Throughout this book I understand the terms "happy" and "unhappy" (and their variants) in scare-quotes. This is not merely my signaling the construction of mental health categories out of a philosophical discourse of happiness but to indicate also that the use of the term is actually taken from the psychological and surgical literature on the topic. Happiness is often paralleled to psychologically distressed. See Robert M. Goldwyn's discussion of "happiness as an objective," in his *The Patient and the Plastic Surgeon* **(Boston: Little Brown, 1981) p. 62 and P. Marcus, "Psychological Aspects of Cosmetic Rhinoplasty,"** *British Journal of Plastic Surgery* **37 (1984): 313—18, here p. 315.**

fig. 4

The nose and mouth operations of Johannes Scultetus (1595—1645). Scultetus was one of the first doctors to perform surgery for purely aesthetic reasons instead of restricting himself to regenerative methods. Source: Typis Combi & La Nou, 1665. National Library of Medicine. Privatarchive Gilman, Chicago

ticipate in the world. This was mirrored in the rise of modern notions of the citizen as well as the revolutionary potential of the individual. Autonomy stands as the central principle in the shaping of aesthetic surgery. "'Dare to use your own reason'" wrote Immanuel Kant (1724—1804) "is the motto of the Enlightenment."[5] (fig. 3) And it is the ability to remake one's self, which is the heart of the matter.[6] Aesthetic surgery is therefore a truly modern phenomenon that demanded not only a set of specific technical innovations in surgery, but also a cultural presupposition that you have the inalienable right to alter, reshape, control, augment, or diminish your body with of course the help of the surgeon. The autonomy that aesthetic surgery represents is truly a modern one: you can act as you desire to become happy, but only with the aid and comfort of the technocrats whose expertise you can employ.

From Pharaonic Egypt to Renaissance

There is no moment in the historical records of medicine where there are not procedures undertaken to improve the appearance of the body. This was true in general surgery. Scarring has always been seen as an undesirable result of the surgical intervention in the body. As early as the Edwin Smith Surgical Papyrus (ca. 1600 B. C. E.) surgeons in Pharaonic Egypt were concerned about the aesthetic results of their interventions.[7] The papyrus is believed to be a copy of an older work from 3000 B. C. E. The Egyptians were careful to suture the edges of facial wounds. Even fractures of the nose-bone were dealt with by forcing them into normal positions by means of "two plugs of linen, saturated

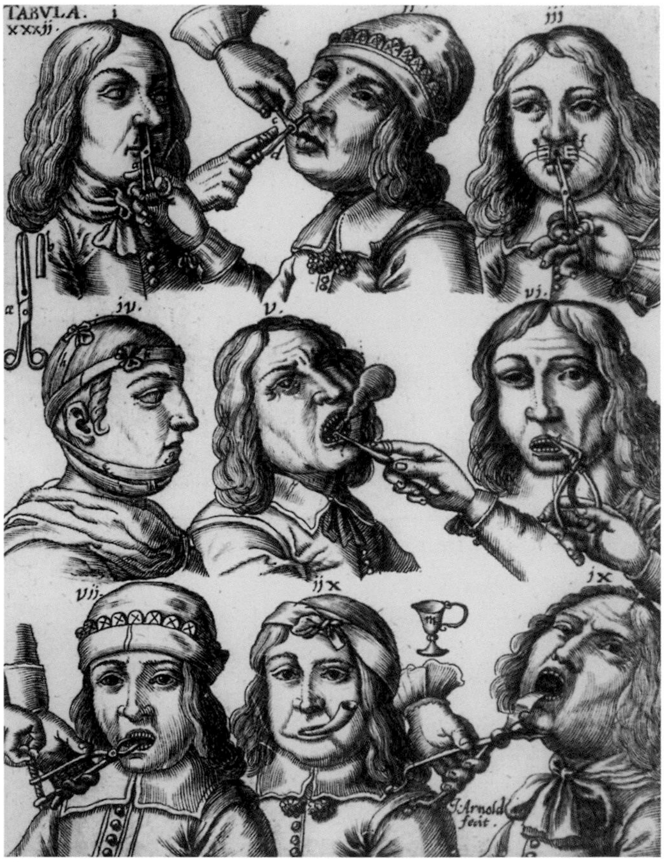

fig. 4

with grease" which were inserted into the nostrils.[8] The Roman encyclopedist Aulus Cornelius Celsus (first century A. D.) stressed the importance of the "beautiful" suture.[9] In ancient China, as in Pharonic Egypt and classical Greece, there are early records, such as the bone oracles (14th century B. C. E.), which mention illnesses of the

5 — Immanuel Kant, "What is Enlightenment?" in Lewis White Beck, ed., *On History* (Indianapolis: Bobbs-Merrill, 1963), p. 3.

6 — Autonomy is a contested concept in modern American thought. See David Riesman, Nathan Glazer, and Reuel Denney, *The Lonely Crowd: A Study of the Changing American Character* (New Haven: Yale University Press, 1950); Robert N. Bellah, et al., *Habits of the Heart: Individualism and Commitment in American Life* (Berkeley: University of California Press, 1985); and, most recently, Willard Gaylin and Bruce Jennings, *The Perversion of Autonomy: The Proper Uses of Coercion and Constraints in a Liberal Society* (New York: The Free Press, 1996).

7 — See the discussion in Walter E. Kunstler, "Aesthetic Considerations in Surgical Operations from Antiquity to Recent Times," *Bulletin of the History of Medicine* 12 (1942): 27—69.

8 — The translation from the Edwin Smith Papyrus on the fracture of the nose is reprinted in Frank McDowell, ed., *The Source Book of Plastic Surgery* (Baltimore: Williams & Wilkins, 1977), pp. 54—64.

9 — Aulus Cornelius Celsus, *De medicina*, trans. and intro. by W. G. Spence. 3 vols. (London: W. Heinemann; Cambridge, MA: Harvard University Press, 1935—38), 3: 339.

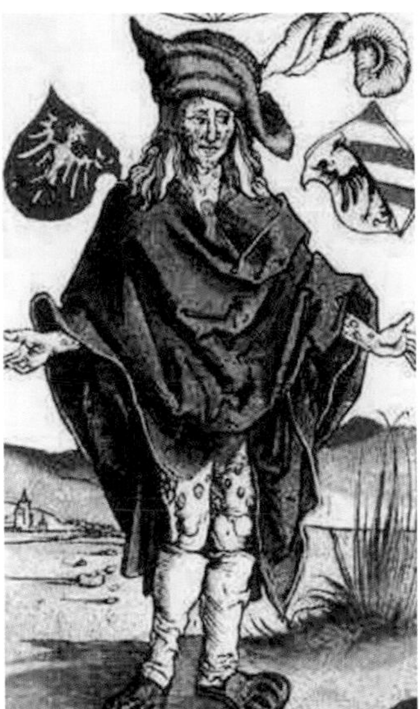

fig. 5

fig. 5

A man suffering from syphilis, as depicted by Albrecht Dürer (1471—1528). After the discovery of the Americas, seafarers brought syphilis to Europe in October 1492. As penicillin did not yet exist, the disease was practically incurable.
© A Med-World AG

fig. 6

In his book "De Curtorum Chirurgia per insitionem", the Italian practitioner Gaspare Tagliacozzi (1545—1599) published 22 wood engravings about aesthetic surgery and surgical implements.
© Columbia University Health Sciences Library. Photo: Dwight Primiano

nose.[10] The chinese physician Bian Que (fifth century B. C. E.) wrote texts in which he describes how he treated the ears and eyes of patients. Likewise the chinese physician Hua Tuo (ca. 150—208 A. D.) documented his treatment of the eyes and ears. The traditional chinese prohibition against opening the body limited all forms of surgical intervention until fairly recently. It is only in the northern T'ang and Gin dynasty in the middle of the 10th century A. D. that medical texts begin to record the reconstructive surgery of the harelip.

But there were also procedures that were clearly to improve the appearance as well as the function of the body. The Alexandrian physician, Paulos of Aegina ( ), developed a procedure in the seventh century to remove breasts in men, a social discomfort that he defined as a medical problem to be cured through surgery. Its technical name is gynecomastia (woman-breast), the presence of breasts on the male and such procedures are still done today, if in different form. Today's liposuction as a cure for obesity is also not new.[11] Pliny the Elder (23/24 A. D. — 79 A. D.) describes a similar "heroic cure for obesity" in an operation on the son of the Consul L. Apronius and in 1190 a surgeon cut open the belly of Count Dedo V von Rochlitz-Groitzsch to remove excessive fat.[12] In the Middle Ages there was no discussion of aesthetic surgery[13] as all surgery was seen to remedy some type of pathology; physical and psychological illnesses were seen as interrelated and inherently connected. And yet noses and other body parts were certainly lost to war, accident, and disease in the Middle Ages[14]. And one can function, if not well, without them. Only with the Renaissance did surgeons begin to speak again of aesthetic or beauty surgery.[15] (fig. 4)

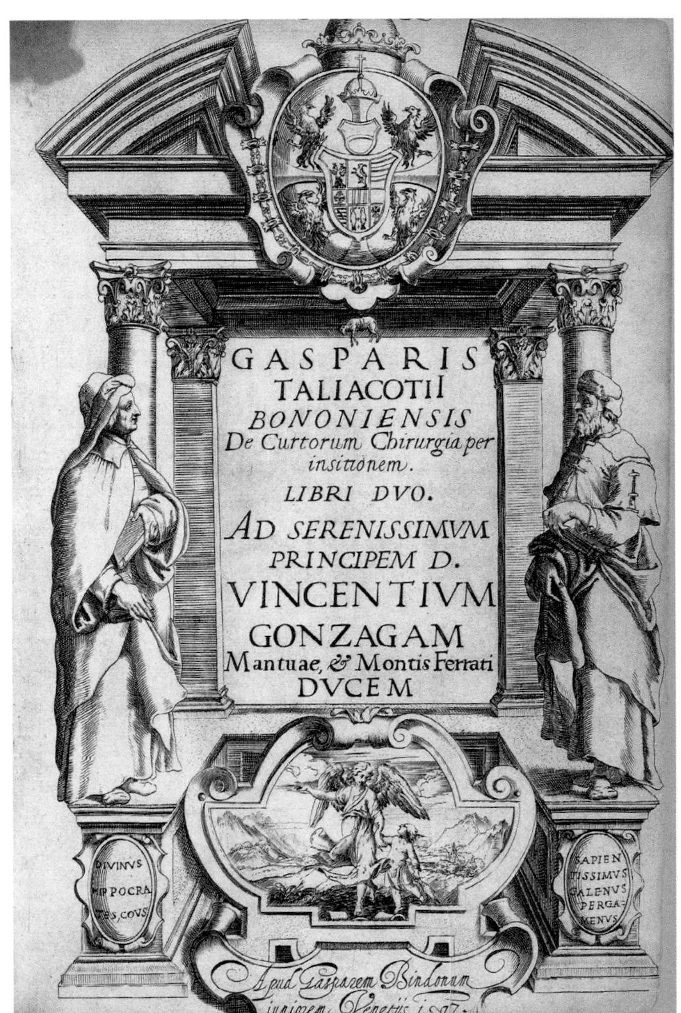

fig. 6

10 — M. Chien Chih Tzu Chu, *Nu Hsing Mei Yung Hsin Chih* (Tai-pei: Kuo chi tsun wen ku shu tien, 1995).

11 — Harvey J. Sugerman, "Obesity Surgery," *Surgical Clinics of North America* 81 (2001): 1001—1198.

12 — Julius Preuss, *Biblical and Talmudic Medicine*, trans. Fred Rosner (New York: Sanhedrin press, 1978), p. 215.

13 — Guy de Chauliac (died 1368), perhaps the most important surgeon of his time, defined the role of surgery as being threefold: *solvit continuum* (separating the fused), *iungit separatum* (connecting the divided), and *exstirpat superfluum* (removing the extraneous). See Guy de Chauliac, *Chirurgia magna* Guidonis de Gauliaco, ed. Gundolf Keil (Darmstadt: Wissenschaftliche Buchgesellschaft, 1976), p. 3.

14 — Marie-Christine Pouchelle, *The Body and Surgery in the Middle Ages*, trans. Rosemary Morris (New Brunswick, N. J.: Rutgers Univ. Press, 1990).

15 — Gaspare Tagliacozzi (1545—1599) made the distinction between *chirurgia curtorum (per insitionem)* (surgery healing by grafts) and *chirurgia decoratoria* (beauty surgery). All references are to Gaspare Tagliacozzi, *La Chirurgia Plastica per Innesto*, trans. and ed., Werner Vallieri. Bologna. Università. Cattedra di storia della medicina. Vita e opere di medici e naturalisti, 3 (Bologna: n. p., 1964) and the standard monograph on him by Martha Teach Gnudi and Jerome Pierce Webster, *The Life and Times of Gaspare Tagliacozzi, Surgeon of Bologna 1545—1599* (Milano: U. Hoepli; New York: H. Reichner, 1950).

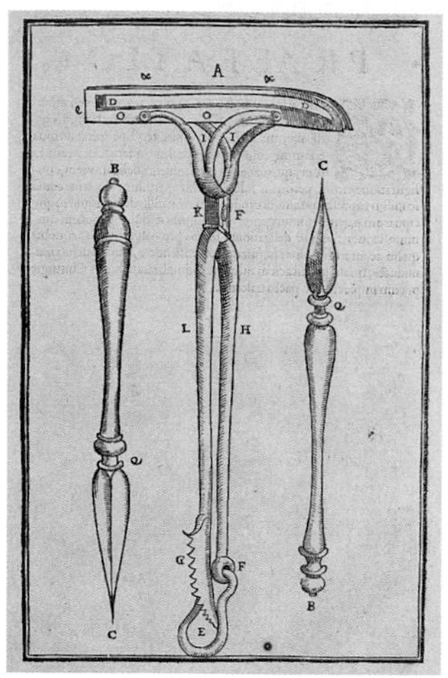

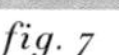

fig. 7

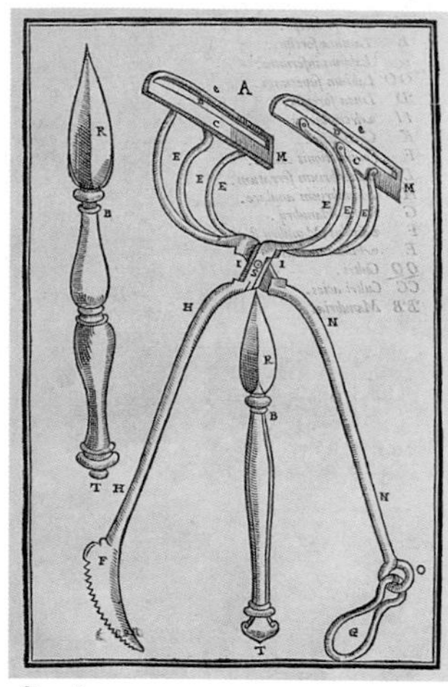

fig. 8

fig. 7 & 8

For his rhinoplasties, Gaspare Tagliacozzi (1545—1599) used differently-sized scalpels for different incision depths, as well as two- or three-pronged braces to manipulate skin flaps.
© Columbia University Health Sciences Library. Photo: Dwight Primiano

fig. 9 & 10

After surgery, the wound was sutured and dressed. The patient was required to wear a support bandage around the head and upper torso, and had to endure a healing period of several weeks — which was frequently prolonged by painful infections. © Columbia University Health Sciences Library. Photo: Dwight Primiano

fig. 11 & 12

Special implements such as rounded needles, knives and pincers were used to sculpt a new septum between the tip of the nose and the upper lip, for example. Models of noses, attached to the patient's head with strings, were used to outline and protect the operative site.
© Columbia University Health Sciences Library. Photo: Dwight Primiano

The Rise of Syphilis in the 16th Century

The rise of aesthetic surgery at the end of the 16th century is rooted in the appearance of epidemic syphilis. (fig. 5). Syphilis was a highly stigmatizing disease from its initial appearance at the close of the 15th century, an import from the newly discovered Americas. The role of a new *chirurgia decoratoria* was to rebuild the noses of syphilitics so that they could become less visible in their society. An early historian of aesthetic surgery, the German Otto Hildebrand (1858—1927), himself a reconstructive surgeon, noted the relationship between the new aesthetics of the Renaissance, the outbreak of syphilis, which caused defects of an "unaesthetic" nature, and the rise of aesthetic surgery.[16]

The First Documented Illustrated Nose Job in 1597

Decorative surgery was a proprietary trade secret and was usually passed on from father to son. Heinrich von Pfalzpaint (born after 1400 — death before 1465), a knight of the Teutonic Order, described the use of the connected arm flap to provide a graft with which to repair the nose as early as 1460.[17] According to his account he learned it from a foreigner and it enabled him to earn very much money.

It is, however, only with the Italian Renaissance and the work of Gaspare Tagliacozzi (1545—1599), professor of surgery at the University of Bologna, that the relationship between the missing or flattened nose and the unhappiness of the patient is first articulated. Tagliacozzi's most important innovation was the development of a means of replacing the missing nose, for a person without a nose is bound to be unhappy and this unhappiness could well make him or her (physically) ill. It also marked that person as not only diseased but also infectious, whether or not actual infection, as we know it, was present. The stigma was indeed real enough! They were polluted and polluting.

In the 1597 Gaspore Tagliacozzi introduced or at least documented for the first time in his book "De curtorum chirurgia" per insitionem in words and illustrations the use of pedicle flap grafts for the reconstruction of the missing nose because of trauma or syphilis.(fig. 6)

But such flaps evidently had been used in the West in the early modern period. F. e. the Branca family in 15th century Sicily employed such technique. The father used a flap of skin taken from the cheek (*ex ore*) to rebuild the nose; his son, Antonius Branca, used a flap from the upper arm, which left less of a visible scar on the face. The son's procedure demanded that the flap, still attached to the arm, be joined to the now abraded stump of the nose for as long as 20 days. Unlike the much less cumbersome and much less complicated operation, which took the flap graft from the cheek, it created no further scars on the face.[18]

Here the problem of the relationship of reconstructive surgery (regaining function) to aesthetic surgery (creating improvement) appears at the very origin of aesthetic surgery. It seems self-evident that any one without a nose will be unhappy, and the reconstruction of the nose will make one happier and therefore healthier. Tagliacozzi recognized this. In chapter eleven of his book "De curtorem Chirugia per insitionem" he discusses the means of replacing the missing nose by the use of a pedicle flap graft.[19]

16 — **Otto Hildebrand,** *Die Entwicklung der plastischen Chirurgie* **(Berlin: August Hirschwald, 1909), p. 8.**

17 — **Christoph Weisser, "Die Nasenersatzplastik nach Heinrich von Pfalzpaint: Ein Beitrag zur Geschichte der plastischen Chirurgie im Spätmittelalter mit Edition des Textes," in Josef Domes, et al., eds.,** *Licht der Natur: Medizin in Fachliteratur und Dichtung* **(Göppingen: Kümmerle, 1994), pp. 485—506.**

18 — **"Ex ejusdem lacerto detruncabat, ita ut nulla deformitas oris sequeretur." Ernst Gurlt,** *Geschichte der Chirurgie und ihrer Ausübung; Volkschirurgie, Alterthum, Mittelalter, Renaissance.* **3 vols. (Berlin: Hirschwald, 1898), 2: 489.**

19 — **Gaspare Tagliacozzi,** *Gasparis Taliacotii.... De curtorem chirurgia per insitionem; libri dvo. In quibus ea omnia, quae ad huius chirurgiae, narium scilicet, aurium, ac labiorum per insitionem restaurandorum cum theoricen, tum practicen pertinere videbantur, clarissima methodo cumulatissime declarantur. Additis cutis traducis instru-*

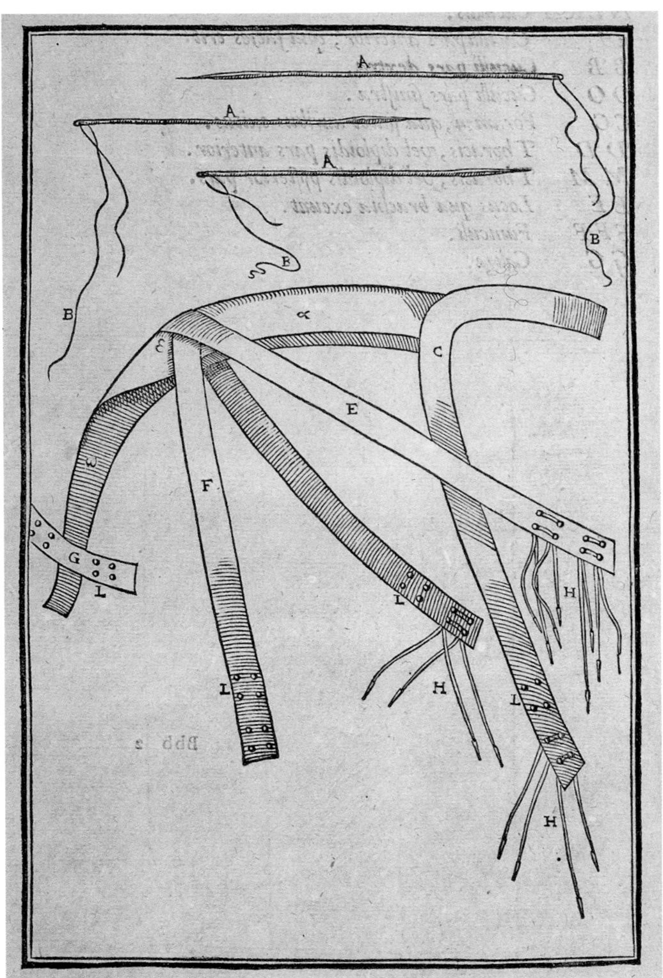

fig. 9

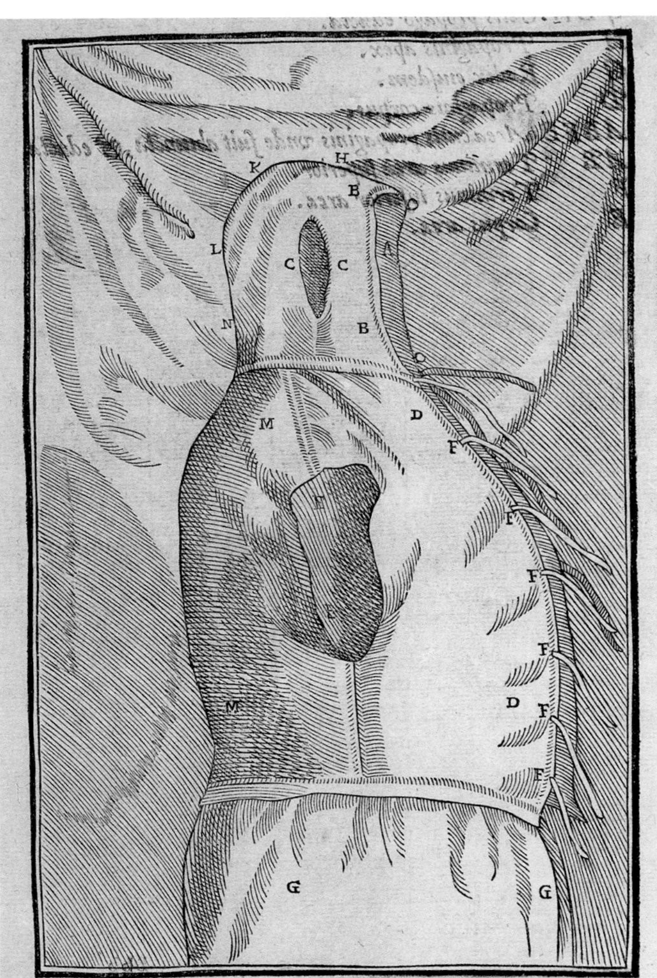

fig. 10

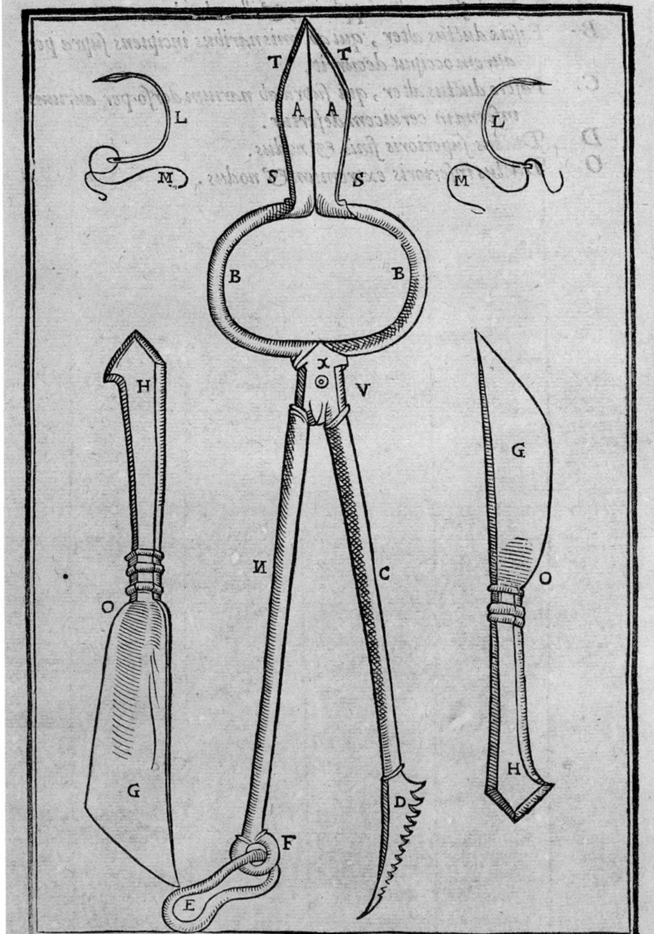

fig. 11

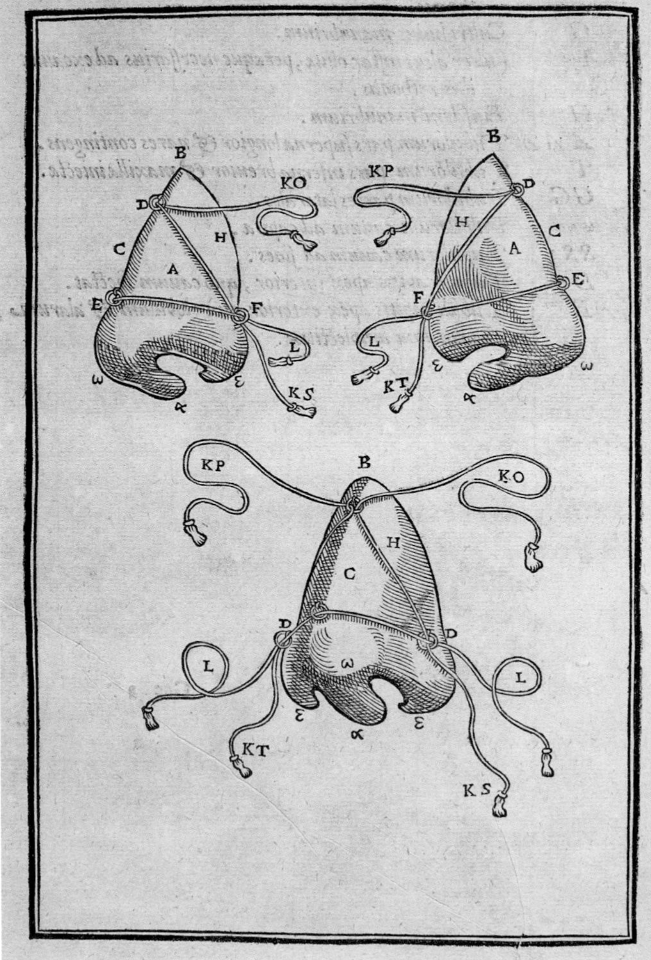

fig. 12

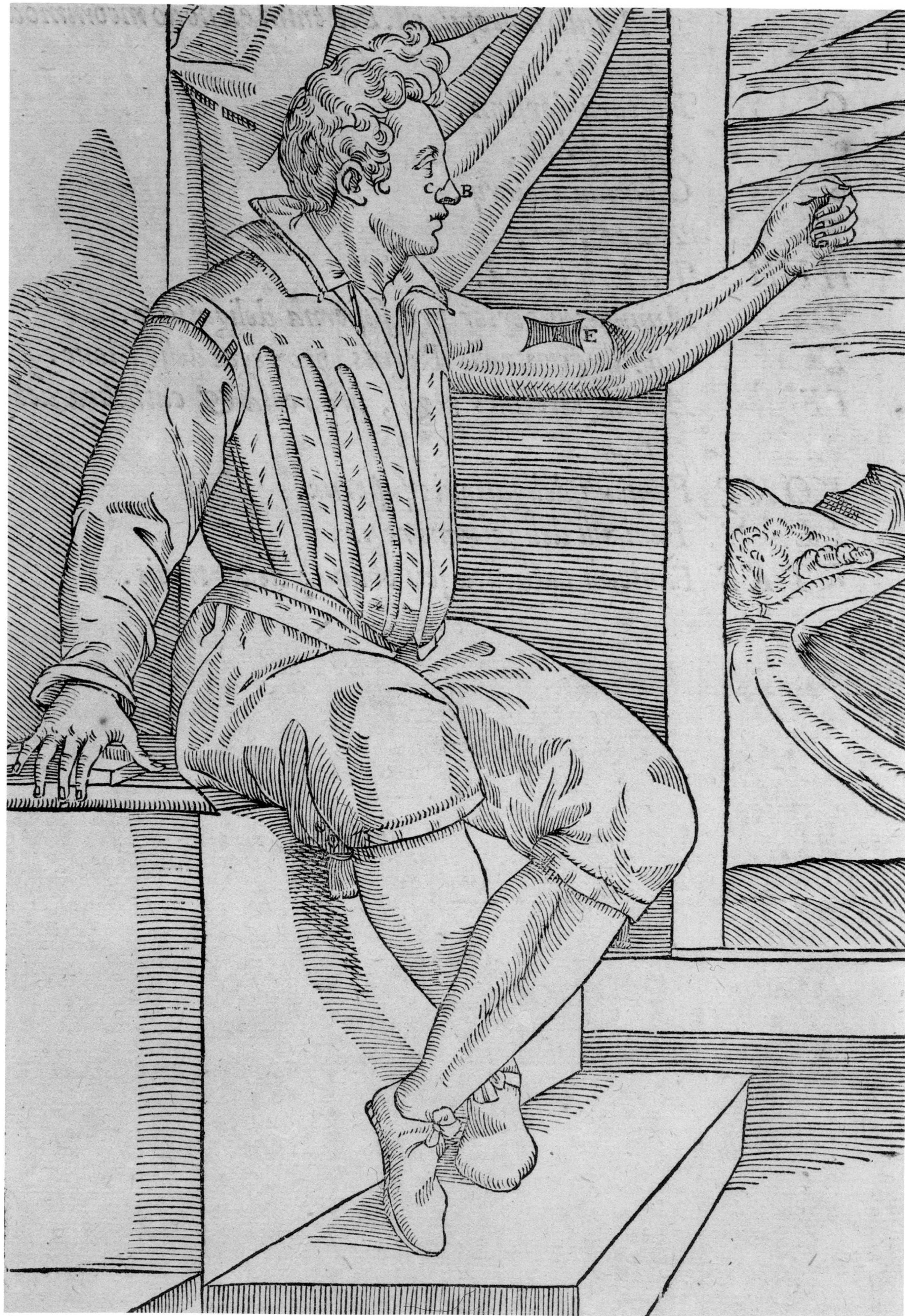

fig. 13

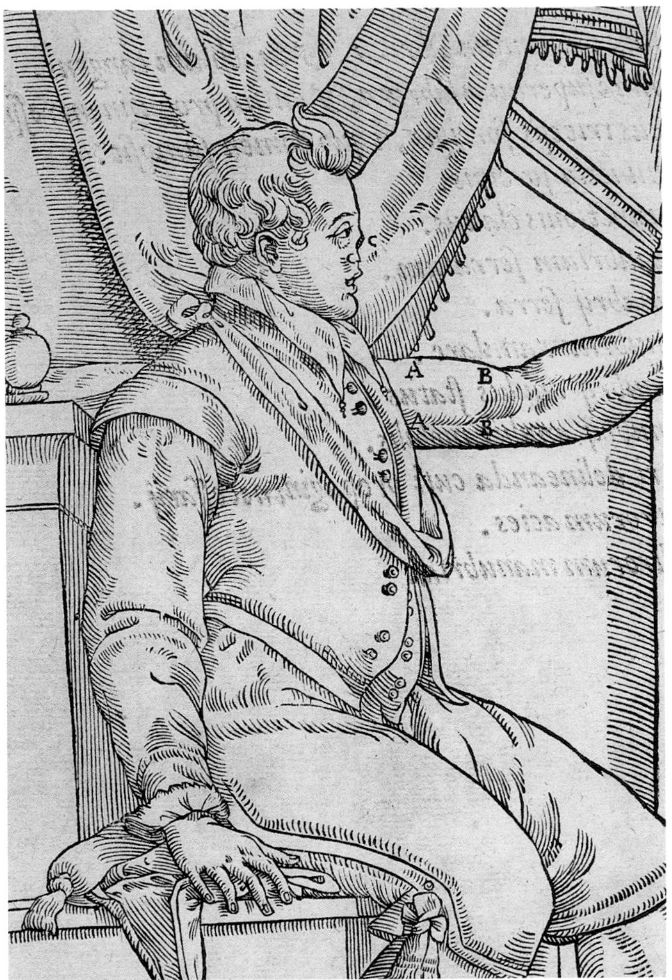

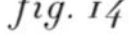
fig. 14

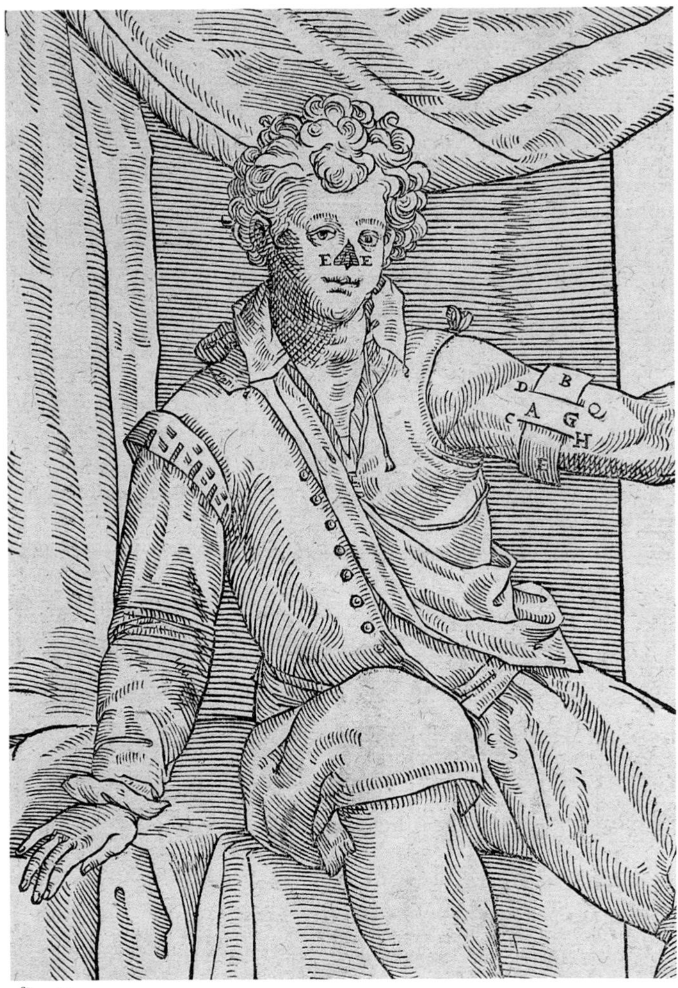

fig. 15

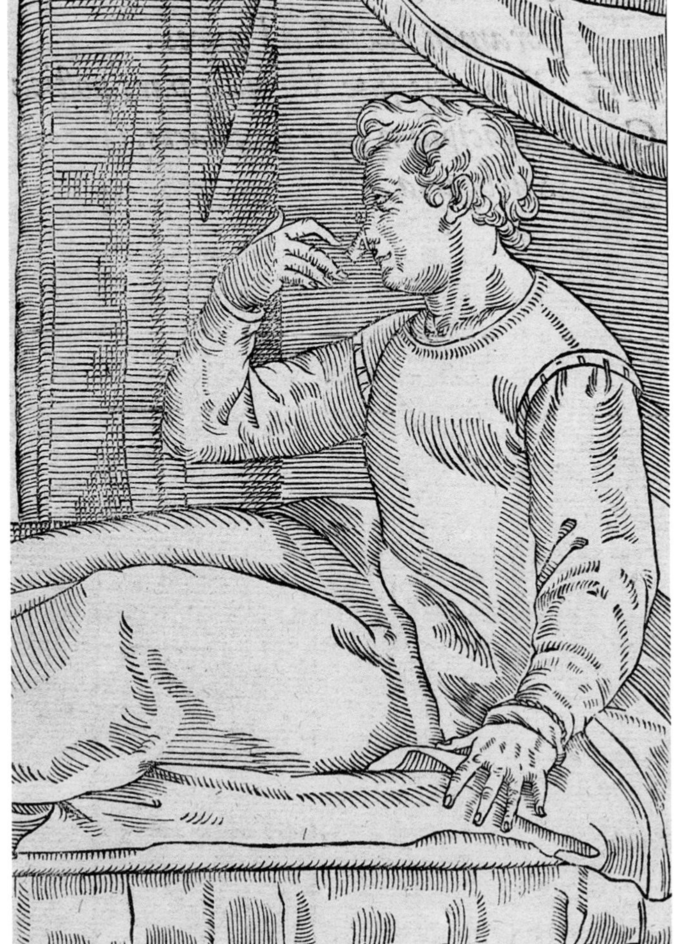

fig. 16

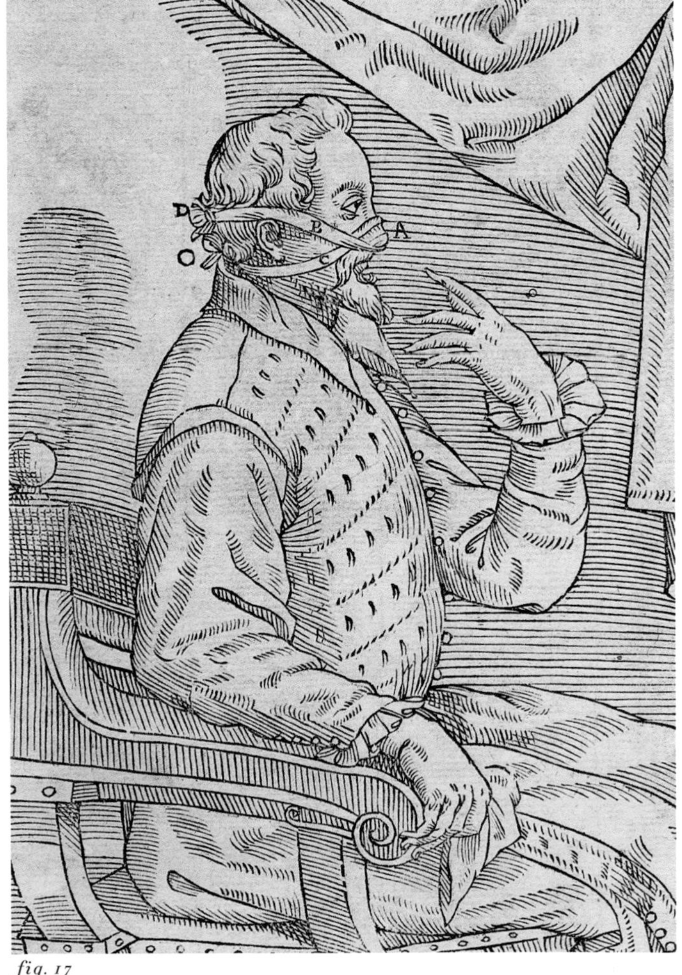

fig. 17

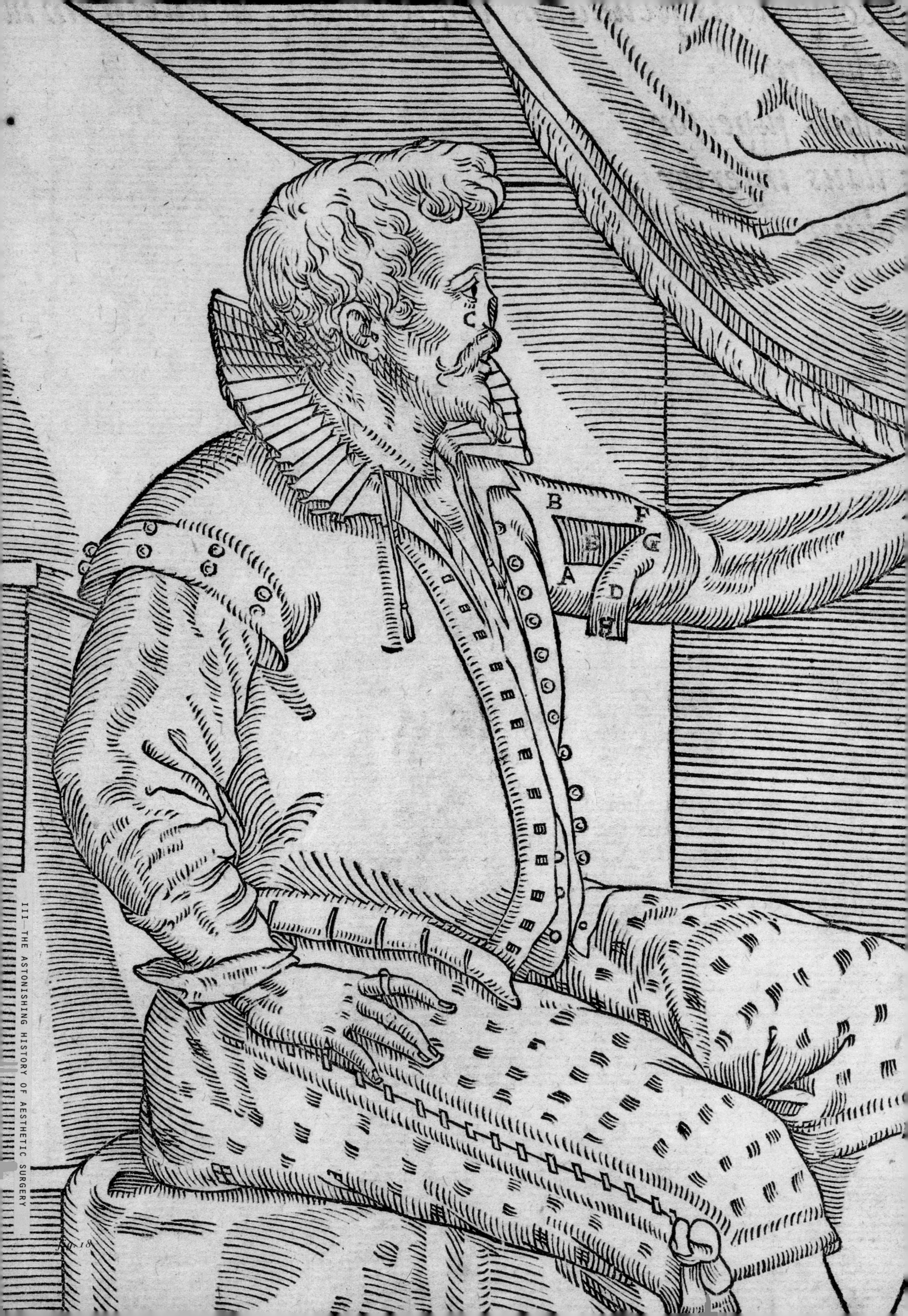
B
F
E
C
A
D
Fig. 18

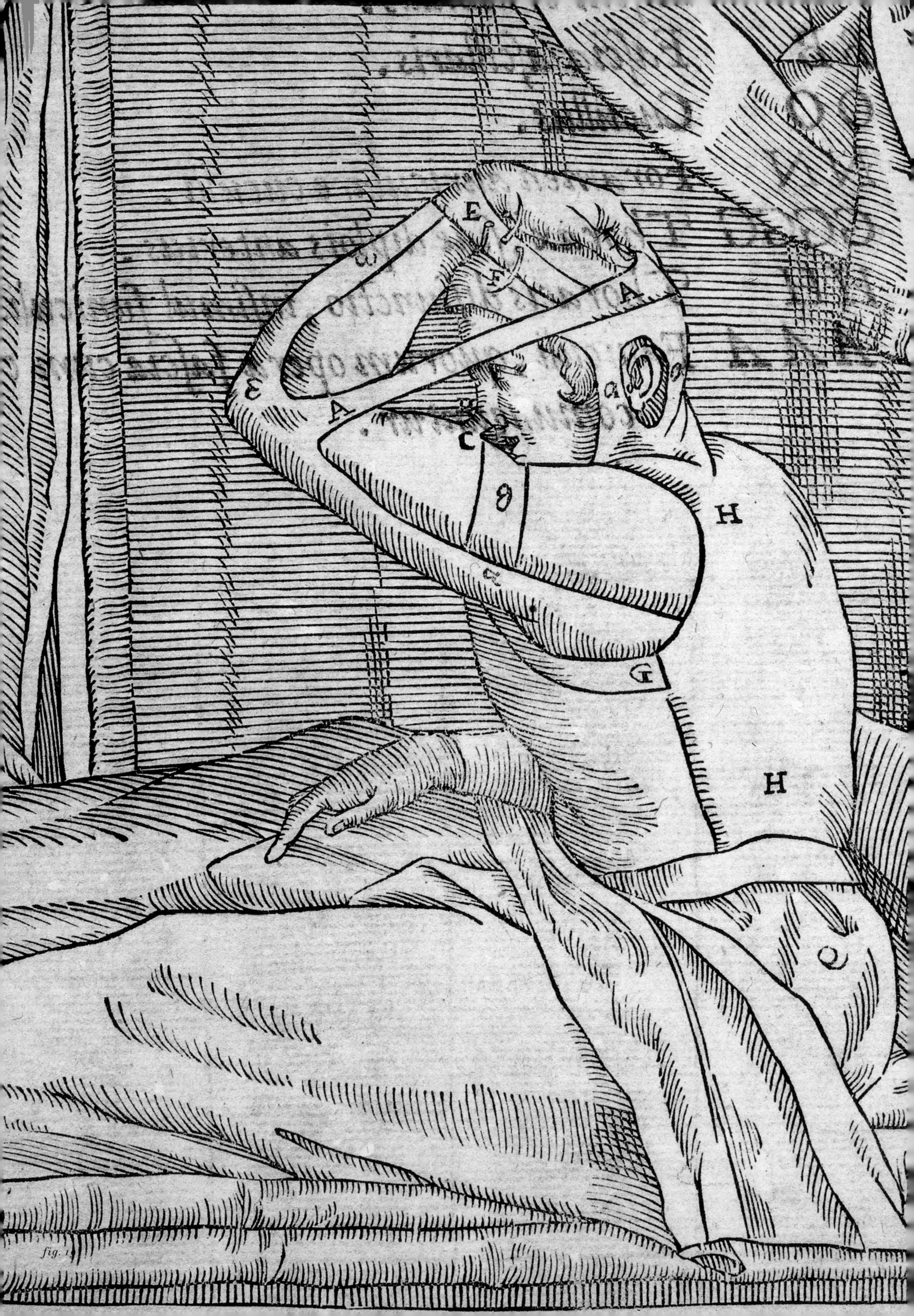

fig. 1

fig. 13–17

To create a new nose, Gaspare Tagliacozzi (1545—1599) transplanted a skin graft from the inner upper arm to the face — the outline of the incision already suggests the shape of the new nose. The skin flap was positioned, reshaped and sutured. After the procedure, the surgeon fitted a support bandage around the patient's head and upper torso. © Columbia University Health Sciences Library. Photo: Dwight Primiano

fig. 18 & 19

A skin flap was taken from the patient's left arm and transplanted to his deformed nose. Subsequently, the arm and head needed to be stabilised by a support bandage — a lengthy healing period with sustained physical discomfort. © Columbia University Health Sciences Library. Photo: Dwight Primiano

fig. 20

In October 1794, an article about an Indian rhinoplasty appeared in "The Gentlemen's Magazine" (London), the first such report to be published in Europe. The operation performed on the patient, whose name was Cowasjee, involved a skin graft being cut out of the brow to create the new nose. © Columbia University Health Sciences Library. Photo: Dwight Primiano

fig. 21 a+b & 22 a+b

After Tagliacozzi und Carpue, Carl Ferdinand von Graefe (1787—1840) was one of Europe's most renowned aesthetic surgeons. Depicted here are a cut nose (severed during fencing), which Graefe reconstructed using the Italian method, and a nose destroyed by cancer, reconstructed with the Indian method. © Columbia University Health Sciences Library. Photo: Dwight Primiano

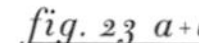

fig. 23 a+b

A rhinoplasty by Eduard Zeis (1807—1868). The first drawing shows the face immediately after the operation — the skin graft for the new nose was taken from the brow and the nose still looks very flat. In the second drawing, the face is shown one day later; the nose's colour and shape have improved considerably. © Columbia University Health Sciences Library. Photo: Dwight Primiano

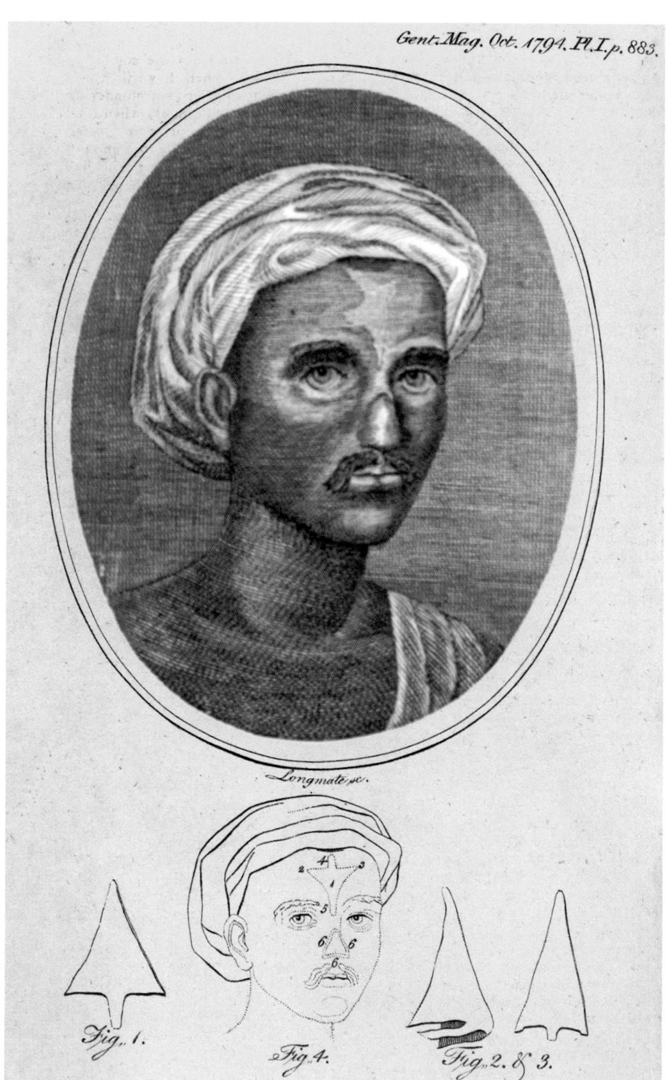

fig. 20

Like the younger Branca he chose to use the skin from the arm. He made two parallel incisions over the biceps, loosened the skin between these two cuts, and placed linen dressing under the skin. This he left untouched for four days and then dressed the wound daily so as to encourage scar formation under the loosened skin. On the 14th day he cut the flap at one end. Two weeks later he abraded the stump of the nose and grafted the attached flap onto the nose, holding the arm in place with a strong halter. 20 days later he cut the flap free from the arm and two weeks after this began to shape a nose and attach this nose to the upper lip. Six procedures (at least) and more than a month later, a rudimentary nose was present. The risks of infection were great and the pain and discomfort excruciating. (fig. 7—19)

A Nose Job in India in 1794

The Catholic Church did not like the notion that one could surgically rectify the scarring and distortion that syphilis caused its sufferers. Tagliacozzi's innovations were forgotten or ignored as they presented a human intervention into the realm of divine punishment. It was only in 1794, with the establishment of the British colonial power in India, that the first detailed account of the reconstruction of a nose was published in the West following the disappearance of Tagliacozzi's procedures into literary legend. Appearing under the initials B. L. in the Gentlemen's Magazine in London[20], the anonymous article — most probably written by the British surgeon Coly Lyon Lucas — documented "the ... very curious, and, in Europe, unknown chirurgical operation," which was the use of a connected skin-graft from the forehead to reconstruct or rather to replace the nose.[21]

The patient, a Parsi bullock-driver named Cowasjee, had been in the service of the British when he was captured by the rebellious Tipu Sultan, Fath Ali, Nawab of Mysore (1753—1799), who had Cowasjee's nose and one hand amputated.

mentorum omnium, atque deligationum iconibus, & tabulis .... **(Venetiis: Apud G. Bindonum iuniorem, 1597).**

20 — I am indebted to the work of Ann Laura Stoler, *Race and the Education of Desire: Foucault's History of Sexuality and the Colonial Order of Things* **(Durham: Duke University Press, 1995) as well as to David Arnold,** *Colonizing the Body: State Medicine and Epidemic Disease in Nineteenth-Century India* **(Berkeley: University of California Press, 1993). No commentator, however, has remarked on the transmission of rhinoplasty as a sign of the medical infiltration of the "homeland" and its physiognomy from the colonial sphere.**

21 — Reprinted in McDowell, *Source Book*, **op. cit., pp. 75—77.**

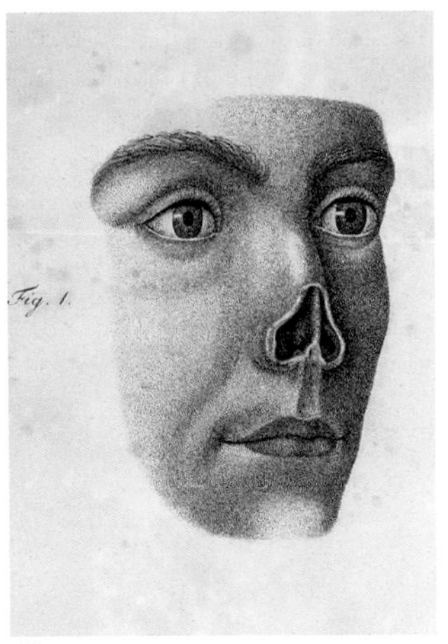

fig. 21 a

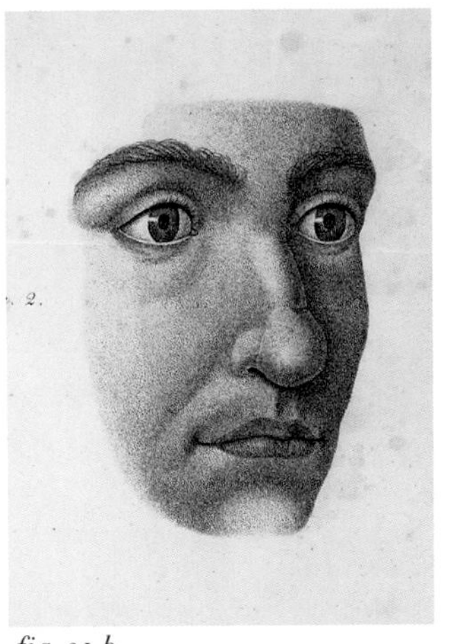

fig. 21 b

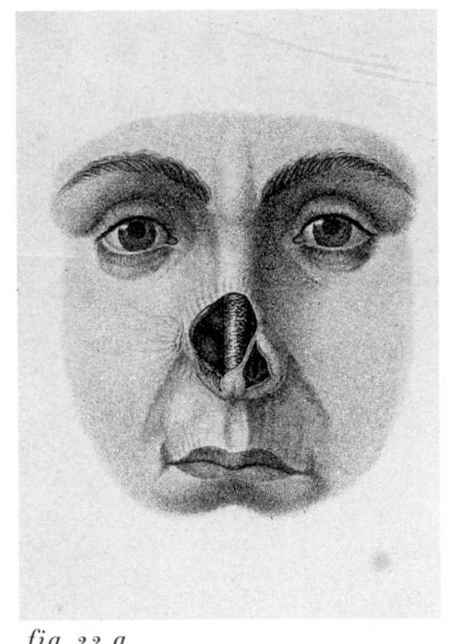

fig. 22 a

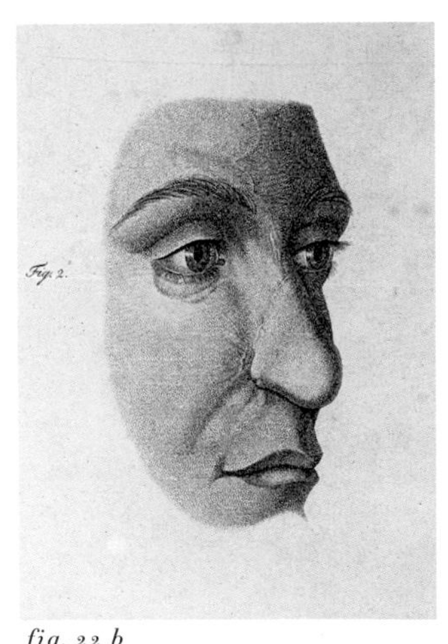

fig. 22 b

When twelve months later, Cowasjee minus his nose and hand rejoined the British army in Bombay, he went to a "member of the Brick maker caste" to replace his nose. The procedure began by tracing a replacement using a wax model onto Cowasjee's forehead and loosening the skin from the forehead. Leaving a connecting flap, the brick maker abraded the stump, twisted the graft around and formed the nose. 25 days later, he cut the remaining bridge and Cowasjee had his new nose. This version of the pedicle skin-flap had the advantage over Tagliacozzi's arm flap in that it did not encumber the patient with a brace for a long period, but alternately left an extensive scar on the forehead. An army surgeon who may well have read of it in the local Madras paper in March of 1794 reported this procedure. There was a portrait of Cowasjee by James Wales included which appeared and was reprinted in all of the subsequent versions of this tale. This portrait shows a much diminished scar and a nose, which appears aesthetically normal. (fig. 20)

However, according to this 1794 account in the British press, the "oriental" and "barbaric" practices of amputating the nose were the impetus for the development of the reconstructive rhinoplasty aspect of traditional Indian medicine, as opposed to the earlier, lost Western European cure for the syphilitic nose. Following the British model, which he knew well, the German surgeon Eduard Zeis (1807—1868), wrote in 1838, that it "owes its origin to the custom of punishing thieves, deserters, and, particularly, adulterers by cutting off their noses and ears, which was practiced in olden times, and is still practiced today. It is no wonder that the art of making noses developed much later in Europe, where such a grisly custom did not exist...."[22] The barbarism of the orient led to the development of reparative procedures, according to this narrative.

22 — Eduard Zeis, *Handbuch der plastischen Chirurgie* **(Berlin: G. Reimer, 1838). All citations from this will be to the translation by T. J. S. Patterson,** *Zeis' Manual of Plastic Surgery* **(Oxford: Oxford University Press, 1988), p. 53.**

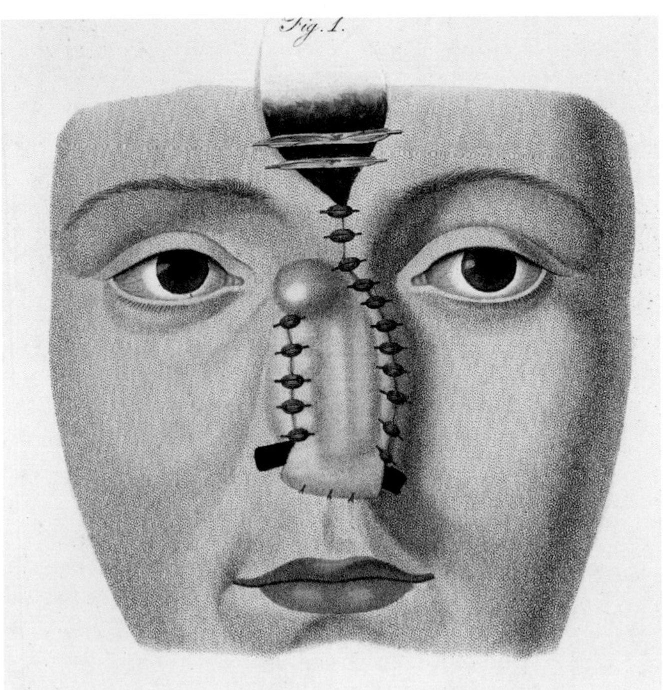

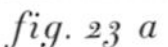

fig. 23 a

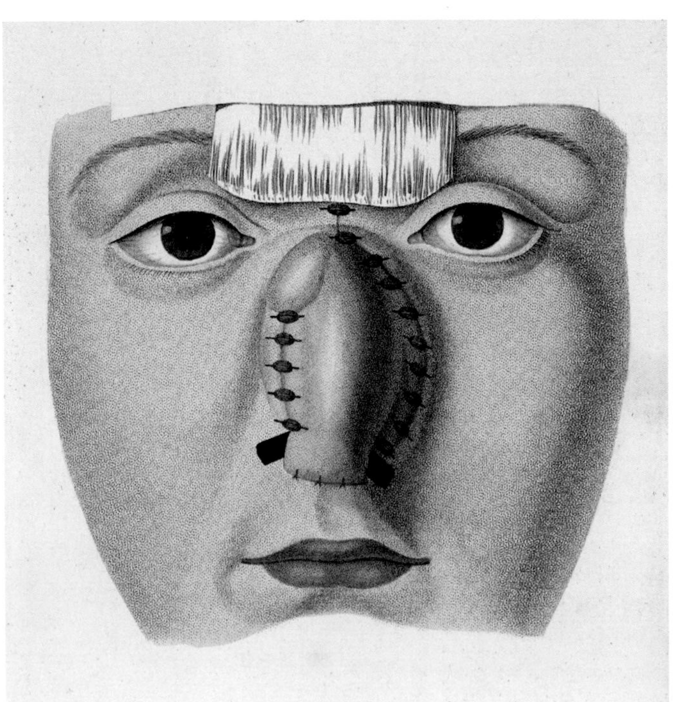

fig. 23 b

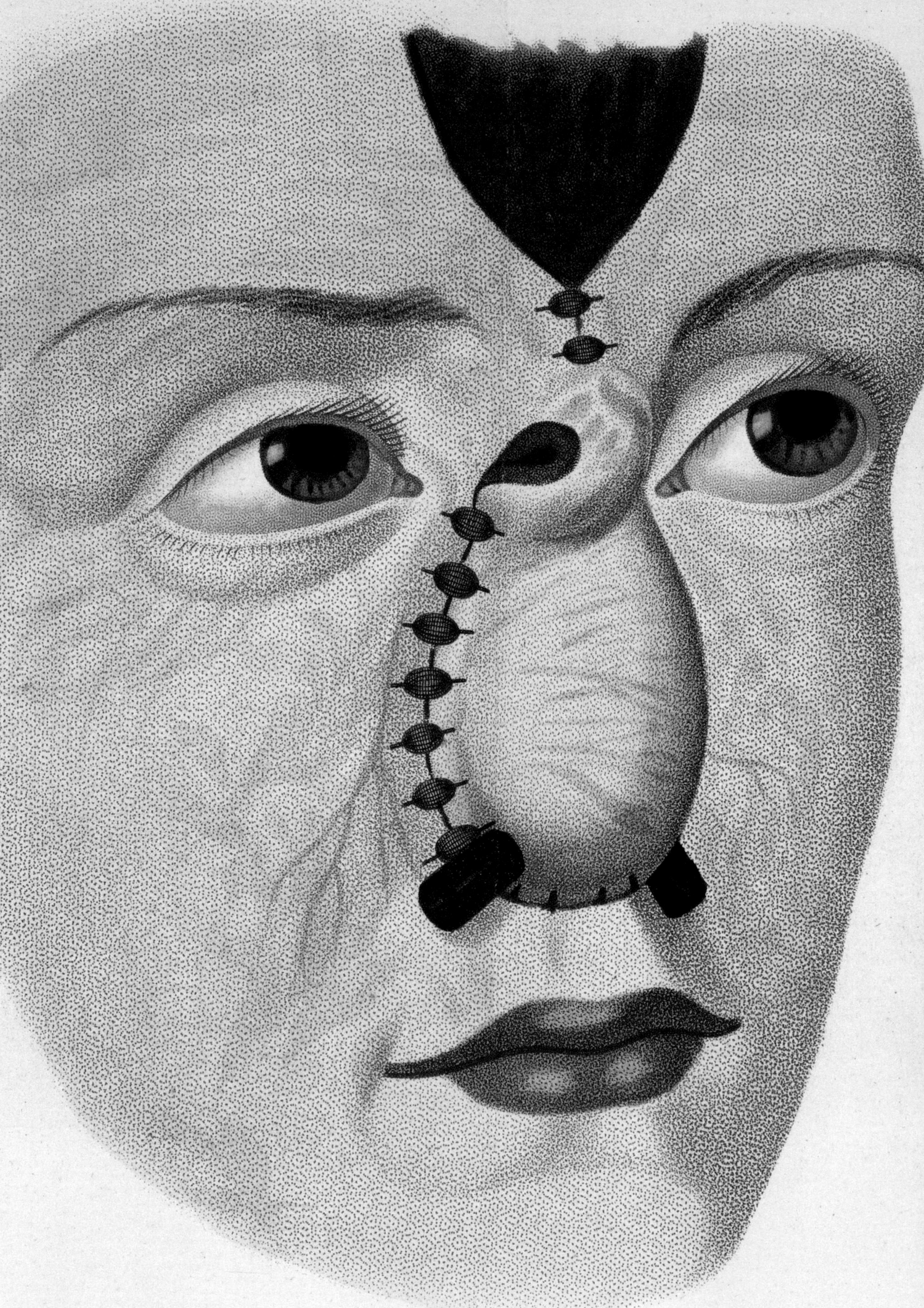

fig. 24 a

Fig. 4.

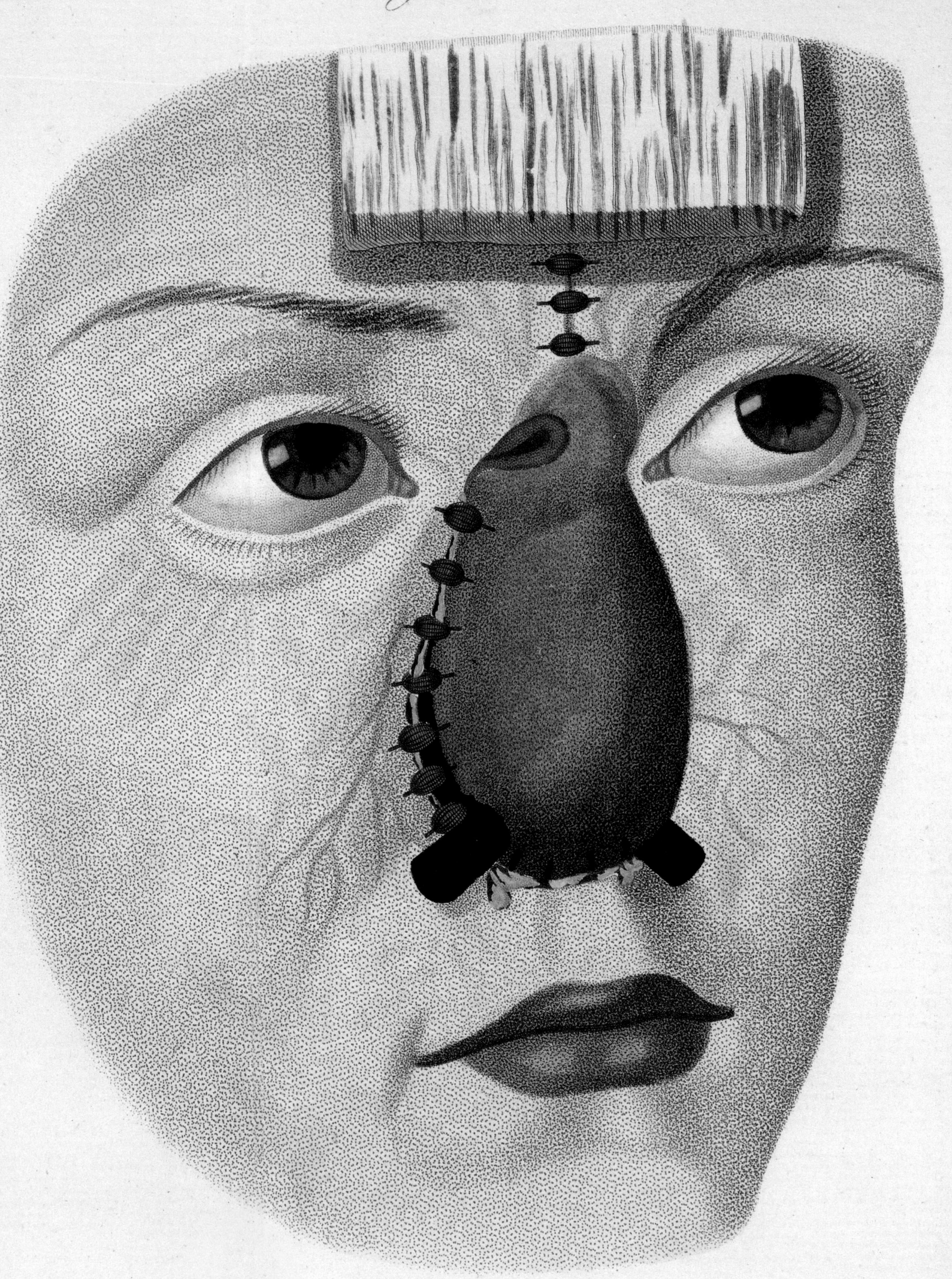

fig. 24 b

fig. 24 a+b

On the second day after the operation, the nose looks much less healthy already. The skin has an unnatural colour, there is significant scarring, and the skin graft is in danger of being rejected by the patient's body. Eventually, the suture wound is suppurating strongly and there are scabs — "It looks as if all is lost," states surgeon Eduard Zeis in his diagnostic report (c. 1832).
© Columbia University Health Sciences Library. Photo: Dwight Primiano

fig. 25

The healing process following a rhinoplasty, as performed by Hermann Eduard Fritze (1811—1866). The drawings are from the book "Rhinoplastic operations; with some remarks on the antoplastic methods unusally adopted for the restoration of parts lost by accident or disease" by Jonathan Mason Warren (1811—1867) (Boston: Clapp, 1840) © Columbia University Health Sciences Library. Photo: Dwight Primiano

But the adoption in England and then on the continent of this specific procedure was also contingent on the meaning ascribed to India in the 18th century. In Europe, the primary application for this procedure would be for the syphilitic nose, and not reparations for barbaric behaviour, and yet, there were still complications with even this form for reconstructive surgery. (fig. 23 a+b, 24 a+b)

The Princess and the Golden Nose

Remember, all of this surgery hurt terribly over a long period of time, there was a high risk of infection, and the driving force was the anxiety about stigma coupled with the functional difficulties of the syphilitic nose. Thus when a Dr. von Klein writing in a Heidelberg medical journal at the beginning of the 19th century tells us the rare story of one of his patients who requested his help in acquiring a "more beautiful" nose it is a tale fraught with pain, danger, and unpleasantness.[23] She was a young princess of less than 20 who had what is technically called a saddle nose, a nose that sagged at the bridge. The princess suggested to her physician that a bridge of gold be inserted to build up and straighten the nose. The bridge had to be inserted through the skin and could leave scars. So she also proposed that the procedure first be tried on some poor individual to see whether infection and ugly scarring would result. Dr. von Klein proceeded to the local pauper's hospital, found an individual to volunteer — based on the payment of a thaler and the promise that he could keep the gold bridge once it was removed. To the doctor's surprise

23 — Dr. v. Klein, "Über Rhinoplastick," *Heidelberger Klinische Annalen* 2 (1826):103–11.

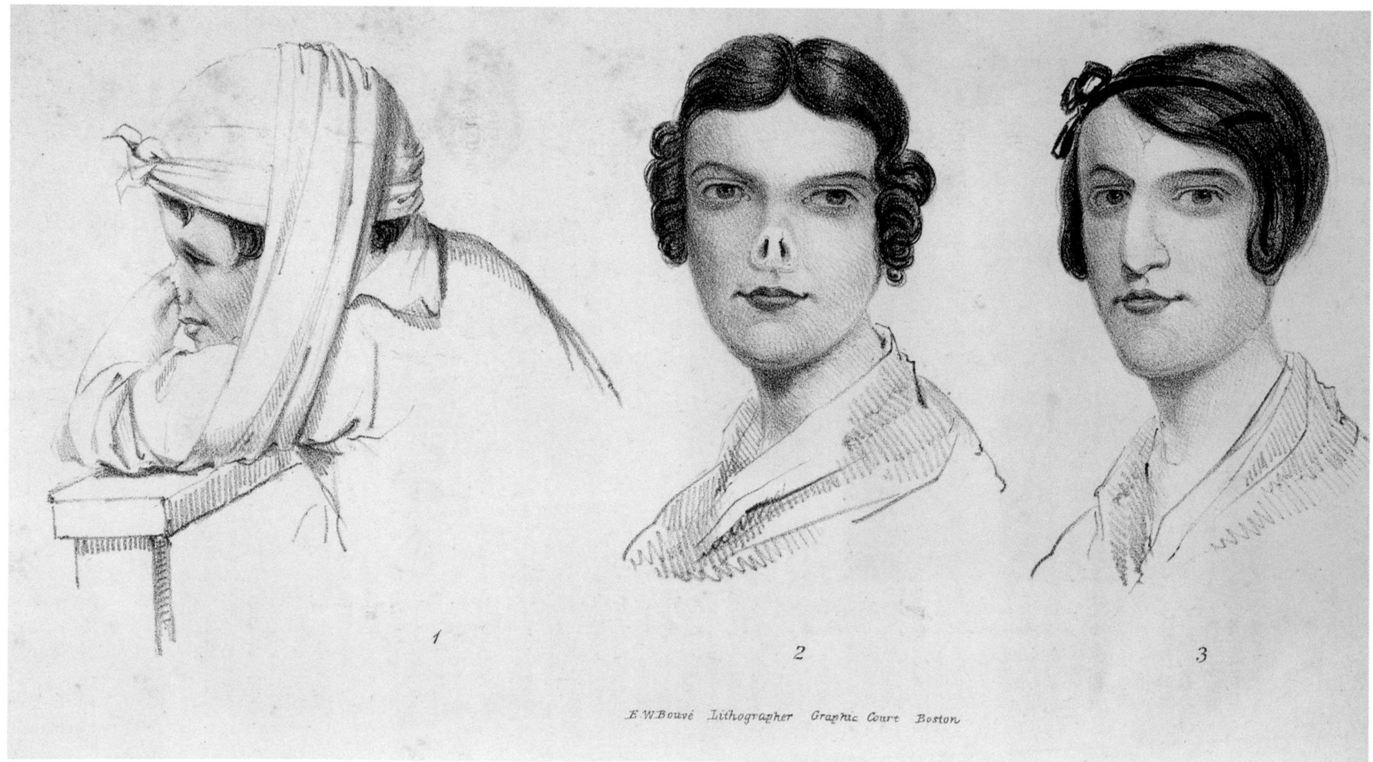

fig. 25

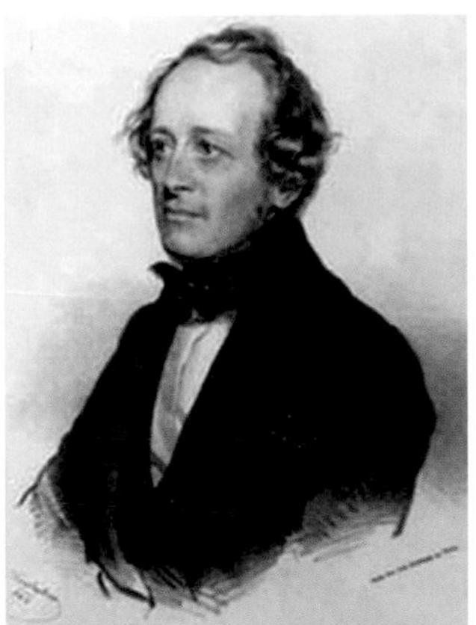

fig. 26

In the 19th century, Berlin aesthetic surgeon Johann Friedrich Dieffenbach (1792–1847) was regarded as the best in the field. He specialised in rhinoplasty.

fig. 26

the operation was a success — no infection and a very small scar. But his original patient, the princess, vacillated once confronted with the possibility of such a procedure — without any general or even local anesthetics. At one point she actually got up and ran away with the chair to which she had been strapped for the procedure.

Dr. Klein's insertion of a gold bridge would have scarred the nose. Scars tell the world the patient's secret. They are the shadow presence of what the patient wished to hide. In the tale of the princess, she is a young woman who sees herself as ugly and devises her own treatment. To do this, the princess turned to an expert from the world of medicine. Although his patroness did not in the end permit herself to be operated upon, von Klein reveals why she felt herself to be ugly and wanted surgical treatment — such an operation, he noted, should be thought of for those who had lost their noses through the pernicious actions of scrofula, lupus, or syphilis. The moral fault here, however, is not that of the princess but rather a sign of the collapse in morality of the aristocracy. Born with a sunken nose she was the victim of her infected parents whose legacy to her was hereditary syphilis.

The Father of Plastic Surgery: Johann Friedrich Dieffenbach from Berlin

By the middle of the 19th century, the surgical techniques that were to make modern aesthetic surgery possible had been developed in the attempt to reconstruct the face and the body. But it was disease and the anxiety about its public recognition that drove patients to undertake painful and dangerous procedures. The Berlin surgeon Johann Friedrich Dieffenbach (1792–1847) (fig. 26), the central figure in 19th century facial surgery, wrote in 1834 that "... a man without a nose [arouses] horror and loathing and people are apt to regard the deformity as a just punishment for his sins. This division of diseases, or even more their consequences, into blameworthy and blameless is strange.... As if all people with noses were always guiltless! No one ever asks whether the nose was lost because a beam fell on it, or whether it was destroyed by scrofula or syphilis."[24]

Dieffenbach had pioneered the sort of procedure that Klein undertook on the pauper. In the early 19th century Dieffenbach made the repair and replacement of missing body parts, such as the nose, a major part of his focus in reconstructive surgery. He developed a method of using external excisions to raise a flattened or depressed nasal tip as well as to reduce an overly large nose.[25] Dieffenbach proposed the total rebuilding of the nose both to restore function and to create a more human visage. He did not envision removing all traces of disease and treatment — visible scars would remain to alert healthy people against unwitting contact with carriers of venereal disease. But the syphilitic's extreme isolation and suffering would be lessened.

Dieffenbach also suggested the use of a gold bridge for a sunken nose. The case that Dieffenbach recounts, the only one in which he attempted to rebuild the bridge of the nose through the use of a gold insert, is that of a man who had lost the bridge of his nose through syphilis and the contemporary cures for syphilis, such as mercury. As with Dr. von Klein's patient, Dieffenbach's attempt seemed to be successful. Even following the incision made on the exterior of the nose, the person's appearance was surprisingly

24 — Cited from Johann Friedrich Dieffenbach, *Chirurgische Erfahrungen, besonders über die Wiederherstellung zerstörter Theile des menschlichen Körpers nach neuen Methoden.* 4 vols. (Berlin: Enslin, 1829–34), 3: 39.

25 — Johann Friedrich Dieffenbach, *Die operative Chirurgie.* 2 vols. (Leipzig: Brockhaus, 1845), 1: 312–92 on plastic surgery of the nose. See also Richard Lampe, *Dieffenbach* (Leipzig: J. A. Barth, 1934); Wolfgang Genschorek, *Wegbereiter der Chirurgie: Johann Friedrich Dieffenbach, Theodor Billroth* (Leipzig: S. Hirzel, 1982); U. Ulrich and C. Lauritzen, "Johann Friedrich Dieffenbach, 1792–1847: 'Vater der plastischen Chirurgie' in Deutschland," *Deutsche medizinische Wochenschrift* 117 (1992): 1165–1167; F. E. Mueller, "Der Chirurg Johann Friedrich Dieffenbach und sein Einfluss auf die Entwicklung der Plastischen Chirurgie," *Chirurgie* 63 (1992): 127–131; H. Wolff, "Das chirurgische Erbe: zum 200. Geburtstag von Johann Friedrich Dieffenbach," *Zentralblatt für Chirurgie* 117 (1992): 238–243. On the institutional history of reconstructive surgery in Berlin see Paul Diepgen and Paul Rostock, eds., *Das Universitätsklinikum in Berlin: Seine Ärzte und seine wissenschaftliche Leistung* (Leipzig: Barth, 1939) on Dieffenbach, pp. 66–80; Gerhard Jaeckel, *Die Charité: Die Geschichte eines Weltzentrums der Medizin* (Bayreuth: Hestia, 1963), on Dieffenbach, pp. 231; 238–47.

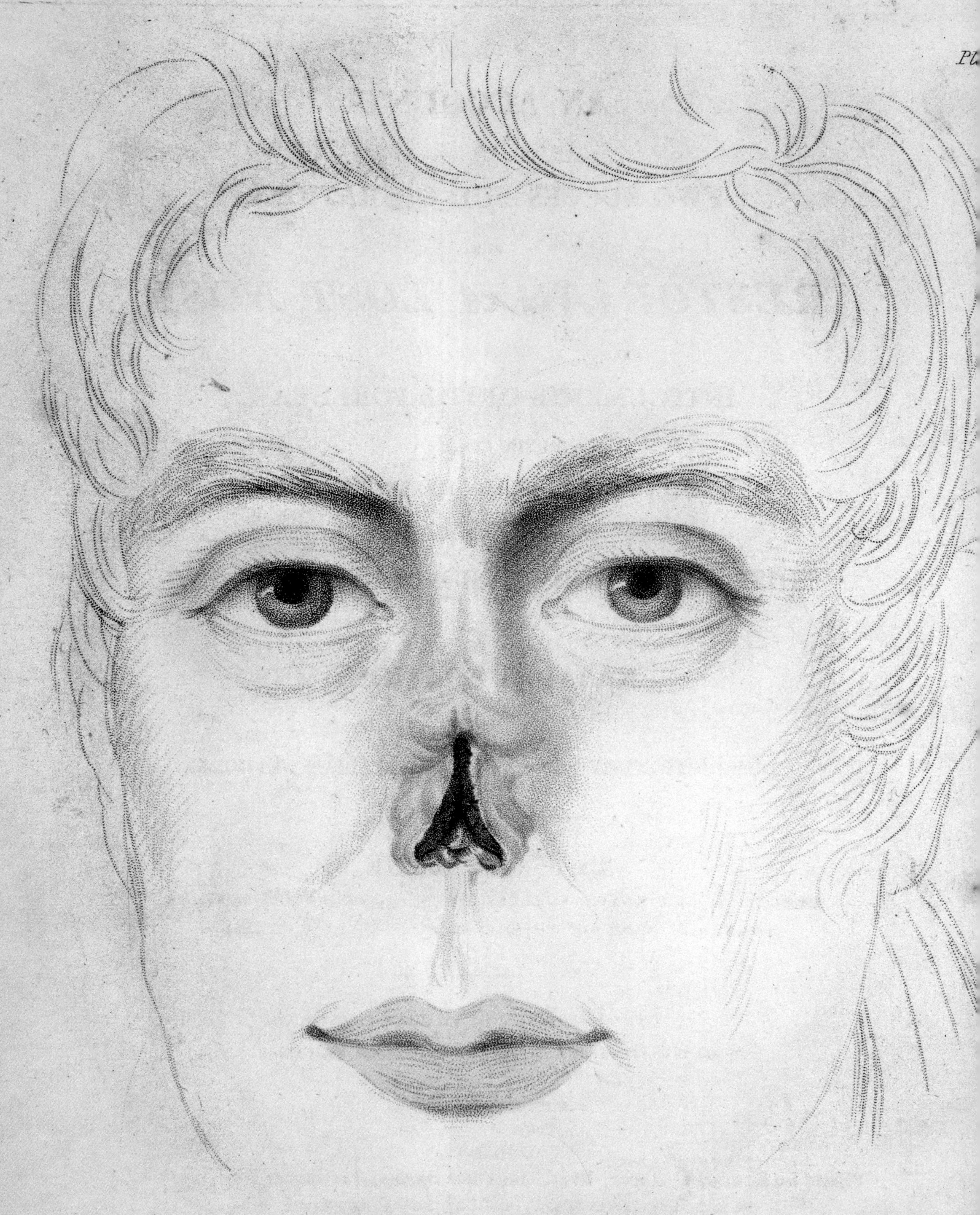

C. Turner

London, Published October 20th 1815 for the Proprietors by C. Turner, No. 50 Warren Street, Fitzroy Square.

fig. 27 a

Plate

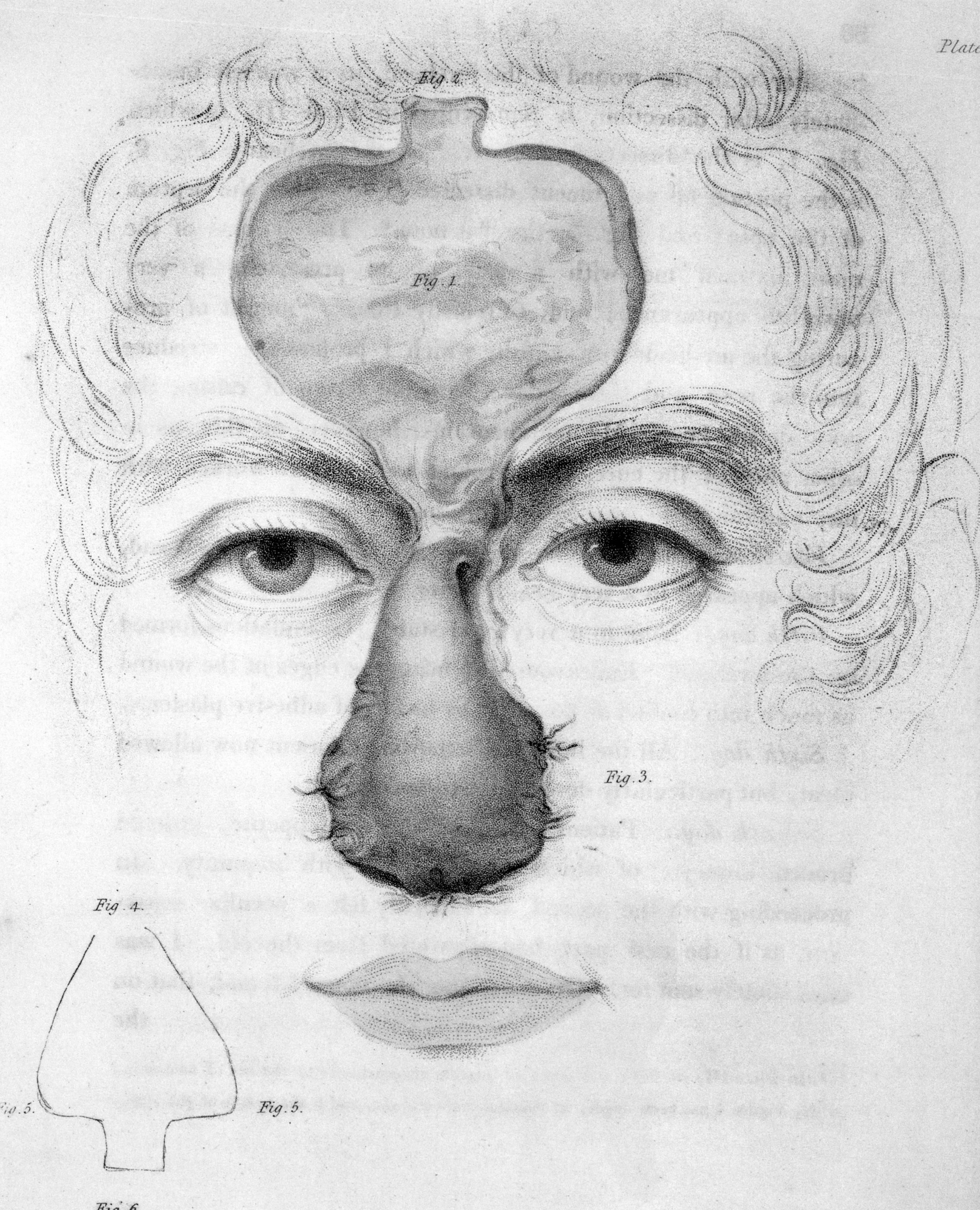

C. Turner fecit

London, Published October 20th 1815 for the Proprietors, by C. Turner, No. 50 Warren Street, Fitzroy Square.

fig. 27 b

Fig. 1.

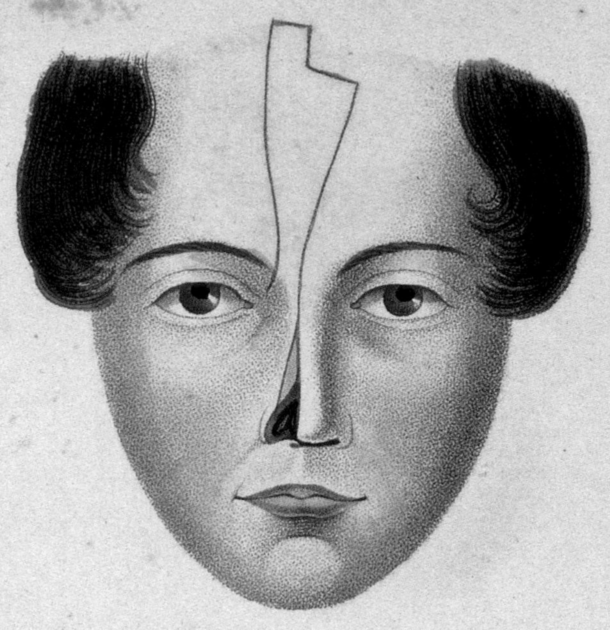

Fig. 2.

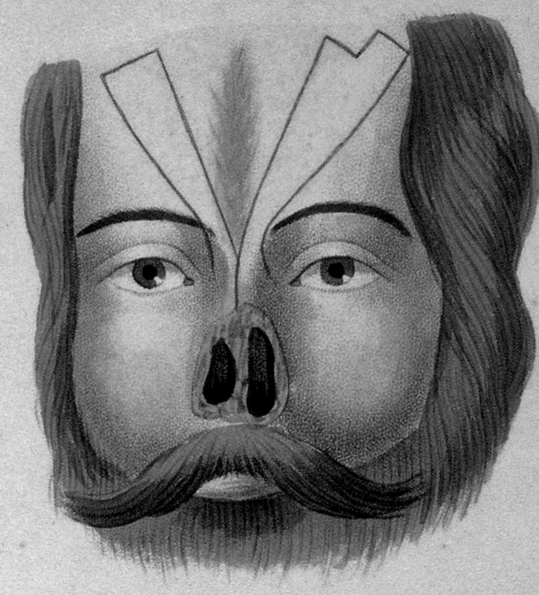

Fig. 5.

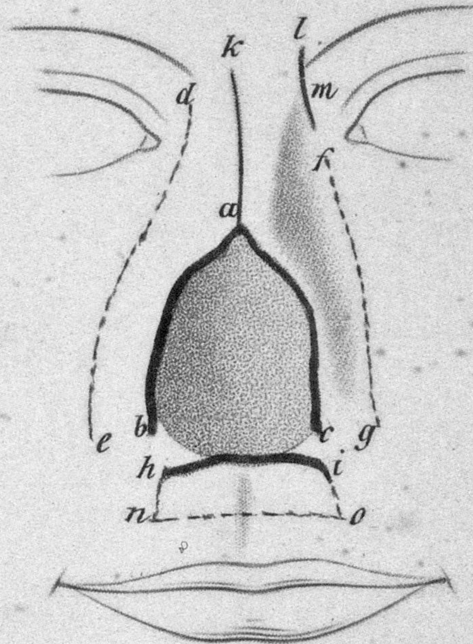

Fig. 6.

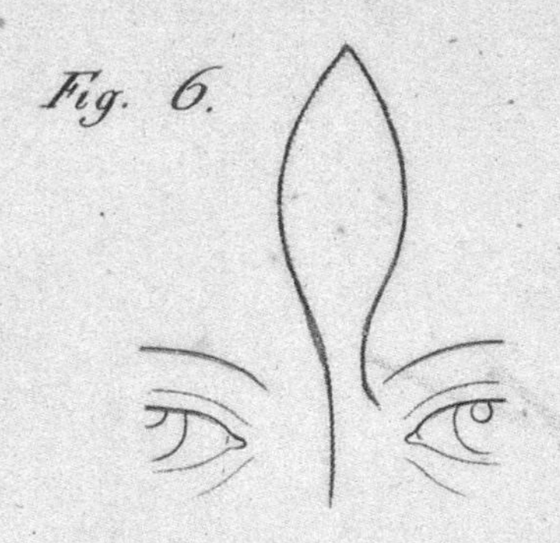

Fig. 8.

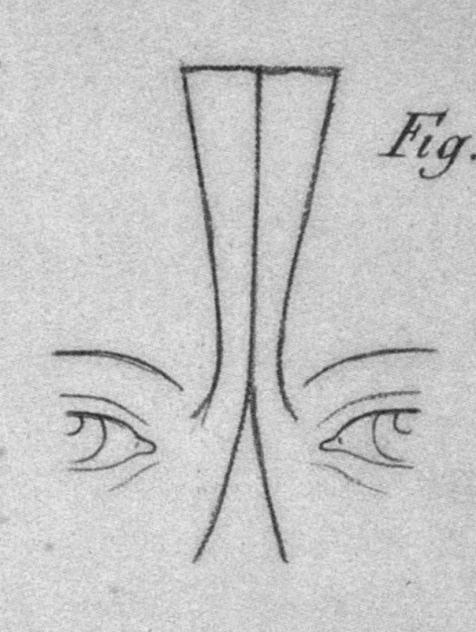

Fig. 3.

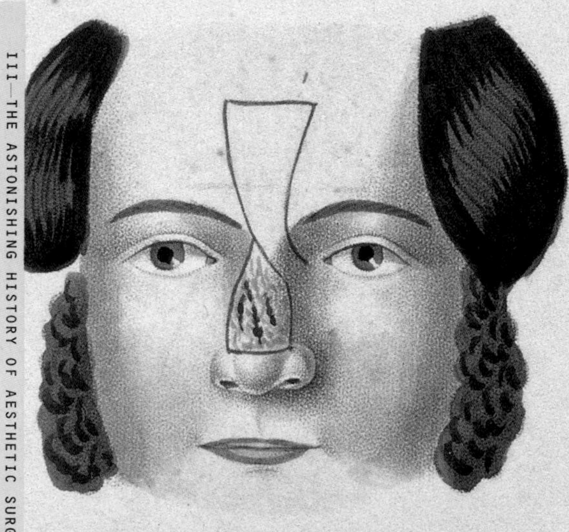

Fig. 7.

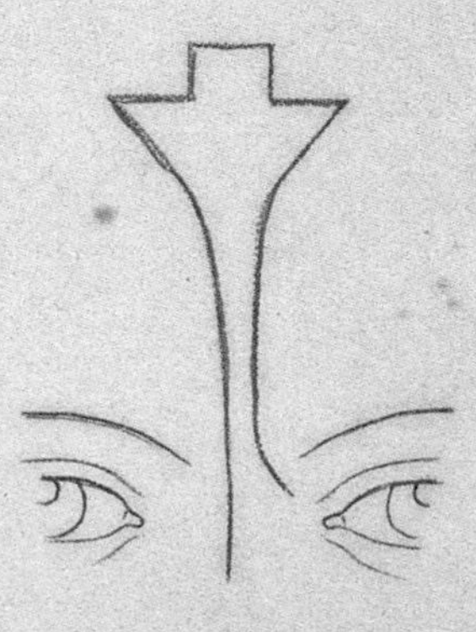

Fig. 4.

fig. 28

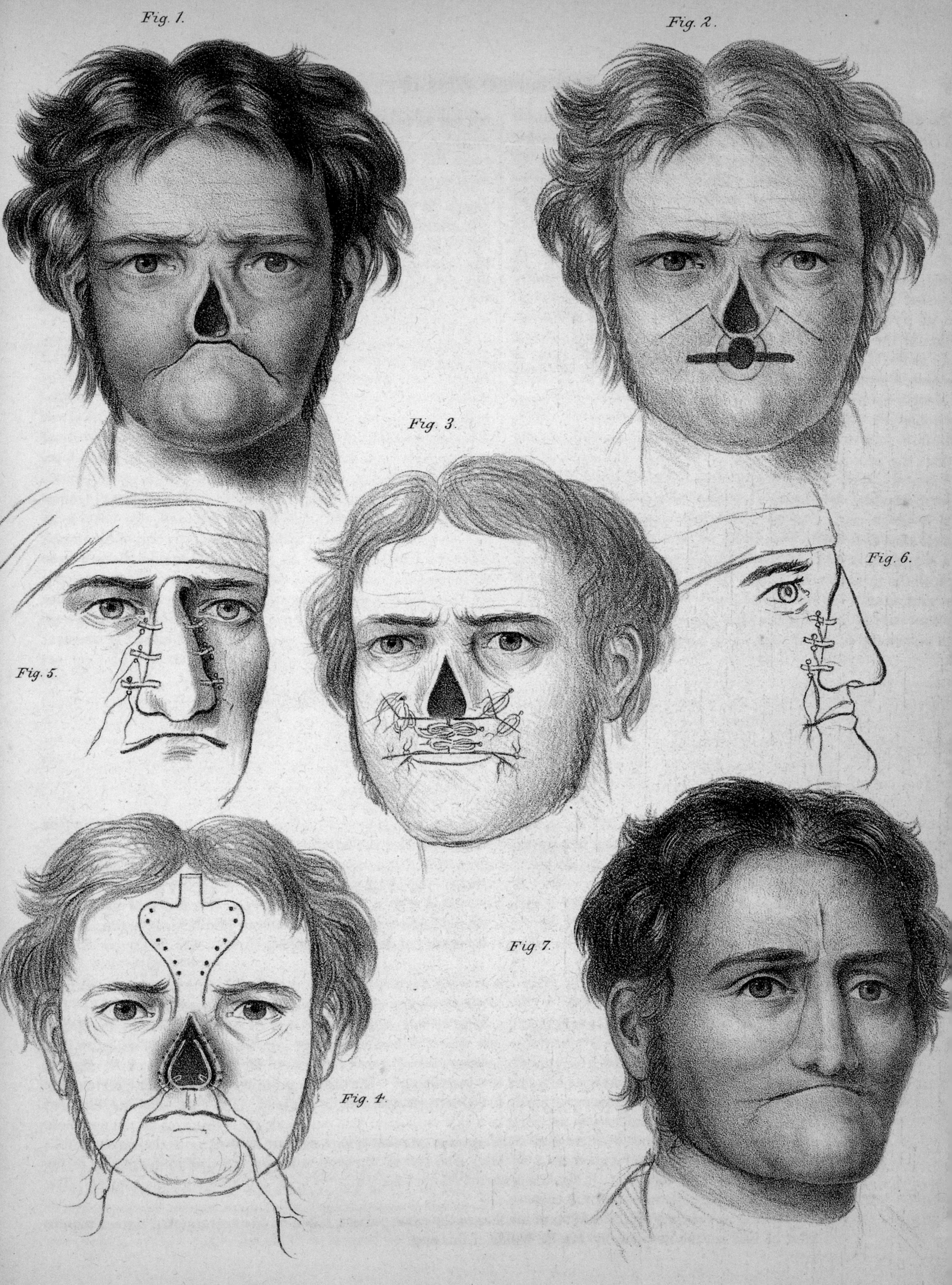

fig. 29

On Stone by A. Newsam. Philadelphia, Published by Carey & Hart. P. S. Duval, Lith. Phil.

fig. 27 a+b

The reconstruction of a nose, as performed by Joseph Constantine Carpue (1764–1846). The surgeon's work and his book, "An Account of Two Successful Operations for Restoring a Lost Nose", were seminal to the onset of modern plastic surgery. © Columbia University Health Sciences Library. Photo: Dwight Primiano

fig. 28

Sketches of rhinoplasties performed by Jonathan Mason Warren (1811–1867). Warren had adopted Tagliacozzi's technique. His study was published in 1840 in the book "Rhinoplastic operations; with some remarks on the antoplastic methods unusally adopted for the restoration of parts lost by accident or disease" by Jonathan Mason Warren (1811–1867) (Boston: Clapp, 1840) © Columbia University Health Sciences Library. Photo: Dwight Primiano

fig. 29

Illustration of a rhinoplasty by Joseph Pancoast (1805–1882). It was published in 1846 in the book "A Treatise on Operative Surgery" — the first American reference work with comprehensive sections on plastic surgery. © Columbia University Health Sciences Library. Photo: Dwight Primiano

fig. 30 a+b

In the rhinoplasty technique developed by Hermann Eduard Fritze (1811–1866), the new nose is sculpted from skin flaps taken from the upper lip or the cheek. Fritze, who also operated on harelips, was a student of Johann Friedrich Dieffenbach, similarly based in Berlin. © Columbia University Health Sciences Library. Photo: Dwight Primiano

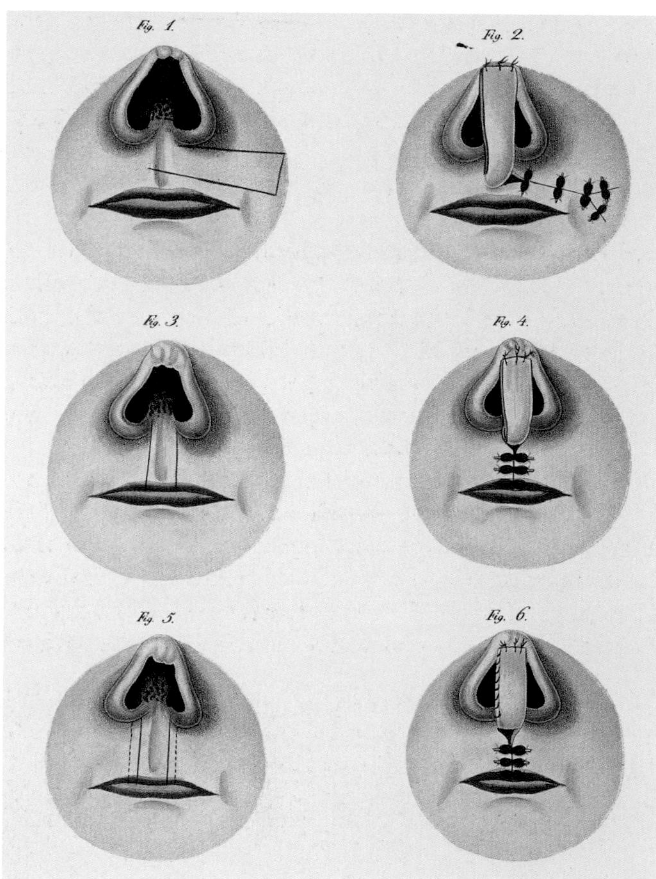

fig. 30 a

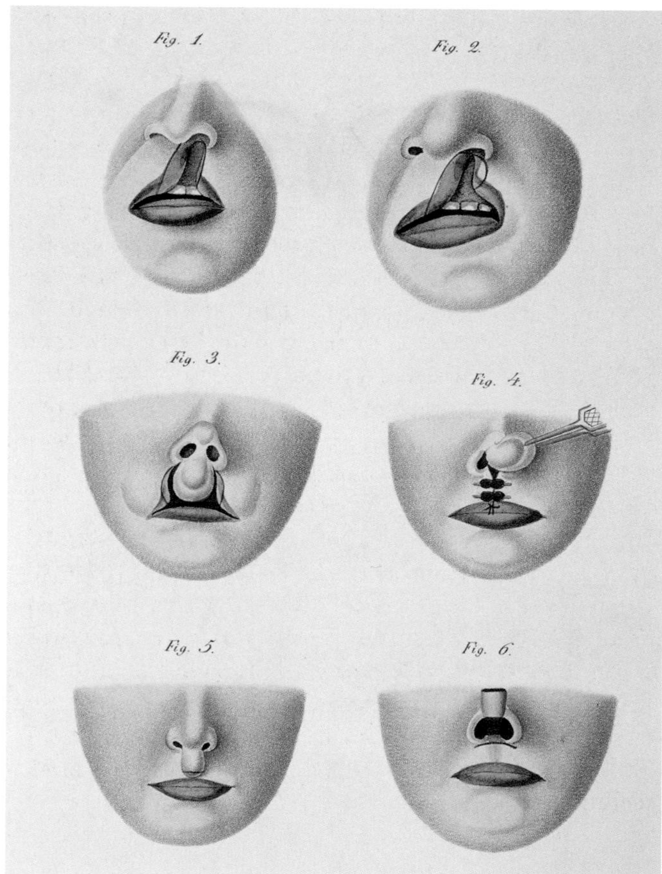

fig. 30 b

natural. However, soon the bridge began to shift to one side and then to the other and eventually vanished into the nasal sinus. It had to be removed and a skin graft used to close the incision in the nose.

Dieffenbach rarely discusses the psychology of his reconstruction of the face and body in any detail. He writes of meeting an 18-year-old Polish woman whose face was the most horrible he had ever seen: "I trembled, for a death's head, of the sort I have never seen on a living body, stood before me." Her face had been eaten away by scrofula (tuberculosis). He undertook to restore her nose using a flap graft from her upper arm and after a successful transplant spent six months undertaking smaller corrective procedures to shape the nose. "The success of the operation gave this unhappiest of people her life again, so that she could boldly go among people, visited the theatre with flowers in her hair and was able to leave Berlin with a happy heart ..." The happy heart of his patient was paralleled by Dieffenbach's immense popularity in Berlin. The populace sang the following ditty:

Who doesn't know Doctor Dieffenbach
The Doctor of all the Doctors
He takes from your arm and leg
And makes you new noses and ears.[26]

26 — **Walter Hoffmann-Axthelm, et al.,** *Die Geschichte der Mund-, Kiefer- und Gesichtschirurgie* **(Berlin: Quintessenz Verlag, 1995), p. 225.**

fig. 31

On May 15, 1899, Baltimore surgeon Howard A. Kelly (1858—1943) performed the first documented abdominoplasty. He liberated his patient, who had weighed 129 kilogramms, from a skin and fatty tissue strip 90 centimetres long, 31 centimetres wide, and seven centimetres deep. Source: Annals of Surgery 33, 1901. Private archive Gilman, Chicago

The popularity of Dieffenbach was tied not only to his abilities as a surgeon, which were evidently great, but to the specific types of procedures that he was seen to undertake. Dieffenbach's Polish patient got off relatively well, given the fact that patients regularly died from infection following such procedures. In a case reported by Jacques Lisfranc (1790—1847) in 1828, when a forehead skin flap graft was used in an attempt to reconstruct a destroyed syphilitic nose, the patient died of sepsis on the 13th day.[27] All of these operations took place before the age of antisepsis and anesthesia. They were done, in terms of the latter 19th century, in the most appalling conditions, done quickly, and done at great risk to body and spirit. It is a sign of the power of the stigma associated with the missing nose that patients were willing to risk such procedures for an almost human nose.

With the introduction of anesthetic and antisepsis during the later third of the 19th century, the possibility of having procedures that a patient desired rather than needed was more probable. The movement from operations to correct the horrific results of infection gave way to procedures to disguise ethnic identity and then to mask aging and then to transform sexual anatomy. This development took place over about 40 years and was the result of both patient demands as well as improvements in surgical techniques.

The First Tummy Tuck in 1899

Abdominal apronectomy or dermolipectomy for abdominal panniculus in order to reduce obesity was developed by Howard A. Kelly (1858—1943) in Baltimore. On May 15, 1899 he removed the pendulous abdomen weighing 14.9 pounds from a 285-pound woman.[28] The piece removed was 90 centimetres long, 31 centimetres wide, and 7 centimetres thick and was, according to the surgeon "larger than the ordinary woman's whole belly." (fig. 31) The rebuilding of this obese female body had begun with a breast reduction. In 1896 J. W. Chambers of Baltimore removed 25 pounds of this woman's "large, flabby and ... very pendulous breasts."

Kelly saw the removal of the abdominal fat as a reconstructive procedure analogous to the removal of the pendulous breasts. It is no surprise given the discourse on the racial breast and the racial body that "the woman was a Jewess, Mrs. M., thirty-two years of age ... with the complaint of 'excessive fat over the lower part of the abdomen.'" She also suffered from a "neuralgic headache."

The body, which began the history of the aesthetic surgery of the abdomen, was a Jewish woman's body. One of the most evident visual stereotypes of the Jewish woman at the time was that of the heavy-set female. Thus the racial anthropologist Hans F. K. Günther (1891—1968), in representing the Jewish woman, chooses as a model the painting

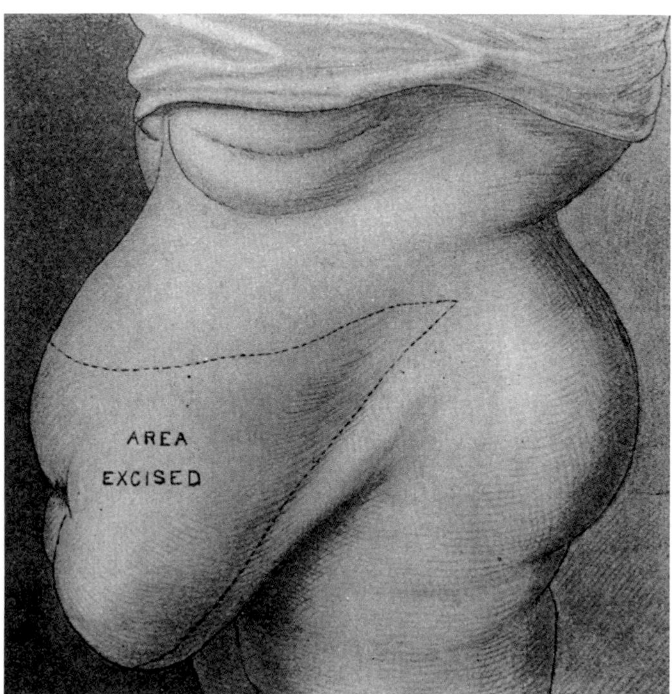

fig. 31

27 — Cited by Blair O. Rogers, "Nasal Reconstruction 150 Years Ago: Aesthetic and Other Problems," *Aesthetic Plastic Surgery* 5 (1981): 283—327, here p. 290.

28 — H. A. Kelly, "Excessive Growth of Fat," *Bulletin of the Johns Hopkins Hospital* 10 (1899): 197. A detailed follow-up on Kelly's patient is to be found in Lindsay Peters, "Resection of the Pendulous, Fat Abdominal Wall in Cases of Extreme Obesity," *Annals of Surgery* 33 (1901): 299—304.

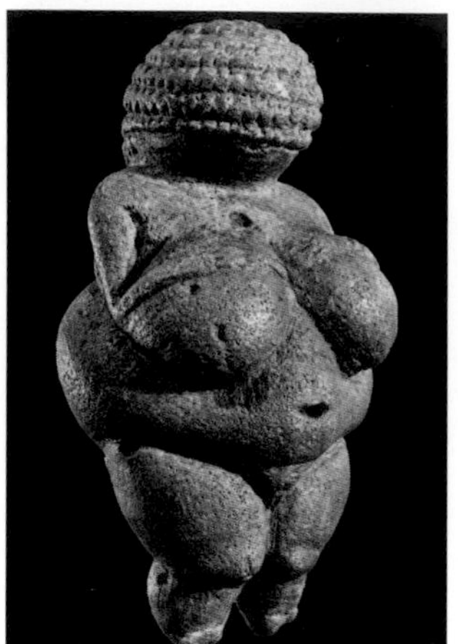

fig. 32

fig. 32

The "Venus of Willendorf," found by the archaeologist Hugo Obermaier (1877–1946) in 1908, he declared her as a symbol for the faceless and fat body frequently associated with Jewish women. As a popular stereotype, it also served well to promote aesthetic surgery. © Archivo Iconografico, S.A. / CORBIS

fig. 33

Radical anthropologist Hans F. K. Günther (1891–1968) used Böcklin's painting "Susannah in the Bath" to illustrate his 'scientific" and highly anti-Semitic view of the supposedly ugly female Jewish body. Source: Rassenkunde des jüdischen Volkes, J. F. Lehmann, Munich 1930. Private archive Gilman, Chicago

by Arnold Böcklin (1827–1901) for his intensely anti-Semitic image of "Susannah in the Bath" with the naked, very large figure of Susannah representing the female Jewish body in a "scientific" context. (fig. 33) He stands in a long German tradition of the ethnological understanding of the Jewish female body. The expansive image of the Jewish woman's body had become a commonplace at the turn of the century. Hugo Obermaier (1877–1946), the German archaeologist who in 1908 discovered the primitive statue he labeled the "Venus of Willendorf" (fig. 32), entered the following note into his diary about it: "a schematically degenerate figure, which represents a higher, exemplary school [of art], such as the Tanagra. No face, only fat and

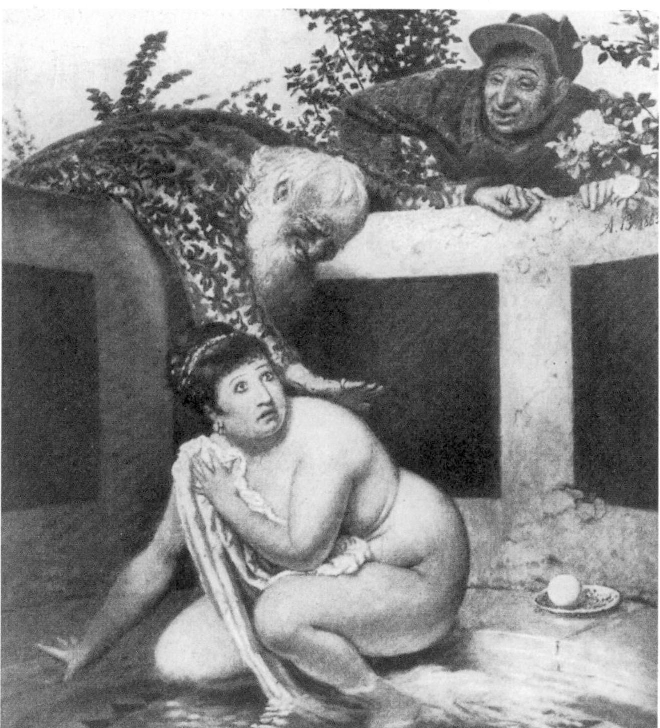

fig. 33

feminine, prosperity, fertility, compare today's lazy / rotten [faule] Jewesses."[29] It is this image which served as the basis for the anxiety about the "primitive" Jewish woman's body.

Such images had particular salience in the melting pot ideology of the United States. The American eugenist Albert Wiggam (1871–1957) complained that the United States was being invaded by ugly women who are "broad-hipped, short, stout-legged with big feet [and] faces expressionless and devoid of beauty."[30] Wiggam also stressed that "good looking people are better morally, on average, than ugly people."

The First Face Lift in 1901

After the turn of the century, the focus of the aesthetic surgeon's innovations becomes the aging face in addition to the ethnic body. The earliest accounts of aesthetic surgery for aging come in the first decade of the 20th century. (fig. 34,35). In 1901, according to his much later account, the German surgeon and cultural historian Eugen Holländer (1867–1932) undertook the first rhytidectomy or face lift on a Polish aristocrat.[31] Holländer's narrative is vital to understanding the role that patients played in initiating treatment by aesthetic surgeons. For just as Jacques Joseph's (1865–1934) patients came to him with complaints about their (or their children's) ears or nose, they also made suggestions as to how these problems should be corrected. It was, of course, the surgeon's role to work out the specific techniques, the incisions, and to visualize the results by evoking aesthetic models.

In Holländer's case the situation was somewhat different but even more exemplary. For the woman who came to him made very specific suggestions. She came with a drawing, which illustrated to her surgeon how, if facial skin were

29 — **Fritz Felgenhauer,** *Willendorf in der Wachau: Monographie der Paläolith-Fundstellen I–VII.* **3 vols. (Vienna: R. M. Rohrer, 1956–59), 1: 11.**

30 — **Albert Edward Wiggam,** *The Fruit of the Family Tree* **(Garden City, N. Y.: Garden City Publishing Co., Inc., 1924), pp. 262, 272.**

31 — **See his accounts in Eugen Holländer, "Die kosmetische Chirurgie," in Max Joseph, ed.,** *Handbuch der Kosmetik* **(Leipzig: Veit, 1912), p. 688 and in his "Plastische (Kosmetische) Operation: Kritische Darstellung ihres gegenwärtigen Standes," in Georg Klemperer and Felix Klemperer, eds.,** *Neue deutsche Klinik: Handwörterbuch der praktischen Medizin mit besonderer Berücksichtigung der inneren Medizin, der Kinderheilkunde und ihrer Grenzgebiete.* **11 vols. (Berlin: Urban und Schwarzenberg, 1928–1932), 9: 1–17.**

fig. 34 a–d

Operations on the upper and lower eyelid, as developed by Joseph Pancoast (1805—1882). Pancoast was a professor at the Jefferson Medical College in Philadelphia and developed numerous surgical techniques. © Columbia University Health Sciences Library. Photo: Dwight Primiano

fig. 35

Cosmetic surgery, June 17th, 1932. The patient wanted to get his lachrymal sacks removed. Since the start of the 20th century, blepharoplasty had become an increasingly popular procedure at surgical clinics. © Getty Images

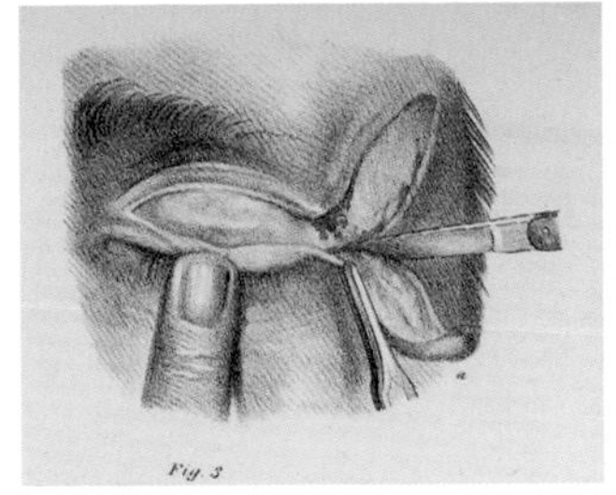

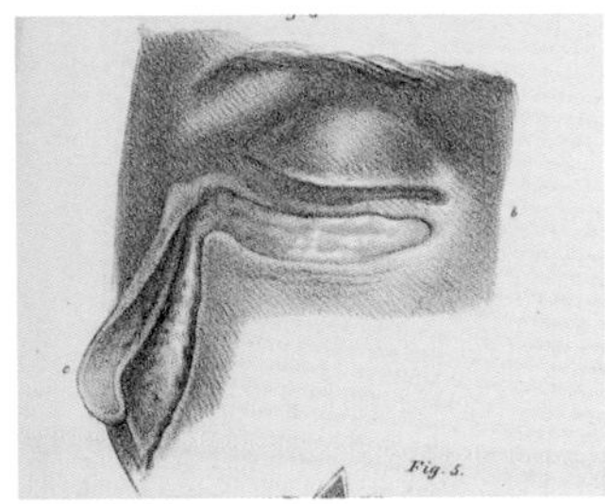

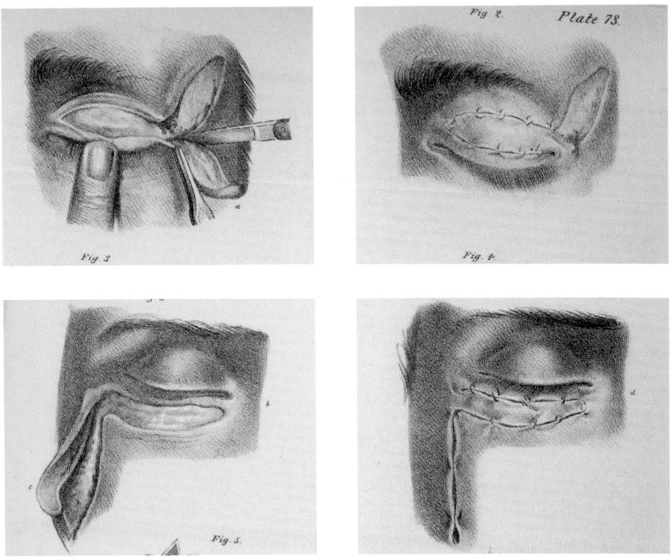

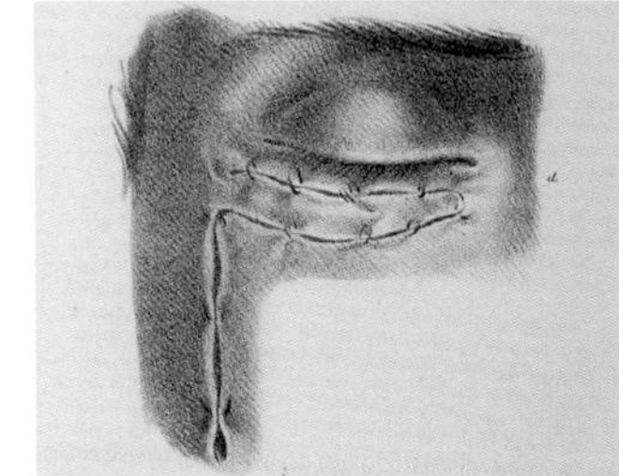

fig. 34 a–d

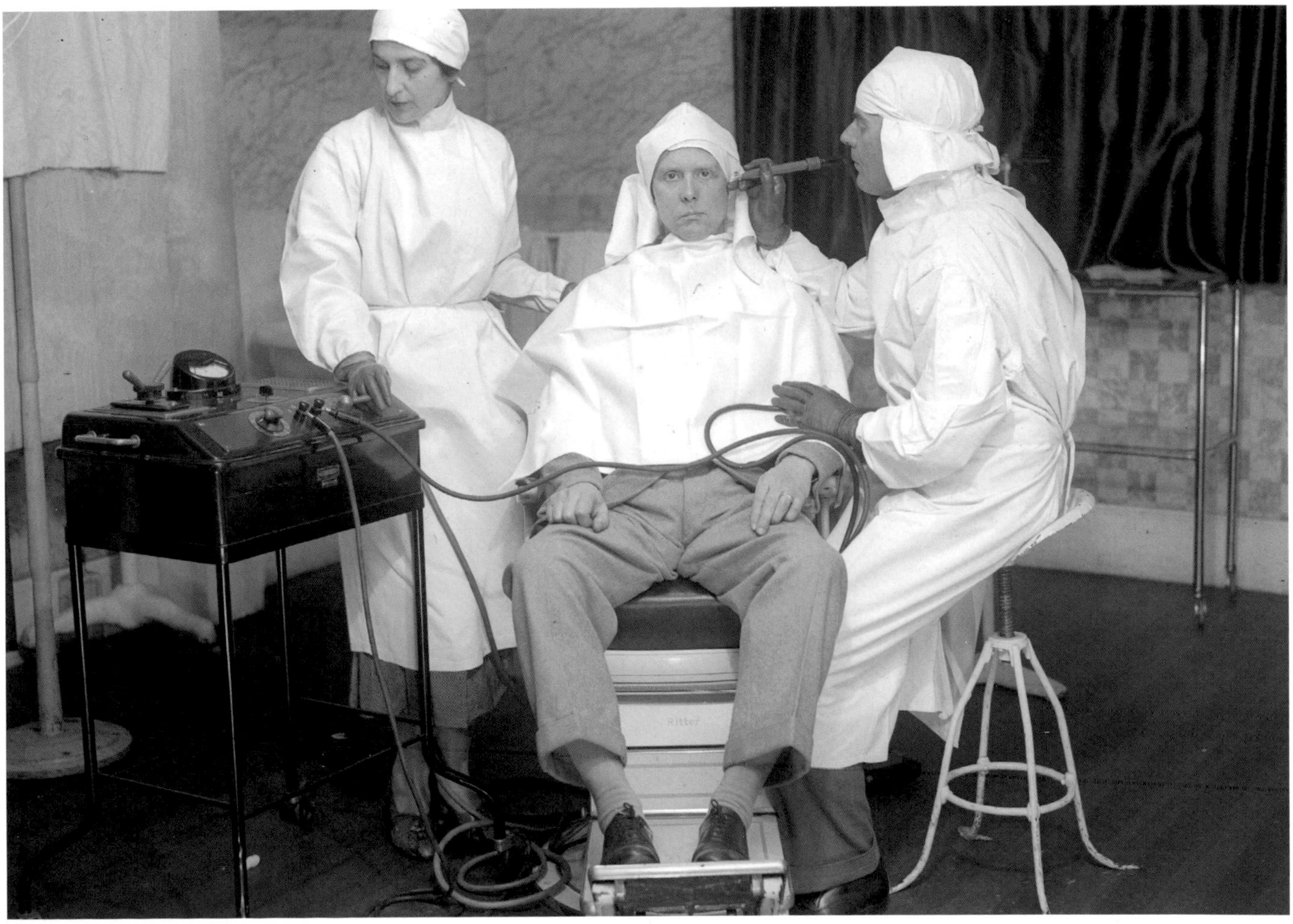

fig. 35

removed at the front of the ear, the nasolabial fold and the corners of the mouth would be tightened. He initially did not want to undertake this but was compelled through "feminine persuasion" to do so. He removed small amounts of skin at the hairline and behind the ear and was able to make some limited changes on the upper face, which he considered inferior but made his patient happy. In 1906 the German surgeon Erich Lexer (1867—1937) also undertook a similar procedure on an actress. His patient had been pulling up the skin of her face by taping her forehead at night and drawing it tight with rubber bands over the top of her skull. This both caused her skin to stretch, creating transverse folds above her zygomatic arches, but also provided a model for how this corrective procedure could be undertaken. Lexer removed S-shaped incisions of skin at the temples, behind the ears and at the hair-line. According to Lexer the result was a success.[32]

32 — Erich Lexer, *Die gesamte Wiederherstellungschirurgie*. 2 vols. (Leipzig: J. A. Barth, 1931), 2: 548.

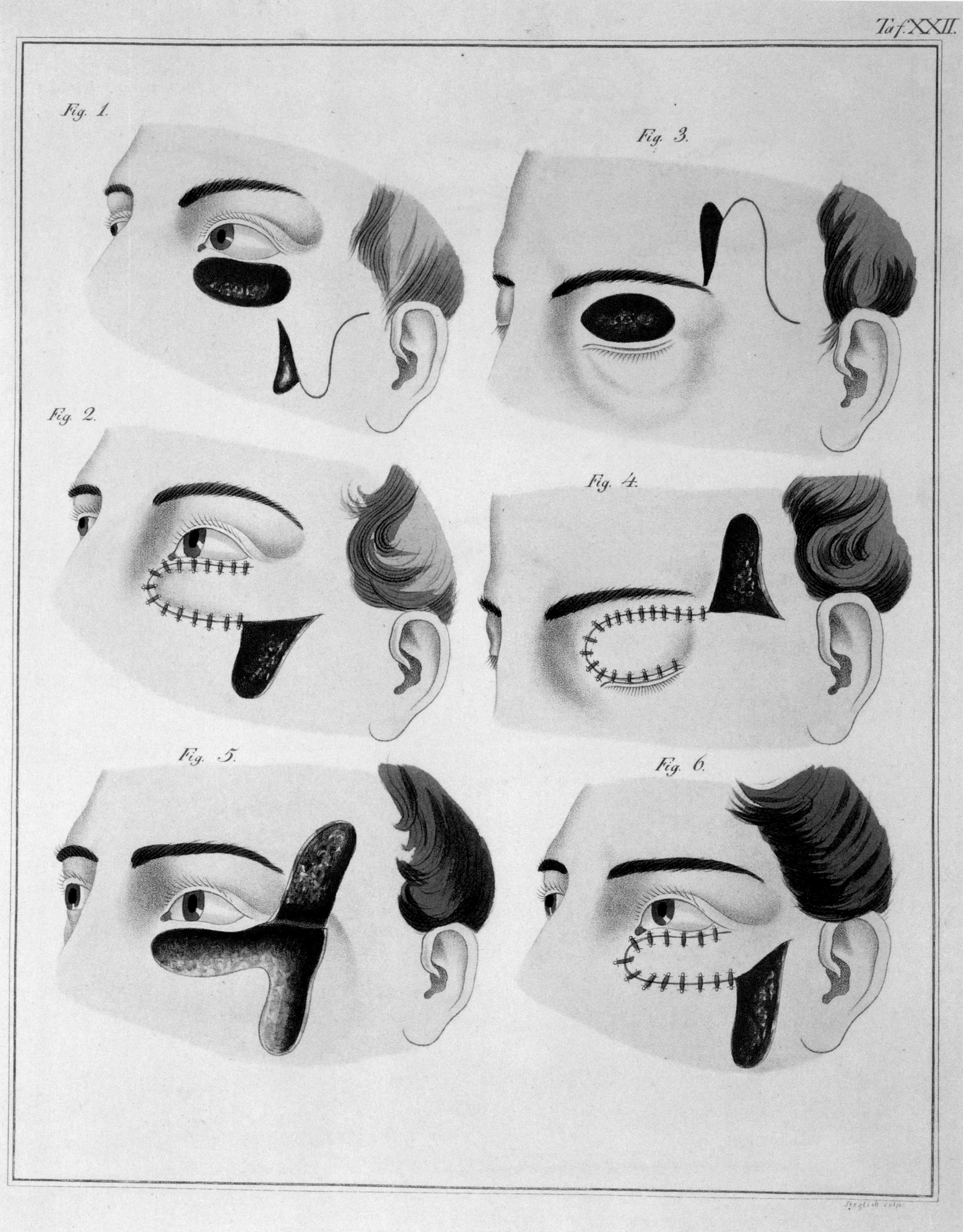

fig. 36

fig. 36

Eyelid lifting techniques developed by Hermann Eduard Fritze (1811—1866). Both the upper and lower eyelids could be operated on — the necessary skin flaps were taken from the cheeks or the temples. © Columbia University Health Sciences Library. Photo: Dwight Primiano

fig. 37

Surgical techniques for correcting the eyelid if it folds inwards or outwards, as developed by Johann Friedrich Dieffenbach (1792—1847). This problem is usually caused by the eyelid becoming lax; it is re-tightened surgically. © Columbia University Health Sciences Library. Photo: Dwight Primiano

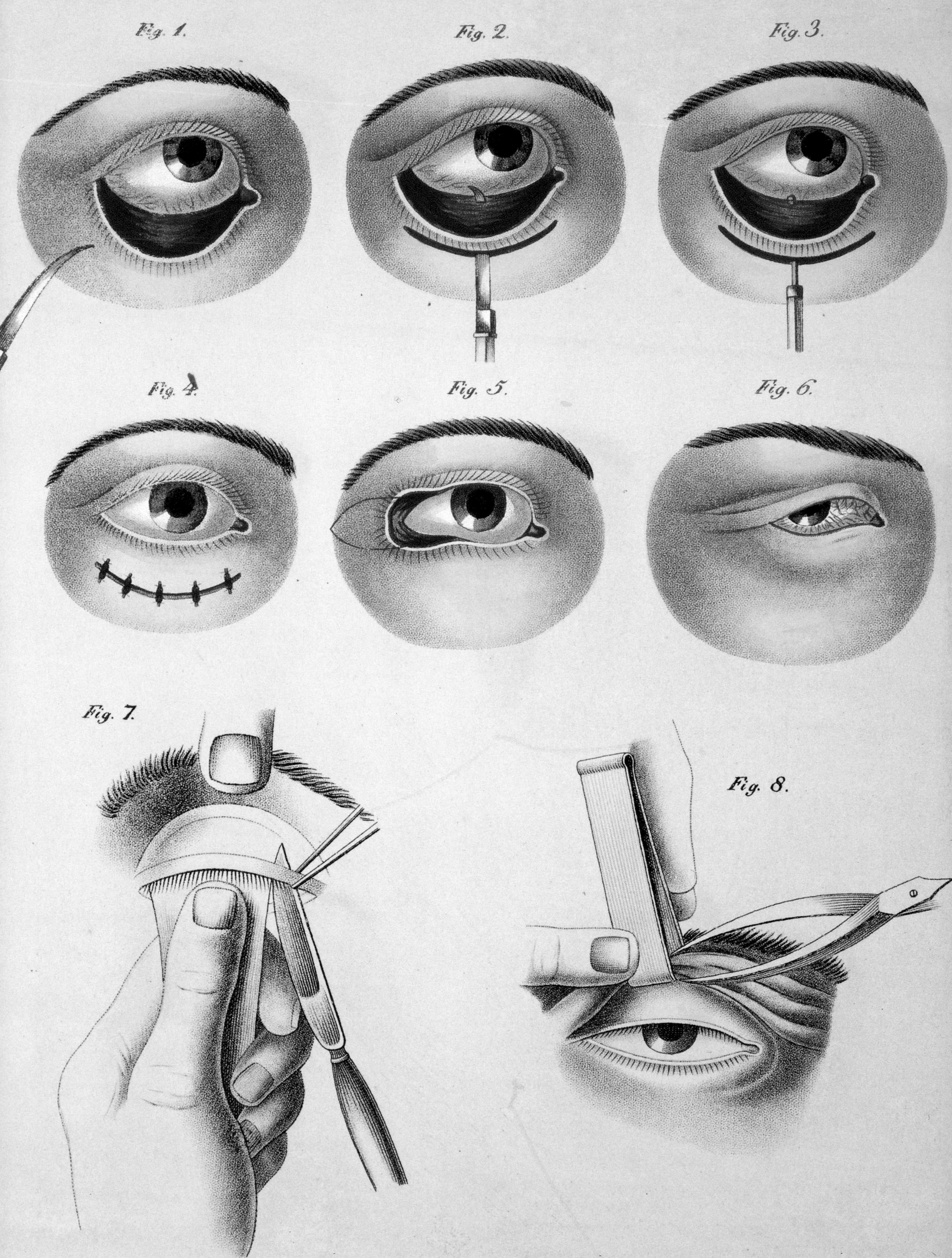

fig. 37

Steglich sculp.t

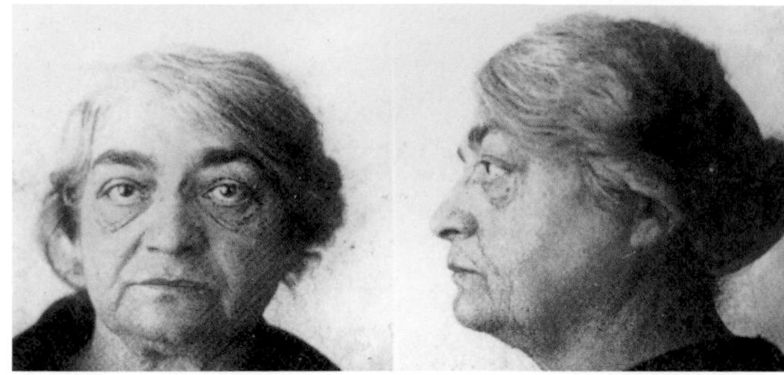

fig. 38 a

fig. 38 a–c

Examples of some of the first facelifts performed by a woman: The French surgeon Suzanne Noël (1878—1954) was the wife of a dermatologist whose work had introduced her to the field of cosmetic surgery. Source: A. Noël, La chirurgie esthétique et son role social, Masson et Cie, Paris 1926. Private archive Gilman, Chicago

fig. 39

Looking into the mirror for the first time: Suzanne Noël's patient is brushing her hair after having received a facelift, still unsure of the effects of the operation. Source: A. Noël, La chirurgie esthétique et son role social, Masson et Cie, Paris 1926. Private archive Gilman, Chicago

fig. 40

Suzanne Noël met Sarah Bernhardt in 1912; Bernhardt had received cosmetic surgery in the US. Thanks to her well-known patients, Noël's reputation grew, as did her patient numbers. She continued to perform surgery well into her old age. Private archive Gilman, Chicago

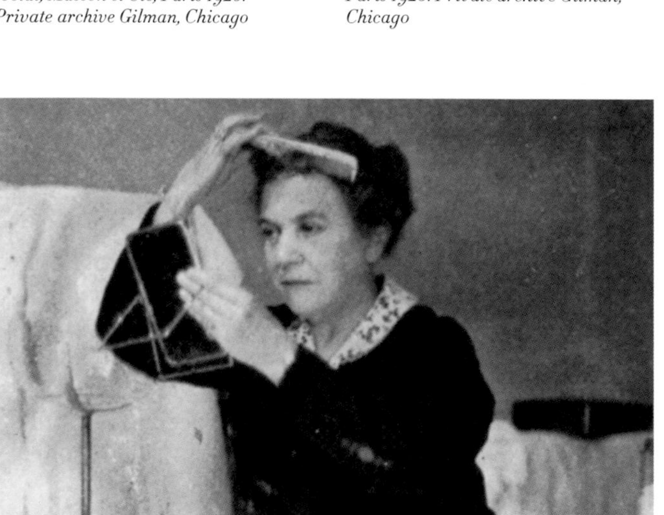

fig. 39

The First Eye Lid Surgery in 1906

In Chicago, Charles Conrad Miller (1880—1950) by 1906 had developed procedures for the removal of "bag-like folds of eyelid skin." Similar procedures had been suggested as early as Aulus Cornelius Celsus, but were either the reconstruction of a missing eyelid which, like the missing nose, was seen as a form of punishment or the removal of a *palpebrae laxioris*, relaxed lid, as the folds of skin were understood to impair vision. The German Surgeon Johann K. G. Fricke (1790—1841) introduced the modern term blepharoplasty in 1829. Numerous approaches to the reconstruction of both the upper and lower eyelid followed him. But Miller's procedure in 1906 was self-consciously aesthetic. Miller is often given credit for having developed the first rhytidectomy, which was then copied by other surgeons of his day. Miller's career was typical for many of the early aesthetic surgeons, as patients (and their families) constantly harassed him when procedures failed to deliver the expected changes in appearance and they could not pass. Eventually he gave up aesthetic surgery and turned to general surgery — feeling that it was "more satisfying to cure disease than to satisfy vanity."

The First Female Aesthetic Surgeon: Suzanne Noël

In Paris, following the lead of Holländer and Lexer in listening to their patients, Suzanne Noël (1878—1954) began to excise excess skin in order to tighten the face and remove wrinkles. (fig. 38 a–c, 39)

She began in 1912 when Sarah Bernhardt returned from America (perhaps from a session with Charles Conrad Miller in Chicago) and showed her the results of the procedures that she had undergone there. (fig. 40) The social

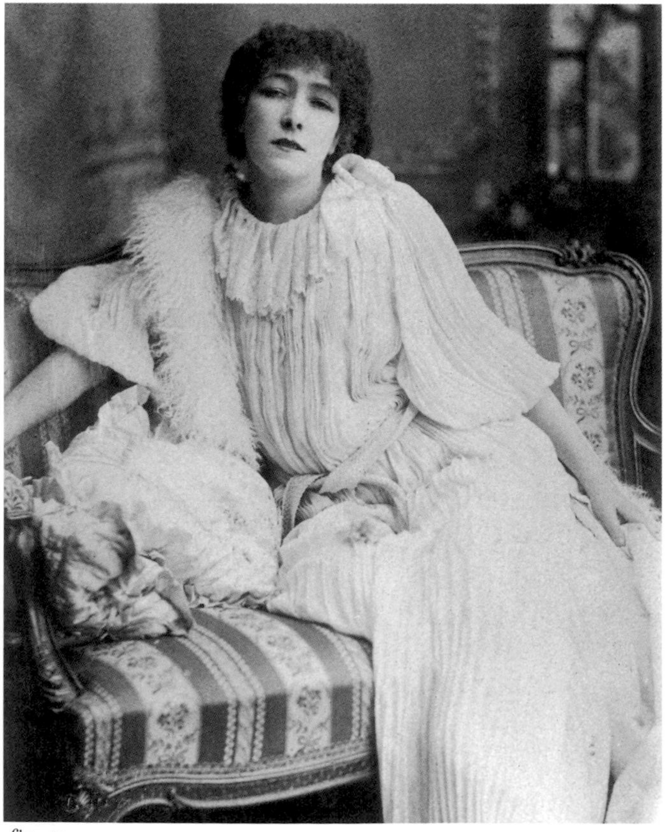

fig. 40

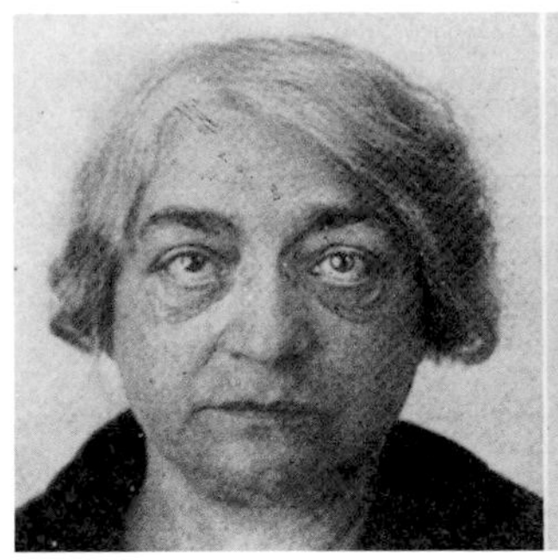
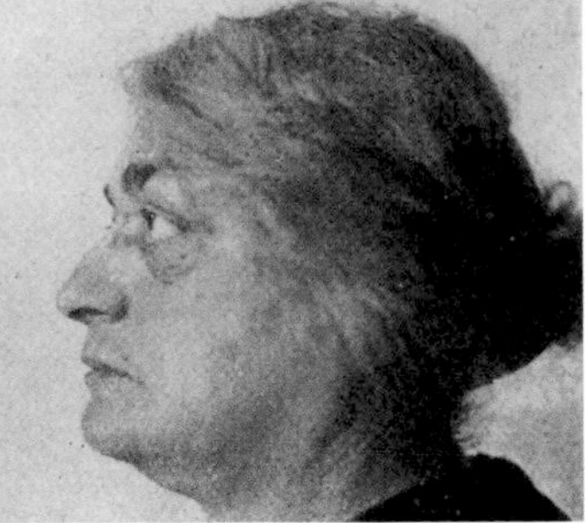

fig. 38 b

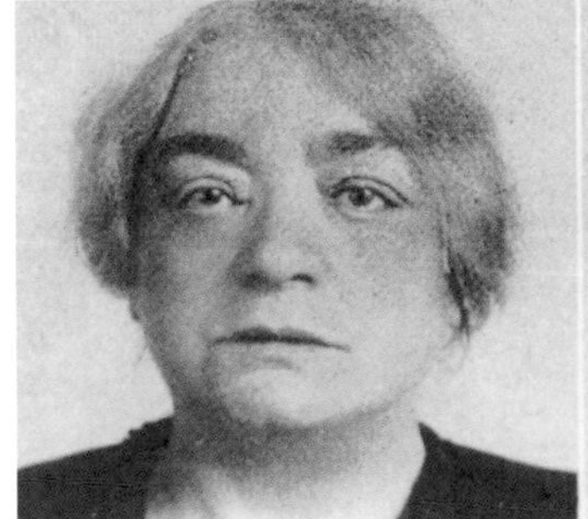
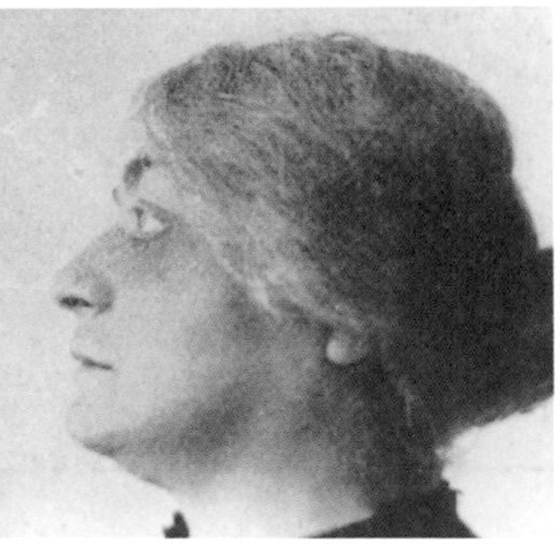

fig. 38 c

fig. 41 a+b

Before and after: On the left, the patient's face is characterised by sagging cheeks and a double chin. On the right, her facial contours have been tightened — thanks to a facelift by London surgeon Charles H. Willi. Source: Charles H. Willi, Facial Rejuvenation: How to Idealise the Features and The Skin of the Face by the Latest Scientific Methods, Cecil Palmer, London 1926. Private archive Gilman, Chicago

stigma of such procedures in Paris was clear: "Women have their operations and do not talk about it," Noël wrote. Silence here is also a mark of consent. While it is evident that she began by operating on what she described as desperate cases such as a woman abandoned by her husband, she quickly had clients who were motivated by their "love of finery and beauty."[33] The fact that they could come to a female surgeon was certainly an aspect of the claim for secrecy.

Suzanne Noël was born Suzanne Blanche Marguerite Gros in 1878 in Laon, France. She married in the 1910s to a dermatologist and in 1905 she began her medical studies in that same field. Dermatology was one of the medical specialties from which aesthetic surgeons came. Indeed the reason we speak of "cosmetic surgery" in medicine was that it had its origin in the subspecialty of cosmetic dermatology.[34] Her husband committed suicide in 1924, by which time she was well established as a surgeon. She worked as a reconstructive surgeon during World War I where she honed her skills. She lived well past World War II, dying in 1954. In her old age she was a prime example of her own art, as a visitor remarked in 1942: "She was sitting at a desk in a consulting room at the Clinique des Bleuets and wearing a black feather hat and black coat. She

33 — A. Noël, *La chirurgie esthétique* (Paris: Masson, 1926), pp. 6–7. See also Jeannine Jacquemin, *Suzanne Noël* (Paris: Soroptomist International, 1988).

34 — See my "Cultural and Socio-economic Background," in Larry Millikan and Lawrence Charles Parish, eds., *Global Dermatology* (New York: Springer, 1994): 20–27 as well as John Thorne Crissey and Lawrence Charles Parish, *The Dermatology and Syphilology of the Nineteenth Century* (New York: Praeger, 1981); Joachim J. Herzberg and Günter W. Korting, eds., *Zur Geschichte der deutschen Dermatologie: zusammengestellt aus Anlass des XVII. Congressus Mundi Dermatologiae, 24.-29. Mai, 1987* (Berlin: Grosse Verlag, 1987).

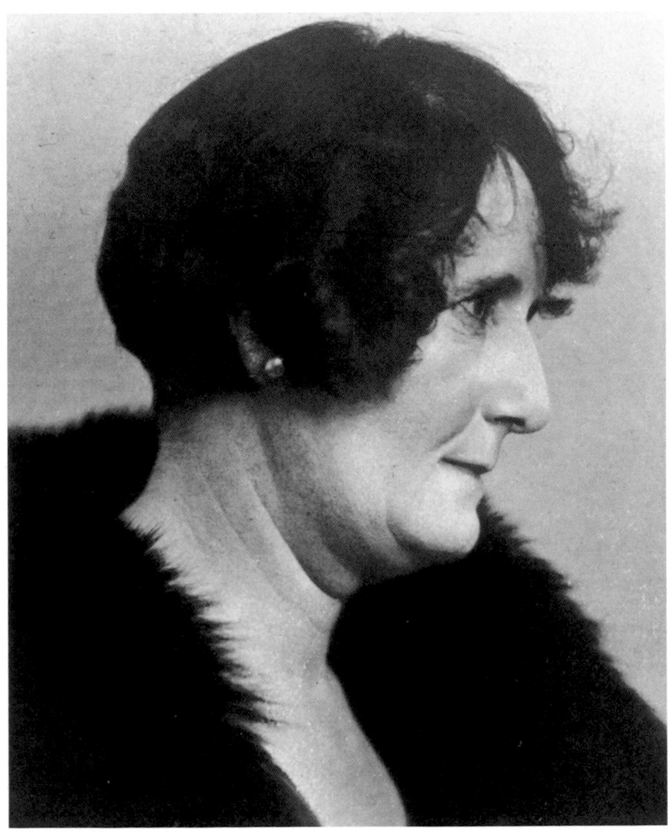

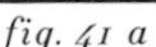

fig. 41 a

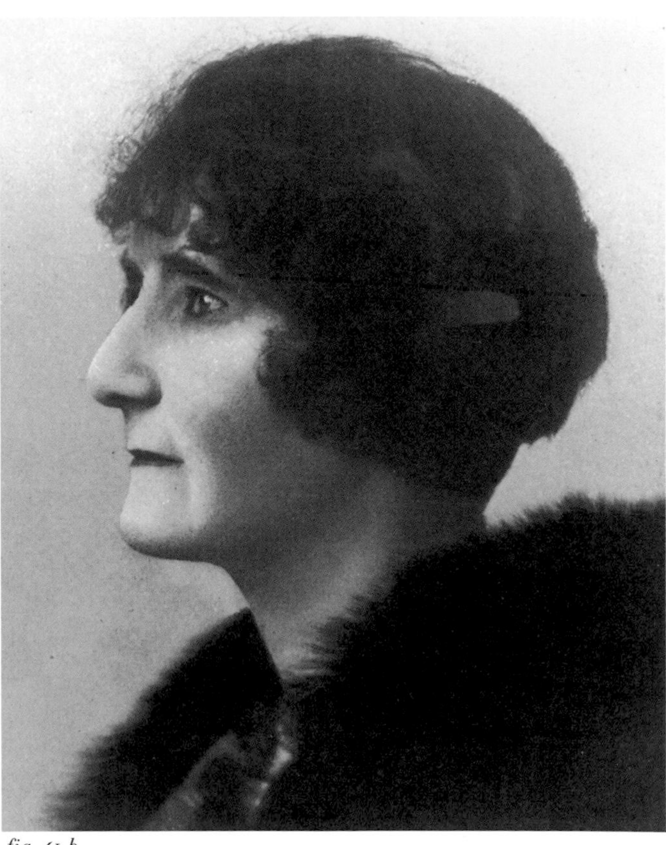

fig. 41 b

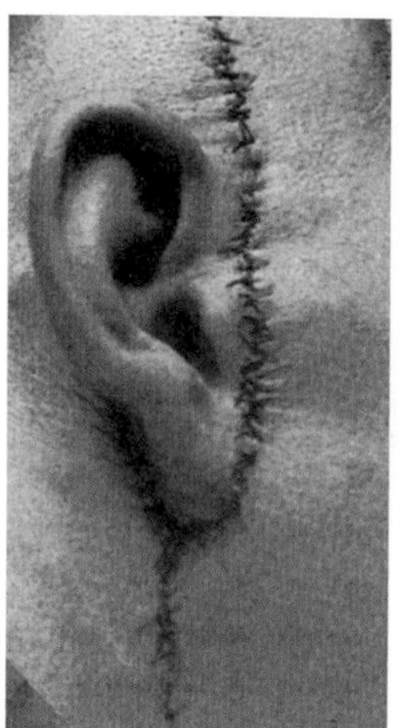

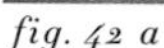

fig. 42 a

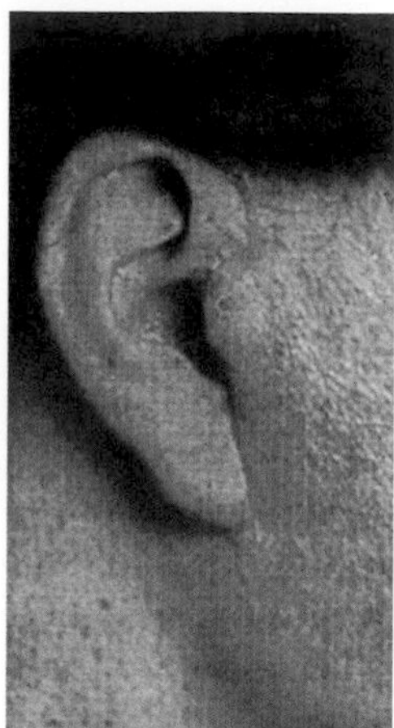

fig. 42 b

fig. 42 a+b

In order to disguise the traces of a cheek lift, Jacques Joseph (1865—1934) revised his surgical technique: Whereas previously there was a prominent scar in front of the ear, the incision was now made behind the ear — and almost completely out of sight. Source: J. Joseph, Nasenplastik und sonstige Gesichtsplastik, Leipzig 1931

fig. 43

Facelifting surgery at Charles H. Willi's London practice, February 24, 1932. Willi no longer used the conventional knife and scalpel but an electrical tool. © Getty Images / Hulton Archive

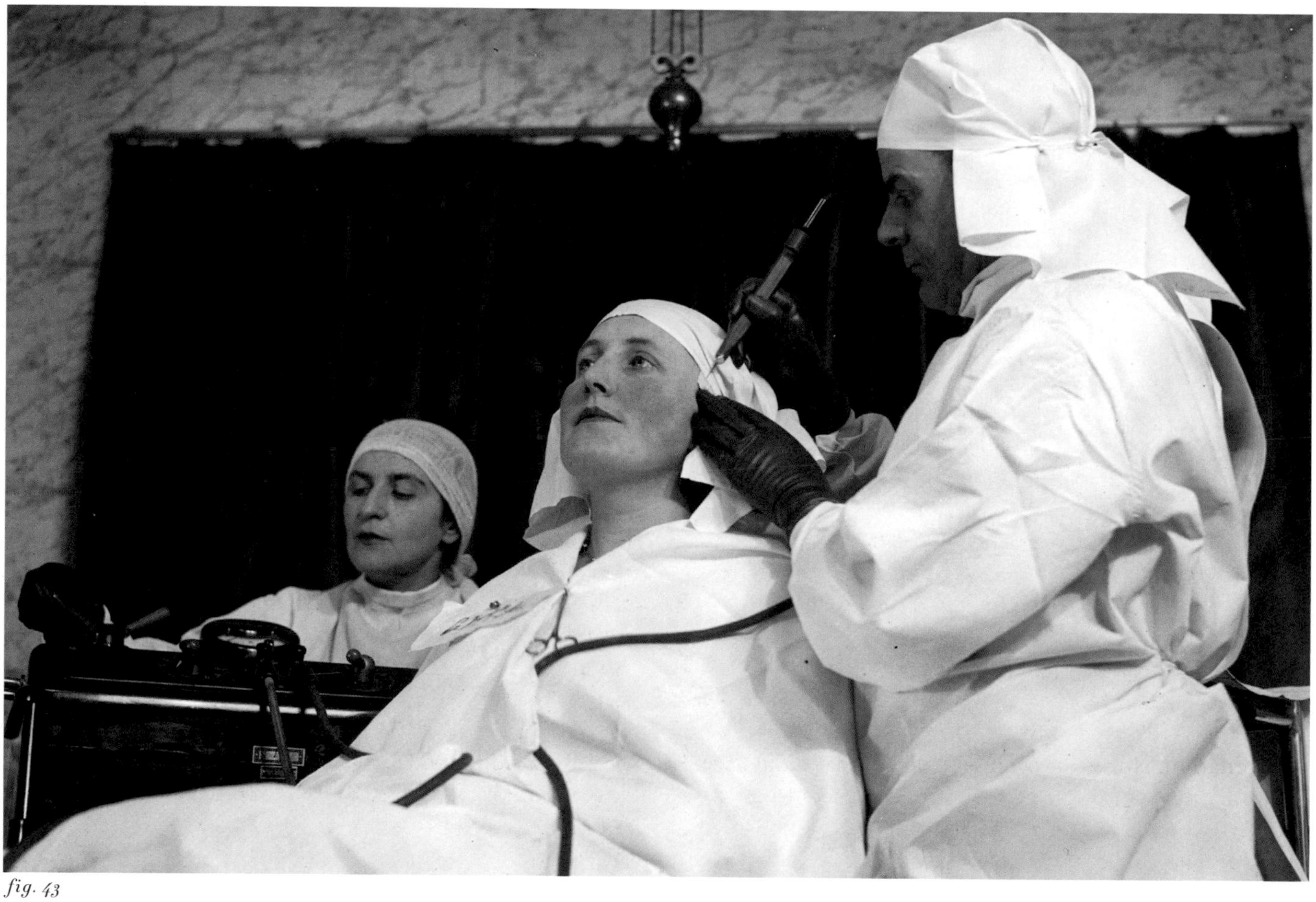

fig. 43

looked exactly as she appears in the picture that is reproduced here. She had a smooth and oval face without a wrinkle — having herself had multiple face lifts and blepharoplasties ... I was impressed by her dignity. She gave, at once, the impression of being a grand lady — although she was no more than five feet four inches high ... her words were simple and direct. They revealed a clear mind ... wisdom, calmness, and self-confidence emerged from her appearance and manner." She was one of the remarkable first generation of aesthetic surgeons produced from the battlefields of France.

Sagging Cheeks and Double Chins in 1912

In 1912 the German surgeon Jacques Joseph (1865—1934) developed a procedure for the tightening of sagging cheeks (*ptosis*), which initially left a small scar in front of the ear (fig. 42 a+b). He modified this as he did with virtually all of his procedures to eliminate the scar.
In 1919 Raymond Passot, a student of Hippolyte Morestin (1869—1919), developed a procedure for the removal of the

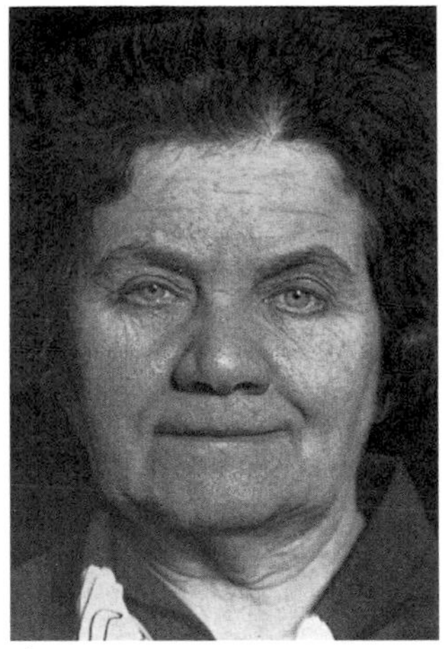

fig. 44 a

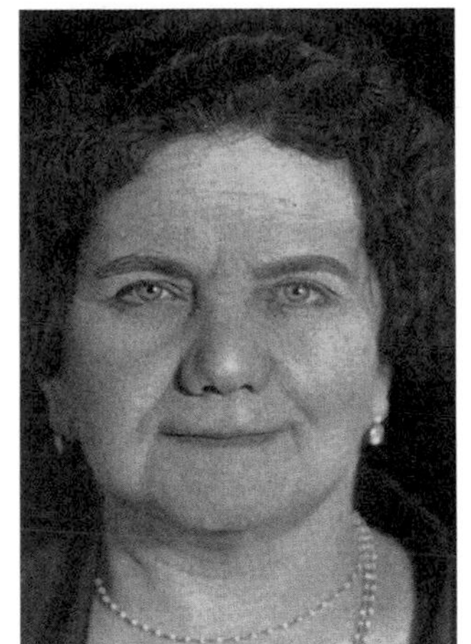

fig. 44 b

fig. 44 a+b

Another cheek lift by Jacques Joseph. These before / after photos were also included in the Berlin-based surgeon's book, "Nasenplastik und sonstige Gesichtsplastik", one of the most important reference works for plastic surgery published in the early 20th century. Source: J. Joseph, Nasenplastik und sonstige Gesichtsplastik, Leipzig 1931

fig. 45 a–c

After the First World War, plastic surgery was also performed on transsexuals, for example at Berlin's Institut für Sexualwissenschaften. Under the guidance of Magnus Hirschfeld (1868—1935), the institute's surgeons transformed male into female genitalia. Source: Felix Abraham, "Genitalumwandlung an zwei männlichen Transvestiten," Zeitschrift für Sexualwissenschaft und Sexualpolitik 28, 1931. Private archive Gilman, Chicago

double chin. Such procedures continued through to the 1970s with numerous small improvements on the placement of incisions and the removal of tissue.(fig. 44 a+b) But alternatives, such as estrogen therapy in the 1980s and 1990s, had begun to take their place as part of facial surgery.

The First Fat Injections in the 1920s

The face-lift came to be a standard surgical procedure to change the surface of the body through the tightening of the skin. The aesthetic surgeons of the 1920s evoked the idea of rejuvenation of the spirit. Charles Willi wrote in 1926 concerning subcutaneous fat injections: "A lady enters the studio with a permanent frown, and a few minutes later the frown has disappeared for ever; she entered with two naso-labial lines cut as with a knife between her cheek and nose, a needle-prick and the furrows are filled for ever; she enters with wrinkles that suggest old age, she goes out a young unwrinkled woman. There is no pain, there is no danger, it is an instantaneous and painless rejuvenation. Nor is it possible to detect that hand of man and not hand of Nature has effected the transformation." (fig. 43) The anxiety about scarring is real in the world of the aesthetic surgeon. For it is the invisibility of the procedures which validates one's appearance. People can not pass if they are scarred in such operations.

Charles Conrad Miller stressed that signs of maturity in women must go. Featural surgeons can do much to perpetuate youthful contour, but usually it cannot be accomplished without a good deal of scarring, for most of the surgical steps which accomplish these effects require the excision of rather large segments of integument. The acceptance of scarring (and the development of procedures which hide or mask or reduce scarring) becomes part of the history of facial surgery, including the history of the rhinoplasty and rhytidectomy.

The First Transsexual Surgeries in the 1920s

After World War I, there is a moment when in Germany, aesthetic surgery moves from the masking of ethnicity and aging to sexual transformation. In the 1920s, primarily through Magnus Hirschfeld's (1868—1935) Institute for Sexual Science in Berlin, a series of surgical interventions were developed by Ludwig Levy-Lenz (1889—1976) and Felix Abraham (1901—1938). (fig. 46) They surgically transformed male genitalia into simulacra of the external female genitalia (without, of course, the ability to reproduce). (fig. 45 a–c)

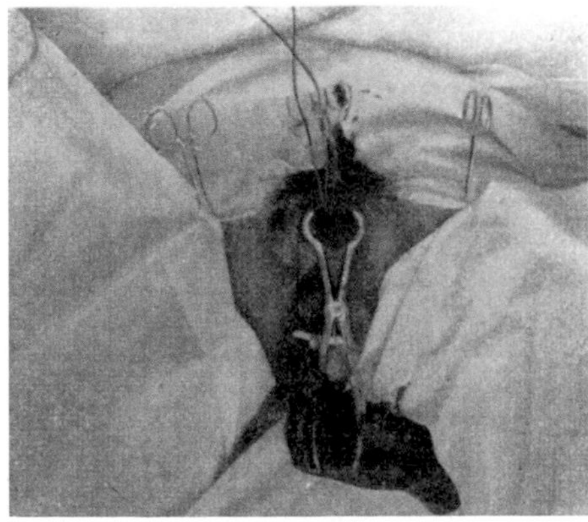

fig. 45 a

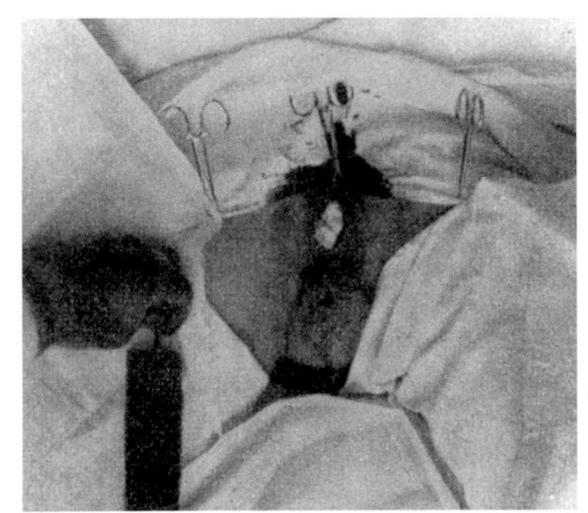

fig. 45 b

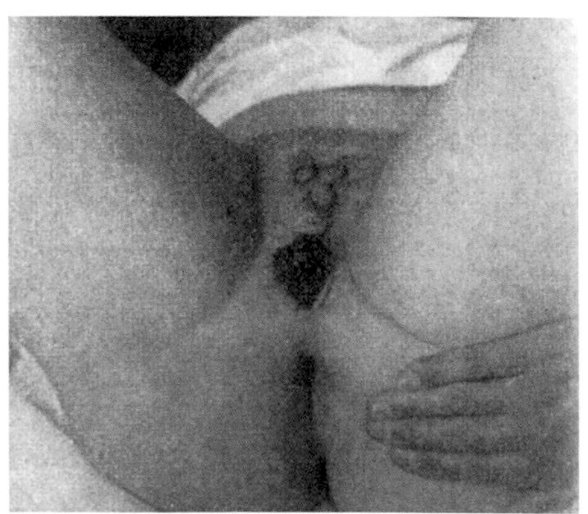

fig. 45 c

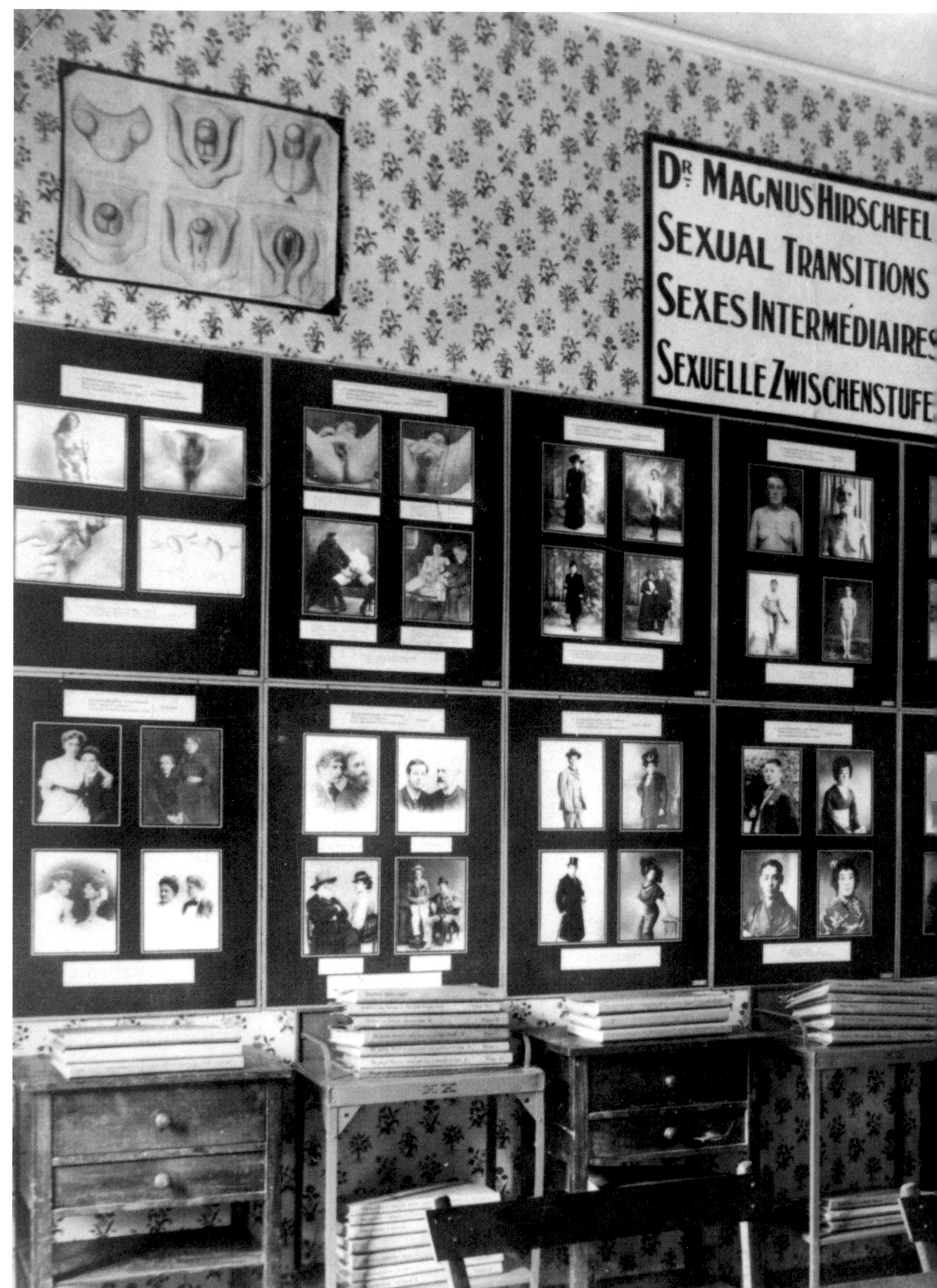
Dr. Magnus Hirschfel
Sexual Transitions
Sexes Intermédiaires
Sexuelle Zwischenstufe

fig. 46

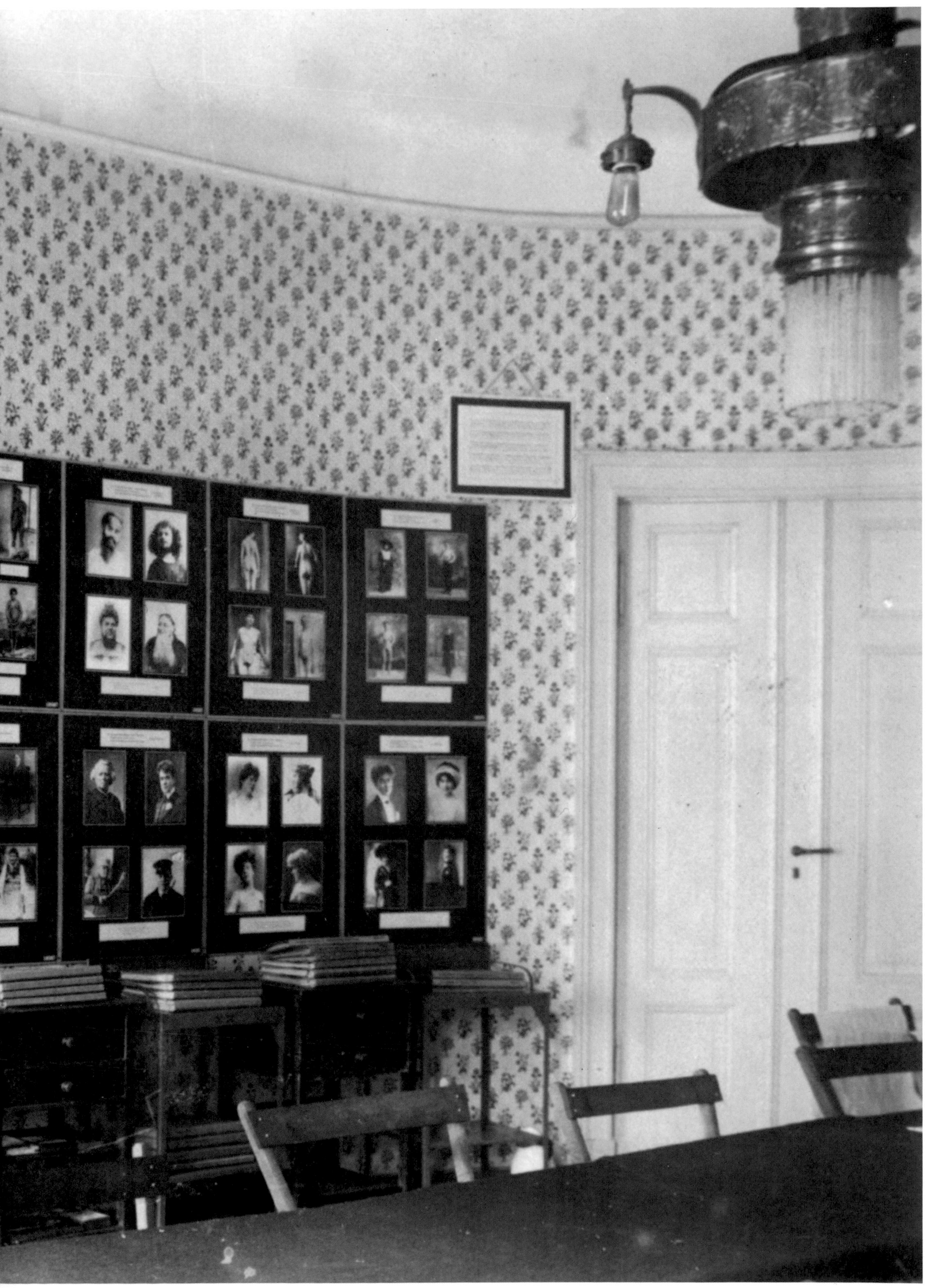

fig. 46

Office of Magnus Hirschfeld (1868–1935). The physician, sexologist and pioneering gay rights campaigne founded the Institute for Sexual Science in Berlin in 1919, the first of its kind in the world. His study Die Homosexualität des Mannes und des Weibes (Homosexuality in Man and Woman) published in Berlin in 1914 was one of the 20th century's milestone works on gender and sexuality. Photo, 1930 © akg-images

fig. 47

On March 13, 1954, the "Picture Post" published the story of Roberta Cowell — a woman who was born a man. Roberta made history as Britain's first fully reoperated transsexual. © Getty Images / Hulton Archive

fig. 48 a+b

A sex change that was incomplete but nevertheless made the patient happy, as stated by the surgical documentation from 1926. Source: Richard Mühsam, "Chirurgische Eingriffe bei Anomalien des Sexuallebens," Therapie der Gegenwart 28, 1926. Private archive Gilman, Chicago

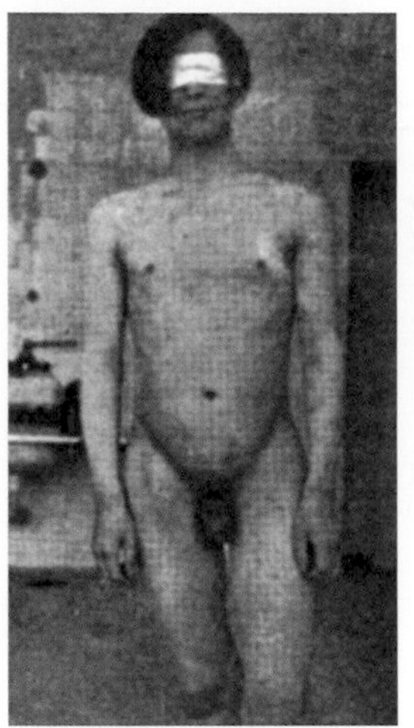

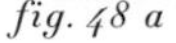

fig. 48 a

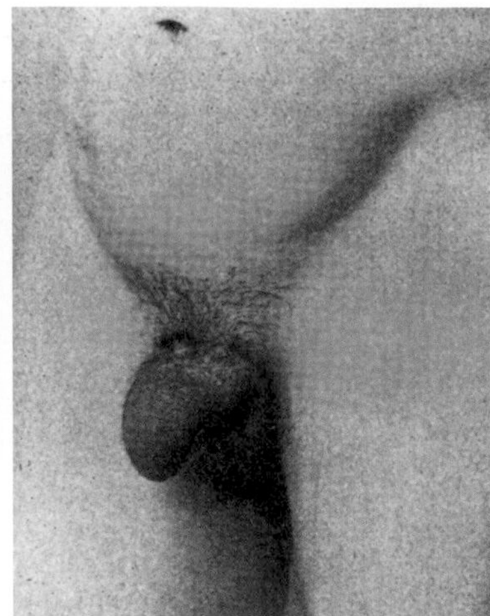

fig. 48 b

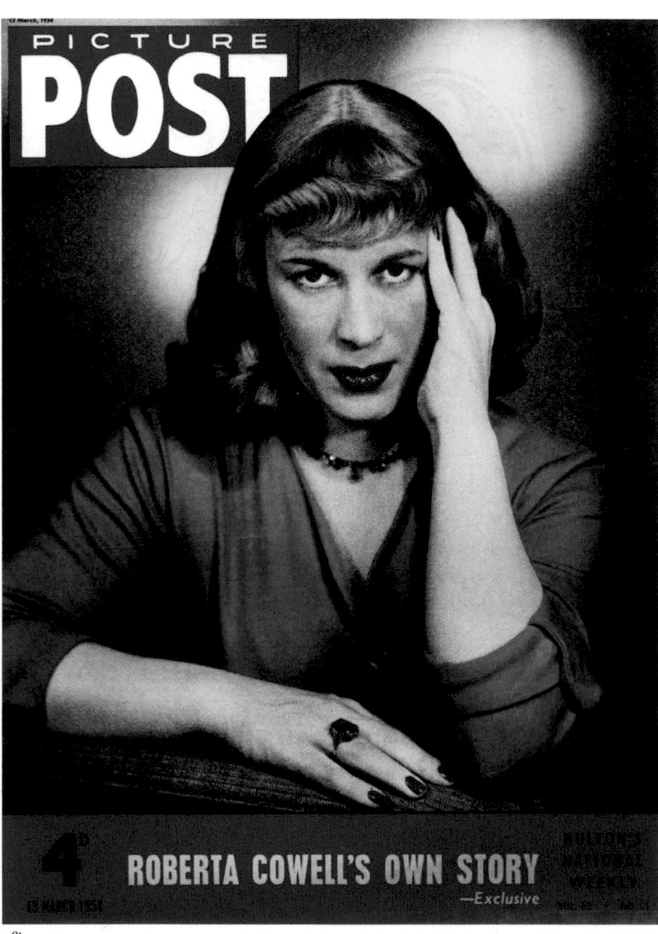

fig. 47

The emphasis in such surgery was the creation of the appearance of female genitals, which could be erotically stimulated. Reproduction was never even imagined as a goal, as the transplantation of ovaries for reproductive purposes was (and has) never been part of the conceptual strategy of becoming female in transsexual surgery.

In an earlier paper, Richard Mühsam (1872–1939) of the City Hospital in Berlin recounts that as early as 1920 a male patient referred to him by Magnus Hirschfeld requested that he be castrated and that in 1921 he removed the ovaries of a female transvestite at her request. One can add that in the 1920s and '30s castration was understood as a medical practice, which was a form of therapy for neuroses, perversions, sexual crimes, sexual abnormalities, mental disease, and even tuberculosis.[35] Mühsam's paper was read by his contemporaries in this broader context. In all of the cases in which Mühsam undertook the removal of the gonads, there was no claim that the patient was either a pseudo — or an actual hermaphrodite. There had been a long history of the surgical reconstruction of "ambiguous" genitalia, usually as female genitalia.[36] Given that one out of a thousand births result in such cases, this was already an established part of reconstructive urology. Indeed the transgender patients all were represented as suffering from psychological difficulties rather than physical anomalies.

Mühsam's first patient, a 23-year-old student, had been dismissed from a military school for "lack of guts." He served as an officer during World War I, testing his manhood, and came to Mühsam after the war when he no longer could function. "He gave up his medical studies ... spent the day in bed and slept most of the day." When he was in public he wore a corset, women's stockings, and high heel shoes. Mühsam's text makes it evident that it was the patient who desired to be castrated and transformed into a woman: "The fate of this man sounds like a novel," Mühsam wrote in 1926, "it shows that the most active fantasy cannot imagine what feelings, wishes, and imaginings one finds with sexual neurotics." On June 21, 1921 the young man was castrated and on June 23, for the first time in a long while, asked for a book and resumed his studies. He requested to have an ovary implanted to generate female hormones rather than for reproductive purposes and this was done in March, 1921 after his castration. Following the surgical interventions, he developed breasts and wore women's clothing in private. He also began to sound feminine. His larynx was examined and revealed a "laryngeal feminine type structure."

Mühsam could not bring himself to amputate the penis so he created a mock vagina into which the penis was placed, so that it could be sexually stimulated. By August 1921 the young man returned to the surgeon and requested that he return his penis to a form more functional for intercourse as he had a new woman friend. After this was done he com-

fig. 49

After the First World War, the significance of reconstructive plastic surgery increased dramatically. This photo shows an injured soldier for whom Jacques Joseph (1865—1934) created a new nose as well as operating on his upper jaw and cheeks. Source: J. Joseph, Nasenplastik und sonstige Gesichtsplastik, Berlin 1931

fig. 50

The war in art: Otto Dix (1891—1969) produced this etching titled "Transplantation" for his cycle of etchings "Der Krieg" (1924), which examined the role of plastic surgery during the First World War. © akg-images

pleted his medical studies and emigrated, informing his physician in a letter that: "My health is well. I am absolutely happy [zufrieden] with myself ... and my work pleases me greatly."

35 — Karl A. Menninger, "Polysurgery and Polysurgical Addiction," *Psychoanalytic Quarterly* 3 (1934): 173–199.
36 — There is a very good survey of the literature that includes many such cases in Franz von Neugebauer, "58 Beobachtungen von periodischen genitalen Blutungen menstruellen Anschein, pseudomenstruellen Blutungen, Menstruatio vicaia, Molimina menstrualia usw. bei Scheinzwitter," *Jahrbuch für sexuelle Zwischenstufen* 6 (1904): 277–326.

World War I

The movement from restorative surgery to mask the ravages of disease to the transformation of ethnicity to the reconstruction of sexuality moves aesthetic surgery into the 1930s. It was the innovations during World War I that made transsexual surgery possible.

The range and sophistication of aesthetic procedures was exponentially increased as a result of many innovations made on and off the battlefield, not just for transsexual surgery.

And yet the social stigma associated with aesthetic surgery increased accordingly as the number of procedures and

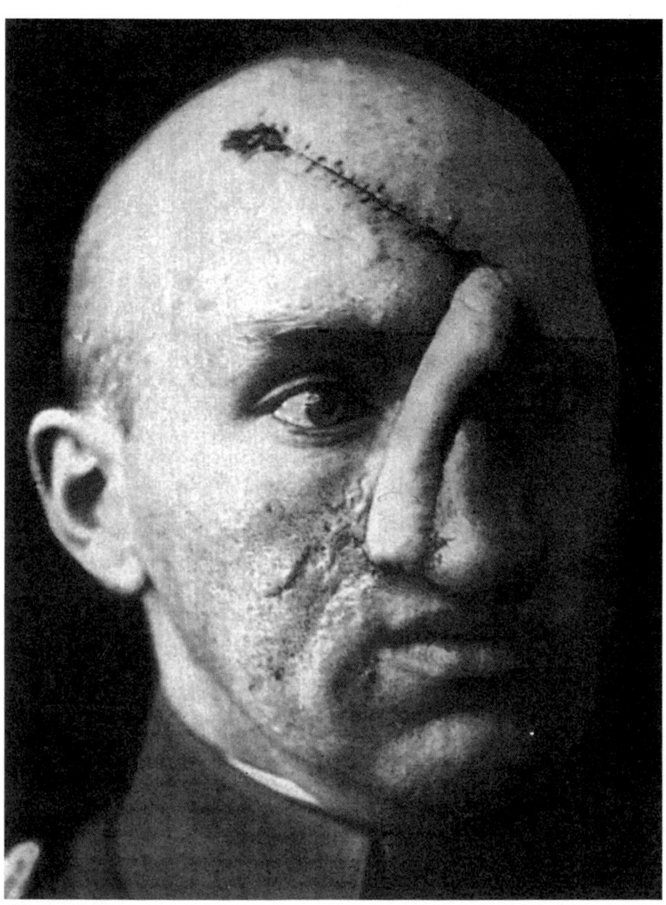

fig. 49

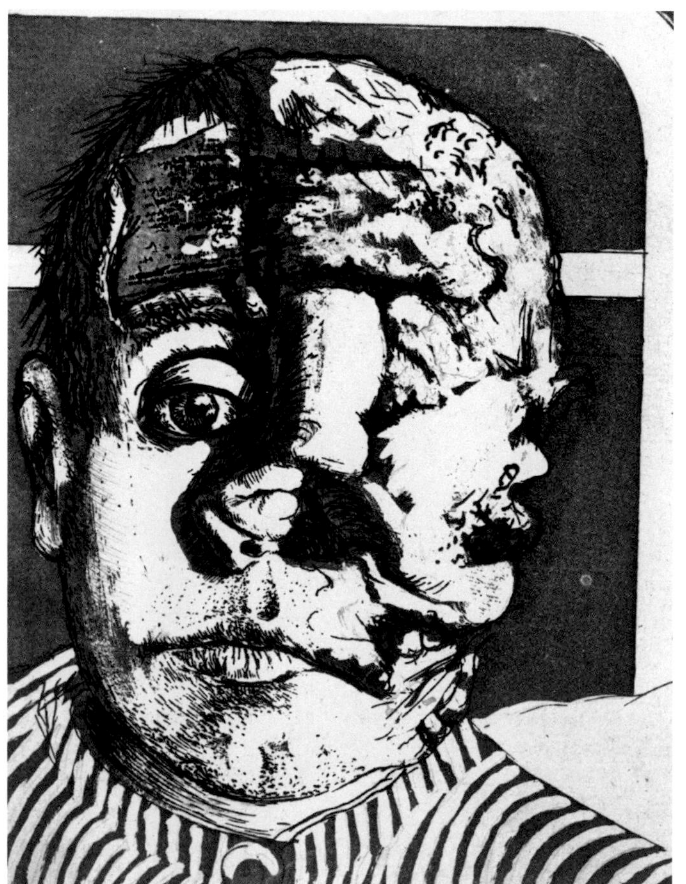

fig. 50

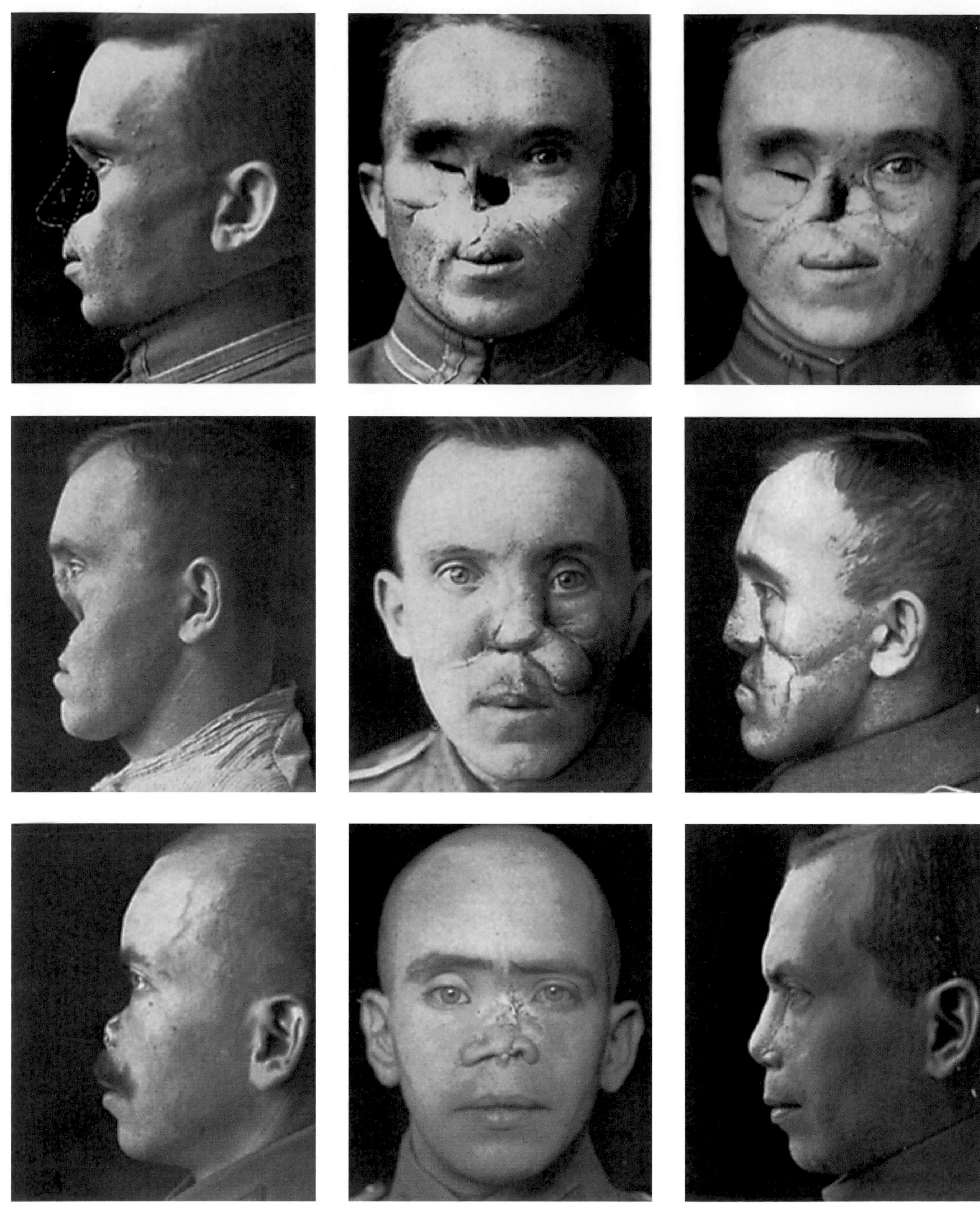

fig. 51 a–r

fig. 51 a–r

Plastic surgery provided a new way of treating and correcting war-related injuries such as skewed or flattened noses, eye injuries, and burns. The surgeons frequently used skin flaps from the brow and bone fragments for their reconstructive operations. All photos: J. Joseph, Nasenplastik und sonstige Gesichtsplastik, Berlin 1931

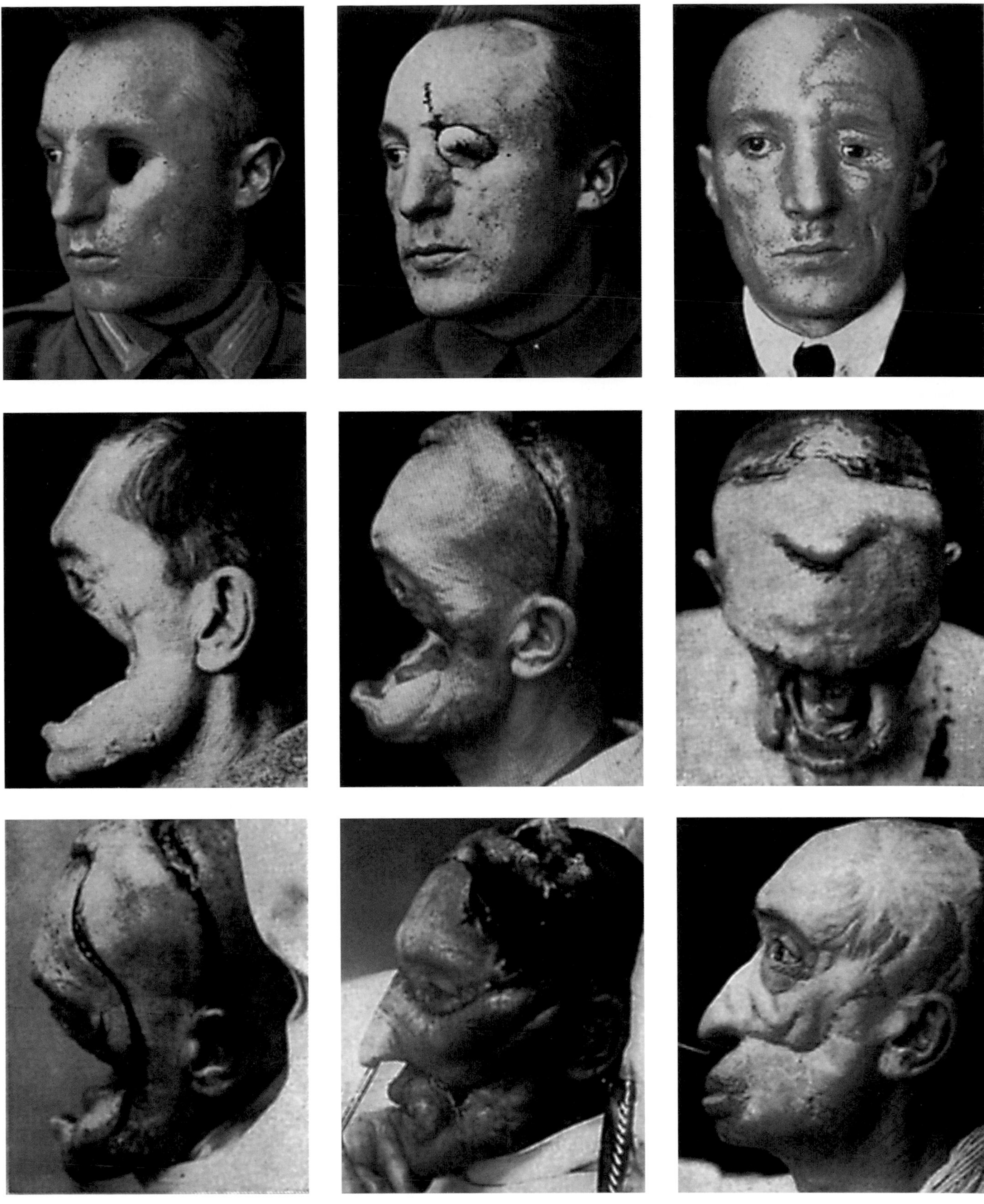

fig. 52 a+b

Even young girls had breast operations: In this case, Jacques Joseph (1865–1934) reduced a 15-year-old's sagging breasts. His doctrine: "The principal aim of an operation is to achieve a significant improvement on the patient's previous condition." Source: J. Joseph, Nasenplastik und sonstige Gesichtsplastik, Leipzig 1931

fig. 53 a–h & 54 a–f

Early illustration of mammaplasty by Jacques Joseph. Source: J. Joseph, Nasenplastik und sonstige Gesichtsplastik, Leipzig 1931

interventions increased. One of the most knowledgeable aesthetic surgeons before World War I, Frederick Strange Kolle (1871–1929), was already puzzled by this. He distinguished between the surgery of the nose applied to "deformities when caused by traumatism, the excision of neoplasms or destructive disease" and "such corrections [which] are made purely with the object of improving the nasal form when the deformity is either hereditary or the result of remote accident." He continued however: "For some unaccountable reason [aesthetic surgery] has not met with the general favor the profession should grant it, yet the results obtained by such specialists as have undertaken this artistic branch of surgery have been all that could be desired, and have consequently added much to the comfort and happiness of the patient."[37] Kolle's distinction between reconstructive and aesthetic surgery is continued in a widely quoted aphorism by the New Zealand-born surgeon Sir Harold Delf Gillies (1882–1960) who understood reconstructive surgery as "an attempt to return to normal; aesthetic surgery as an attempt to surpass the normal."[38] Gillies needed to provide a meaningful continuity between his reconstructive work during World War I and the post-war interest in aesthetic surgery. In doing so he stressed the continuity between two concepts of the "normal." The first is a reconstructive model, restoring function and a somewhat human visage, which can pass as normal, if the range and meaning of the trauma is understood. The second, that of aesthetic surgery, seeks to transcend the given and the normal.

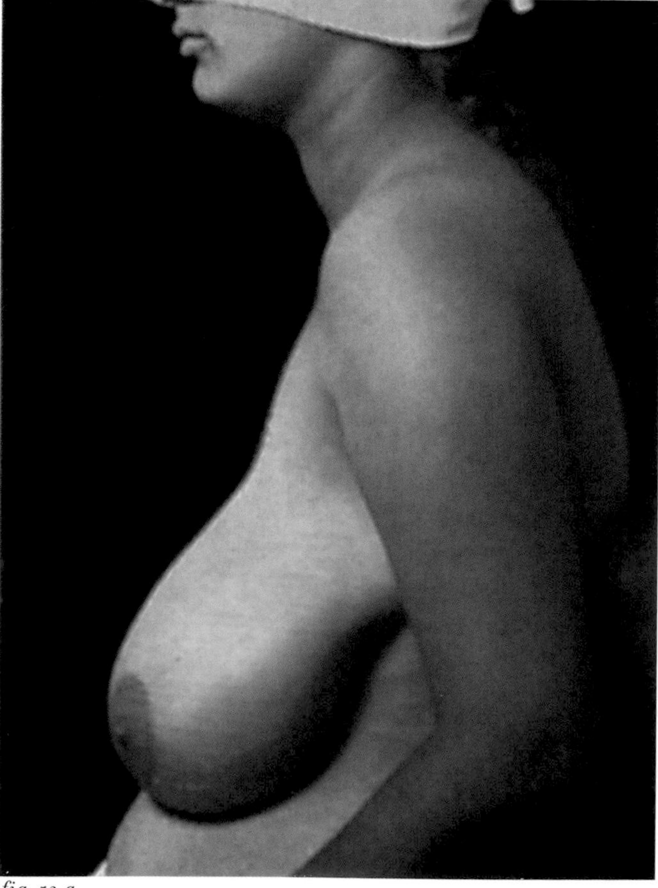

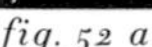

fig. 52 a

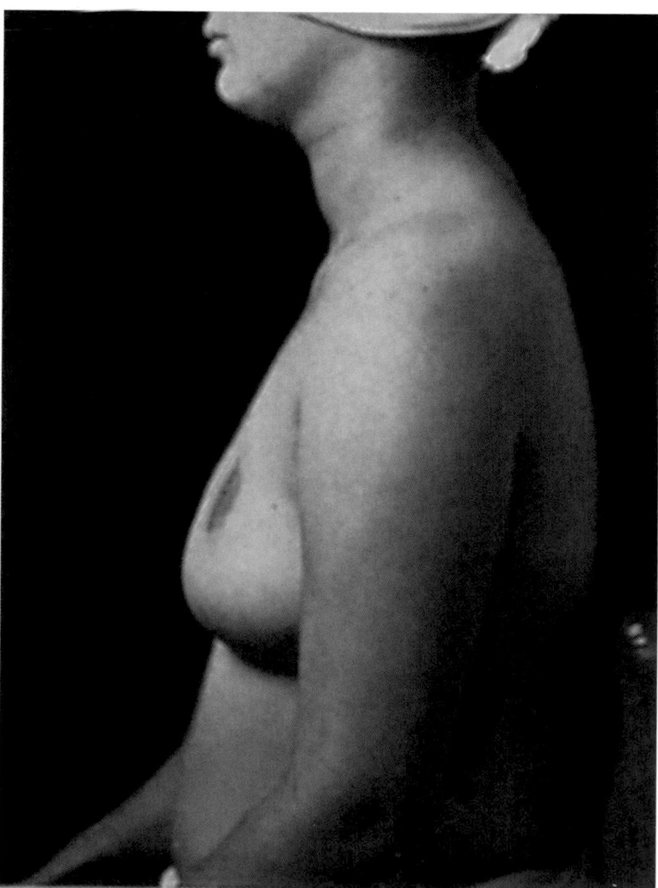

fig. 52 b

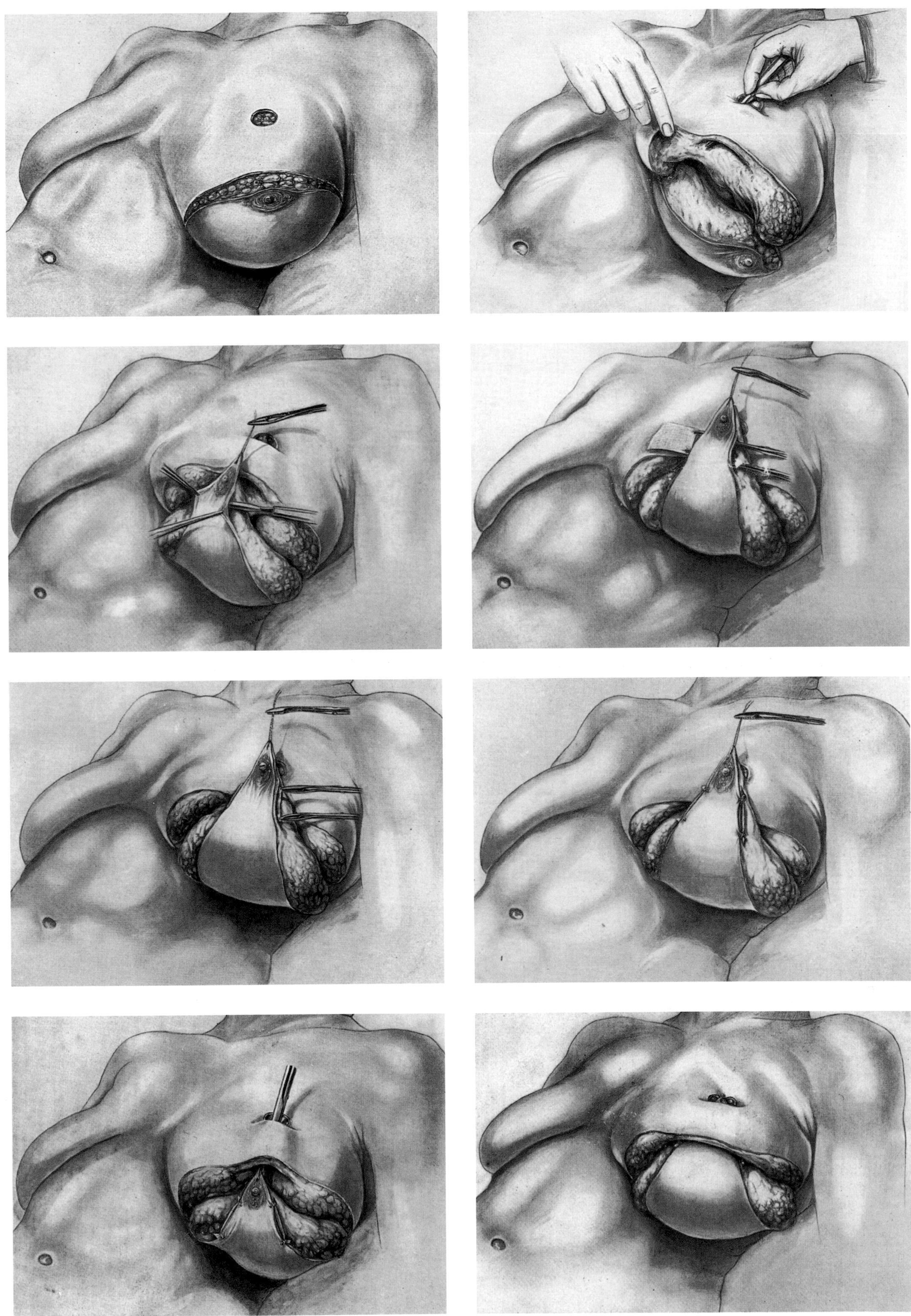

fig. 53 a–h

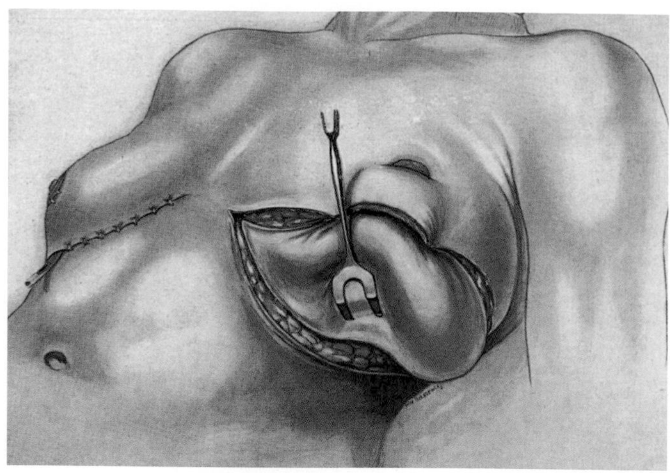
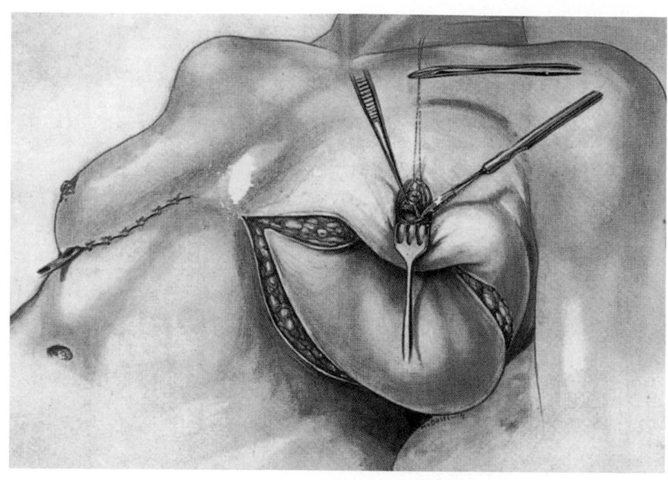
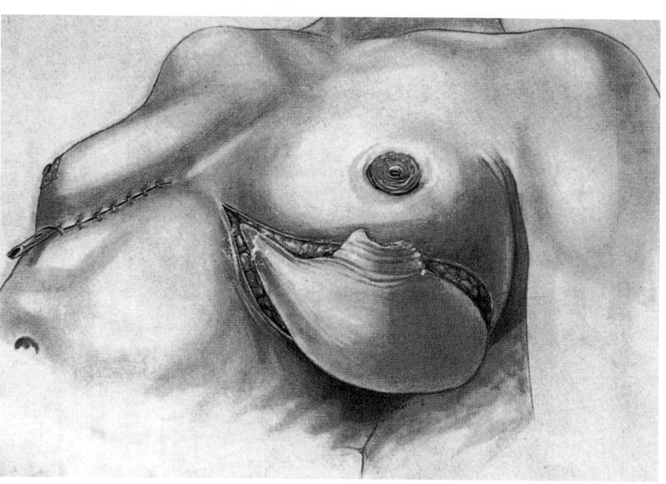
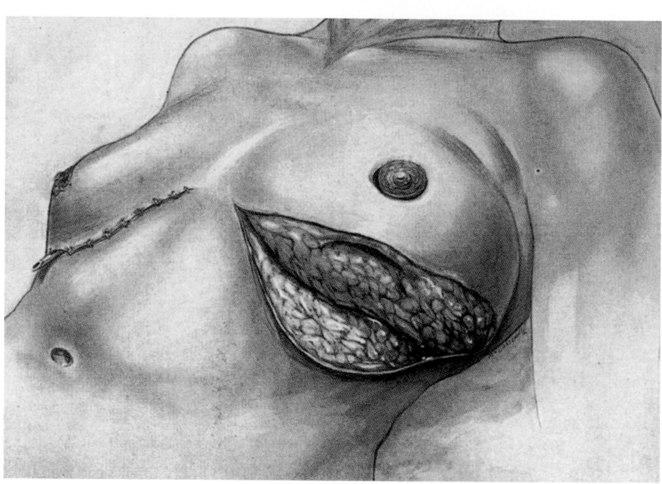
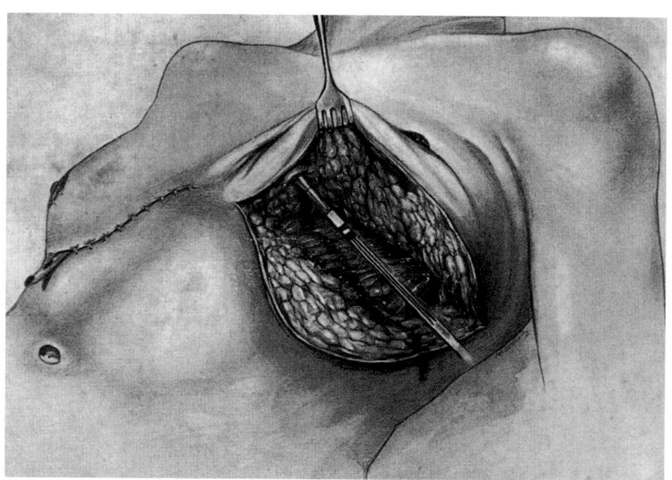
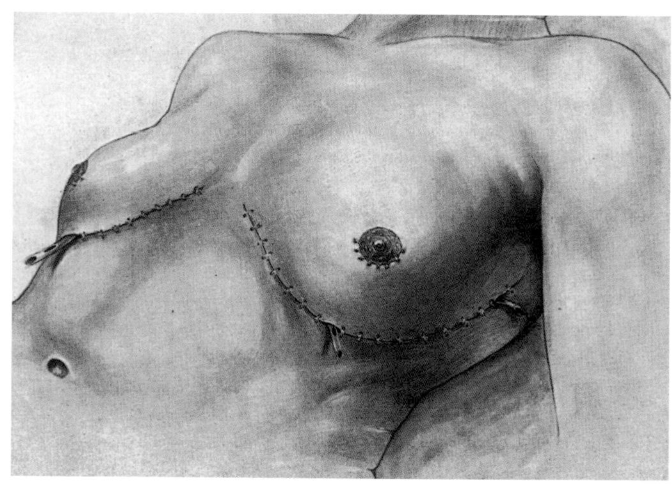

fig. 54 a–f

fig. 55 a+b

Initially, silicone implants were placed on top of the pectoral muscle (left), but only by placing them behind the muscle (right) was it possible to reduce the risk of undesirable side effects, such as hardening tissue. Source: Alan M. Engler, BodySculpture, New York 2000

fig. 56

Buxom Jayne Mansfield was a sex goddess of the 1950s and 1960s, conquering Hollywood with films like "The Girl Can't Help It". Mansfield graced more than 500 glossy magazine covers in the space of her lifetime. © picture alliance

fig. 57 a–d

A suitable model for every type of breast: In the 1990s, a wide range of silicone implants became available, offering a multitude of shapes and sizes. Many of the implants make the augmented breasts look more natural. Source: Alan M. Engler, BodySculpture, New York 2000

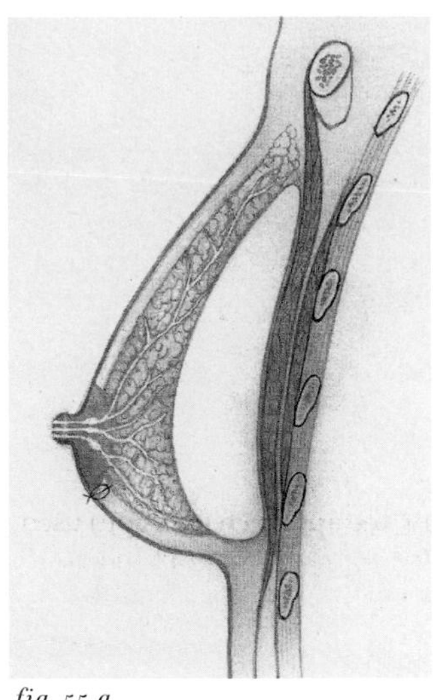

fig. 55 a

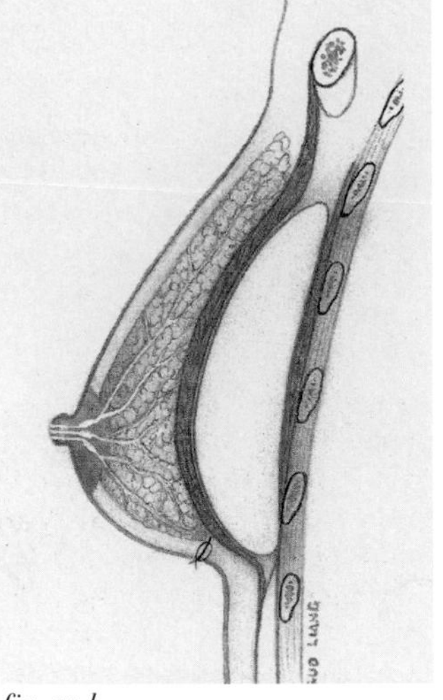

fig. 55 b

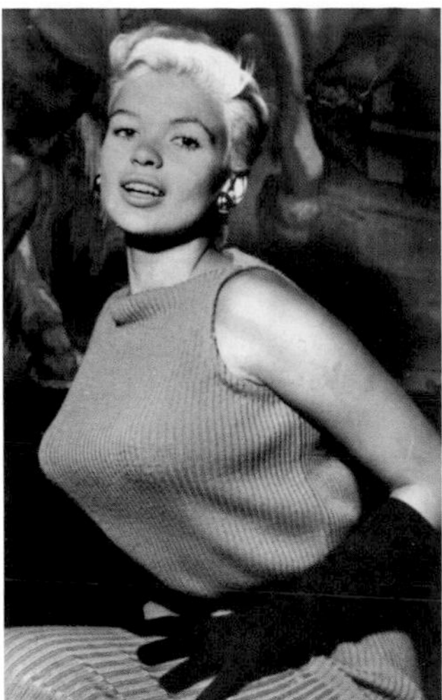

fig. 56

Central to the post World War II expansion of aesthetic surgery are two seemingly contradictory directions that indeed have as their primary audience women. They are breast augmentation and body fat reduction. The latter quickly becomes a procedure of choice for men. Indeed, while the earliest aesthetic surgical patients are generally men, the procedures by the 1920s become strongly identified as beauty surgery for women.

The Increasing Role of Breast Augmentation Since the 1950s

Where in the 1880s breast reduction was part of a culture of de-ethnicizing the body and creating a New (non-ethnic) Woman, by the 1940s breast augmentation was all the rage. The small breasts of the New Woman, which were defined by her function as a sports woman, are replaced by the very breasts the absence of which defined her as new — large breasts. Beginning in the United States in the 1950s, there is a concerted effort to search for cures for this new disease of too small breasts. This becomes medicalized in the 1950s. H. O. Bames observed that "hypomastia causes psychological rather than physical distress. Its correction has been receiving increased interest only since our 'cult of the body beautiful' has revealed its existence in rather large numbers."[39] Here the shift is complete and the too small breasts have been medicalized. Today there are many more women who are persuaded that their breasts are too small than there are those who are persuaded that their breasts are too large. Breast augmentation is now a cure for a psychological problem, the lack of happiness.

37 — Frederick Strange Kolle, *Plastic and Cosmetic Surgery* (New York; London: D. Appleton, 1911), p. 339.
38 — Harold Gillies and D. Ralph Millard, *The Principles and Art of Plastic Surgery*. 2 vols. (Boston: Little, Brown [1957]), 1: 32. See also in: *The Development and Scope of Plastic Surgery* (Chicago: Northwestern University, 1935).
39 — H. O. Bames, "Breast Malformations and a New Approach to the Problem of the Small Breast," *Plastic and Reconstructive Surgery* 5 (1950): 499.

The History of Silicone Implants

Silicone had first been used in the 1950s in the form of subcutaneous injections for body augmentation. Thus injected into the body, it was soon shown to have the risks of migration and infection. Other problems such as hematoma, visible lines of implantation, and, most frequently, capsule contracture (abnormal firmness of the breast to the touch) also were experienced by women who had had silicone injections.[40] Alternative substances were experimented with: Ivalon, a derivative of polyvinylic alcohol in 1949, Polistan, a derivative of polyethelene in 1959, Etheron, a derivative of polymethane in 1960s, and Hydron, a derivative of polyglycomethacrylate in 1961. Each had a spongy texture and was advocated for short periods as the ideal substance for breast augmentation. And each had extremely negative outcomes for the health of the patient.

In 1963 a "silastic gel" prosthesis was developed by the Houston surgeons Thomas Cronin and Frank Gerow, which contained saline and provided a preshaped form and size.[41] Gerow came to the idea of a silicone sack filled with liquid by observing a plastic bag filled with blood used for transfusion. He saw in its form the shape of a breast.

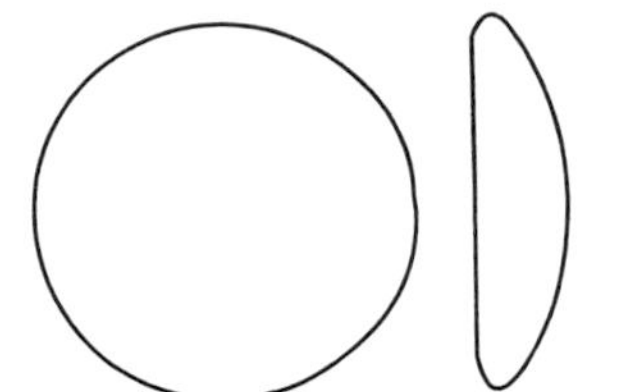

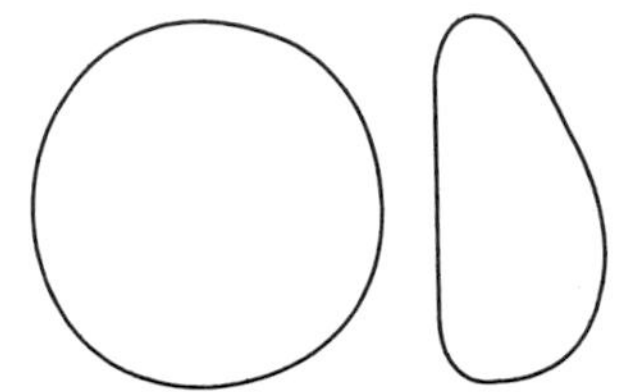

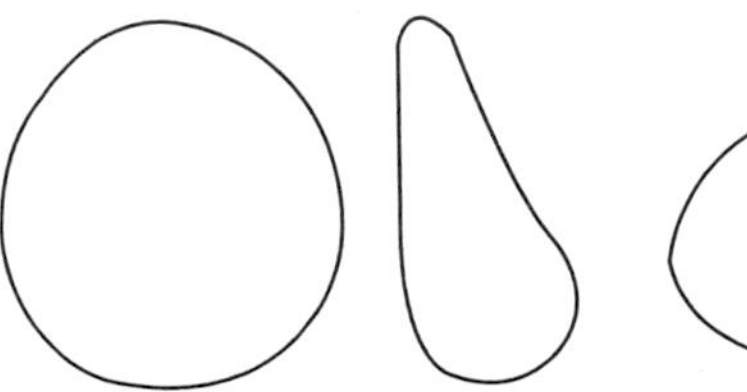

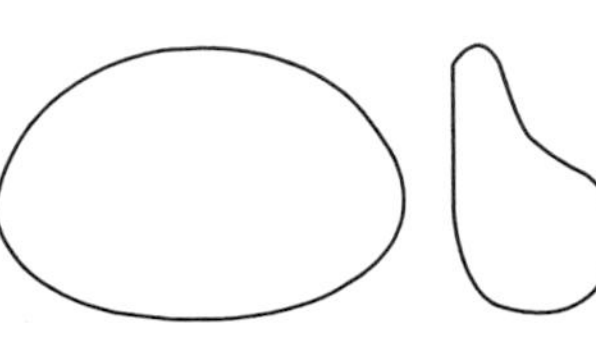

fig. 57 a–d

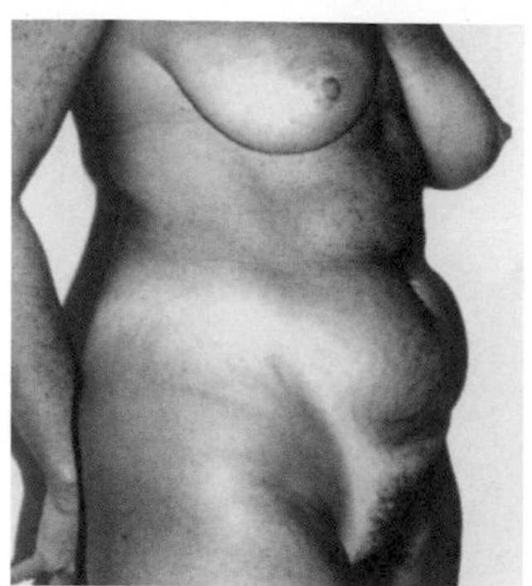

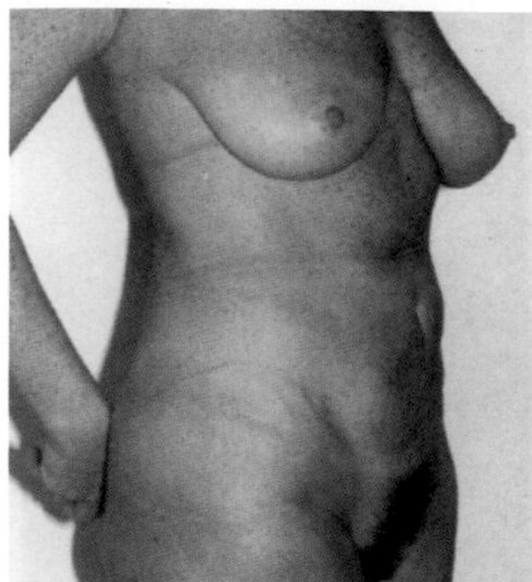

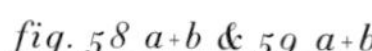

fig. 58 a+b

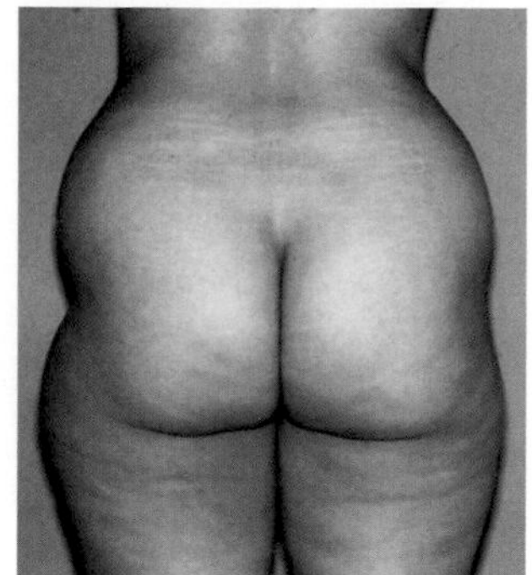

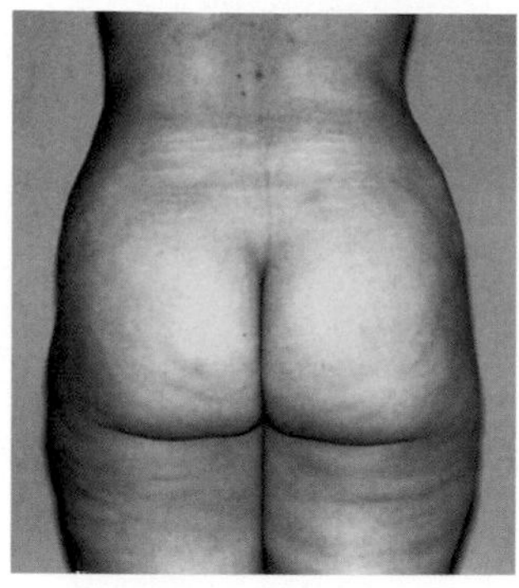

fig. 59 a+b

fig. 58 a+b & 59 a+b

In the 1970s, liposuction methods improved considerably. There was less scarring, and the possibility of new fatty tissue forming in the lifted body parts was reduced greatly. Shown are a 48-year-old patient whose tummy was reduced and a 34-year-old patient with contoured hips. Source: Alan M. Engler, BodySculpture, New York 2000

fig. 60

The term "Rubens figure" is still in use today, but its aesthetic connotations have changed. While voluptuous figures were considered beautiful in the Baroque period, beauty is now more generally associated with slender silhouettes. Peter Paul Rubens (1577–1640) named this weighty masterpiece "The Three Graces." Its home is the Museo del Prado in Madrid.

Thus aesthetic augmentation had its conceptual origin in the context of real surgery. Gerow implanted the first such prosthesis in March, 1962. It broke and released the saline. A week later he implanted a prostheses filled with silicone gel and this was successful. The result was a patient who "was healed and happy," according to one account. Thus the surgeons neglected to pay much attention to the actual, negative outcomes, such as the fact that some of the breasts with the prosthesis became very hard (contracted capsules). The surgeons relied on initial success, ignoring long-term problems until confronted with them. With insertion of the implant under the muscles of the chest wall (submusclar augmentation mammaplasty) and the introduction of Franklin L. Ashley's silicone-gel implant covered with polyurethane foam in the 1970s, which reduced the risk of contracture, many of the initial problems associated with breast augmentation seemed to have been overcome. While improved saline-filled implants reappeared in the 1970s, they remained less attractive until the attack on the silicone implants two decades later. They were felt to be less natural and did not give the illusion of the breast form and texture that physicians and women wanted. Silicone held its own for augmentation of the breast for all purposes.

In 1990 a House committee chaired by Representative Ted Weiss held its first hearings on the safety of silicone implants and this quickly became a major media event. The claim was that the improved procedures still masked long-term major medical problems. By 1991 the first court case was resolved with findings that the silicone implants had caused immune system illnesses in patients. A $7.3 million damage claim was lodged against Dow Corning, the developer of the gel implant. A number of recipients of silicone breast implants then claimed to have developed a wide and divergent set of symptoms ranging from chronic fatigue, to rheumatoid arthritis (and other inflammatory illness of the joints), lupus, damage to the immune system, and scleroderma (a hardening of the skin and internal organs).

The debate about breast implants came to be one about to what degree the government would permit a woman to pass as whole and, therefore, as healthy. If she was missing a breast, went the argument, she would be "unhappy" about her body and would need augmentation surgery to make her happy. This was worth the risk. If she only wanted to be "happy" without having first suffered cancer that was not worth the risk. The reconstruction of the erotic, female body in the first instance was seen as a goal of reconstructive surgery; the construction of the erotic body in the latter was merely aesthetic surgery and a sign of false vanity.

The History of Liposuction since the 1970s

The augmentation of the breast has thus became a topic of debate about the limits of aesthetic interventions: reconstruction versus vanity. This would not have been out of place in the 17th century as women (and men) then also had their body size reduced. A series of procedures to firm and tighten the buttocks to restore youthful contours, including the use of liposuction to remove localized fatty deposits (from other parts of the body as well as the buttocks), has become a relatively common procedure.[42] Until the 1970s the classic method of removing fatty deposits from the buttocks, stomach, and thighs was by "block lipectomy with skin resection," surgery that removed fat tissue as well as excess skin.[43] The result was a slimmer body – but one clearly marked by scars, which often became the loci for new fat deposits! These procedures grew directly out of the reduction operations beginning in 1889 with Howard Kelly's removal of fat and skin from the abdomen and thighs.

Through the 1970s various procedures, including those by Ivo Pitanguy, were developed to hide the scars.[44] The Brazilian aesthetic surgeon Pitanguy developed a but-

40 – A. S. Braley, "The Use of Silicone in Plastic Surgery: A Retrospective View," *Plastic Reconstructive Surgery* 51 (1973): 280–88.

41 – E. S. Truppman and B. M. Schwarz, "Aesthetic Breast Surgery," *Journal of the Florida Medical Association* 76 (1989): 609–12.

42 – C. M. Lewis, "Early History of Lipoplasty in the United States," *Aesthetic Plastic Surgery* 14 (1990): 123–6; B. E. Burnham, "Notes on the History of the Adoption of Liposuction," *Plastic and Reconstructive Surgery* 97 (1996): 258–259.

43 – Francis M. Otteni and Pierre F. Fournier, "A History and Comparison

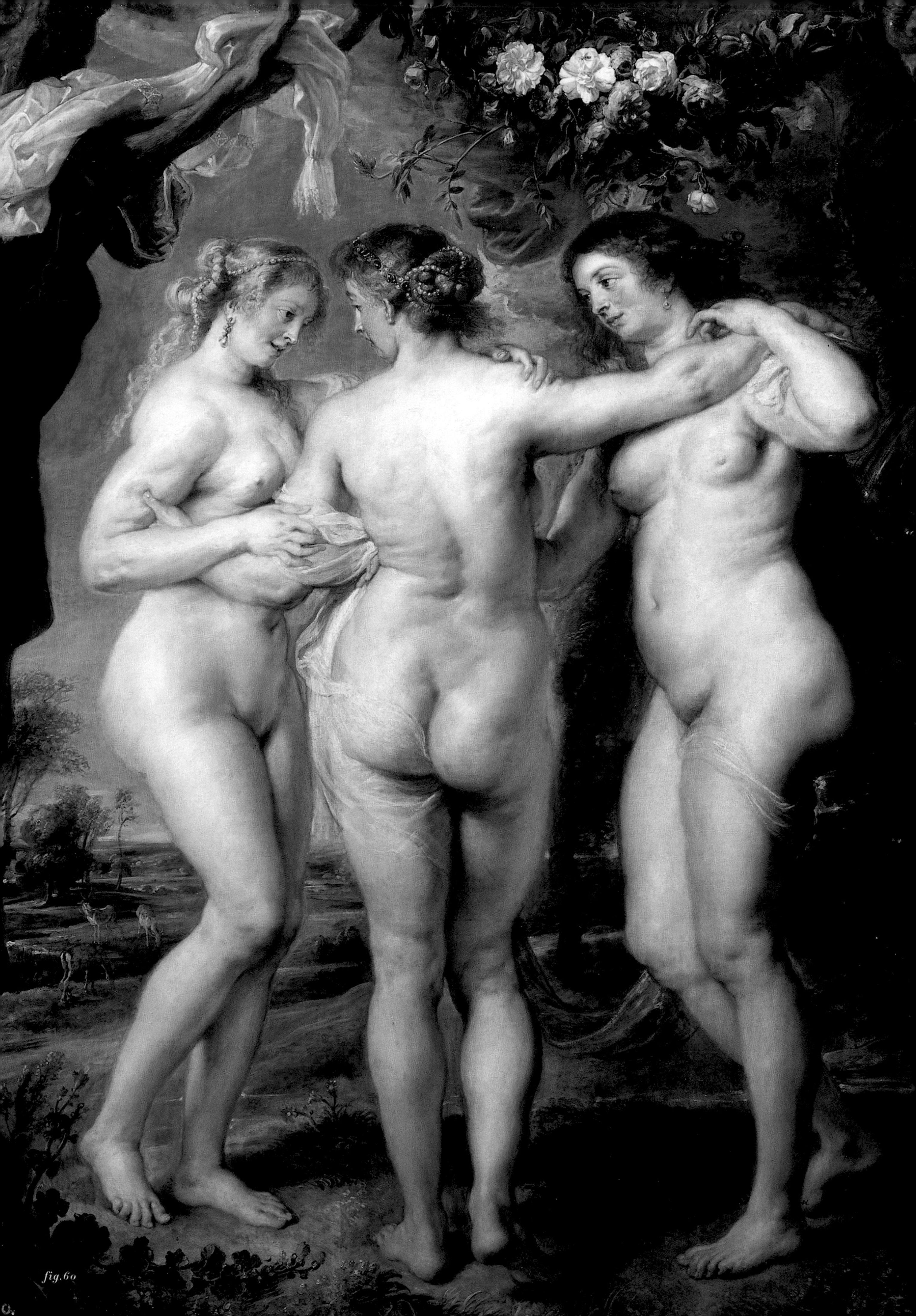

fig. 60

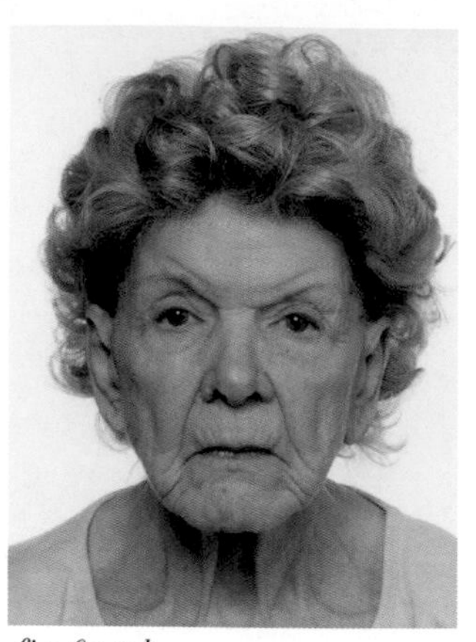

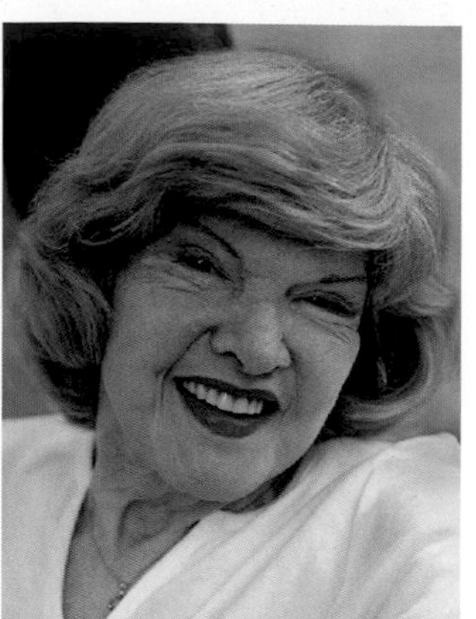

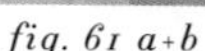

fig. 61 a+b

Phyllis Porter at the age of 79 (left) and 82 (right). Porter is one of America's most celebrated cosmetic surgery patients. As well as a mammaplasty, she has had Botox injections and many other treatments. The price of her new body and battle against age: US$ 25,000. Source: Noel Young, "Is this the most Amazing Cosmetic Surgery Op ever?" Sunday Mirror, June 30th, 2002 © Zed Nelson / IPG / Katz / Studio X

fig. 62

Queen Elizabeth I (1533—1603) was arguably the most painted woman of her time. However, hardly any of the portraits reveal her age — the artists who favoured her cleverly hid her true appearance behind a youthful mask, dazzling garments, and gleaming jewels. © www.bridgemanart.com

tock lift in the 1970s which was widely copied.[45] Pitanguy, who was born in 1926, was trained at the faculty of Medicine in Rio de Janeiro and served on the staff of the Pronto Socorro Hospital, where he did reconstructive surgery.[46] At 22 he left Rio and traveled to the United States to study at Bethesda Hospital in Cincinnati. Later he worked with surgeons in France and the United Kingdom, including Archibald McIndoe in London who taught him rhinoplasty and prepared the way for his encounter with Harold Delf Gillies. Thus the line from Pitanguy's development of aesthetic surgery in Brazil, where he opened his first clinic in Rio 1963, led in straight back to the early days of aesthetic surgery at the beginning of the century. Various methods of subcutaneous surgery were tried to replace the procedures that caused visible scarring. The use of the uterine curette often led to rather catastrophic results, as one was never quite sure what was being removed from under the skin. Thus the first malpractice suit for aesthetic surgery in France was brought against a surgeon who used a curette to reduce the calf of a dancer. He damaged a blood vessel and she had to have her leg amputated.

Modern liposuction, using blunt instruments to create tunnels and to pass between major blood vessels, was developed by Yves-Gérard Illouz in France in 1977 and introduced into the United States in 1981.[47] It quickly became the most popular means of shaping the body, especially the buttocks and thighs. Illouz noted that he wanted to develop a procedure for "removing riding breeches" without scars.[48] His first patient was a young woman who wanted a lipoma removed from her back and did not want to have a scar. He undertook this procedure and there was little scarring but also no excess skin to signal that fat had been removed. It was essentially "invisible" surgery replacing earlier procedures where "the resulting scars did not compensate for the prior deformities."[49]

Aesthetic Surgery Today

From the close of the 19th century to the present, aesthetic surgery has come to be ever more widely practiced. It has also become a standard topic for the on-going criticism of what limits society and the individual can or should set for control over our own bodies and the bodies of others. These debates are often undertaken in complete ignorance of the history of aesthetic surgery.The reality is that aesthetic surgery is a classic product of the modern world, with all of its advantages and disadvantages, including our claim to control our bodies.

In the United States today the debate about cloning seems to be the more serious side of this question. Can we, through the agency of the scientist, replicate another or ourselves and to what purpose? This question, hotly debated both in the halls of power and the laboratories of science, is a further version of the debate about human autonomy that echoed over a century ago with the rise of aesthetic surgery. In our fantasy, we have imagined a world where either the individual had absolutely no autonomy over themselves or where autonomy was imaginable but within severe limitations. With the development of new technology, the potential for human autonomy was unleashed. The invention of the (fill in the bank: astrolabe, microscope, steam engine, etc.) enabled the limits on human autonomy to be slowly lifted and we came to have more and more control of our world and ourselves.

This model is usually bemoaned by political liberals and seen as progress by conservatives. It, of course, had the potential to be both.

The technology of aesthetic surgery, in its modern form, arose out of the anxiety about the visibility of the diseased and damaged body that form its common history with

of Suction Techniques until their Debut in North America," in Gregory S. Hetter, *Lipoplasty: The Theory and Practice of Blunt Suction Lipectomy* (Boston MA: Little, Brown, and Co., 1990), pp. 19–23.

44 — A detailed history of "Thighplasty" with comments is to be found in Hetter, op. cit. and Jerome R. Klingbeil, *Body Image: A Surgical Perspective* (St. Louis: The C. V. Mosby Company, 1980), pp. 238–44, here p. 238.

45 — Ivo Pitanguy, *Aesthetic Plastic Surgery of Head and Body* (Berlin — Heidelberg — New York: Springer, 1981).

46 — Martha Gil-Montero, "Ivo Pitanguy: Master of Artful Surgery," *Americas* 43 (1991): 24.

47 — Lewis, "Early History of Lipoplasty in the United States," op cit., p. 123.

48 — Yves-Gérard Illouz, "The Origins of Lipolysis," in Hetter, op. cit., pp. 25–33, here p. 25. See also his *La sculpture chirurgicale de la silhouette* (Edinburgh; New York: Churchill Livingstone, 1988).

49 — R. Baroudi, M. Moraes, "Philosophy, Technical Principles, Selection, and Indication in Body Contouring Surgery," *Aesthetic Plastic Surgery* 15 (1991).

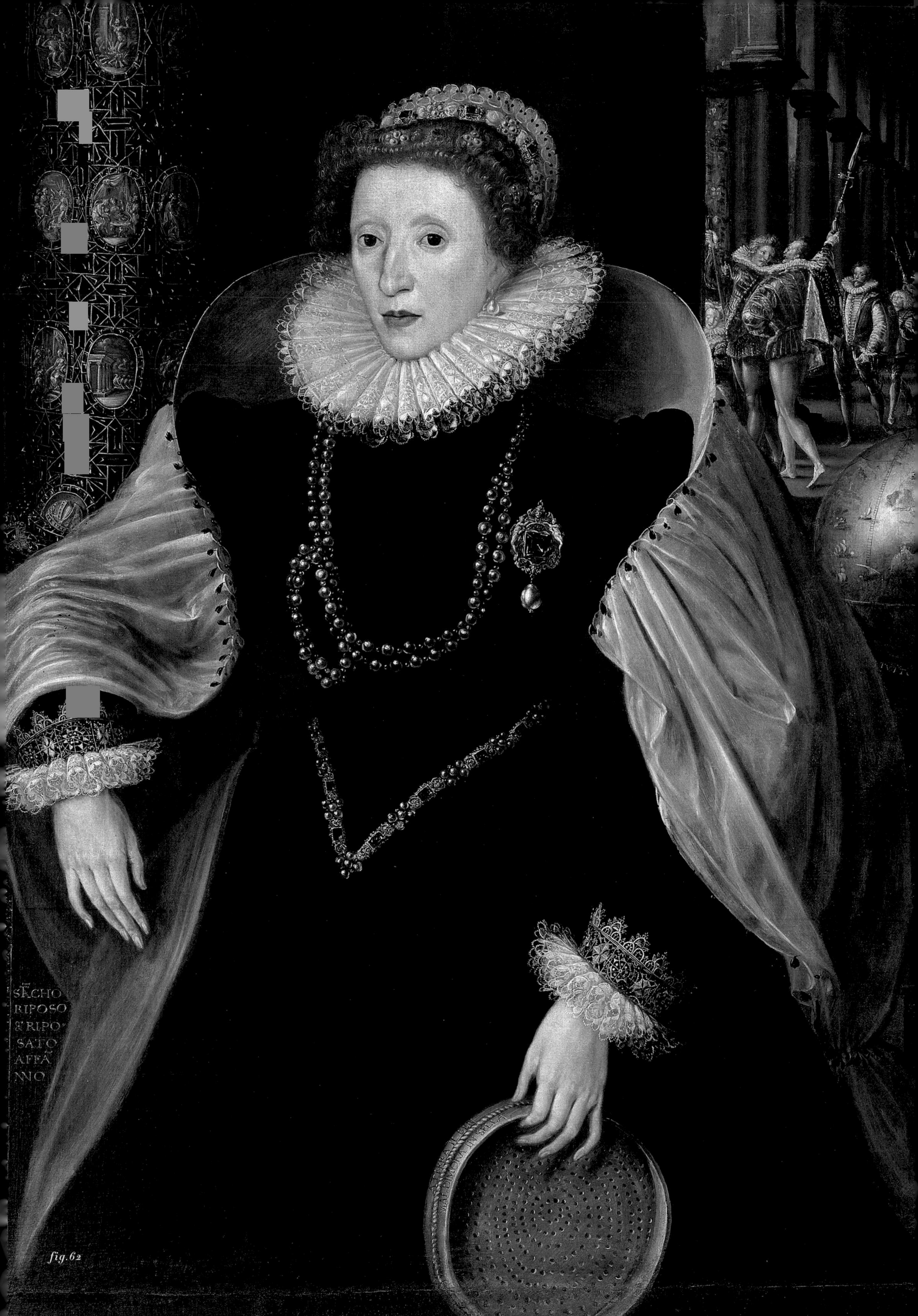

fig. 62

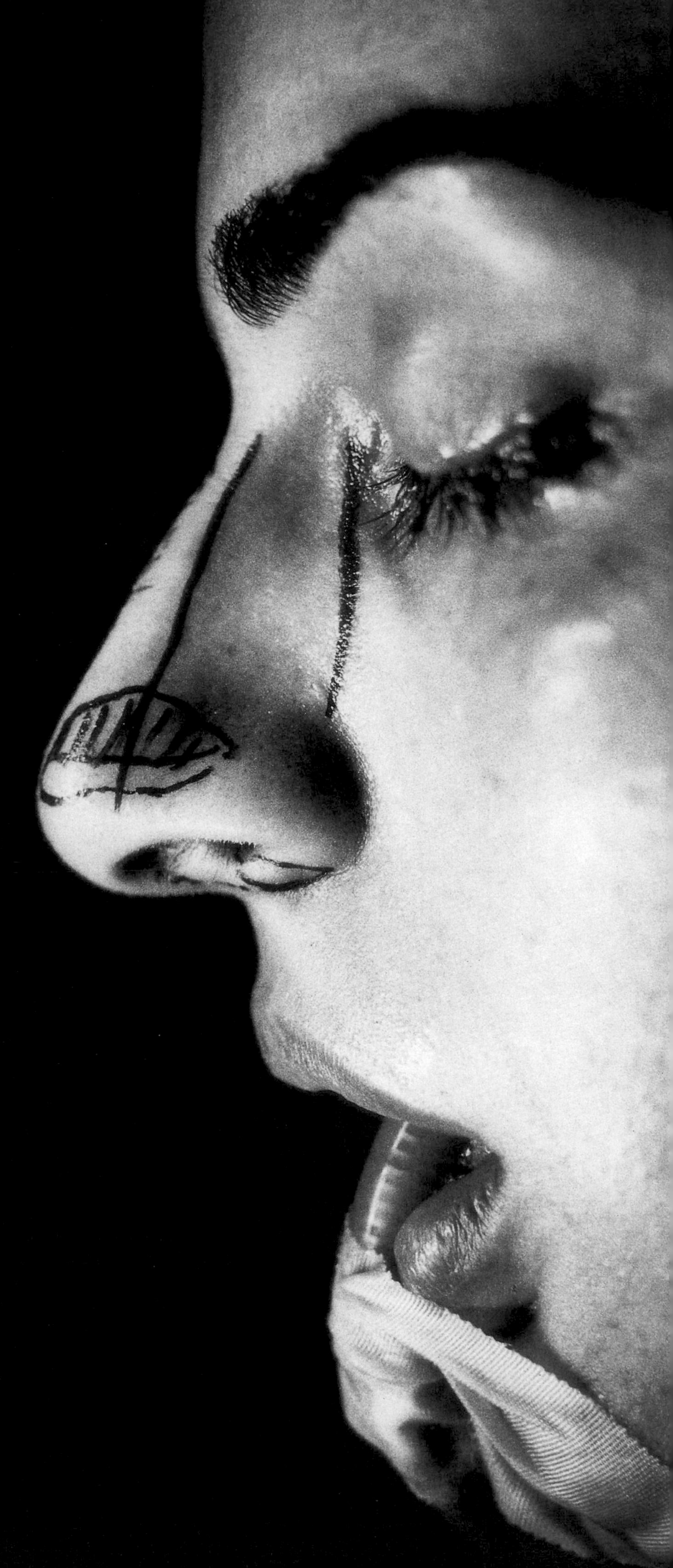

fig. 63

fig. 63

For Iranian women, especially those spending prolonged periods of time in the Western world, a new nose is also an expression of their political and religious views. They don't want their first impression to be one that suggests fundamentalism — which for many Westerners has a stereotypical face.
© Zed Nelson / IPG / Katz / Studio X

reconstructive surgery. Wounds of war, lesions of diseases from syphilis to smallpox, and congenital malformations all formed the background to the beginning of aesthetic surgery at the close of the 19th century. With the introduction of anesthetics in 1846 and antisepsis in 1867, the potential of a single human being, through surgical intervention, to change their bodies as they would have them becomes both imaginable and practicable. From the first patients in the 1870s and 1880s to the millions (perhaps billions) having surgery across the world today, the idea of surgical manipulation of the body has become common place. Yet aesthetic surgery remains contested, as contested as cloning, to which it is closely related both in the roots of aesthetic surgery to the eugenics movement and ongoing fantasies about the transmission of the alteration of the body in some patients. But the anxiety about the ability to alter the body, like that of cloning, rests not only in theological debates about the nature of life, but in cultural assumptions about the transparency of the body.

Alter the body and you obfuscate our ability to read the body. A British gossip columnist in 2002 comments: "Meet Phyllis Porter. On the left aged 79. On the right aged 82. She is America's most famous cosmetic surgery case — the result of seven hours of botox injections, a facelift, lip resculpting, a chemical peel to erase wrinkles and breast implants — all for $ 25,000. In the past five years, the number of facelifts for over-65s in the US have trebled, a trend Phyllis's surgeon calls 'downaging.' Hmmm."[50] (fig. 61 a+b) In the rhetoric of this observation aging is seen as a permanent blemish that should not be corrected. At 80 Phyllis Porter had approached the plastic surgeon Sheldon Sevinor and told him: "I want everything, including a boob job." Subsequently she had the wide range of procedures that amazed the columnist. "I think she is possibly the oldest woman in the world to have that amount of plastic surgery and certainly the oldest to have breast implants," said her surgeon. She was delighted with the result: "I think I look good. I don't care what other people think."[51] What is wrong in Tony Blair's swinging London, as elsewhere, is that, according to the columnist, really old people should, indeed must, look their age. For the aged body is a sign of the absence of desire and desire is for the young. Not for themselves, but because we live in a culture of youth and that is reserved for the young. If you are 82 you dare not look 52! How are we to trust our own authenticity when all about us people are transforming themselves into us!

In the 16th century, Queen Elizabeth I is "continuously painted, not only all over her face, but on her very neck and breast" as she ages.[52] (fig. 62) Ben Jonson in 1619 observed that "Elizabeth never saw herself after she became old in a true glass; they painted her, and sometimes would vermilion her nose."[53]. She suffered from smallpox late in life. Her courtiers avoided commenting on this by praising her beautiful eyes; those who were her enemies stressed the artificial of her aging and scarred face.

Elizabeth may have been the most visible woman of her time but it is not just women who are part of the new and old world of aesthetic surgery. Indeed, I was able to establish that virtually all of the first patients in cosmetic surgery, from breast reductions to ear tucks to nose jobs, were men, whose sense of masculinity was imperiled by their sense of their bodies as not being manly enough. Race impacted on this in the 19th century, as male Jews in Germany wished to vanish into the non-racial world of unracialized men. Today in we have a resurgence in the idea that men (too) desire to shape their bodies through surgery to provide them with new, younger bodies. It is not actually much of a change. Body building culture for men that stressed the muscular, shaped body arises in the 1890s at the same time as the origin of modern aesthetic surgical procedures. Shaping or cutting can reform the male body by the desire of the individual in concert with the professional (either body builder or surgeon).

In the beginning of the 21st century things are not much different as we can see in the case of one Tommy DeMaio

50 — **"The curious world of David Raldall,"** *Independent on Sunday* **(London, July 7, 2002, Sunday): 12.**

51 — **Noel Young, "Is this the most Amazing Cosmetic Surgery Op ever?"** *Sunday Mirror* **(June 30, 2002, Sunday): 19.**

52 — **Quoted in a letter by Father Anthony Rivers (January 13, 1601) from Henry Foley, ed.,** *Records of the English Province of the Society of Jesus* **(London, 1877; New York: Johnson Reprint, 1966): I: 8.**

53 — **Francis Teague, "Queen Elizabeth in Her Speeches," in S. P. Cerasano and**

fig. 64

Hands-on beauty: While digital beauties are only a few mouse clicks away on any computer screen, the current trend towards real-world cosmetic surgery is growing fast – the number of men and women receiving operations for purely aesthetic reasons is steadily increasing. 3D model by Peter Choe, © Somavision.com

who noted that "I didn't like looking at my double chins or the bags under my eyes." He began to have cosmetic procedures 20 years ago when he was 42. Mr. DeMaio, now 62, says he looks and feels 40. And his professional future was a big factor in his electing these procedures. "I have another 40 years to be successful," he said. "Looking well can bring in more business. And even C. E. O.'s are replaced with younger people today."[54]
About the only difference between this case and the cases reported by surgeons at the close of the 19th century is that the patient is willing to unveil his surgery in the public forum. Today even though there is a clear public anxiety about the transformation of the body, those who have had procedures claim their right to change their bodies. And they now claim this right in public. With the explosion of procedures and the general sense that such alterations are part of a claim that we can control our own bodies, more and more men are not only willing to undergo procedures but also willing to speak about them in public.
A columnist in Australia writes in 2002: "What man or woman is ever truly happy with every part of their face or body? Even if you are quite comfortable with your appearance, you probably think there is room for improvement. Cosmetic surgery can be a great adjunct to your health and fitness regime, improving those areas that diet and exercise won't. Whether you'd like a smaller nose, fewer wrinkles or bigger breasts, there is a cosmetic surgery procedure that can help."[55]
Can we truly become happy? And what does that happiness come to mean for us when we achieve it through surgery? We have moved far from the syphilitic face to the reshaped buttocks, and yet these and all other aesthetic procedures demand the ability of individuals to exercise their own autonomy in conjunction with a medical establishment willing to develop and make available new procedures. The history of aesthetic surgery reflects our ability to reimagine every aspect of our bodies as different and improved.
At the beginning of the 21st century, with the development of less intrusive forms of aesthetic improvement such as botox injections to remove wrinkles, men to an even greater degree than women are using aesthetic surgeons' skills. Indeed if the present rate of increase continues, then there will be gender parity in about a decade. And the increase in absolute numbers of people throughout the world having procedures may well mean that those who do not have them will become a minority.

Marion Wynne-Davies, eds., *Gloriana's Face: Women, Public and Private, in the English Renaissance* **(New York: Harvester Wheatsheaf, 1992), pp. 63–78, here p. 63.**
54 – "Men Put Plastic Surgery on the Resume," *The New York Times* **(July 7, 2002, Sunday, Late Edition): Section 3, p. 12.**
55 – Anne Duggan, "Improve on Nature," *Sunday Mail* **(Queensland, April 14, 2002, Sunday): A07.**

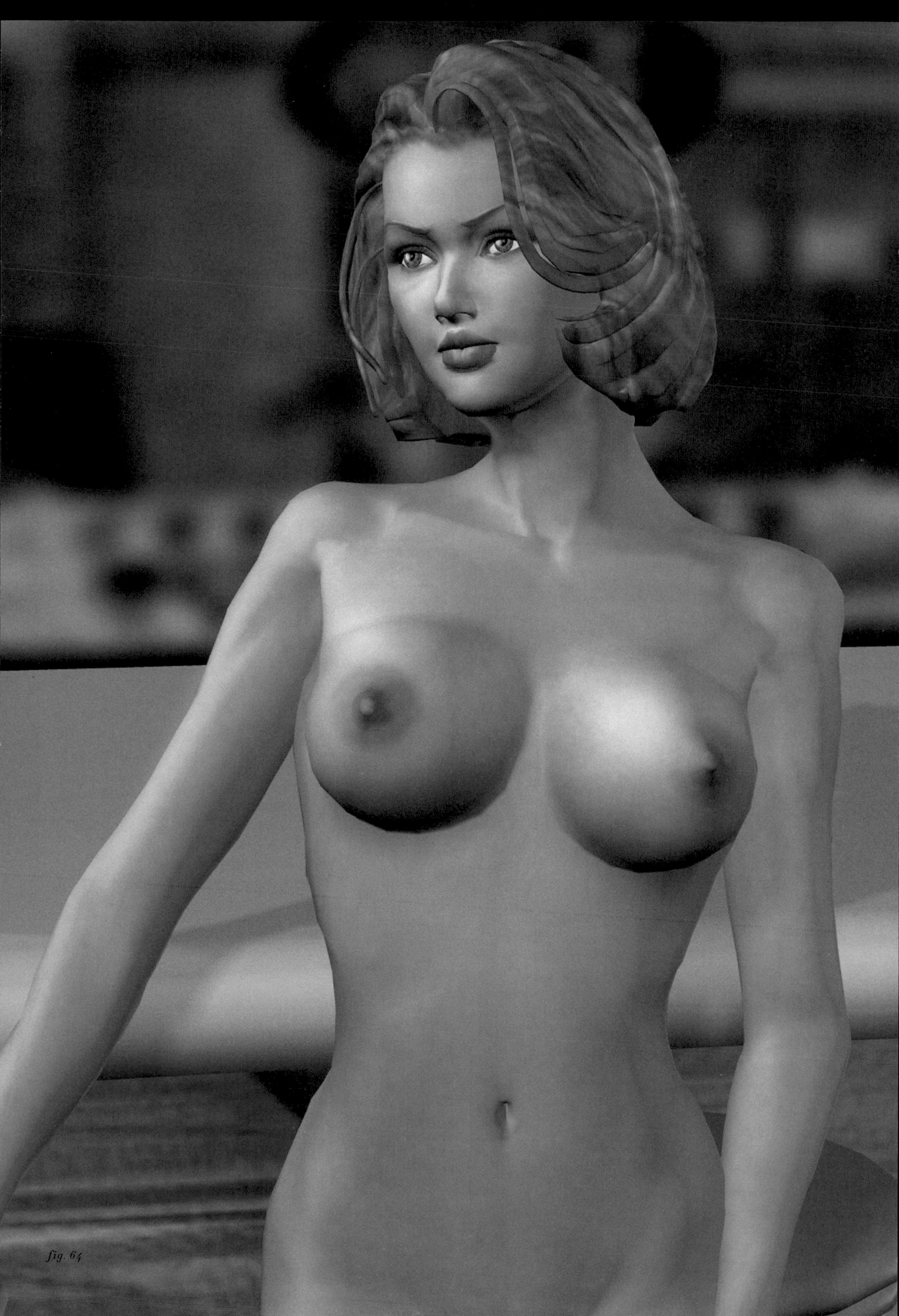
fig. 64

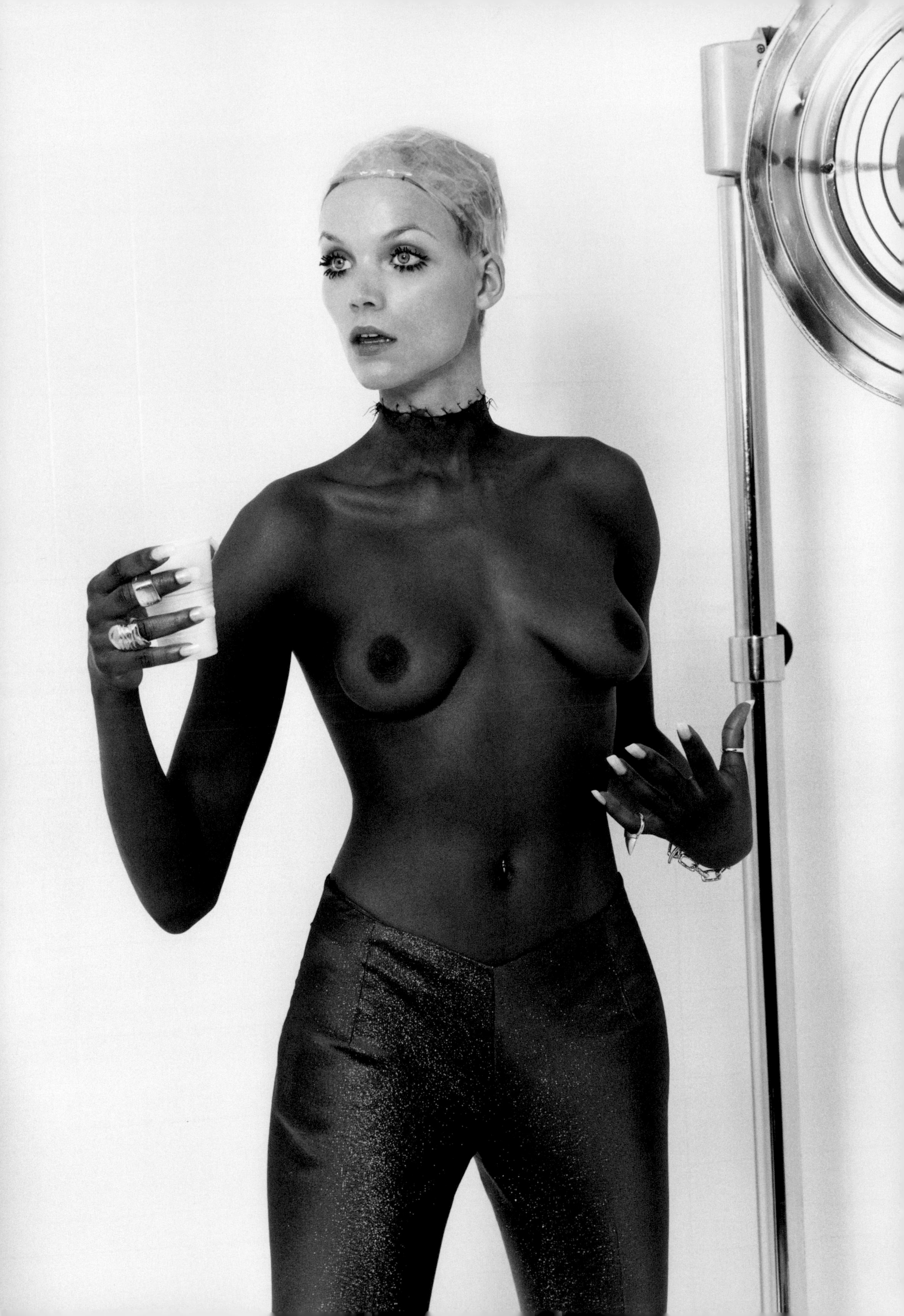

IV.

ETHNICITY AND AESTHETIC SURGERY

Text by

SANDER L. GILMAN

IV.

Ethnicity and Aesthetic Surgery

SANDER L. GILMAN, Chicago

New Bodies, New Identities

How does one become a good citizen of a new land? You must relocate there; you must learn the language; dress according to the style of the country to which you move; learn the rules of etiquette, so that you do not appear conspicuous at the dinner table. But what if that is not enough? What happens when you imagine that not only your actions but your very body needs to be transformed so that you can "pass?" Altering the body in order to become a "real" citizen becomes imaginable at the close of the 19th century. Aesthetic surgery in its modern form begins at that moment in Europe and the United States among those groups that desire a true physical transformation so as to become like the citizens of their new country. How one does this differs from nation to nation and group to group. This is the history of aesthetic surgery within ethnic groups, however defined, across the world.

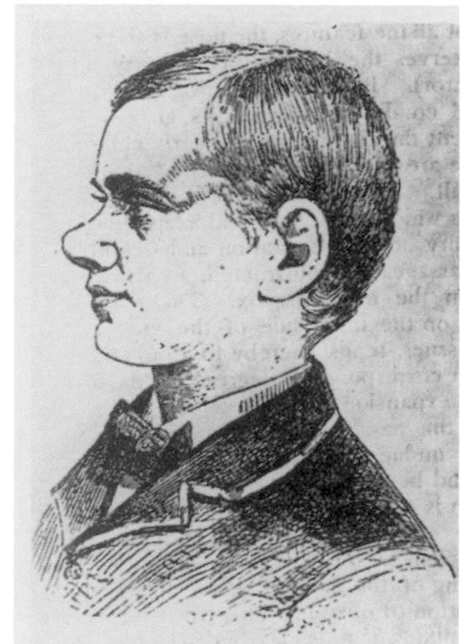

fig. 2 a

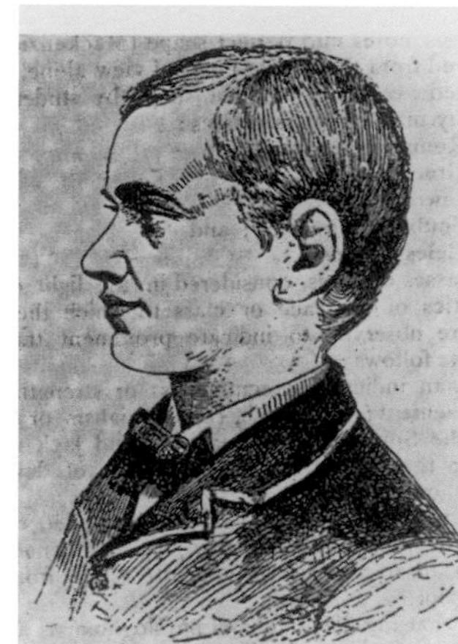

fig. 2 b

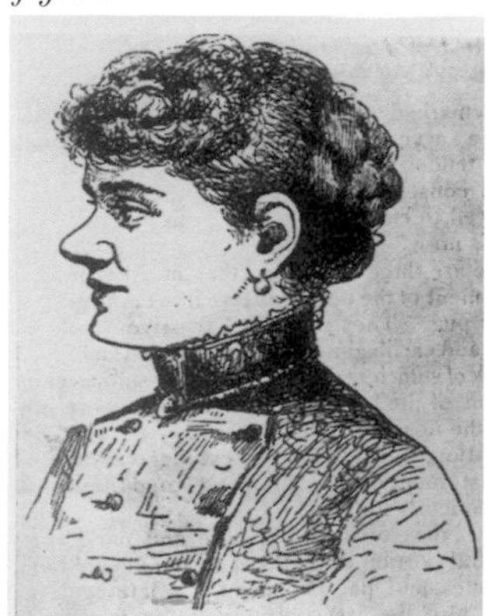

fig. 2 c

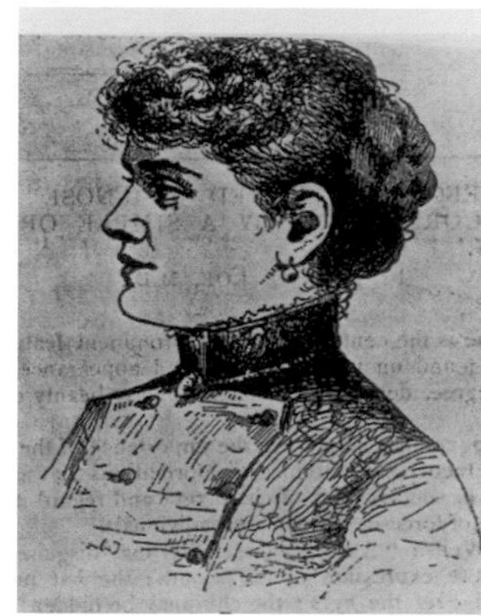

fig. 2 d

Assimilation of Irish Immigrants: Pug Noses and Bat Ears

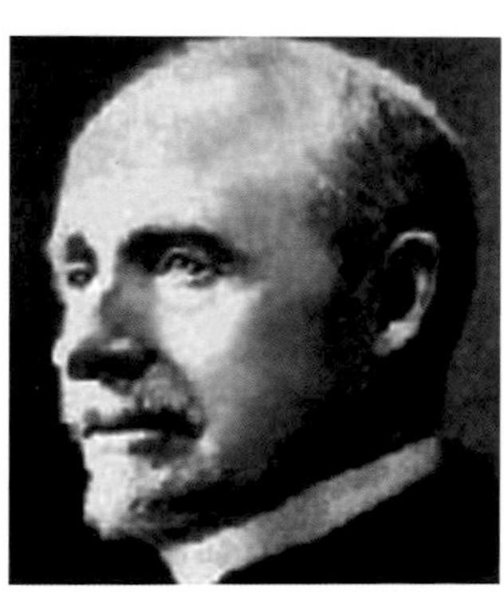

fig. 1

In the 1880s, John Orlando Roe (1848–1915) in Rochester, New York, performed an operation to "cure" the "pug nose."[1] (fig. 1) The too small nose he corrected was not the syphilitic nose; rather, he intervened to create new "American" noses out of the noses of Irish immigrants. Their new noses did not mask the sexual sins of the parents, but the fact that one's parents came from elsewhere, in the case of the pug nose, from Ireland. (fig. 2 a–d) Roe's innovation was not only to transform his patients from "Irish" into "Americans", but also to do so without the tell-tale scars that revealed the work of surgeons repairing or replacing syphilitic noses. They were no longer marked in terms of contemporary racial science as Celts but could truly pass as Anglo-Saxons.

These operations, even to visibly alter the surface features for cosmetic reasons, did not come without potential physical and emotional peril. Aesthetic surgery of the nose as practiced by such surgeons as Johann Friedrich Dieffen-

1 – John O. Roe, "The Deformity Termed 'Pug Nose' And its Correction, by a Simple Operation," *The Medical Record* 31 (June 4, 1887): 621–23; reprinted in Frank McDowell, ed., *The Source Book of Plastic Surgery* (Baltimore: The Williams & Wilkins Company, 1977), pp. 114–19, here p. 114.

fig. previous pages

Is it possible to "think" white and "act" black or vice versa? David LaChapelle's photographic manipulations are titled "Make-Over (Surgery Story)." © David LaChapelle, New York

fig. 1

John Orlando Roe (1849—1915) specialised in correcting the pug noses of Irish immigrants to the United States. He was one of the first surgeons to operate without leaving any visible scars. © facial-plastic-surgery.org

fig. 2 a–d

Two examples of Roe's rhinoplasty technique. Before their operations, contemporary racial science would have classified these patients as Celts — with their corrected noses, they could now pass as "true" Anglo-Saxons. Source: John Orlando Roe, The Deformity Termed 'Pug Nose' And its Correction, by a Simple Operation, The Medical Record 31 (June 4, 1887). Private archive Gilman, Chicago

fig. 3 a–c

The classic Greek profile of the Venus of Milo and the Roman profile of Julius Caesar. According to surgeon Jacques Joseph (1865–1934), the ideal facial profile is a combination of Greek and Roman characteristics — as displayed here by his wife (right). Source: Jacques Joseph, Nasenplastik und sonstige Gesichtsplastik, Leipzig 1931

fig. 4

Edward Talbot Ely (1850—1885) pinned back this 12-year-old's bat ears. The boy had been ridiculed by his American playmates. Source: Edward Talbot Ely, An Operation for Prominence of the Auricles, Archives of Otology 10 (1881). Private archive Gilman, Chicago

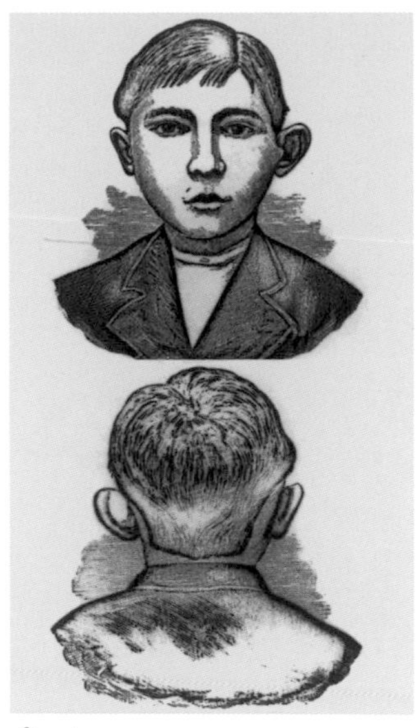

fig. 4

bach (1792—1847), before the introduction of anesthesia in 1846 and antisepsis in 1867, left scars and placed patients' lives at risk because of the dangers of shock and infection. With the introduction of antisepsis and anesthesia, the scar itself remained the only major danger for patients.[2] Scars showed that a medical intervention had taken place and what patients came to fear most was having an operation which revealed that they had done so. This powerful innovation was to change the course of aesthetic surgery. Not only was his surgical procedure innovative in the United States, but so too was the nose on which he operated.

Roe provides us with substantial information about his theory of appearance and its meaning. Based on the profile, Roe divided the image of the nose into five categories: Roman, Greek, Jewish, Snub or Pug, and Celestial. Each type of nose indicated qualities of character, following Samuel Roberts Wells' (1820—1875) phrenological / physiognomic theories: "The Roman indicates executiveness or strength; the Greek, refinement; the Jewish, commercialism or desire of gain; the Snub or Pug, weakness and lack of development; the Celestial, weakness, lack of development, and inquisitiveness." For Roe the snub-nose is "proof of a degeneracy of the human race." Roe sees this as a sign of congenital pathology that must ultimately be racially based. Thus, the short nose announces the degenerate race.

In New York, Irish immigrants had their ears pinned back by Edward Talbot Ely (1850—1885) so that this sign of their "degenerate Irish nature" vanished and they could pass as American. Edward Talbot Ely corrected a "bat ear deformity" on a twelve-year-old boy in 1881. (fig. 4) Ely undertook the procedure because the child had been "ridiculed by his companions,"[3] and he felt it was potentially within his power as a surgeon to help him. In contemporary Eire, the use of aesthetic surgery continues as a means to remedy Irishness. Today, not rhinoplasty but the ear pin-back is the operation of choice. Michael Earley, an aesthetic surgeon based in Children's University Hospital Temple Street, Dublin, says he treats a number of children for "what is called bat ears here, or Football Association Cup ears in England, a Celtic feature which some children get badly teased about."[4] This is also a permanent part of the Victorian representation of the "jug-eared Irish."[5] It is not surprising that it has maintained its importance in Ireland, while losing it in the United States, where the Irish became "white." Although "the removal of tattoos would not be considered medically necessary for instance" and most

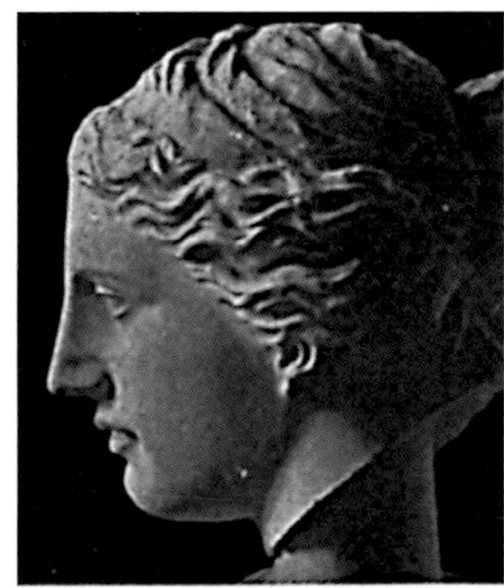

fig. 3 a

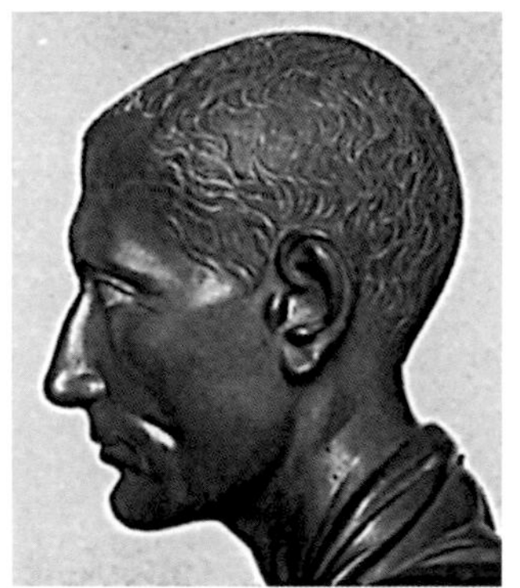

fig. 3 b

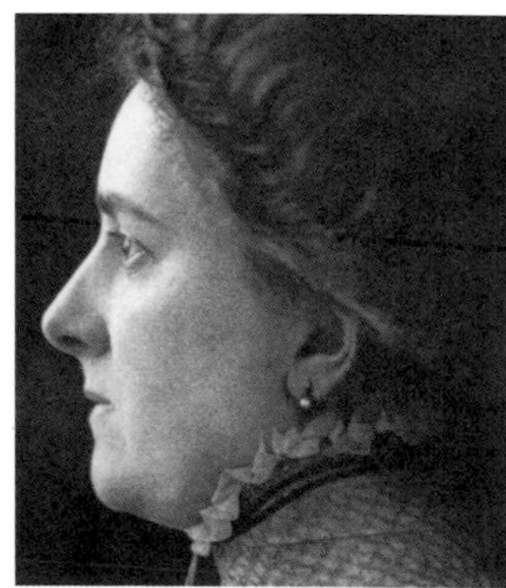

fig. 3 c

2 — Robert F. Weir commented in the late 19th century on procedures developed by the Berlin surgeon James Israel, the chief surgeon of the Jewish Hospital in Berlin. Israel's procedures were developed to cure the saddle nose. Weir noted that "the scar ... is the unavoidable result of this operation" and that the failure of the procedure sometimes reproduces the deformity. Weir, "Restoring Sunken Noses without Scarring the Face," cited from McDowell, *Source Book*, op. cit., p. 137.

3 — Edward T. Ely, "An Operation for Prominence of the Auricles," *Archives of Otology* 10 (1881): 97; reprinted in McDowell, *Source Book*, op. cit., pp. 346–49.

4 — Sylvia Thompson, "Facing up to a Face Lift," *The Irish Times* (August 22, 1994): 10.

5 — Lewis Perry Curtis, *Apes and Angels: The Irishman in Victorian Caricature* (Washington DC: Smithsonian Institution Press, 1971). For images of big, protruding ears see pp. 49, 54, 63, 67, 80; on jaws and noses see pp. 20–1., 29–30, 45.

6 — Yetti Redmond, "Holding Back the Years," *The Irish Times* (June 8, 1992): 8.

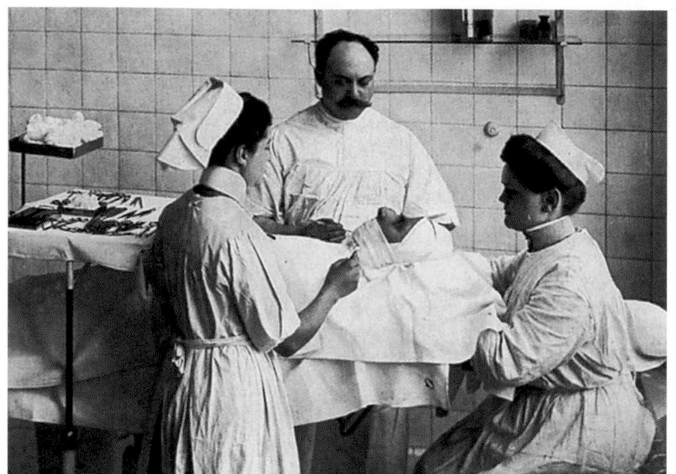

fig. 5

fig. 5

Jacques Joseph (1865—1934) prepares for a rhinoplasty. The patient's head needed to be elevated slightly. All surgical implements and swabs were arranged on a "silent assistant," the small table seen to the left. Source: J. Joseph, Nasenplastik und sonstige Gesichtsplastik, Leipzig 1931

fig. 6 a+b

As anti-Semitism became a potent political force in Germany, Jacques Joseph, himself a Jew, developed the first technique to correct "Jewish" noses. These two photos show the correction of a nasal hump and the septolabial angle, a thin flap of skin between the tip of the nose and the upper lip. Source: Jacques Joseph, Nasenplastik und sonstige Gesichtsplastik, Leipzig 1931

fig. 7 a+b

One of the procedures Jacques Joseph had learnt from his acclaimed teacher Julius Wolff (1836—1902) was the correction of the saddle nose. A piece of ivory was implanted in this patient's nose. Source: J. Joseph, Nasenplastik und sonstige Gesichtsplastik, Leipzig 1931

fig. 8 a+b

When operating on "jug" or "bat" ears, skin and cartilage frequently needed to be removed. These photos depict one of Jacques Joseph's corrections. Source: J. Joseph, Nasenplastik und sonstige Gesichtsplastik, Leipzig 1931

aesthetic surgery is not covered by the Department of Health "things like bat ears would be done on the medical card."[6] The coverage of the medical card for such a procedure accurately displays the notion that in modern Ireland, psychological afflictions caused by physicality are considered to be just as important as other physical afflictions. One can make people happy by correcting the visibility of their ears and in this way they become less "Irish" and more "beautiful."

Too, too Jewish: The Jewish Nose and Ears

In Germany in the 1890s there was Jacques Joseph (1865—1934). Joseph had been a highly acculturated young German Jewish surgeon practicing in *fin-de-siècle* Berlin. Born Jakob Joseph, he had altered his too-Jewish name when he studied medicine in Berlin and later also in Leipzig. Joseph developed the first procedure of reducing the size and shape of the "Jewish" nose at the moment when political anti-Semitism first became a potent force in Germany. (fig. 6 a+b)

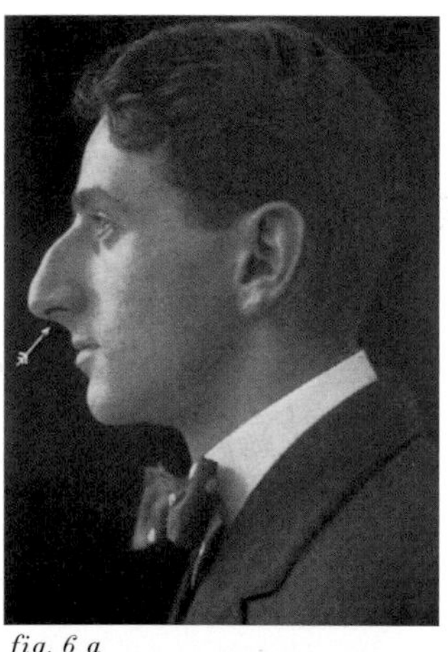

fig. 6 a

fig. 6 b

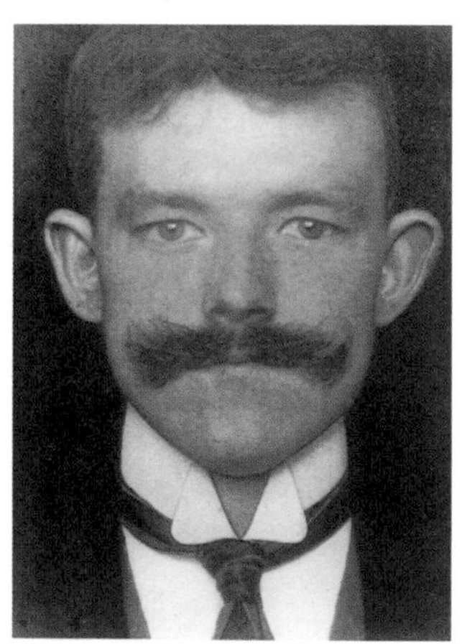

fig. 8 a

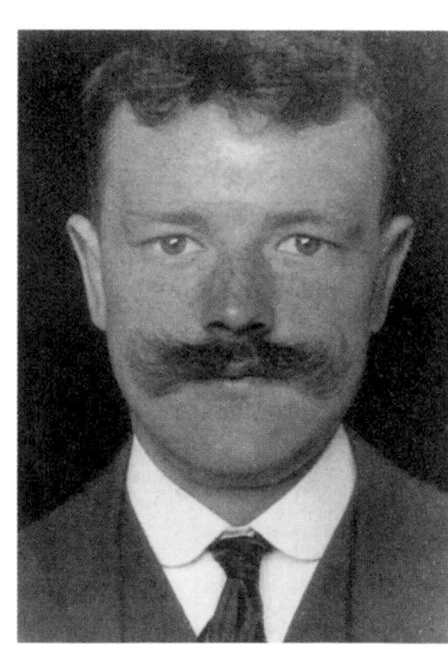

fig. 8 b

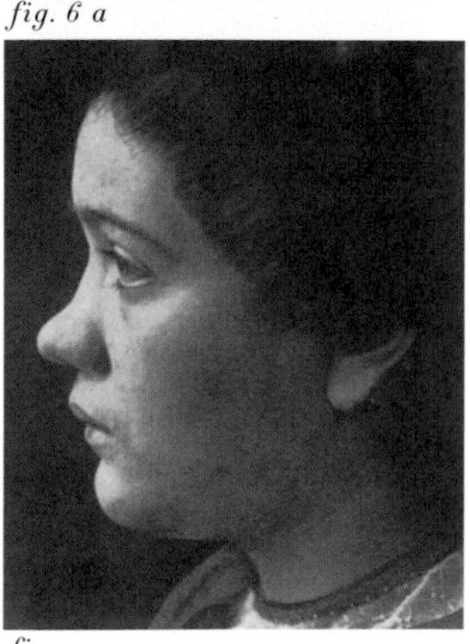

fig. 7 a

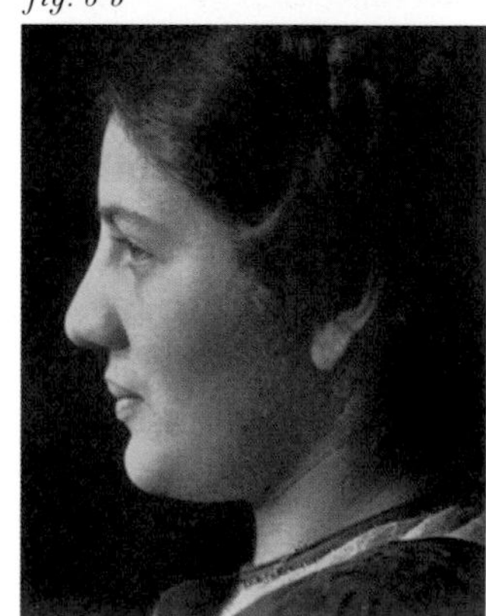

fig. 7 b

Jacques Joseph was trained as an orthopedic surgeon under Julius Wolff (1836—1902), one of the leaders in that field. In 1893 Julius Wolff developed a surgical procedure to correct the saddle nose, which followed up James Israel's (1848—1926) earlier work repairing the syphilitic nose in the mid 1880s (fig. 7). Wolff's major surgical innovation was not cutting the graft from the forehead, thus avoiding a telltale scar.[7] Wolff's wide-ranging contributions to the practices of his day included developing a therapeutic pro-

7 — **Friedrich Trendelenburg**, *Die ersten 25 Jahre der Deutschen Gesellschaft für Chirurgie: Ein Beitrag zur Geschichte der Chirurgie* **(Berlin: Julius Springer, 1923), p. 197.**

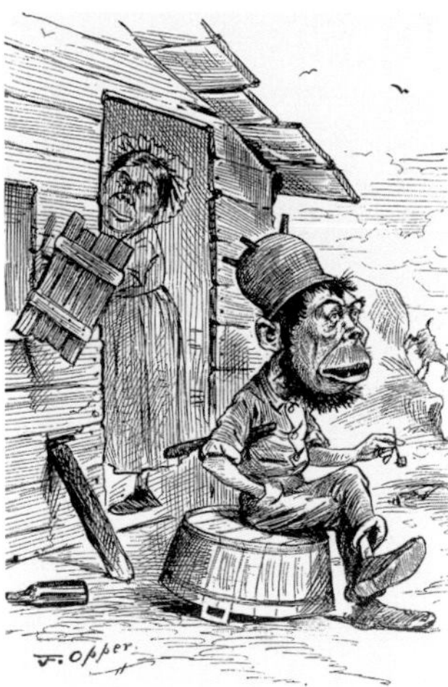

fig. 9

fig. 9

At the turn of the century, the Irish were a subject of ridicule for American cartoonists. In his sketch "Paddy as the King of Ashantee and his wife", Frederic B. Opper (1857—1937) depicts an Irish couple in the manner of the "savages" of the West African kingdom. For added insult, the figure of Paddy also features "Jewish" ears. Source: Puck 10 (February 15, 1882). Private archive Gilman, Chicago

fig. 10

In late 19th century anti-Semitic literature, it was common to describe facial and bodily traits perceived as "Jewish" — including "nervous, suspicious eyes," "big lips and sharp rats' teeth," or even just "round knees" and "flat feet." Source: Telemachus Thomas Timayenis, The Original Mr. Jacobs (New York: The Minerva Publishing Co., 1888). Private archive Gilman, Chicago

cedure for correcting a club foot with the use of a specialized dressing which altered the very shape of the foot.[8] Orthopedics, more than any other medical specialty of the period, presented the challenge of altering the visible errors of development so as to restore a normal function.

Joseph's interests did not lie with the foot, even though the feet were thought to be another sign of Jewish inferiority, but elsewhere in the anatomy. In 1896 he undertook a corrective procedure on a young child with protruding ears, that, while successful, caused him to be dismissed as Wolff's assistant. Joseph's procedure was his own, but it paralleled the work of the previously mentioned American otorhinolaryngologist Edward Talbot Ely who operated on "Irish" ears. According to the child's mother, he had suffered from humiliation in school because of his protruding ears. It was the child's unhappiness with being different that Joseph (and Ely) was correcting. Abnormally big and protruding ears alone might account for the child's unhappiness. But it was the specific cultural meaning of protruding ears at the close of the 19th century that really added insult to injury.

An old European trope about the shape of the Jew's ears can be found throughout the anti-Semitic literature of the *fin de siècle*. The racial anthropologist Hans Friedrich Karl Günther (1891—1968) summarizes the turn-of the-century view that Jews, especially the males, have "fleshy ear lobes" and "large, red ears" more frequently than other peoples do. They have "prominent ears that stick out." According to Günther, prominent ears are especially prevalent among "Jewish children; one refers to them in Austria as 'Moritz ears.'"[9] Moritz (Morris) was a typical Jewish name of the day. They are the "elongated ears" which appear as the "ill-shapen ears of great size like those of a bat," according to an English-language anti-Semitic text of 1888.[10] (fig. 10)

In his major paper of 1910 on the correction of prominent ears, William H. Luckett (1872—1925), a surgeon in New York, comments obliquely about the "odium attached to these ears."[11] In the American context, these may have been the jug-ears which dominated the caricatures of the Irish in American culture (and which, as we have seen, Irish aesthetic surgeons continue to treat aggressively in mod-

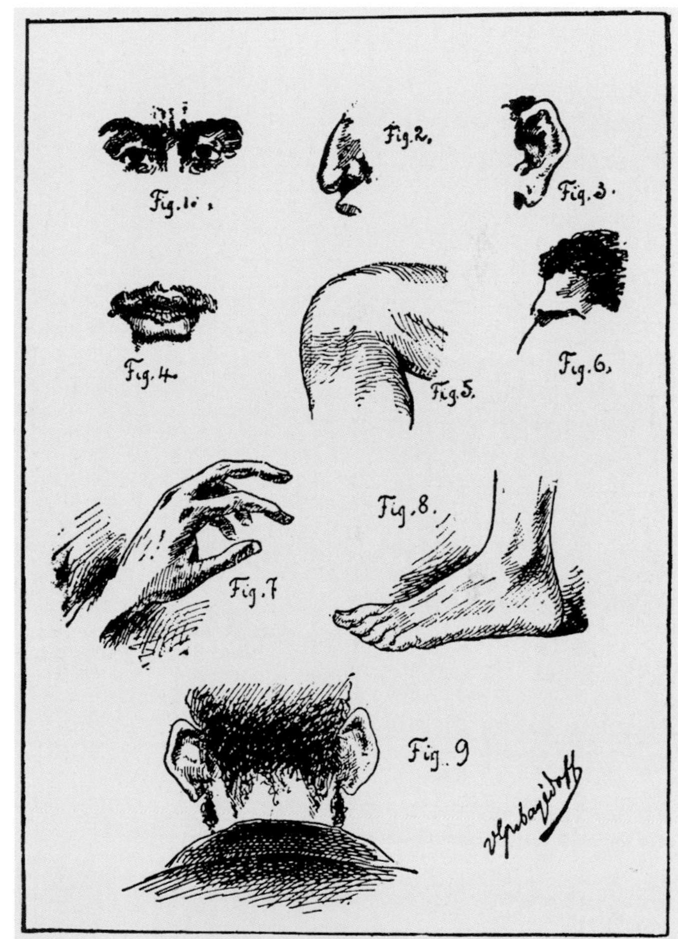

fig. 10

ern Eire). However, they may also have been the ears of the Jewish immigrants on the Lower East Side. The stigma they evoke is repugnance at a visible sign of difference; a

8 — **Bruno Valentin**, *Geschichte der Orthopädie* **(Stuttgart: Georg Thieme, 1961), pp. 101–2.**

9 — **Hans F. K. Günther**, *Rassenkunde des jüdischen Volkes* **(München: J. F. Lehmann, 1930), p. 218.**

10 — **Telemachus Thomas Timayenis**, *The Original Mr. Jacobs* **(New York: The Minerva Publishing Co., 1888), p. 21. See Michael Selzer, ed.**, *"Kike!": A Documentary History of Anti-Semitism in America* **(New York: World Publishing, 1972), plate 16.**

11 — **William H. Luckett, "A New Operation for Prominent Ears Based on the Anatomy of the Deformity,"** *Surgical Gynecology & Obstetrics* **10 (1910): 635–37; reprinted in McDowell,** *Source Book*, **op. cit., pp. 351–3, here 351.**

fig. 11

In 1898, Jacques Joseph (1865–1934) performed his first reduction rhinoplasty. The patient had complained that people constantly stared at him because of his ungainly nose, and that he was the target of insulting remarks. After the operation, the patient was able to enjoy his life again. Source: "Über die operative Verkleinerung einer Nase (Rhinomiosis)", Berliner klinische Wochenschrift 40 (1898): 882–85. Private archive Gilman, Chicago

fig. 12 a+b

According to Jacques Joseph (1865–1934), the prime objective of plastic surgery was to heal the patient's psychological state of depression. These photos, taken in the postoperative stage, were meant to demonstrate that an emotional improvement was evident soon after the procedure. Source: Jacques Joseph, Nasenplastik und sonstige Gesichtsplastik, Leipzig 1931

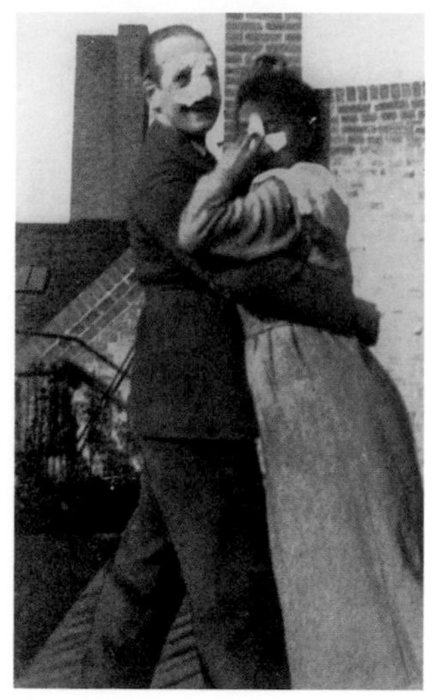

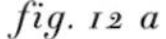

fig. 12 a

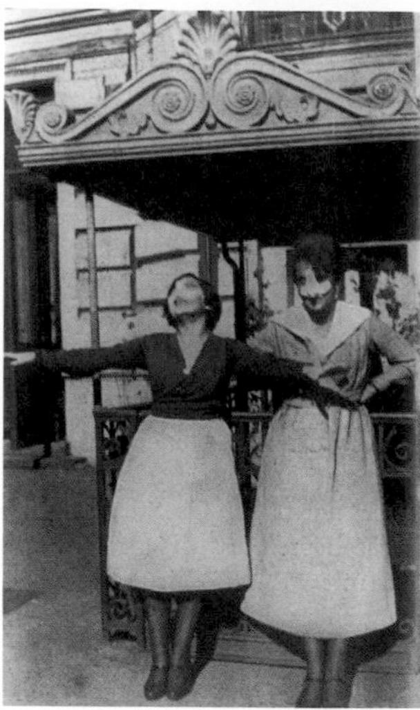

fig. 12 b

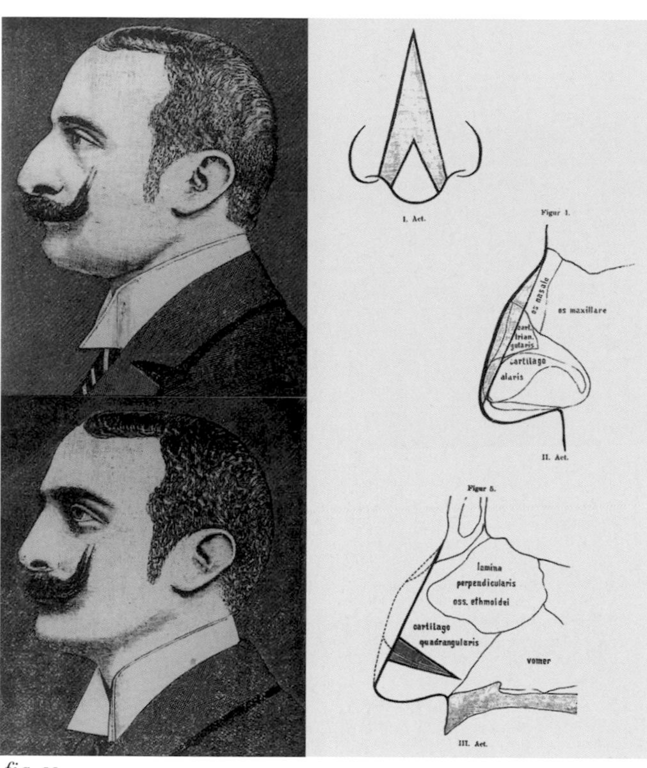

fig. 11

difference ascribed to the character as well as to the body. In January 1898, a 28 year old man came to him, having heard of the successful operation on the child's ears. He complained that "his nose was the source of considerable annoyance. Wherever he went, everybody stared at him; often, he was the target of remarks or ridiculing gestures. On account of this he became melancholic, withdrew almost completely from social life, and had the earnest desire to be relieved of this deformity."[12] The psychological symptoms were analogous to those of the young boy whose ears Joseph had repaired.

Joseph took the young man's case and proceeded to perform his first reduction rhinoplasty, cutting through the skin of the nose to reduce its size and alter its shape by chipping away the bone and removing the cartilage. On May 11, 1898 he reported on this operation before the Berliner Medizinische Gesellschaft. In that report Joseph provided a detailed "scientific" rationale for performing a medical procedure on an otherwise completely healthy individual: "The psychological effect of the operation is of utmost importance. The depressed attitude of the patient subsided completely. He is happy to move around unnoticed. His happiness in life has increased, his wife was glad to report; the patient who formerly avoided social contact now wishes to attend and give parties. In other words, he is happy over the results."[13] Yet he had left scars, which pointed to the procedure itself, and this became a major concern of Joseph's. He warned his colleagues that, "disclosure to the patient on the problem of scarring is very important. Many patients, however, will consider even simple scars too conspicuous...."[14] He raised the specter of a court case in which the "unsightly scar might represent

12 — **"Über die operative Verkleinerung einer Nase (Rhinomiosis),"** *Berliner klinische Wochenschrift* **40 (1898): 882–85. Translation from Jacques Joseph, "Operative Reduction of the Size of a Nose (Rhinomiosis)," trans. Gustave Aufricht,** *Plastic and Reconstructive Surgery* **46 (1970): 178–81, here 178; reproduced in McDowell,** *Source Book*, **pp. 164–67. See also Paul Natvig,** *Jacques Joseph: Surgical Sculptor* **(Philadelphia: W. B. Saunders, 1982), pp. 23–24. C. Walter, D. J. Brain, "Jacques Joseph,"** *Facial Plastic Surgery* **9 (1993): 116–124; S. Milstein, "Jacques Joseph and the Upper Lateral Nasal Cartilages,"** *Plastic and Reconstructive Surgery* **78 (1986): 424; D. J. Hauben, "Jacques Joseph (1865–1934),"** *Laryngologie, Rhinologie, Otologie* **62 (1983): 56–7; T. Gibson, D. W. Robinson, "The Mammary Artery Pectoral Flaps of Jacques Joseph,"** *British Journal of Plastic Surgery* **29(1976): 370–6; Paul Natvig, "Some Aspects of the Character and Personality of Jacques Joseph,"** *Plastic and Reconstructive Surgery* **47 (1971): 452–3. On the general history of rhinoplasty see Blair O. Rogers, "A Chronological History of Cosmetic Surgery,"** *Bulletin of the New York Academy of Medicine* **47 (1971): 265–302; Blair O. Rogers, "A Brief History of Cosmetic Surgery,"** *Surgical Clinics of North America* **51 (1971): 265–88; H. Rudert, "Von der submukösen Septumresektion Killians über Cottles Septumplastik zur modernen plastischen Septumkorrektur und funktionellen Septo-Rhinoplastik,"** *Hals-Nase-Ohren* **32 (1984): 230–3; D. J. Hauben, "Die Geschichte der Rhinoplastik,"** *Laryngologie, Rhinologie, Otologie* **62 (1983): 53–5; P. A. Adamson, "Rhinoplasty—Our Past,"** *Facial Plastic Surgery* **5 (1988): 93–6; C. Walter, "The Evolution of Rhinoplasty,"** *Journal of Laryngology and Otology* **102 (1988): 1079–85; I. Eisenberg, "A History of Rhinoplasty,"** *South African Medical Journal* **62 (1982): 286–92; A. B. Sokol and R. B. Berggren, "Rhinoplasty. Its Development and Present Day Usages,"** *Ohio State Medical Journal* **68 (1972): 556–62.**

13 — **Joseph, "Operative Reduction," p. 180.**

14 — **Jacques Joseph,** *Nasenplastik und sonstige Gesichtsplastik, nebst einem Anhang über Mammaplastik und einige weitere Operationen aus dem Gebiete der äusseren Körperplastik: ein Atlas und ein Lehrbuch* **(Leipzig: C. Kabitzsch, 1931). All quotations are from the translation by Stanley Milstein, Jacques Joseph,** *Rhinoplasty and Facial Plastic Surgery with a Supplement on Mammaplasty and Other Operations in the Field of Plastic Surgery of the Body* **(Phoenix: Columella Press, 1987), here p. 34.**

fig. 13

In order for the patient to retain the use of her right hand, Jacques Joseph used a skin graft from the left arm for this augmentation rhinoplasty. Source: Jacques Joseph, Nasenplastik und sonstige Gesichtsplastik, Leipzig 1931

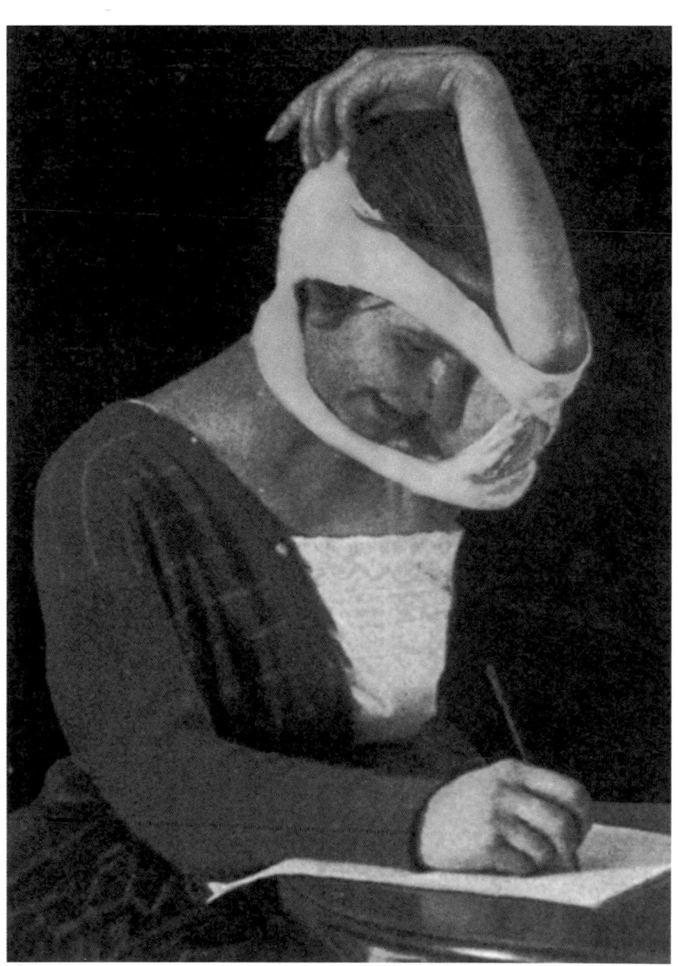

fig. 13

a greater degree of disfigurement than the enlarged cartilage [of the nose] presented previously." More centrally though, surgical scars, unlike scars obtained through socially acceptable and manly activities such as dueling, reveal the inauthencity of the body and the effort to "pass" via medical intervention.

The Invisible Scar and Happiness: Nose Job since 1904

On April 19, 1904 Joseph undertook his removal of a hump from within the nose using cartilaginous incisions. He retrospectively commented that in 1898 he had used the extranasal procedure which "caused a scar, but this scar will be hardly visible after a short time, assuming that the incision is sutured exactly."[15] But hardly visible was not sufficient. Even the slightest scar was enough to evoke a visual memory of the too big nose. The invisibility of the patient hinged on the elimination of the scar. Patients needed to become (in)visible to pass. And Joseph had learned that only (in)visibility left his patients happy.

Joseph's claim to fame was that he solved the problem of the visible scar. Instead of the practiced extranasal operation, his procedure to remove the bone and cartilage from within the patient's nose is still used today as are the surgical tools he developed to carry out the procedure. In his summary paper on the reduction of the size of the nose published in 1904, Joseph commented on the psychology of his male patients: "The patients were embarrassed and self-conscious in their dealings with their fellow men, often shy and unsociable, and had the urgent desire to become free and unconstrained. Several complained of sensitive drawbacks in the exercise of their profession. As executives they could hardly enforce their authority; in their business connections (as salesmen, for example), they often suffered material losses.... The operative nasal reduction — this is my firm conviction — will also in the future restore the joy of living to many a wretched creature and, if his deformity has been hindering him in his career, it will allow him the full exercise of his aptitudes."[16] According to Joseph the patient "is happy to move around unnoticed." The visibility of the Jew made it impossible for

15 — Cited by Blair Rogers, "John Orlando Roe — Not Jacques Joseph — the Father of Aesthetic Rhinoplasty," *Aesthetic Plastic Surgery* 10 (1986): 63–88, here p. 81.

16 — Jacques Joseph, "Nasenverkleinerung (mit Krankenvorstellung)," *Deutsche Medizinische Wochenschrift* 30 (1904): 1095. See also his "Nasenverkleinerungen," *Verhandlungen der deutschen Gesellschaft für Chirurgie* 33 (1904): 112–20, as well as *Eine Nasenplastik, ausgeführt in Lokalanaesthesie* (Berlin: G. Stilke, 1927).

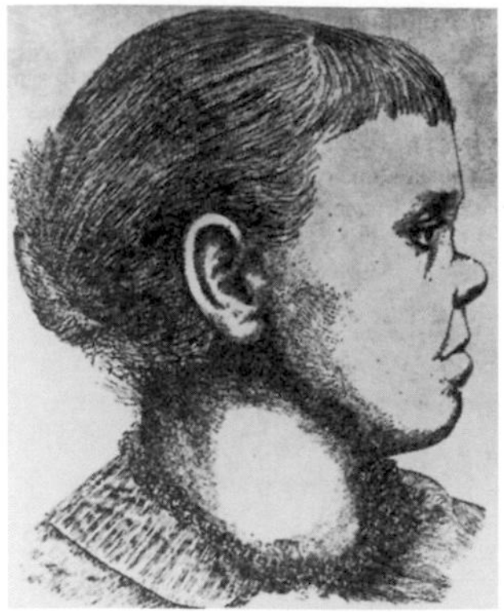

fig. 14 a

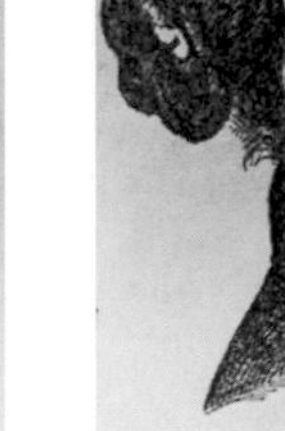

fig. 14 b

fig. 14 a+b

Robert F. Weir (1838–1894) developed a surgical technique that left no scars. Shown here are the before-and-after drawings of a patient whose saddle nose was corrected with an implant. Source: Robert F. Weir, "On Restoring Sunken Noses without Scarring the Face," New York Medical Journal 56 (1892). Private archive Gilman, Chicago

fig. 15 a+b

Jacques Joseph (1865–1934) operated on this boy's shortened saddle nose. As the young skin was still flexible, all that was needed to even out the profile was a bone graft taken from the tibia. Source: Jacques Joseph, Nasenplastik und sonstige Gesichtsplastik, Leipzig 1931

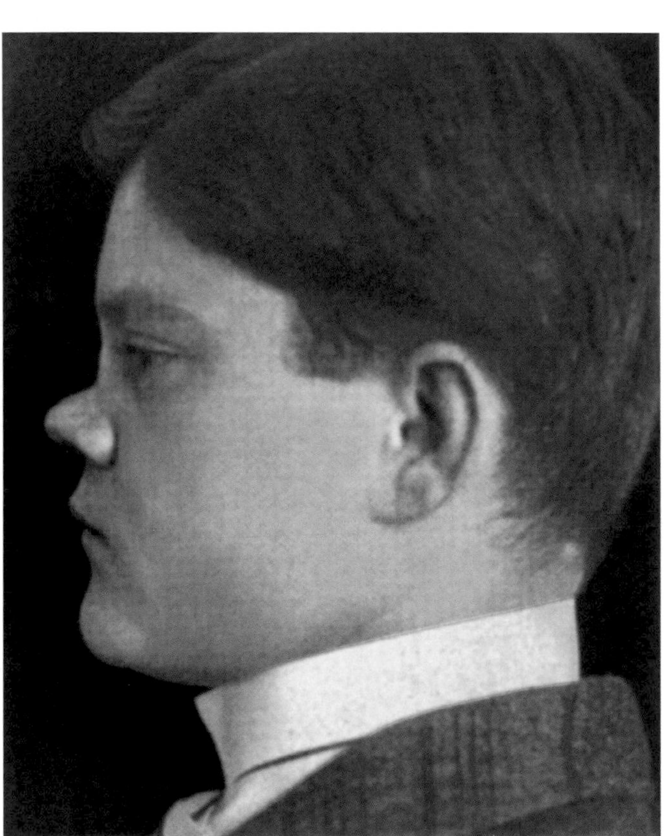

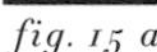

fig. 15 a

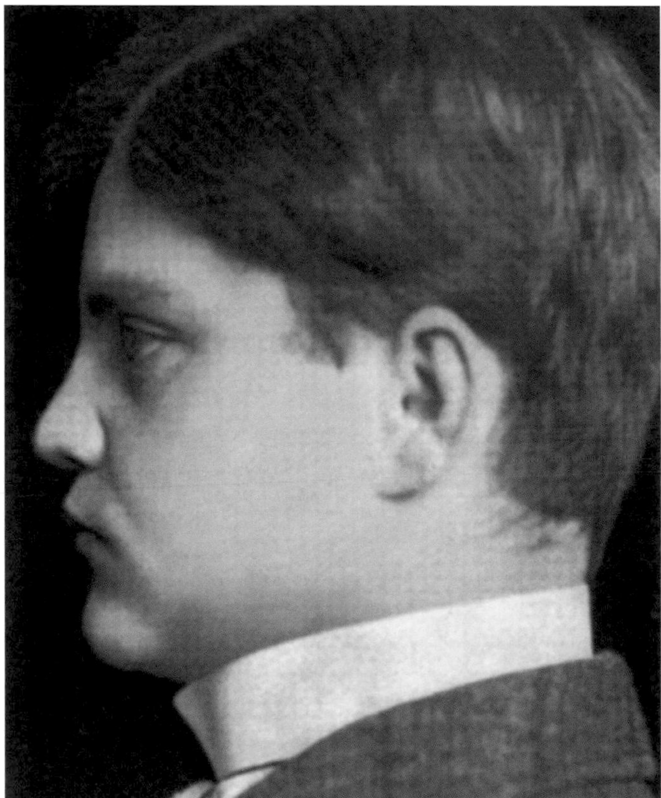

fig. 15 b

him to compete equally with the non-Jew in the economic world at the turn of the century due to stigmatization. The Viennese-Jewish poet Fritz Löhner, famed for his poetry and his opera libretti (such as Franz Lehár's "Land of Smiles") summarized this response in his extraordinary poem of 1908 entitled "Jewish." In it, the speaking voice addresses the doctor asking what he had meant when he said that there was very much Jewish about her. The doctor lists the speaker's best attributes: her satin eyes, her lustrous hair, the bright mouth, as Solomon sings about in the "Song of Songs." But, the speaker says, what is truly Jewish about you, that which "burns the deepest wounds in me" is that "you deny that which is Jewish in you and that is too, too Jewish." ("Missachten, was man 'jüdisch' nennt, / Ist leider, leider jüdisch!")[17] The experience of the Jew of his or her own body was so deeply impacted by the anti-Semitic rhetoric that even when that body meets the expectations for perfection set by the community in which the Jew lived, the Jew experienced his or her body as flawed, as diseased.[18]

Such a transition became possible in late 19th century Germany when the legal restrictions, which limited the Jew (and especially the Jewish male), were lifted. Jewish women were still bound by the limitations applied to women in

17 – **"Beda" [i.e., Fritz Löhner],** *Israeliten und andere Antisemiten* **(Vienna and Berlin: R. Löwit, 1919), p. 32–33. (By this edition the volume had sold 15,000 copies.)**

18 – **On the cultural background for this concept see Jacob Katz,** *Out of the Ghetto: The Social Background of Jewish Emancipation 1770–1870* **(Cambridge, MA: Harvard University Press, 1973) and Rainer Erb and Werner Bergmann,** *Die Nachtseite der Judenemanzipation: Der Widerstand gegen die Integration der Juden in Deutschland 1780–1860* **(Berlin: Metropol, 1989).**

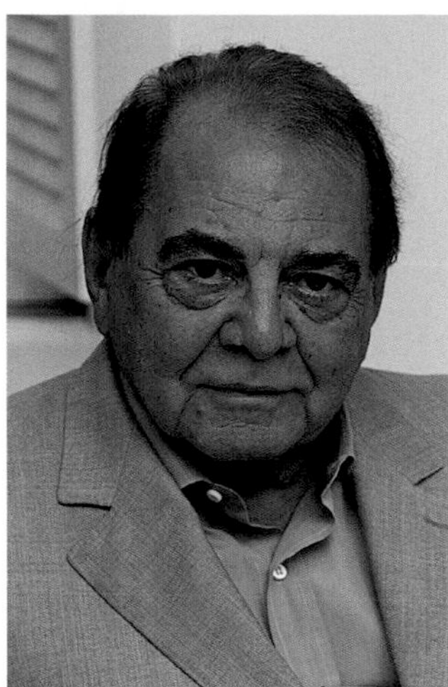

fig. 16

Ivo Pitanguy is Brazil's most prolific cosmetic surgeon. He works in a country where the population presents a broad racial mix — which sometimes causes inherent physical dissonances. Brazilians have been using plastic surgery for more than 150 years. © Tuca Reinés

fig. 16

19th century Europe, but Jewish males generally could enter into the world of masculine endeavors as long as they were not too evidently Jewish. No law bound them (unlike African-American males in the United States at the same moment) from becoming officers, doctors, lawyers, or businessmen in the general society, but the powerful social stigma associated with the Jews continued in spite of civil emancipation. Thus one did not want to appear Jewish – one needed to be able to pass as German. A contemporary commentator notes about Joseph's procedures that: "Even today, 70 years later, one often hears the erroneous remark that rhinoplasty is an operation for vanity's sake. That is not true. Vanity is the desire to excel. The average rhinoplasty patient wishes to be relieved of a real or imagined conspicuousness of his nose."[19]

African and Caucasian Americans

In the United States of America the situation for African-Americans was ever more oppressive after the Civil War. Light-skinned African-Americans had their lips thinned and their noses rebuilt so that they could cross the color line. And if they were too dark, they looked for having their skin lightened.

The origin of the correction of the black nose is masked within the medical literature. No reputable surgeon in the United States wanted to be seen as facilitating crossing the color bar in the age of post-Reconstruction "Jim Crow" and "miscegenation" laws. This is very different from the situation, as discussed earlier, of the Jews in Germany, whose civil emancipation and legal status had been clarified (if not accepted) by the same period. In 1892, the New York surgeon Robert F. Weir (1838–1927) proposed a procedure for the restoration of "sunken noses without scarring the face." [20] This procedure altered the sunken nose through the introduction of an implant and deals quite explicitly with syphilitic noses. Weir also discussed the alteration of the nasal alae (wings). The operation resulted in a "parrot nose" which made his patient look "black." A further surgical intervention to shave the nostrils remedied this problem. When Jacques Joseph in 1931 reports on Robert Weir's paper, he describes it as a "method of correcting abnormally-flared nasal alae (Negroid nose) by means of sickle-shaped vertical excisions ... "[21] Robert Weir's procedure to reconstruct the syphilitic nose was thus also seen as an intervention to enable black noses to "pass."[22] (fig. 14 a+b)

The history of the racial nose and early aesthetic surgery in the United States is one of understatement and dissimulation. In 1934 Jacques W. Maliniac (1889–1976) noted that "the nose has strong and easily discernible racial characteristics. In an alien environment these may be highly detrimental to its possessor. A Negroid nose is a distinct social and economic handicap to a dark-skinned Caucasian."[23] Or, one might add, to someone desiring to cross the color bar. The counter-case was also true. Henry Jurius Schireson noted that one of his patients, a nurse, had massive freckles. She wished to have her freckles removed: "... the excess pigmentation in the lower layers of her otherwise perfect skin was interfering with her work. In a dim light she looked to some of her patients like a mulatto."[24] Perhaps she was indeed someone trying to cross the color bar.

19 – **Blair Rogers, "Roe," op. cit., p. 84.**

20 – **Weir, "On Restoring Sunken Noses without Scarring the Face," cited from McDowell,** *Source Book* **op. cit., p. 139.**

21 – **Jacques Joseph,** *Nasenplastik und sonstige Gesichtsplastik, nebst einem Anhang über Mammaplastik und einige weitere Operationen aus dem Gebiete der äusseren Körperplastik: ein Atlas und ein Lehrbuch* **(Leipzig: C. Kabitzsch, 1931). All quotations are from the translation by Stanley Milstein, Jacques Joseph,** *Rhinoplasty and Facial Plastic Surgery with a Supplement on Mammaplasty and Other Operations in the Field of Plastic Surgery of the Body* **(Phoenix: Columella Press, 1987), p. 83.**

22 – **The Negroid nose isseen as one of the categories which warranted surgical intervention in contemporary Brazil today. One does not want to be seen as "too black." See Aymar Sperli, "Exo-Rhinoplasty: A New 'Old Approach' in Aesthetic Rhinoplasty," and Edwaldo Bolivar de Souza Pinto, "Rhinosculpture: Treatment of the Nasal Tip, Columella, and Lip Dynamics," in the on-line** *Brazilian Journal of Plastic Surgery* **(October 31, 1996) [www.plasticsurgery.orgtet. Both of these essays list "Negroid nose" as one of nasal forms to be "repaired."**

23 – **Jacques W. Maliniak,** *Sculpture in the Living: Rebuilding the Face and Form by Plastic Surgery* **(New York: Romaine Pierson, 1934), p. 55.**

24 – **Henry J. Schireson,** *As Others See You: The Story of Plastic Surgery* **(New York: Macaulay, 1938), p. 276.**

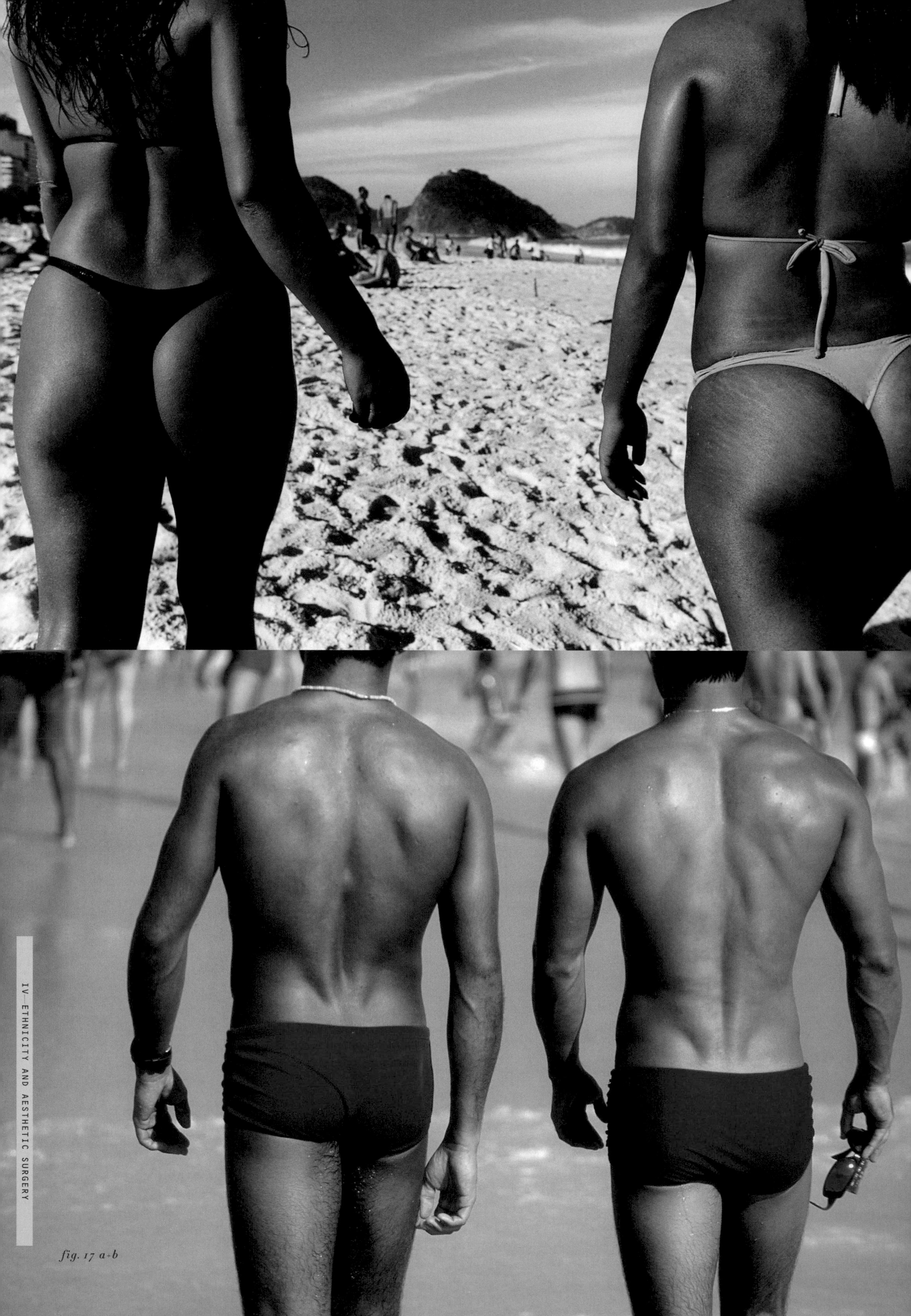

fig. 17 a+b

fig. 17 a+b

Tall and tan and young and lovely ... Whether in Ipanema, Copacabana or anywhere else in Brazil, physical beauty is valued very highly — many girls get a breast reduction for their 16th birthday. Liposuction and injections against wrinkles are also very common. Regardless if they're male, female, rich, or poor — Brazilians are having more plastic surgery, and it's becoming more affordable. © *laif*

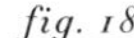

fig. 18

Silicone pads for the buttocks, the breasts, and even the scrotum. © *laif*

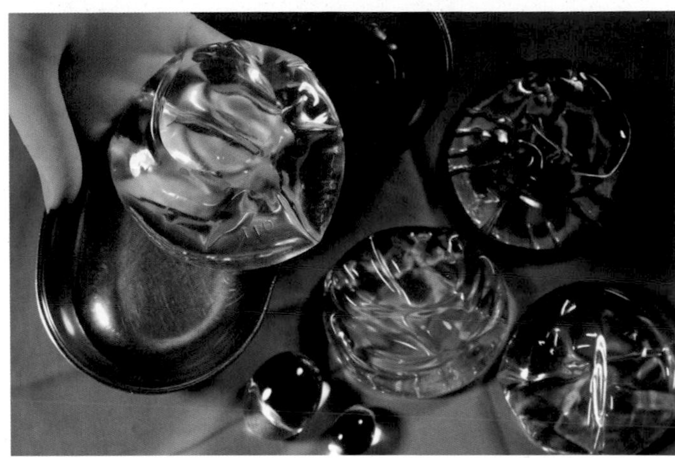

fig. 18

Brazilian Mix and Match

In nations where there is a strong African presence, the very nature of that black body is often drawn into question. Brazilian aesthetic surgery can justifiably claim a history of more than 150 years.[25] Farid Hakme, the former President of the Brazilian Plastic Surgery Society, attributes Brazil's fascination with aesthetic surgery in the 1990s to "the country's mix and match of different races, which can create physical disharmonies. 'What happens is the nose sometimes doesn't match the mouth or the buttocks don't match with the legs,' he said."[26] Such fantasies about symmetry and balance reflect a Brazilian anxiety about looking "too black."[27] And one of the typical characteristics of this is the pendulous [primitive] breast. "The women who want to reduce their breasts here [in Brazil] would probably want to increase them in the United States," Oswaldo Saldanha, the General Secretary of the Brazilian Plastic Surgery Society, noted. His explanation for this avoids the specificity of race; rather, for him, "beauty ideals and cultures are different in every country." The healthy and erotic body in Brazil is not the black body. As with rhinoplasties among Jews in the United States during the 1950s and '60s, Brazilian breast reductions are often "sweet sixteen" birthday presents. Such gifts enable their daughters silently as Brazilians to de-emphasize the breasts while overemphasizing the buttocks, as any decrease in a certain physical proportion will highlight other, more pronounced, features. According to one of its leading practitioners, Ricardo Baroudi, the emphasis on the "culture, genetics, and race" of the patient in Brazil also shaped the Brazilian's attitude toward "the concept of beauty, body fat distribution, and body weight."

In Brazil in the 1990s breast reduction had become common-place among upper middle class families, so as to distinguish their daughters from the lower classes, who are imagined as black, to pass as members of a cohort and find appropriate mates.[28]

Yet by the year 2002, breast augmentation had increased so as to displace breast reduction as the operation of choice on the breast. Sandra dos Santos is "tall, thin, and elegant but the 23-year old says she is missing something that could make her a real beauty — larger breasts."[29] Even the poor like Sandra dos Santos are having breast enlargements. "This is true democracy at work," says Ivo Pitanguy, Brazil's greatest surgeon (fig. 16). "I think more surgeons are beginning to believe what I have known for a long time: Plastic surgery can be important for self-esteem for any one and should be available." Pitanguy had pioneered such procedures for the poor 40 years ago when the operation of choice was breast reduction. At the Annual Meeting of the American Society for Aesthetic Plastic Surgery (ASAPS), in May 2001 in New York, the American aesthetic surgeon Renato Saltz noted this change: "Ideals of beauty traditionally have been somewhat different in the various regions of the world. This goes beyond the obvious differences in racial and ethnic features. For example, breast reduction surgery has been far more common than breast enlargement in Brazil. That's because Brazilian women have preferred to be small on top, and even those with average size breasts often have surgery to make them smaller. Only very recently are Brazilian surgeons reporting that breast augmentation is gaining popularity in their country."[30] Now, in an age of globalized notion of the erotic, breast augmentation is the procedure of choice rather than an emphasis on correcting the appearance of race.

25 — Ricardo Baroudi, "Why Aesthetic Plastic Surgery Became Popular in Brazil?" *Plastic Surgery* **27 (1991): 396–397.**

26 — Simona de Logu, "Plastic Surgery gets Boost in Brazil," *Reuters* **(December 6, 1996).**

27 — Michael George Hanchard, *Orpheus and Power: The Movimento Negro of Rio De Janeiro and São Paulo, Brazil, 1945–1988* **(Princeton: Princeton University Press, 1994) and Gregor Burkhart,** *Die Kinder Omulús: der Einfluß afrobrasilianischer Kultur auf die Wahrnehmung von Körper und Krankheit* **(Frankfurt am Main; New York: P. Lang, 1994).**

28 — Aesthetic surgery in the United States continues to be a sort of holiday present, if just to oneself. The American Academy of Facial Plastic and Reconstructive Surgery found its members performed 7,140 nose jobs nationwide in the last two weeks of 1993, compared with 3,920 in the average two-week period. The increase has been attributed to the seasonal vacation time, but it has also to be seen in terms of the idea of aesthetic surgery as a gift. "Outliers: Asides and Insides on Healthcare," *Modern Healthcare* **(January 6, 1997): 60.**

29 — Patrice M. Jones, "Plastic Surgeries Changing the face of an Eager Brazil," *The Chicago Tribune* **(July 9, 2001): 1, 4.**

30 — Press release, "International Surgeons Bring Unique Perspectives to Cosmetic Surgery Meeting," May 3, 2001, American Society for Aesthetic Plastic Surgery.

fig. 19

At the end of the 19th century, the Japanese began to view the Western double eyelid as a desirable feature. In 1896, the Japanese surgeon M. Mikamo (Daten) operated on a patient whose left eye already had a double eyelid, correcting her right eyelid to match. Source: Y. Shirakabe, T. Kinusgasa, M. Kawata, T. Kishimoto et al., "The Double Eyelid Operation in Japan: Its Evolution as Related to Cultural Change," Annals of Plastic Surgery 15 (1985). Private archive Gilman, Chicago

fig. 20

M. Mikamo's technique employed three silken threads, sewed in above the edge of the eyelid and pulled through the conjunctiva. After four to six days, the new double eyelid emerged. 32 blepharoplasty methods have been based on this technique since. Source: Y. Shirakabe, T. Kinusgasa, M. Kawata, T. Kishimoto, "The Double Eyelid Operation in Japan: Its Evolution as Related to Cultural Change," Annals of Plastic Surgery 15 (1985). Private archive Gilman, Chicago

fig. 21

The print "Three beauties of the present day" by Kitagawa Utamaro (1750—1806) depicts the traditional Japanese concept of beauty: small eyes with flat eyelids, a straight nose, and a receding chin. This aesthetic changed as the influence of Western medicine grew.

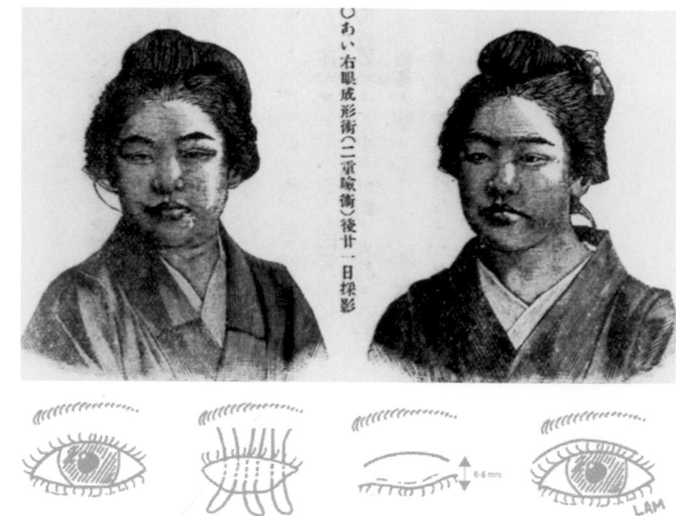

fig. 19 & 20

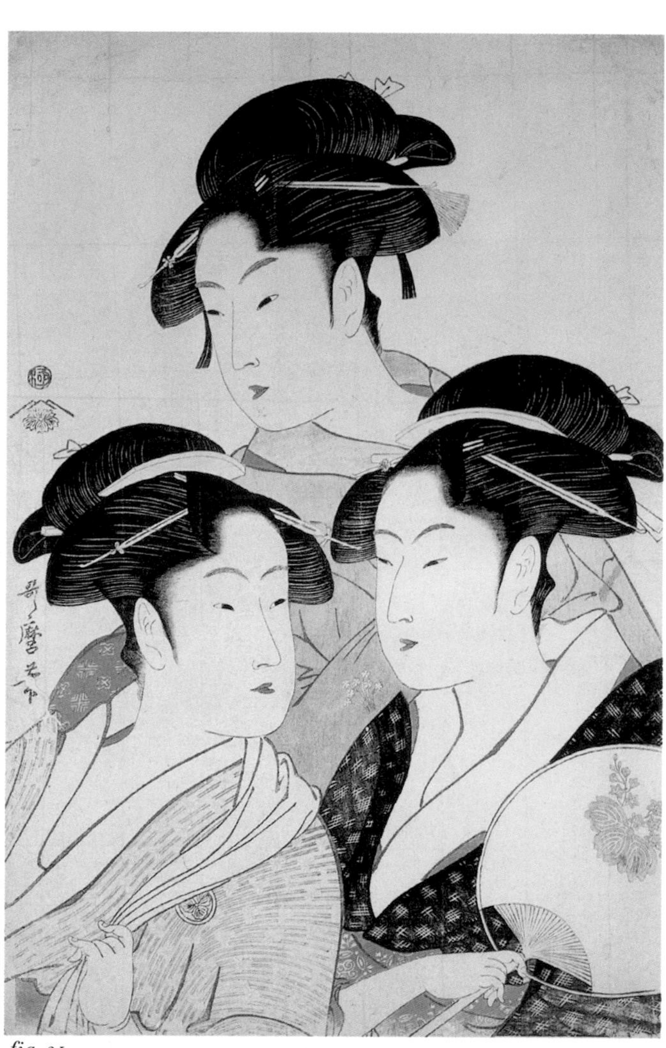

fig. 21

Looking West: The Japanese Eyelid

Globalized notions of what is considered to be beautiful arise in the latter decades of the 19th century with the increased visibility of Western culture in other areas of the world. These are alterations for ethic or rational reasons that are not motivated by a need for "passing" as one of the dominant culture, but rather to simply look more like them and thus be more accepted within their own culture. Breast reductions, ear tucks, nose jobs, skin lightening, are all part of the first generation of modern, Western procedures. In Japan as early as 1896, under the domination of Western medicine, M. Mikamo introduced a non-incision procedure to create a double eyelid, mimicking that of the Western eye.[31] He complained that the single eyelid contributed to a "monotonous and impassive" countenance. (fig. 19, 20) His procedure was developed to create symmetry in a patient who had a single double eyelid. Indeed, he argued that the single eyelid was a "true defect" and that often such an eyelid was produced after an infection in someone who had a double eyelid. Its impetus was reconstructive though evidently its import and influence was aesthetic. In fact, he concludes his essay of 1896 noting that his intent is to have "natural looking eyes."[32] These natural looking eyes were the eyes of the new Japanese — eyes that looked west. From 1896 to the present some 32 different procedures were developed in Japan for purely aesthetic surgery of the eyelid. The desire, well before the defeat of Japan in 1945 and the occupation of the country by the Americans, was "to have a well-defined nose; a clear-cut, double eyelid fold; and larger, more attractive breasts." One must add that plastic surgery was recognized as a medical sub-specialty in Japan only in 1975 and aesthetic surgery only in 1978. All of these procedures existed on the boundaries of official medical practice.[33] This was quite similar to the situation of aesthetic surgeons in Europe and North America.

The procedures to alter the look of the eye did not change the total image of the Japanese visage. During this peri-

31 — Y. Shirakabe, T. Kinusgasa, M. Kawata, T. Kishimoto, T. Shirakabe, "The Double Eyelid Operation in Japan: Its Evolution as Related to Cultural Change," *Annals of Plastic Surgery* **15 (1985): 224–41.**

32 — K. Mikamo, "Plastic Operation of the Eye," *Journal Chugaii Jishimpo* **17 (1896): 1197.**

33 — See the discussion by Naoyuki Ohtake and Nobuyuki Shioya, "Aesthetic Breast Surgery in Orientals," in Nicolas G. Georgiade, Gregory S. Georgiade, and Ronald Riefkohl, eds., *Aesthetic Surgery of the Breast* **(Philadelphia: W. B. Saunders, 1990), pp. 639–53, here 639.**

34 — Yukio Shirakabe, "The Development of Aesthetic Facial Surgery in Japan: As Seen through a Study of Japanese Pictorial Art," *Aesthetic Plastic Surgery* **14 (1990): 215–221.**

fig. 22

Yoshikiyo Koganei (1858—1944), the Head of Anatomy at the Tokyo Medical School, distinguished the "real" Japanese face from the "primitive" face of the Ainu. The Ainu, originally a hunting and gathering people of northern Honshu, typically had long noses and round eyes. Shown here is an Ainu woman with a tattooed-on beard.
© akg-images

od the ideal form of the face as captured in Japanese traditional portraiture shifted. Traditional portraiture had emphasized the "straight eyes and nose, flat, single eyelids, and receding chin."[34] (fig. 21 & 26) There are specific meanings associated with the oriental eye and nose diametrically opposed to that of the occidental eye and nose. The rather wide variations in the Japanese visage, running from the Japanese visage to that of the Ainu, was evidently idealized as a pan-Japanese face in traditional portraiture. Japanese physicians and anthropologists, such as Yoshikiyo Koganei (1858—1944), the Head of Anatomy Department at the Tokyo Medical School at the end of the 19th century, were obsessed with distinguishing "real" Japanese faces from those of the "primitive" Ainu, a hunting and gathering population of northern Honshu[35]. Central to their concern were the long noses and round eyes of the Ainu— features which had virtually vanished by the late 19th century through intermarriage. In 1990, 20.000 Ainu were considered racially distinct. (fig. 22) While Western scientific medicine was determining the "true" nature of the Japanese visage, Western surgical techniques were making that visage not too Japanese.

In 1923 T. Nishihata and A. Yoshida presented the first study of augmentation rhinoplasty using ivory implants to alter the shape of the Japanese "sunken" nose.[36] Indeed, as traditional, non-surgical medicine was transformed into a subordinate form of Western medicine in Meiji Japan, surgery of the eye-lid and nose became common place signs of the advantages of Western clinical practice. The constitution of a new aesthetic ideal, that of Western art representing the Western face, meant the alteration of the eyelids in order to add the superior palpebral fold between the eyelid and brow which is absent or indistinct in about half the population of Asia. The additional introduction of augmentation rhinoplasty was an innovation which radi-

35 — **Yoshikiyo Koganei**, *Beiträge zur physischen Anthropologie der Aino. I. Untersuchungen am Skelet; II. Untersuchungen am Lebenden. Miteilungen aus der medicinischen Facultät der Kaiserlich-Japanischen Universität zu Tokio* **2 (1893).**

36 — **T. Nishihata and A. Yoshida, "Augmentation Rhinoplasty Using Ivory,"** *Clinical Photography* **7 (1923): 8–10.**

37 — **Frank Dikötter,** *The Discourse of Race in Modern China* **(London: Hurst, 1992).**

38 — **Emiko Ohnuki-Tierney,** *Illness and Culture in Contemporary Japan: An Anthropological View* **(Cambridge: Cambridge University Press, 1984), pp. 51–66.**

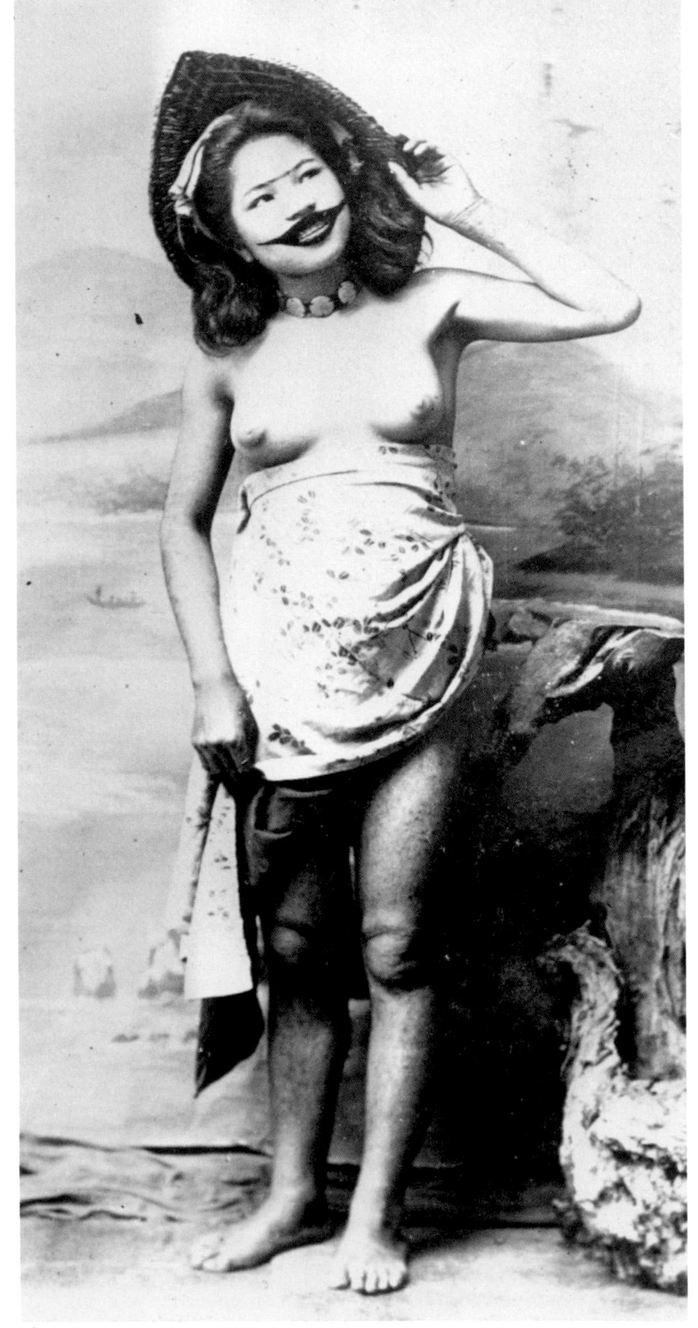

fig. 22

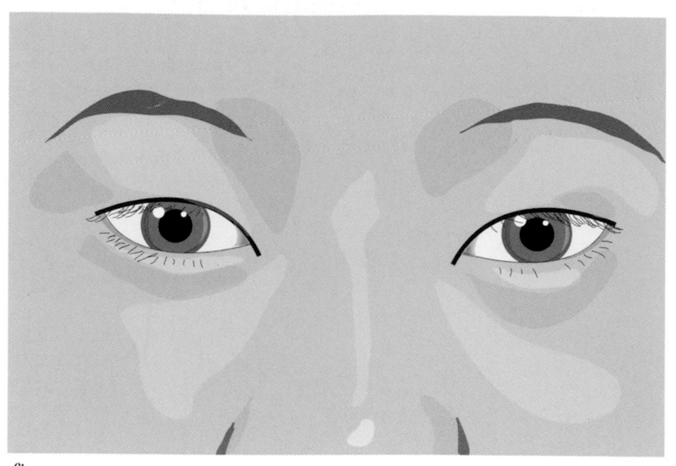

fig. 23

fig. 23

As well as the flat eyelid, the palpebral fold is a typical characteristic of the Asian eye: At the root of the nose, the upper eyelid reaches below the end of the lower eyelid. © Blue Brain Belgium

fig. 24 a+b

Cross-sections of a Western eyelid (left) and an Eastern eyelid (right). The anatomical differences are obvious — for example, the Asian eyelid contains much more skin and fatty tissue. © Blue Brain Belgium

fig. 25 a–c

After the skin, muscle, and fatty tissue are removed, a suture is used to create a new eyelid — giving the Asian eye a more "Western" look. © Blue Brain Belgium

fig. 26

This image of a Japanese woman powdering her neck was produced by Kitagawa Utamaro (1750—1806) in 1795—6. Today, the old traditions no longer offer Japanese women what they want, and they readily talk about their experiences with cosmetic surgery.

cally changed the morphological characteristics of the Japanese face. (fig. 24 a+b, 25 a+b) Following the lines of the Chinese creation of a unified *Han* racial typology in the course of the 19th century, the Japanese created and then reconstituted idealized faces and bodies.[37]

The introduction of aesthetic surgery was likewise in Japan an attempt to cure unhappiness, *jibyo*, that amorphous sense of being unwell that haunts the Japanese medical world.[38] The traditional conception of the individual in *kampo* (traditional) Japanese medicine was one who possessed *taishitsu*, an inborn constitution. Certain constitutions manifested various forms of *jibyo*. Can one alter one's *taishitsu*? Certainly one can intervene through tonics and medicines, but changing one's constitution through aesthetic surgery became possible only when another model, that of Westernized medicine after the Meiji Restoration of 1868, superseded the traditional categories of *kampo* medicine. Unable to open the body, traditional medicine was relegated to second-class status with the Medical Act of 1874, which demanded that all new physicians be trained in Western medicine.[39] Western medicine and surgery were given privileged status to alter and open the body and its *taishitsu*.

Following World War II and the American occupation of Japan, a resurgence of interest in creating "Western" eyes and bodies in Japan led to further developments of such procedures as well as breast augmentation using silicone injections. This responded to the introduction of the Western notion of the larger breast as a sign of the erotic. Traditional Chinese and Japanese portrayals of the female breast, even such as in Kitagawa Utamaro's (1750—1806) 19th-century images of nursing mothers, stress the flat-chested look, which "carried the implication that a woman should be modest in her appearance."[40] As late as 1952 paraffin injections and then in 1958 silicone injections were used for breast augmentation, with devastating nega-

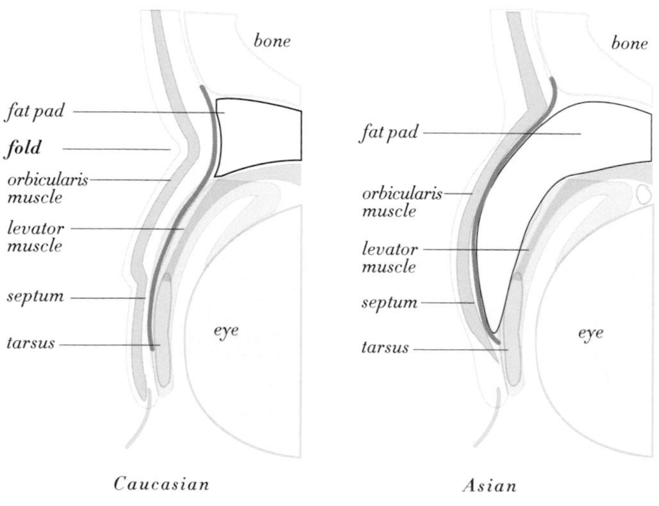

fig. 24 a+b

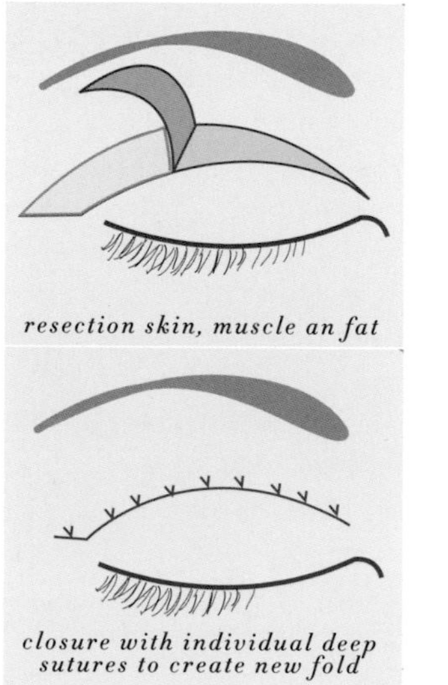

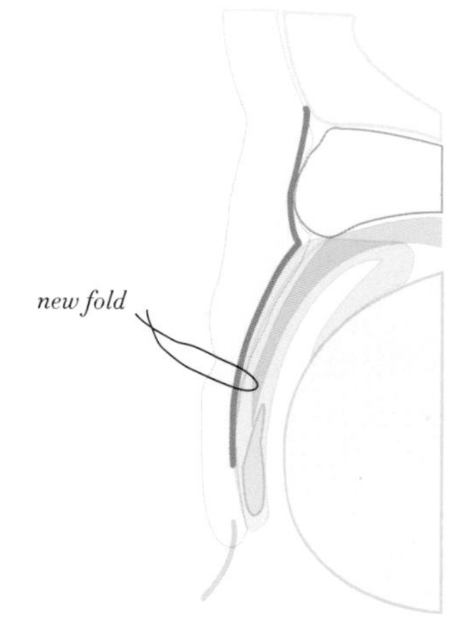

fig. 25 a-c

39 — **Shizu Sakai, "The Impact of Western Medicine and the Concept of Medical Treatment in Japan," in Yoshio Kawakita, Shizu Sakai, Yasuo Otsuka, eds.,** *History of Therapy. Proceedings of the 10th International Symposium on the Comparative History of Medicine — East and West* **(Tokyo: Tanaguchi Foundation, 1990), pp. 157–171.**

40 — **Naoyuki Ohtake and Nobuyuki Shioya, "Aesthetic Breast Surgery in Orientals," in Nicolas G. Georgiade, Gregory S. Georgiade, and Ronald Riefkohl, eds.,** *Aesthetic Surgery of the Breast* **(Philadelphia: W. B. Saunders, 1990), pp. 639–53, here 639.**

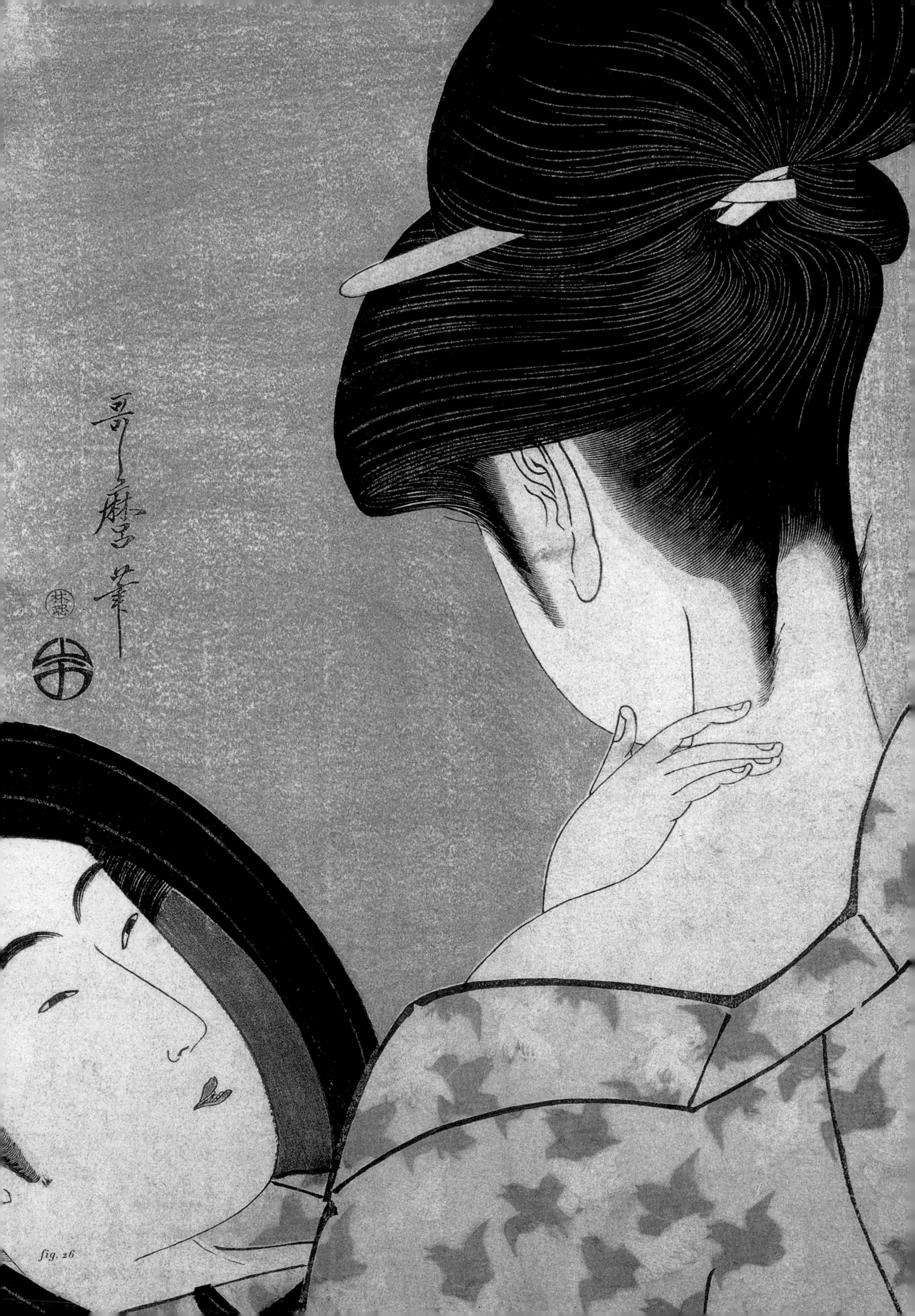

fig. 26

fig. 27

A bus stop in Bangkok. A woman wearing a bandage after rhinoplasty is sharing the bench with two monks. © *laif*

fig. 28

A Chinese woman recovering from an operation to make her eyes look bigger. In Asia, the popularity of cosmetic surgery has extended to include even teenagers: Before the start of a new school year, the clinics and surgery parlours are booked out for weeks. © *sinopix / laif*

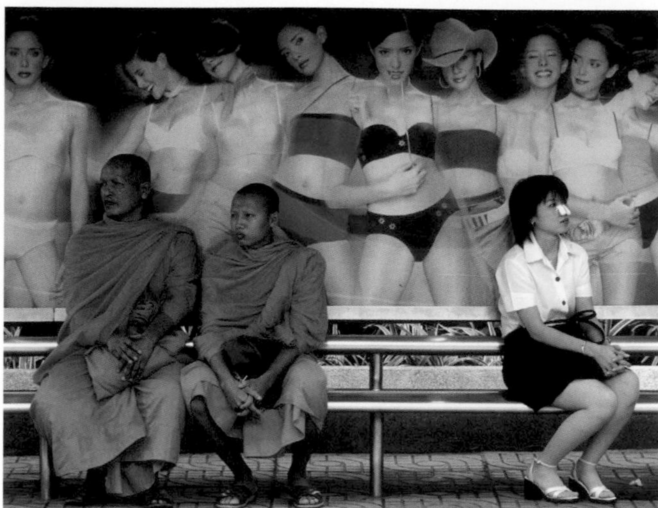

fig. 27

tive results. Taichiro Akiyama actually produced a silicone breast prosthesis as early as 1949.[41] In today's Japan the explosion of interest in aesthetic surgery is related closely to the argument about whether aesthetic surgery can indeed create happiness in banishing the negative *jibyo*. As elsewhere in Asia, the search is not limited to the world of authorized medicine. Thus there are now "aesthetic salons [which] cater to Japanese women seeking a new look, a new face or a new body ... Yet unlike in the past, women who pay for services at these controversial places are not afraid to talk about it. Most seem to believe that cosmetic surgery will open career doors and put a sparkle into their social life."[42] One case report can suffice: "One 22-year-old woman, who asked to be identified only as Mariko, said she had cosmetic surgery six months ago to widen her eyes, lift her nose and chin, and slim her cheeks. She explained that since she was a teenager, she had 'hated' her own face and

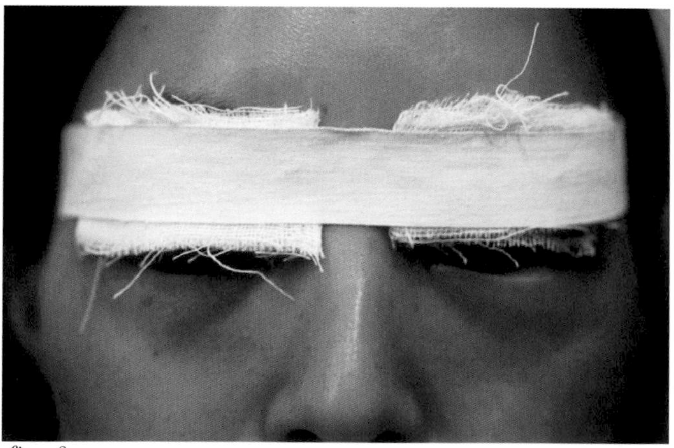

fig. 28

had been working to save money for cosmetic surgery. She put ¥1 million (ca. $ 7300) toward the ¥1.5-million (ca. $ 11000) operation and is paying off the rest in installments. Her decision to go under the knife was also prompted partly by a desire to land a job as a receptionist, and she thought having better looks would improve her chances. After the operation, she promptly got a job. A photograph of her before surgery showed a different woman, at least from the chin up. Some friends complimented her on her new look, but others pointed out the inevitable: beneath the surface, she had not changed. Her father, she claims, did not even notice that she had had surgery." Ichiro Kamoshita, a physician who is the director of the Hibiya Kokusai Clinic, Tokyo believes that women patients "are being duped by cosmetic surgery and aesthetic salon advertising that appeals to a woman's inferiority complex about her looks. Many women believe that if they improve their looks their personal relations with other people will also improve. They are seeking a sense of social achievement while wishing to be lovely as a woman." Nachiko Morikawa, director of another medical clinic, noted that, "they don't have a clear vision of what happiness is." The skeptical attitude of the medical profession mirrors a generation shift of attitude toward aesthetic surgery in Japan. The changes are mirrored to a great extent in not only cultural presuppositions but in the new gender politics. The on-going popularity of aesthetic surgery in Japan has led "an increasing number of Japanese mothers [to] take their straight-A-15-year-old daughters to a cosmetic surgeon"[43] There is now a pattern of presenting procedures as gifts from parents to children, especially those seen to be "hindered by small eyes, a flat nose or a big face." In April and May, at the beginning of the school year, there is a run on aesthetic surgery for teenagers. "It was just amazing to see this many young girls at my clinic all of a sudden. I felt there was something funny going on around mid-March, so I asked my assistant to go through the files. The number [of customers], by the end of the month, had tripled [in

41 — Y. Mutou, "Augmentation Mammaplasty with the Akiyama Prosthesis," *British Journal of Plastic Surgery* 23 (1970): 58–62.

42 — Kyoko Ishimara, "Young Women Turn To Plastic Surgery"; "But Is A New Face Really What They're Looking For?" *The Nikkei Weekly* (December 28, 1992 / January 4, 1993).

43 — Yoshiko Matsushita, "Mama, He's Making Eyes for Me .... And a New Chin," *Asia Times* (May 19, 1997): 1.

44 — One can add that precisely the same scenario can be played out in regard to young men in today's Japan. It seems clear that the shift in attitude toward aesthetic surgery is a generational one. In a recent issue of the teenage magazine *Bart* (March, 10, 1997): 98–103, there was an article on young men in their late teens undergoing cosmetic procedures which cost them as much as ¥ 350,000 (ca. $ 2600) for a nose job and ¥ 300,000 (ca. $ 2200) for an eyelid procedure. This essay, accompanied by before and after photographs, chronicled the masculine drive for happiness through the Western aesthetic alteration of the too Japanese body.

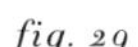

Even Japanese cartoon heroines look like Europeans or Americans — this is the doll-eyed "Princess Knight" from a Manga comic by Osamu Tezuka.
© Tezuka Productions

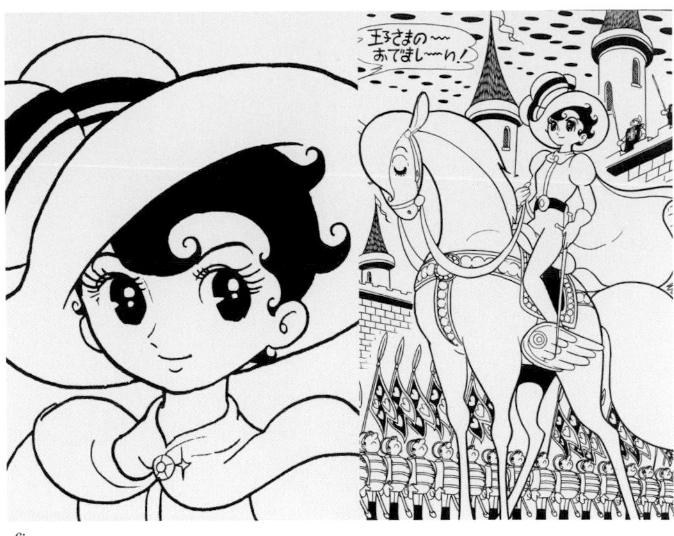

fig. 29

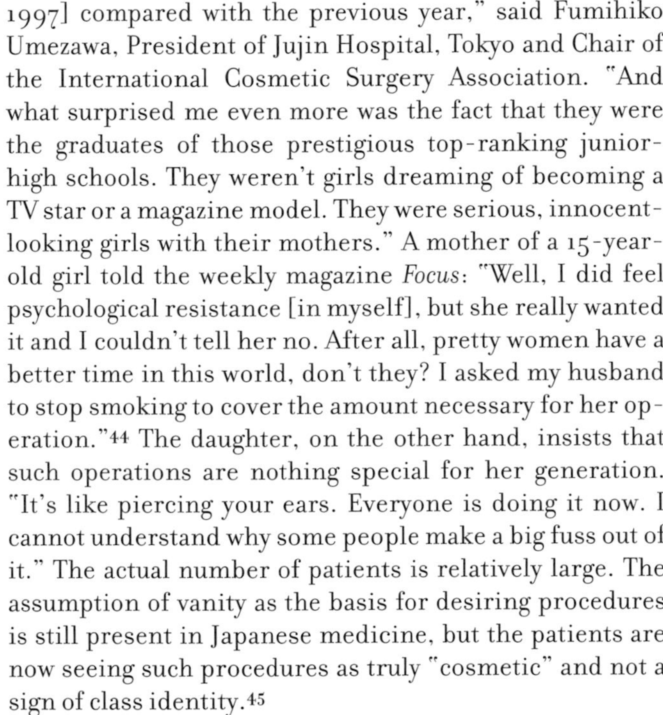

1997] compared with the previous year," said Fumihiko Umezawa, President of Jujin Hospital, Tokyo and Chair of the International Cosmetic Surgery Association. "And what surprised me even more was the fact that they were the graduates of those prestigious top-ranking junior-high schools. They weren't girls dreaming of becoming a TV star or a magazine model. They were serious, innocent-looking girls with their mothers." A mother of a 15-year-old girl told the weekly magazine *Focus*: "Well, I did feel psychological resistance [in myself], but she really wanted it and I couldn't tell her no. After all, pretty women have a better time in this world, don't they? I asked my husband to stop smoking to cover the amount necessary for her operation."[44] The daughter, on the other hand, insists that such operations are nothing special for her generation. "It's like piercing your ears. Everyone is doing it now. I cannot understand why some people make a big fuss out of it." The actual number of patients is relatively large. The assumption of vanity as the basis for desiring procedures is still present in Japanese medicine, but the patients are now seeing such procedures as truly "cosmetic" and not a sign of class identity.[45]

Political Power: Vietnam's Face and Body Imagery

Body imagery follows the lines of political and cultural power. In Vietnam, after the American withdrawal in 1973 and the reunification of the country, a detailed physiognomic study determined the relative facial dimensions of the Vietnamese so as to provide an adequate, non-Westernizing model for the relationship among the features, including the form and shape of the eyes, for aesthetic surgeons.[46] This was clearly in response to the explosion in aesthetic surgery, which remade the faces and breasts of the young women of Vietnam into "Western" faces and bodies. While there was a lively aesthetic surgery industry in Saigon until 1975, it virtually vanished after the end of the war.

In contemporary Vietnam, the function of aesthetic surgery has become normalized. Indeed, in reports from Hanoi, even the criminals are claimed to undergo aesthetic surgery.[47] The nose and the eye remain at the center of concern with the reconstitution of the face in today's Vietnam. "It is the opposite of the Europeans," Nguyen Huy Phan, one of the leading aesthetic surgeons in Hanoi stated to an interviewer, "Here plastic surgery increases the size of the nose, Europeanizing it. We make a superior double eyelid, with a groove, to give a livelier appearance and to awaken the glance."[50] The costs of such procedures are quite low. To have a nose rebuilt in Hanoi costs about $100, "westernizing" the eyelids, $40. Such procedures, however, are no assurance of successful transformation of the psyche. "We only operate when it's reasonable, otherwise we have to send them to the psychiatrist," Nguyen Huy Phan said.

Today in Ho Chi Minh City (formerly Saigon) there are a dozen mini-clinics, sometimes masquerading as barber shops and staffed by lay surgeons. Their patrons are most often men. Clinic owners say that the most popular operations are for the nose, chin, the eyes, and the buttocks. One

45 — The physiognomy of the contemporary *manga* (and the *anime*, the animated film), however, is rooted in the animated work of Osamu Tezuka (1928–1989) from the 1950s. Influenced by American animated cartoons, such as those of Walt Disney, Tezuka "developed some of the characteristics of *manga* ... noting that he drew the princess with big, round eyes in exotic, foreign settings." ("Manga's Appeal not Limited to Japanese Fans," *The Daily Yomiuri* [December 11, 1996]: 3; see also Frederik L. Schodt, *Manga! Manga! The World of Japanese Comics* [Tokyo: Kodansha, 1986].) In post-war Japan such de-racialized ("Western") eyes came to be representative of the physiognomy of the *manga* and were read as a way of imagining a new, exotic, and happy body. The *manga* in this tradition (especially those for girls) have depicted the characters as outrageously Western. This is certainly related to the modern tradition of the "girls' opera" (known as *Takarazuka*, after a city near Osaka) which represents a fictional Western (actually nowhere) world with an all-female cast (with the male characters played by the young actresses.) Takarazuka presents a world analogous to the occidentalist girls' comics in Japan with "neutral" (read: Western) physiognomies. Recently there have appeared very "Japanese" *manga* and *anime*, such as those by Katsuhiro Otomo. His best known work is *Akira*, a near-future science fiction where Japanese characters are depicted with Japanese eyes.

46 — Le Gia Vinh, "Study of Facial Dimensions in Vietnamese Young People: their Application into Aesthetic and Plastic Surgery," *Anthropologie* 27 (1988): 113–5.

47 — Nguyen Man Phuong, "Vietnam: As Confucianism and Socialism Erode, Crime Thrives," *Inter Press Service* (October 1, 1996).

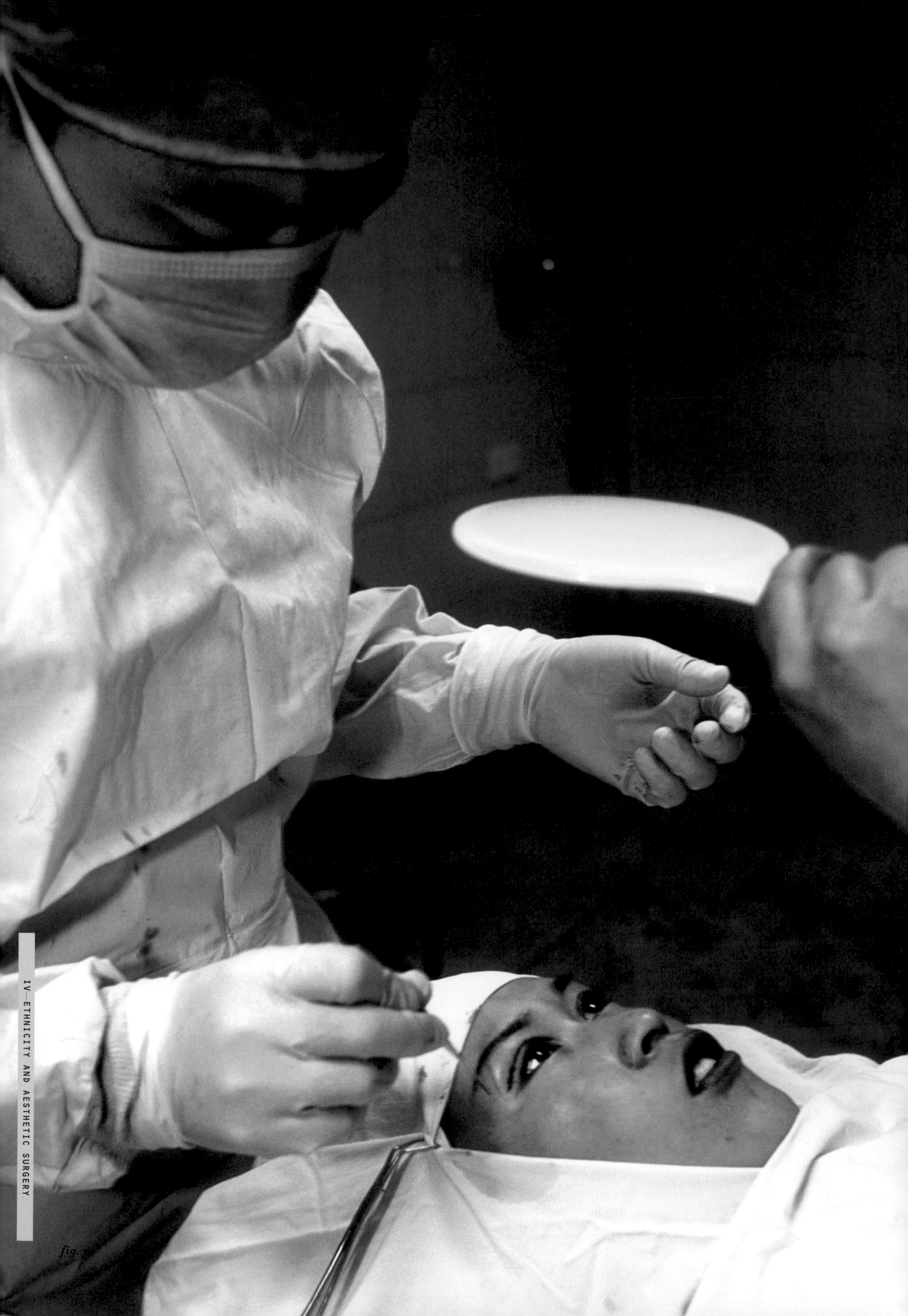

fig. 3

fig. 30

In China, the era of aesthetic surgery didn't begin until after the death of Mao Tse-tung in 1976. Before long, the most popular procedure was the augmentation rhinoplasty — a procedure where a bone graft harvested from the hip or a rib is implanted in the nose. © sinopix / laif

fig. 31 & 32

Blepharoplasty is also in great demand in China — with a Westernized look, the Chinese hope for better job and marriage prospects. © sinopix / laif

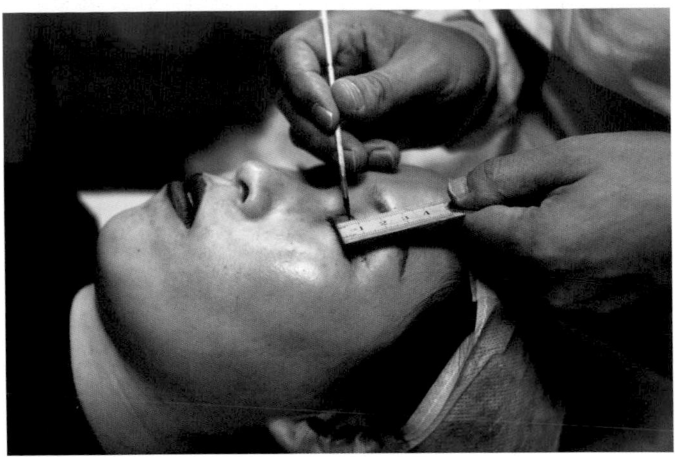

fig. 31

man even asked surgeons to bulk up his chest, which he believed would make him more attractive to women. A popular operation in southern Vietnam, too, is to have the eyes widened by creating the Western eyelid (the superior palpebral fold). Such procedures are especially popular

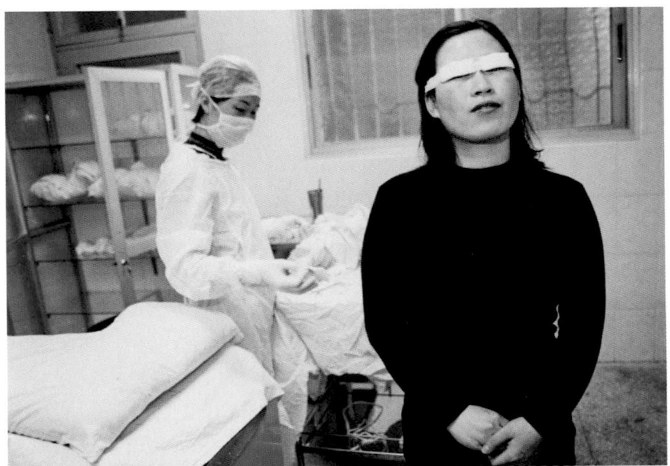

fig. 32

with male stage performers. Nguyen Thu Huong, who owns one of the "beauty salons," claimed that 80% of the young performers of a popular drama style known as *cai luong* have had this procedure done and some singers have paid her a visit for Westernizing procedures.[48]

The New Chinese Capitalist and Aesthetic Surgery

The function which aesthetic surgery has as a marker of the shift to a market economy with its claims of individual autonomy (as opposed to state control) can also be measured in the People's Republic of China with the liberalization after the death of Mao Tse-tung. Ruyao Song, former President of the Chinese Plastic Surgery Society, noted in 1994 that "altering eyelids is the most popular cosmetic surgery practiced at [my] Institute of Plastic Surgery in Peking, which with 400 beds is among the largest plastic surgery hospitals in the world."[49] The explosion of interest in aesthetic surgery in the People's Republic is to no little degree a sign of the increasing affluence of the general population. It has fueled an explosion of "beauty parlours [which] offer cheap cosmetic surgery promising miraculous outcomes but often mutilating their customers."[50] Ten cosmetic surgery parlours were set up in Shanghai in the early months of 1996, but when 800 beauty parlours opened in Sichuan province's capital city, Chengdu, in a year the municipality began to try and regulate them after numerous patient complaints.[51] In the southeastern city of Shenzhen a "quack" named Hu Jinsong performed breast augmentation surgery in 1995 and 1996.[52] According to his account, he used a "sophisticated and top quality" procedure, which removed body fat by liposuction and injected it into the breasts. This was supposed to reduce obesity while enhancing breast size. "The operation is simple," the ads said. "There is no hospitalization or scars and the surgery does not affect normal life and work afterwards." His patients wound up hospitalized when the procedures went horribly awry. Hu had gone to university but had no medical credentials. The most popular aesthetic surgical procedures in these new clinics are the "double eyelid operation" and nose-bridge surgery, in which a bone graft is shaved from a patient's hip or rib to augment the existing nose. Unlike at the Institute of Plastic Surgery, aesthetic surgery in these establishments is undertaken by marginally qualified or unqualified practitioners. Even though China's cabinet-level State Council has recently put beauty parlours under the management of public health departments, abuses continue to mount. The local hospitals also participate in the beauty business as hospital beauty centre do not need to even register with local industry and commerce administrative departments. Aesthetic surgical procedures to modify the Chinese eye had been widely carried

48 — Le Thang Long, "Vietnamese Men line up for a Nip and Tuck," *Agence France Presse* (June 7, 1996).

49 — Dean Lokken, "Doctor Says Cosmetic Surgery Makes Gains In China," *U. S. News & World Report* (October 17, 1994).

50 — "Blinded woman Sues Beauty Parlor," *U. P. I.* (October 14, 1996, BC cycle).

51 — Alison Dakota Gee "The Price of Beauty," *Asiaweek* (August 2, 1996): 38.

52 — *United Press International* (May 1, 1996, BC cycle).

fig. 33–36

To conform to the Western look as much as possible, some Chinese people even get their legs surgically extended. In this complex procedure, an artificial epiphysis is created and the leg is stretched to extend by eight to ten centimetres. In some cases, an extension of up to 16 centimetres has been reached. The X-ray images (34 and in the background of 36) show a leg before and during the procedure. © sinopix / laif (34, 35), Zed Nelson / IPG / Katz / Studio X (33, 36)

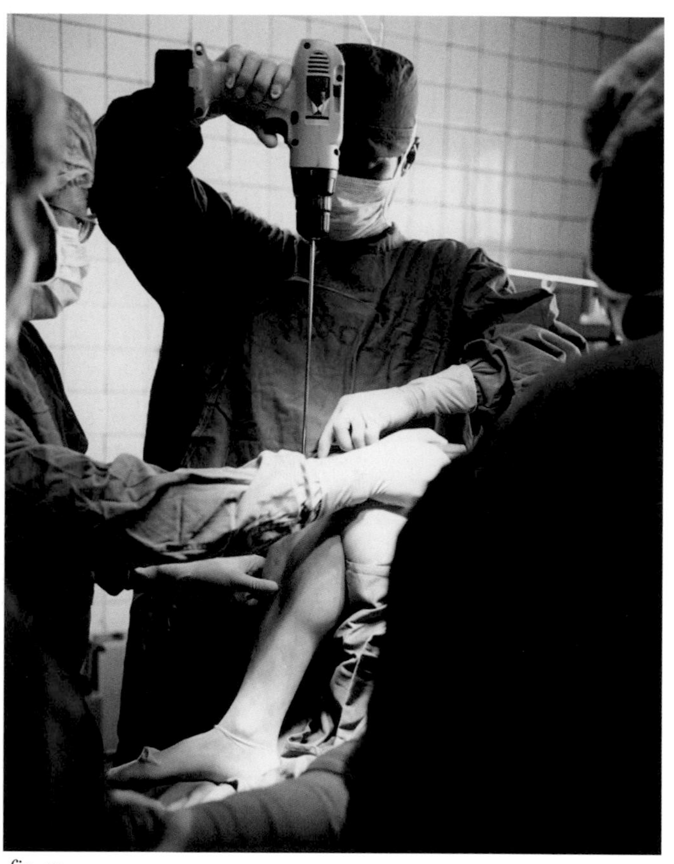

fig. 33

out elsewhere among Chinese communities in Asia. Khoo Boo-Chai is the Singaporean surgeon who developed the modern double eyelid modification about 40 years ago in the midst of the American occupation of Japan and the Korean War. He stitched along the eyelid to create a fine line of scars, which provided the appearance of a supratarsal fold. He wrote in 1963 that: "Our Eastern sisters put on Western apparel, use Western make-up, see Western movies and read Western literature.
Nowadays, there even exists a demand for the face and especially the eyes to be Westernized."[53] The specific reason for such aesthetic surgical procedures was the ability to increase one's income or marriagability by looking more Western and thus to insure personal happiness.[54] In Beijing today Zhou Xiaoling, one of the chief plastic surgeons in the Chinese capital, increases the size of Lang Wenyu's nose. She is a slight 26-year-old woman who "wants to become beautiful" so that she can "find a boyfriend." And you do that by looking like the "modern" Chinese models you see in magazines and television. This is not limited to younger Chinese women: "If I have a bigger nose, I think I will find a wife," said Wen Biao who is 26. "I already have a good job. My family thinks it's a great idea," he added, pointing out that his mother did not begin to wear makeup until the 1980s, when she was past 50, because of worries that she would be criticized as bourgeois. "They're all interested in bigger noses."[55] The new Chinese capitalist looks like the Westerner — and therefore is the better citizen of his or her new country.

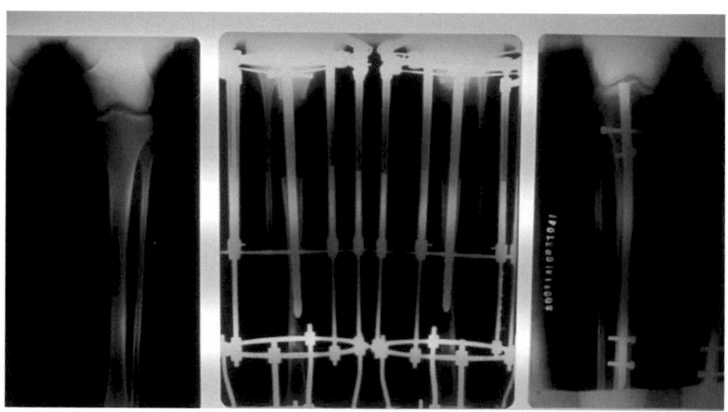

fig. 34

Asian-Americans: Flexibility of Identities

The Asian development of aesthetic surgery as a sign of the modern is paralleled by the focus on the alteration of the body among the new immigrants labeled by American census law as Asian-Americans. Thus among Vietnamese in the United States a similar fascination with the newest and latest developments in aesthetic surgery exists. The fascination with skin lightening, nose lengthening, and eye reshaping in Japan and Vietnam today reflects the globalization of standards of beauty rooted in Euro-American stereotypes. In the case of the youth of Japan and Vietnam,

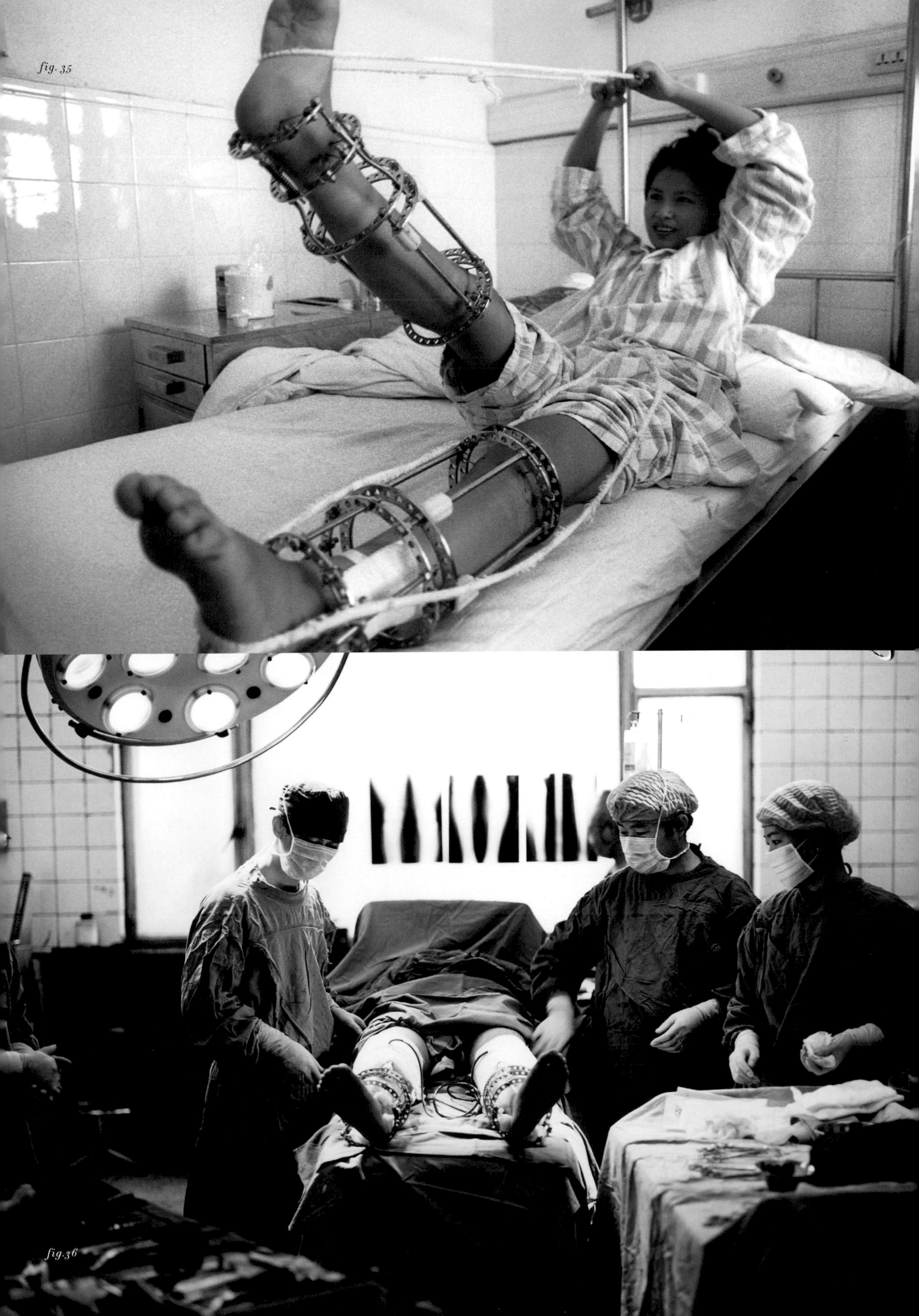

fig. 35

fig. 36

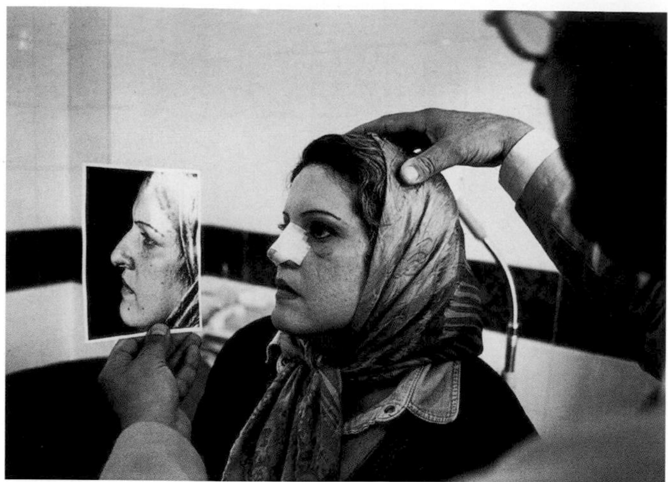

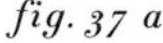

fig. 37 a

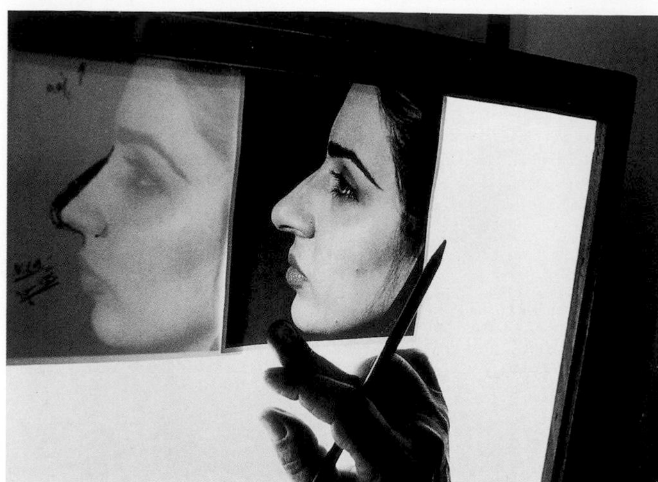

fig. 37 b

the ideal is not to be "too Asian." In the United States, this desire is more directly shaped by the notion of fitting into a niche of an acceptable American physiognomy. As with many of the ethnic specific procedures, they are undertaken by ethnic surgeons who would more fully appreciate their patients' desired outcome. A parallel development can be found in The Republic of Korea (South Korea) which has the largest single group (430) of aesthetic surgeons to be found in Asia in the 1990s.[56] The alterations of the nose and eyelid have become a major source of income for the physicians of the new economies of Asia. With the movement of Korea on to the global scene during the 1980s, the globalization of Korean advertising brought images of the Western face into the culture as part of the new middle-class ideal. In the United States, Korean Americans, like other groups of new immigrants, began to offer eyelid surgery to their teenage children "to make their eyes look 'more American.'"[57] Such ideals seem less present in Korea (or Vietnam or Japan) among the middle class. There aesthetic surgery is a sign of middle class rather than American identity, though one could argue that there is a fatal parallelism between these two ideas of imagining oneself as different. Thus among Asian-Americans in California double eyelid surgery has become "the gift that parents offer their daughters when they graduate from high school or college."[58] This parallels the experience of Jewish Americans in the 1960s. For the Vietnamese and Koreans in America, aesthetic surgery becomes a means of defining the flexibility of identity as opposed to its permanence.

The Covered Body: The Importance of Noses in Iran

It is not merely acculturation that determines how we want to be seen. In a culture in which the body is mostly clothed and the face is covered but for the nose, nose jobs are big business. "It just like women's clothing — things go in and out of fashion," said Ali Akbar Jalali, a leading plastic surgeon in Tehran who spent the summer getting laser training in Cleveland. "And what's in fashion right now is getting the nose done. After that come facelifts. Only a small percentage of women want body work because there are so few opportunities in Iran to see women's bodies. No seashore, no swimming pools — except for women only. So if women do body work, it's for their husbands. The face is really the only part that can be seen." Today in Theran Ali Akbar Jalali will make women more beautiful for $1000, an enormous sum in contemporary Iran. He, like all surgeons, uses a variant of Jacques Joseph's procedures. As one of the mothers of a patient said: "We did her nose so she could become more beautiful and enjoy her face for the rest of her life. I could see that she had a flaw in her face, and I was very glad we could get rid of it." Another young woman has a computer image of herself that her fiancé had made for the doctor — with red hair and blue eyes and without the bump on her long nose.[59] Two Turkish sisters, one living in Berlin, the other in Istanbul, both have their noses redone. The first because she wants to look "less Turkish" in her new home; the second, because she wants to look more Western in a world threatened by fundamentalism, which has a very specific "face."

53 — Khoo Boo-Chai, "Plastic Construction of the Superior Palpebral Fold," *Plastic and Reconstructive Surgery* 31 (1963): 74. See also his "Augmentation Rhinoplasty in the Orientals," *Plastic and Reconstructive Surgery* 34 (1964): 81.

54 — The beautiful as it is understood in contemporary Chinese culture remains the symmetrical. Indeed, it defines the beautiful for the clinical practice of aesthetic surgery. See X. Wang and Z. Zhang, "[Three Dimensional Analysis of the Facial Lateral Region with Beautiful Appearance of Chinese and its Clinical Value]," *Chung-Hua Kou Chiang i Hsueh Tsa Chih / Chinese Journal of Stomatology* 30 (1995): 131–3, 191. The search for happiness comes to be the search for the beauty present in the perceived symmetry of the Western face or at least of the Asian face now reconfigured as neither Western nor too Oriental. Naree Krajang, a Thai jazz singer, who had fat removed from her upper eyelids to make them look rounder and a nasal implant inserted in her "too small" nose, stated that "Westerners have perfect figures, beautiful faces and shapes ... We want to be beautiful, like foreigners." (Shiela McNulty, "Asians Bear the Knife for Western Look," *San Jose Mercury News* (February 21, 1995]: A: 1.) The foreigners, by implication, are truly happy, but would everyone want to be able to cross that border into the world of the beautiful, the happy, the healthy, and the well-to-do?

55 — John Pomfret, "Chinese Aspire to the 'Big Nose' Look," *The Washington Post* (January 11, 1999).

56 — Steve Glain, "Cosmetic Surgery Goes Hand in Glove With the New Korea," *Wall Street Journal* (November 23, 1993): A1.

57 — Elaine T. Matsushita, "Americans, Too. For Asian Americans, As For Other Minorities, Full Assimilation into the American Mainstream is a Bittersweet Process," *Chicago Tribune* (April 29, 1992): C6.

fig. 37 a+b

In Iran, women cover up their bodies when in public — their face is the only part that can be seen. The most popular cosmetic procedure is therefore the rhinoplasty, a lucrative business for Iranian doctors and surgeons. © Zed Nelson / IPG / Katz / Studio X

fig. 39

Many Iranian girls are sent into the operating theatre by their mothers. The corrected nose is meant to grant them a happy life — at the side of a good husband. © Zed Nelson / IPG / Katz / Studio X

fig. 38

Teheran surgeon Ali Akbar Jalali bases his techniques on the methods of Jacques Joseph (1865—1934). His patients pay around a thousand dollars for getting a new nose and a perfect facial silhouette — a considerable sum of money in contemporary Iran. © Zed Nelson / IPG / Katz / Studio X

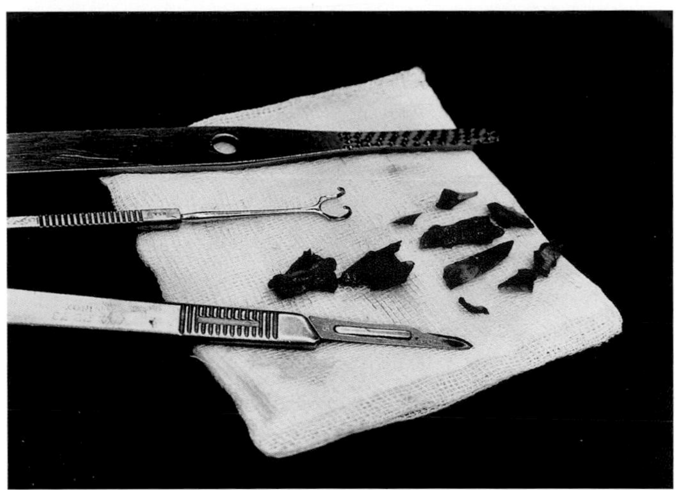

fig. 38

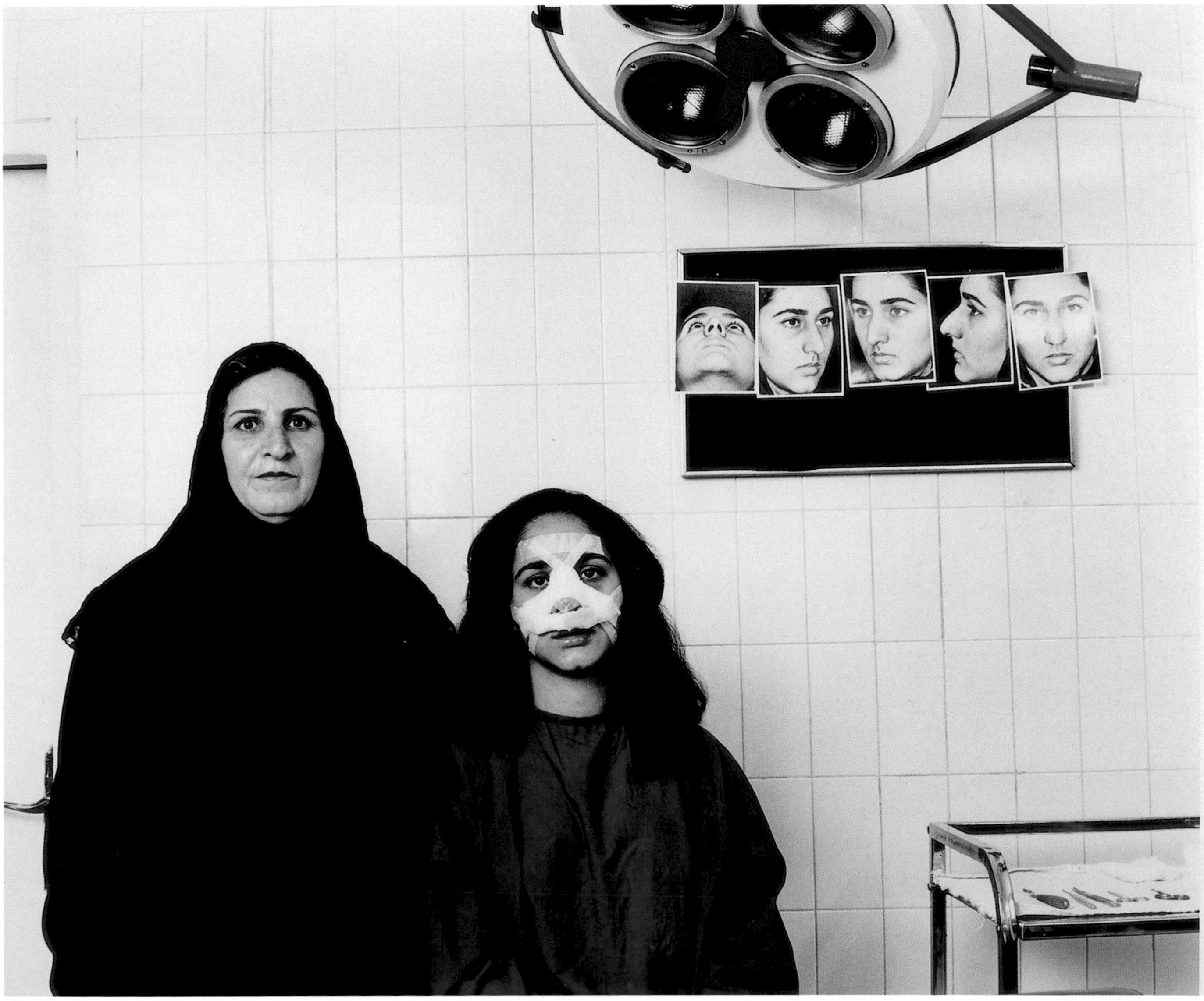

fig. 39

fig. 40

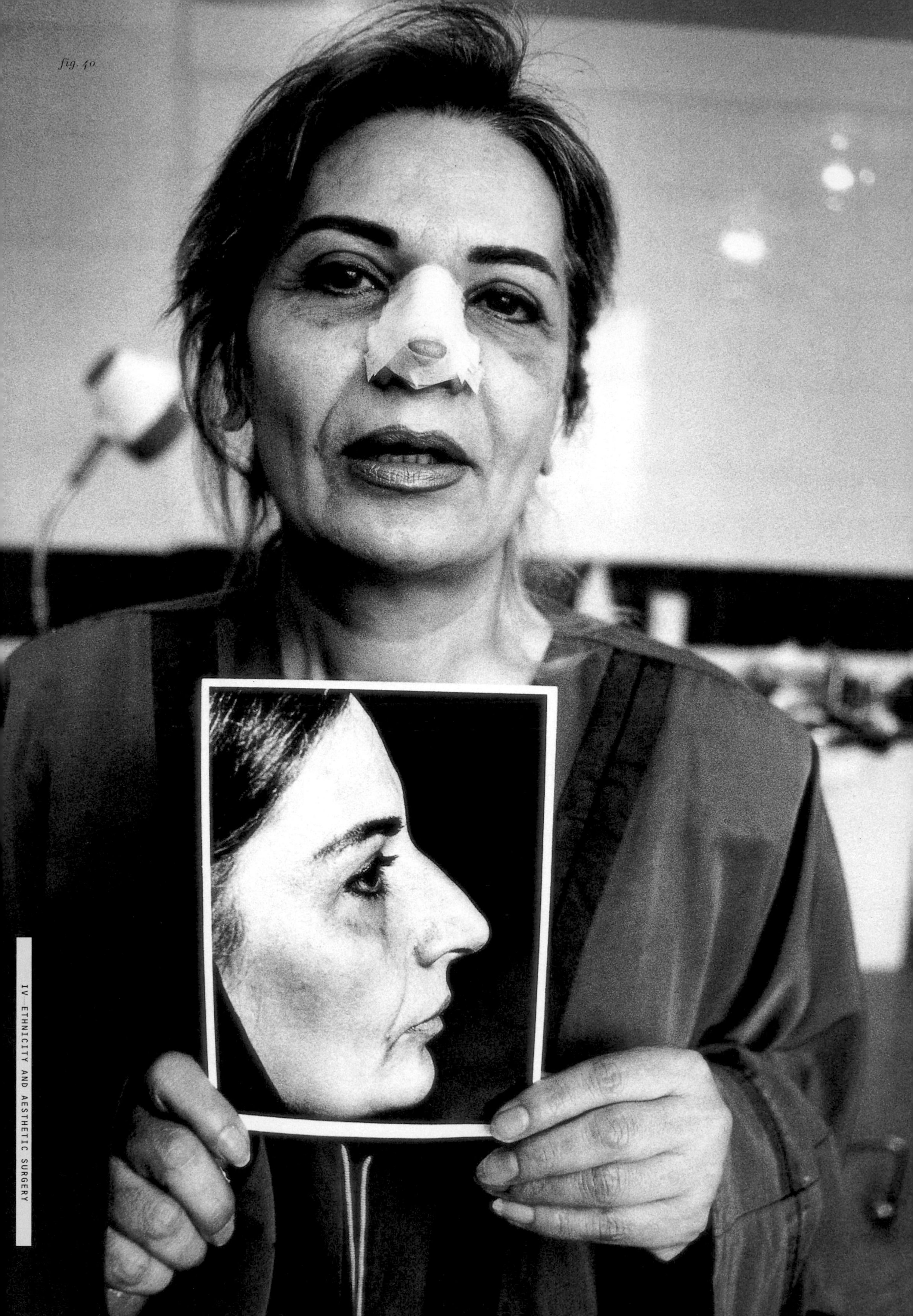

fig. 40

For Iranian women, especially those spending prolonged periods of time in the Western world, a new nose is also an expression of their political and religious views. They don't want their first impression to be one that suggests fundamentalism — which for many Westerners has a stereotypical face.

fig. 41 a+b & 42 a+b

Two examples of reduction rhinoplasties performed on African-Americans. It remains an ongoing subject of discussion if procedures such as these should be regarded like any other aesthetic surgical correction, or if they are inseparable from their ethnic implications. Source: Steven M. Hoefflin, Ethnic Rhinoplasty, Springer Verlag New York, 1998

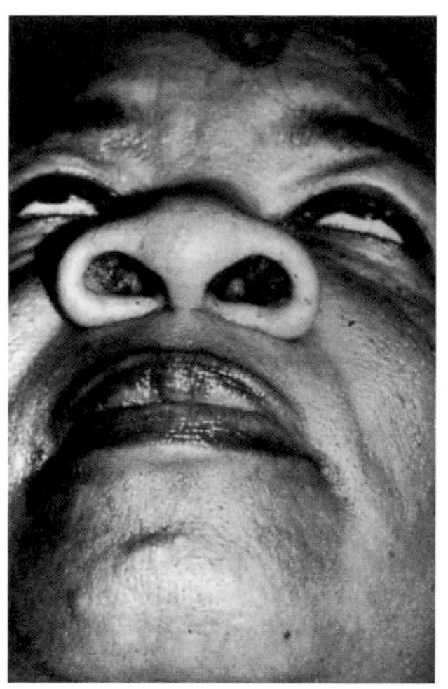

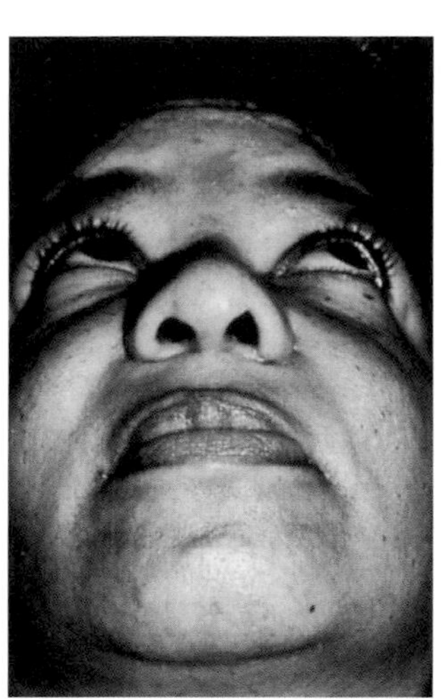

fig. 41 a+b

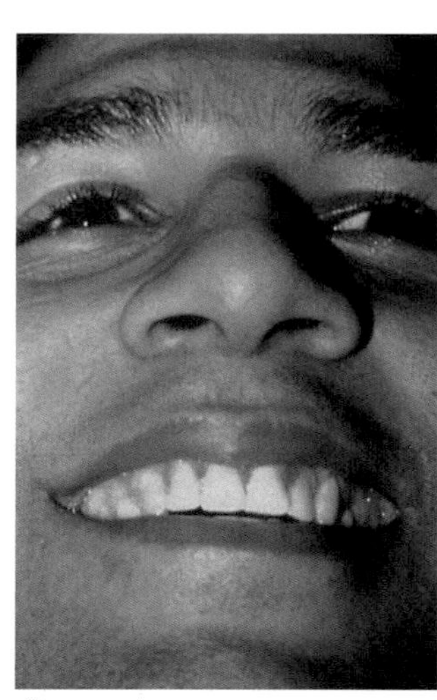

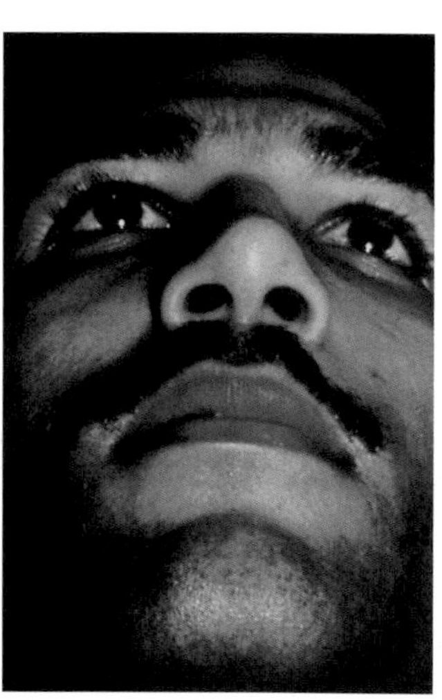

fig. 42 a+b

Ethnic Identity and the Globalization

Like them, Jacques Joseph's patients became "German" at least in their own perception through the alteration of the shape of their noses. Thus Joseph's patients passed into German society. They desired to forget their bodies, to become one with those they imagined to have no worries about the acceptability of their bodies. Whether they succeeded or not, they at least tried to do so. This is the essence of "passing" and it sets the model for a radical rethinking of how we imagine our bodies as responding to our desires to pass. Over the past two decades aesthetic surgeons have been advocating surgery not to obliterate ethnic identity but, as in many of the cases above, to ameliorate it. "My nose is just a nose, not a symbol of my racial identity," says Joseph, an African-American man who recently sought surgery to have his nose narrowed. "The procedure gave me a stronger, more refined nose but maintains an authentic Afro-American appearance." Keisha, who had a lip reduction procedure and a chin implant, agrees. "White people don't hesitate to seek facial plastic surgery to improve their appearance," she asserts. "Why should I hold back simply because I'm African-American? I'm proud of my heritage. I just wanted to look better and feel more confident about my appearance."[63] It is fine to argue that black (or Jewish or Irish or Chinese) is beautiful but one does not want to be too black, or Jewish or Irish or Chinese. Ethnicity is no longer a blemish as long as it is not too pronounced. The tensions between the global standards of beauty that are mid-Pacific or mid-Atlantic still exist. The development of global standards of beauty make it more rather than less likely that aesthetic surgery will be employed to achieve these goals. Today the goal is as much to become a citizen of the new global culture as to become a citizen of any given nation.

58 — **Laura Accinelli, "Eye of the Beholder,"** *Los Angeles Times* **(January 23, 1996): E1.**
59 — **Elaine Sciolino, "In Iran, a Hot Market for Nose Jobs,"** *The New York Times* **(September 22, 2000).**
60 — **"Facial Plastic Surgery Enhances Ethnic Features,"** *Facial Plastic Surgery Today* **10 (1996): 1.**

fig. 43

Is it possible to "think" white and "act" black or vice versa? David LaChapelle's photographic manipulations are titled "Make-Over (Surgery Story)." © David LaChapelle, New York

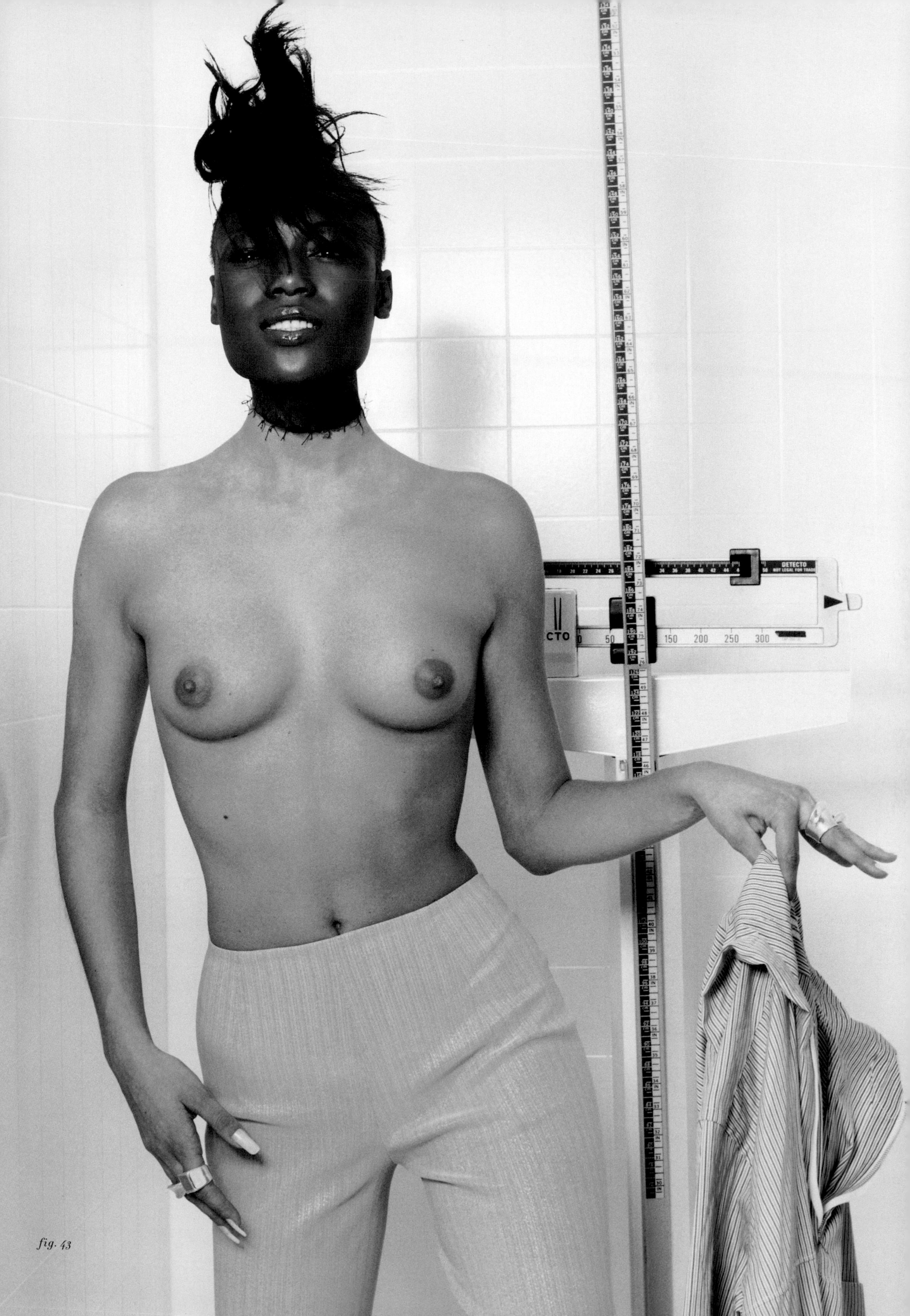

fig. 43

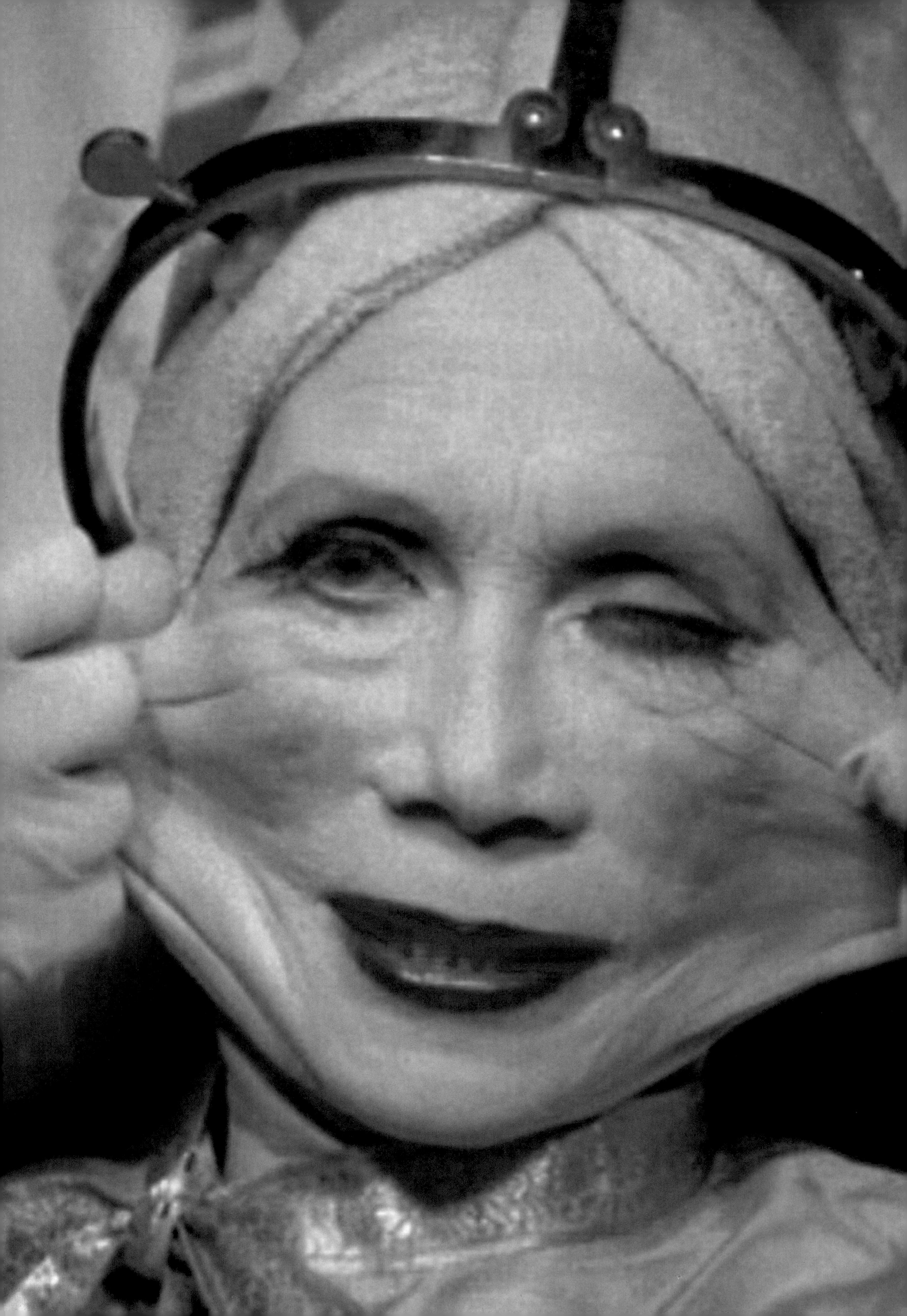

V.

PLASTIC SURGERY IN THE MOVIES

Text by

JUERGEN MUELLER

Plastic Surgery in the Movies

JUERGEN MUELLER, Dresden

Modern men and women are prisoners — prisoners caged by time and thought. To escape the inevitable restrictions of our earthly existence, we have managed to create a number of diversions, albeit temporary ones. Among the most striking and effective of these are cinema — and plastic surgery. As different as the two may seem at first glance, they in fact have plenty in common: both transcend ordinary reality, both can turn back the clock, both pretend to elude the inevitabilities of life and mortality. The perfect embodiment of both is the film star — a person who never ages once captured on celluloid, living on in our imagination unaltered. The stars present us with a taste of eternity, and gratefully we let them live on in our memories.

It thus comes as no surprise that the subject of plastic surgery comes up time and again in cinema and is taken as an opportunity to engage in self-reflection. Of course, a fair portion of irony is involved when such self-reflection becomes entertainment, and in film, the idea of plastic surgery has more often than not been a source of mockery, fear and criticism. Few are the directors who have seriously attempted to give us a complex perspective on plastic and aesthetic surgery and its role in society, respectively presenting it as a medical necessity or an opportunity for social invention. In most cases, the theme is a means to an end — it is used to dramatise or reflect on the essence of identity, typically in the context of symbolising the decadence of modern society.

Plastic surgery made an early entrance into film history, first appearing as a popular subject in gangster films, thrillers and horrors. A gender-specific attribution of the topic can be noted from the start: the women usually need to be made more beautiful, whereas the men "only" need a new identity. The new face serves as a mask or disguise for criminals and fugitives, allowing them to pass through the world unrecognised and escape the seemingly inescapable. The operation itself may well be included in the narrative explicitly, or treated as a "blind spot". In this case we only find out about the surgery indirectly, which can provide additional dramatic tension.

In an attempt to trace an iconography, the following chapter will present a number of examples from film history that address the topic of aesthetic or facial surgery. How are the operations depicted? How do the characters experience them? And what image is created of the cosmetic surgeon? In short — how is aesthetic surgery judged by these films?

Interior and Exterior

In William Wyler's *Dead End* (1937), the surgeon's scalpel opens a doorway to the protagonist's past. After having undergone facial surgery (the operation itself precedes the film's narrative), "Babyface" Martin, a gangster, returns to New York, the setting of his youth. As an anonymous stranger, he now has the chance to meet his mother and teenage love afresh. It soon becomes apparent that this hardened criminal — whose nickname no longer suits his mask-like, motionless face — will never be able to escape his true identity. His mother condemns his past deeds and rejects him, and his erstwhile lover has become a prostitute. While a face can be operated on, time cannot be reversed.

The theme of aesthetic surgery is commonly intermingled with the issue of personal identity; the face plays a crucial role in this, acting as both the proof and the expression of a personality. In this context, a look in the mirror brings with it the question of identity, of whether inside and outside still correspond. The face both displays and conceals the person's interplay of exterior and interior, of outward appearance and true character. The look in the mirror is thus a central allegory in many of the films. By perceiving its mirror image, the figure will find its identity reflected, or know that it has changed forever. The mirror is an ambiguous reflection of the truth — it shows both the identity gained and the identity lost – the latter is more likely to be the case.

In George Cukor's *A Woman's Face* (1941), the protagonist Anna Holm (Joan Crawford), rejects and forbids any type of mirror within her house. Her face is disfigured by a scar — viewed from the right angle, however, her stunning beauty is still apparent. This symbolises the Janus-faced personality of this character. Initially, the embittered woman is presented to us as a ruthless blackmailer who finds it difficult to display any human qualities at all. This changes

fig. previous pages

Aesthetic surgery as art performance: in Terry Gilliam's futurist fantasy Brazil *the high society does not collect art anymore – rather, the ladies have turned themselves inter objects of art with competing surgeons waging a bizarre concourse.*

fig. 1

At the beginning of his career, Humphrey Bogart was frequently typecast as the bad guy. William Wyler's Dead End *(1937) stars Bogart as the gangster "Babyface" Martin. Martin has forced a surgeon to change his facial features, and for the first time since his youth, he visits his mother...*

fig. 2

... who promptly slaps him in the face when he reveals his true identity. To her, the new face symbolises the ruthless thug Martin has become. Any remaining ties to his childhood are now irrevocably severed.

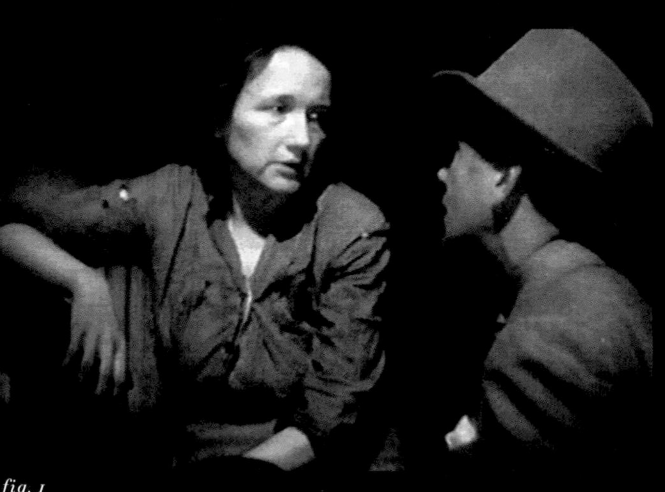

fig. 1

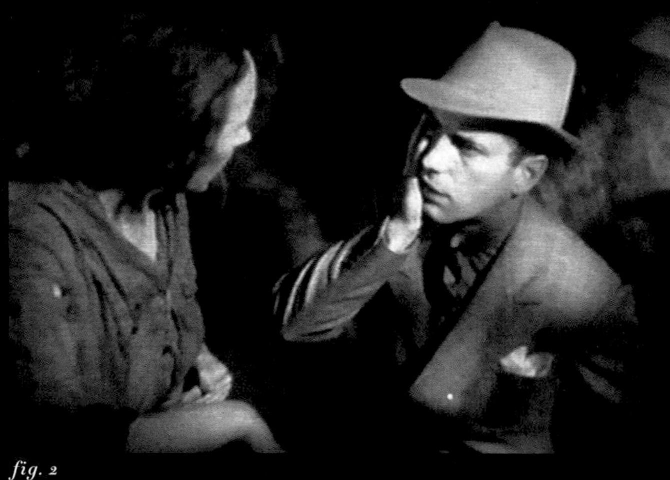

fig. 2

when the aesthetic surgeon Dr. Gustaf Segert (Melvyn Douglas), offers to help her. This character is an exception to the usual depiction of the aesthetic surgeon in films of the time. Here, he is a true benefactor, able and willing to change the lives of the disfigured and outcast. What his patients make of the second chance given to them, however, is ultimately beyond his control. "I will create a monster," he says to Anna before her operation, "with a beautiful face and a heart of stone."

Initially, Anna is entirely under the destructive influence of her lover, the first man she had ever felt accepted by despite her disfigurement. Out of greed, he incites her to pose as a nanny and murder a young boy. The message of this film is unusual for the iconography of the topic: Anna was made evil not only by her accident, but also by her superficial, appearance-focused environment. The operation helps her finally to become herself.

In one of the key scenes, Cukor masterfully shows how this finding of identity is a process both interior and exterior. When Anna — and with her the camera — looks to the surgeon for a reaction after the operation, his eyes are devoid of any emotion. She is handed a mirror but we merely see the back of the mirror, not her face. It is only *she* who knows if she has become a different person, if the exterior change has indeed affected a corresponding change in character.

A different, arguably opposite approach to the identity issue is presented by Frank Capra's *Arsenic and Old Lace* (1944). This comedy shows us that failed attempts to disguise a personality with an artificial face can also be a humorous affair. It presents us with a typical example of the clichéd caricature of plastic surgeons prevalent in many early films.

Surgeon Dr. Einstein (Peter Lorre), is a drunkard. Even his name is a joke on serious science. The character displays overtones of the "mad scientist" stereotype, which are enforced by Dr. Einstein's German ancestry and his doctoral title, supposedly gained in Heidelberg.

As a result of the doctor practicing his arts whilst intoxicated, his buddy Jonathan (Raymond Massey) is horribly disfigured. When the two thugs, the police hot on their heels, break into the house of Jonathan's aunts carrying a dead body, the negative effects of the botched operation become apparent immediately. The aunts don't recognise their nephew but are quick to tell him that they know his face from the movies — Frankenstein's monster! And the first thing Jonathan's much-despised brother Mortimer (Cary Grant) asks him upon seeing him is "Where'd you get that face? Hollywood?" The change of identity has obviously failed; the patient's true character is not disguised, but rather emphasised by the operation. The idea that surgery is a shady business is not only suggested by the clichéd

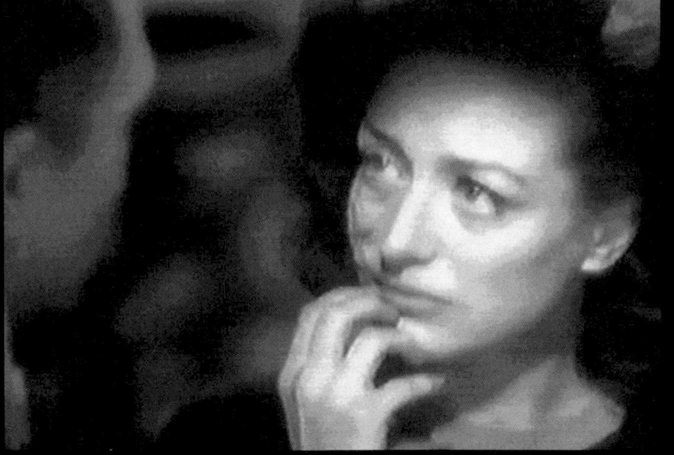

fig. 3

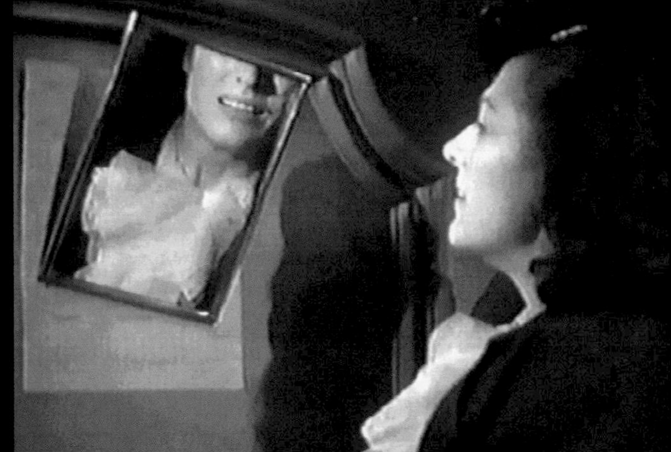

fig. 4

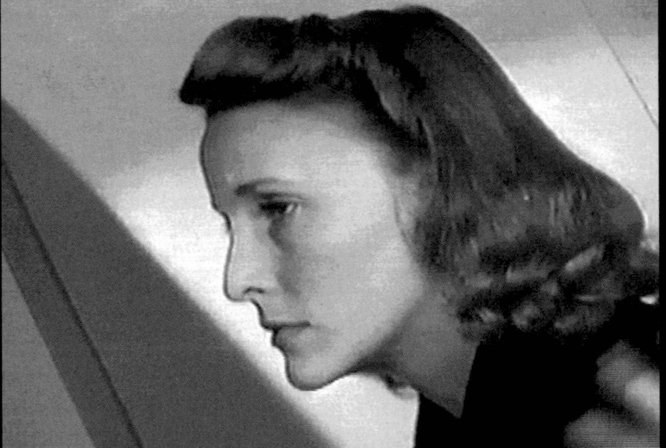

fig. 5

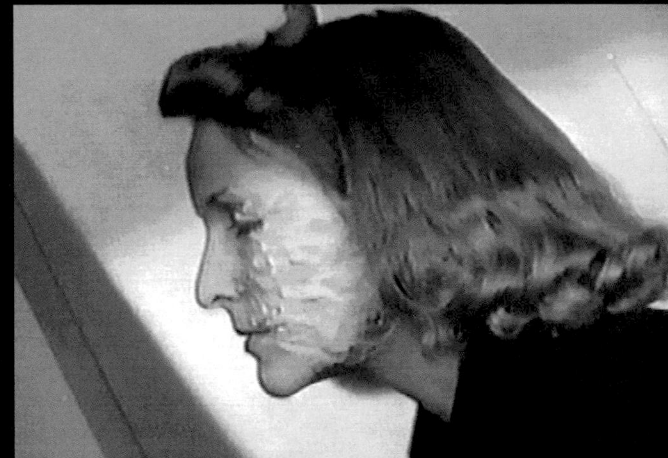

fig. 6

fig. 3 & 4

Joan Crawford was one of the most glamorous stars in the golden age of Hollywood. In George Cukor's A Woman's Face *(1941), her face is so horribly disfigured by a scar that she cannot bear to look at herself in the mirror.*

fig. 5 & 6

Before and after, beautiful or hideous: These two photos of the same woman, shown to Crawford's character, Anna, by a plastic surgeon, convince her of the effectiveness of cosmetic surgery.

fig. 9

The magic of the mirror: Infinite reflections symbolise the danger of losing one's identity — a problem Crawford had to face throughout her career.

fig. 7 & 8

After the operation has been completed, the film plays on the curiosity of the viewer: The back of a mirror hides the "new face" from us.

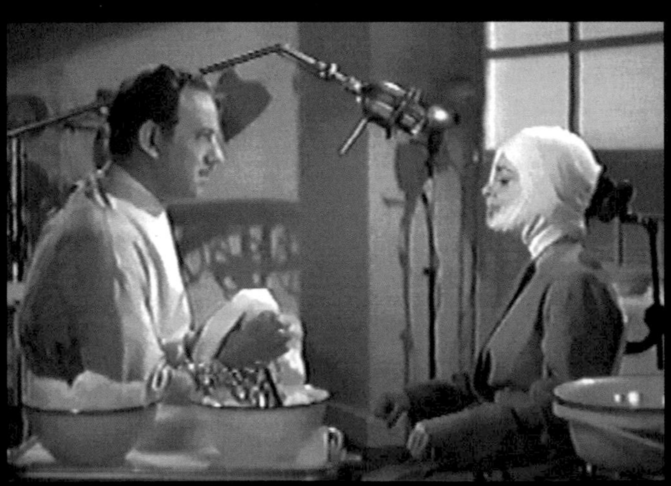

fig. 7

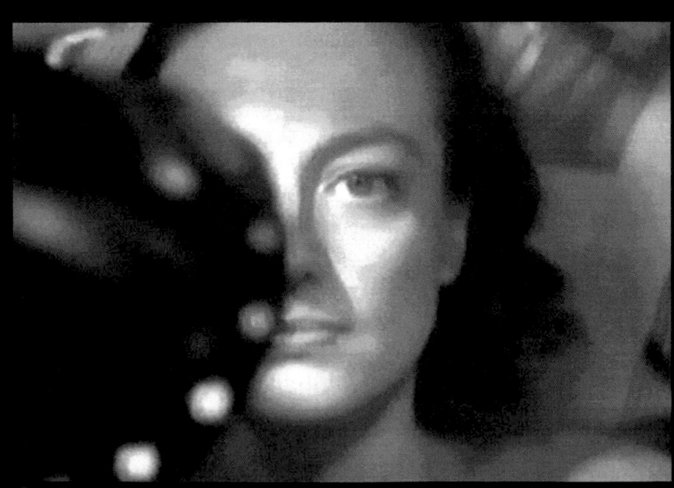

fig. 8

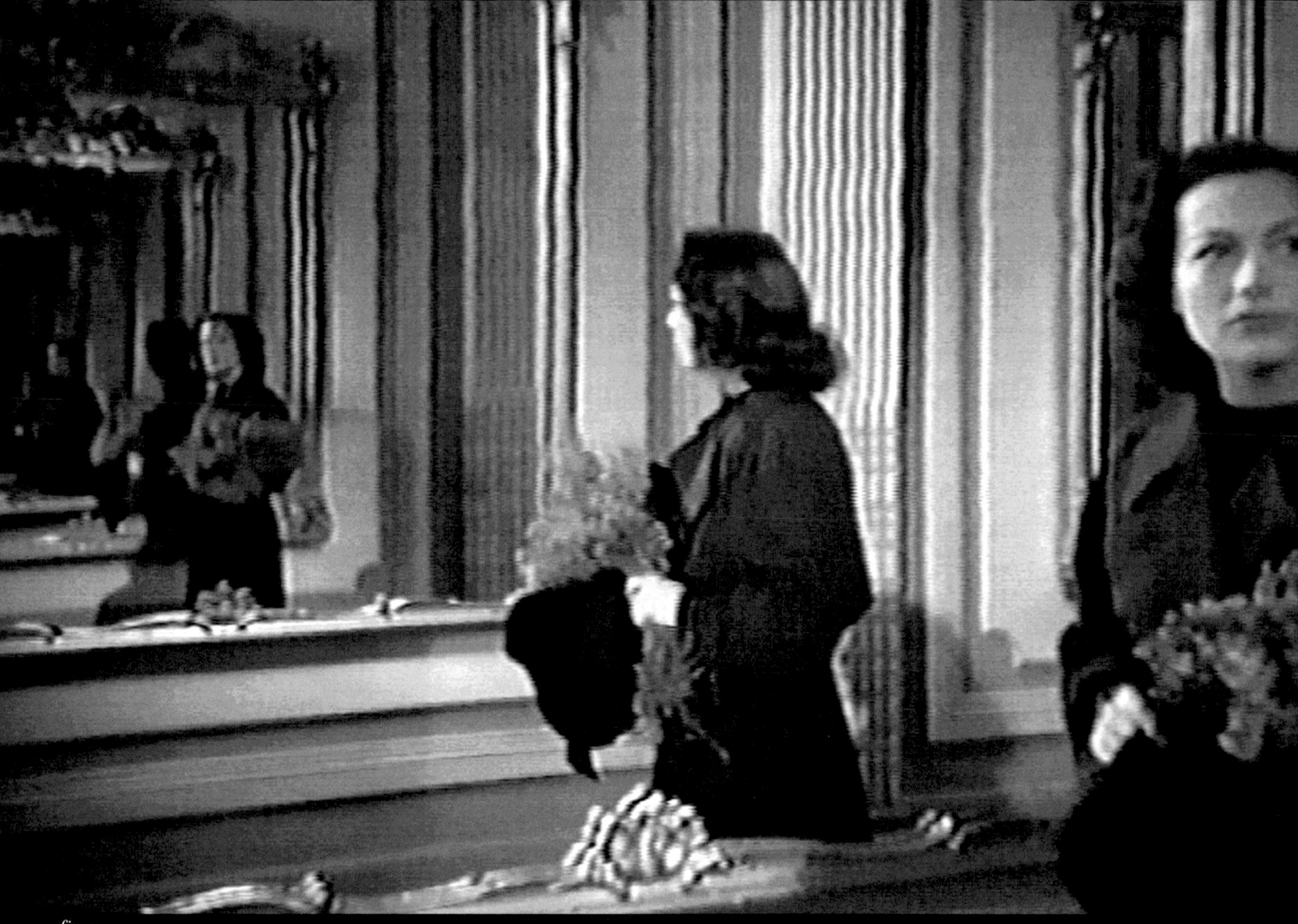

fig. 9

figure of the quack, but also by a scene in which the two criminals are planning to murder Mortimer. We see how Jonathan puts on the surgical gloves with much glee, and proceeds to open the doctor's briefcase containing some very nerve-racking instruments.

Through the Eyes of Another

In *Dark Passage* by Delmer Daves (1947), the camera initially takes the perspective of an escaped prisoner. For the first part of the film, the audience never sees the prisoner's face or body. Vincent Parry (Humphrey Bogart), was sentenced to jail after being found guilty of murdering his wife. For us, the only way to judge this character is through the reactions displayed towards him — the other characters act as mirrors that reflect his personality back at us. This filmic device of the subjective perspective is aesthetically intriguing and an effective way of creating dramatic tension — if this man really is a dangerous criminal, we are his accomplices by force of perspective.

Gradually, it is revealed that Parry is searching for the true murderer of his wife. After his escape, he convinces a taxi driver to help him with his unlikely task. Taking pity on Parry, the taxi driver aids the alleged criminal's getaway and takes his passenger to a plastic surgeon who he knows will give him a new "identity."

The portrait of this cosmetic surgeon is heavily formed by an artist stereotype first encountered in the 19th century — the free thinker who has exiled himself from bourgeois society. "Walter Coley, Specialist," as the surgeon is described on his door plate, musters his visitor with great interest and some disdain, as if presented by an object that will only be worth anything once he, the artist, has sculpted it to perfection. Very much in the guise of an artistic genius — arms folded, smoking a cigarette — Dr. Coley assesses his "object" with the eyes of a specialist, muttering about the philosophical ramifications of the operation he is about to perform. Which, despite its entirely unartistic occasion, is obviously an aesthetic affair.

The doctor is a wronged genius who was thrown out of the medical council because of his bold new surgical techniques. The obligatory slice of insanity this stereotype comes with does not go amiss; Dr. Coley's deliberations on how he could make his enemies look like bulldogs or monkeys have a profoundly unsettling effect on his patient. While under anaesthetic during the operation, Parry hears this sentence resound in his head over and over.

The operation is staged as a cinematic fantasy, told from the perspective of the narcoticised patient in a series of surreal, kaleidoscopic images. The chloroform haze acts as a backdrop to the flashbacks Parry is experiencing, replaying the events and people of his recent past. When the surgeon covers Parry's face with a warm cloth, we only see the model of a human head without its skin — in the context of the narrative, a symbol for the question of identity.

"Well, I've done a nice job," claims Coley when we get to see the protagonist from an external perspective for the first

fig. 10

Frank Capra's black comedy Arsenic and Old Lace *(1944) depicts the grotesque outcome of a botched operation: It serves to emphasise, rather than hide, Jonathan's mean streak. His family members are instantly reminded of Frankenstein's monster...*

fig. 11

...and with fittingly monstrous intentions, Jonathan and his charlatan pal "Einstein" are planning to use their shiny surgical implements on the unsuspecting Mortimer.

fig. 12

A play on perspective: In Delmer Daves' Dark Passage *(1947), a rather dubious cosmetic surgeon eyes up the viewer much like his next patient.*

fig. 13

In limbo: Bandaged Vincent Parry (Humphrey Bogart) has given up his previous identity and awaits a new face.

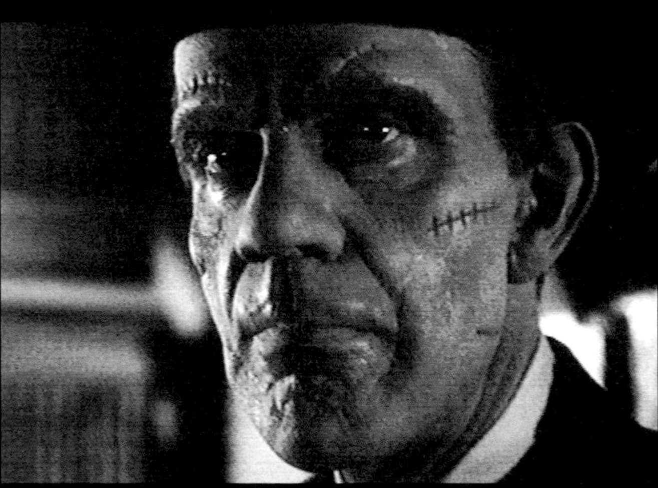

fig. 10

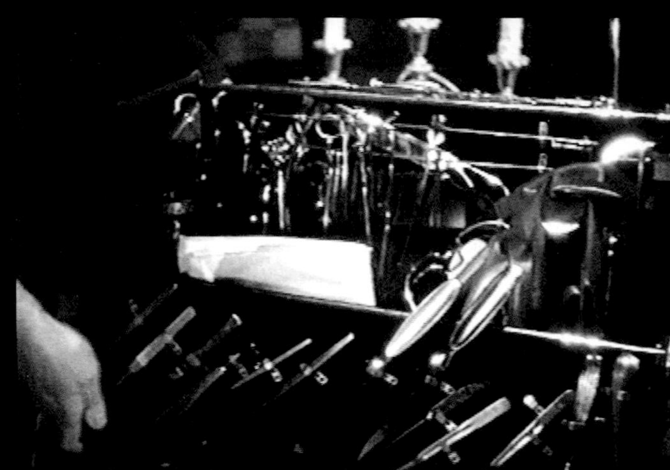

fig. 11

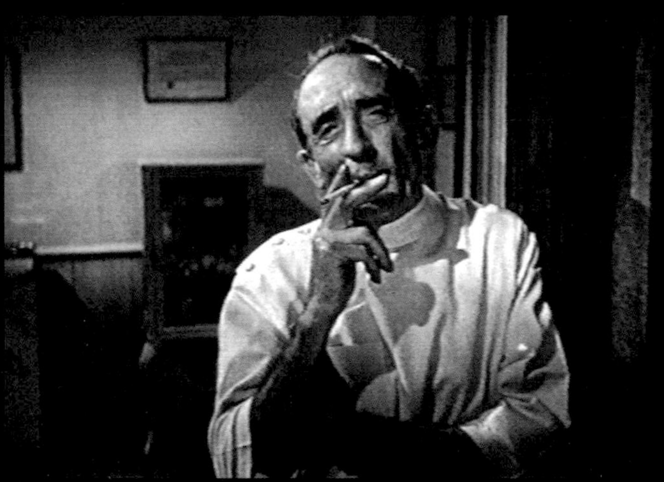

fig. 12

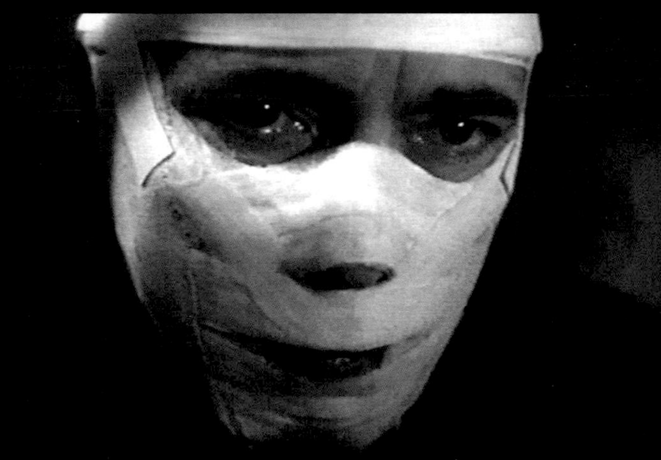

fig. 13

time, "... the artist in me wishes to see what a nice job I've done." Parry's face, however, is still covered in bandages. The filmic device of the subjective perspective, which is finally broken at this point, further demonstrates the potential for cinematic self-reflection offered by the topic and presentation of plastic surgery. One of the central possibilities of film narrative is to shift from an interior to an exterior perspective — no other medium can show us more vividly that we are simultaneously the subject and the object of perception and thought.

Cinema's convincing realism wouldn't be possible without tapping into this existential experience of self-perception; as well as depicting external reality, it can interpret this reality for us through the eyes of others.

An Image of the Soul

In Georges Franju's 1959 horror flick *Eyes Without a Face* (*Les yeux sans visage*), we encounter a scientist (Pierre Brasseur) who has lost control over his life. A renowned surgeon, whose daughter's (Edith Scob) face has been horribly disfigured in an accident, kidnaps young women to remove their facial skin and graft it onto his daughter's face. All the gruesome operations fail; in the end, the daughter frees the last victim, kills her father's malicious assistant and finally her father himself.

Eyes Without a Face is an unforgettable cinematic experience, not so much due to its narrative as to the nightmar-

fig. 14

The skinless face as a further metaphor for the loss of identity: In a kaleidoscopic array of flashbacks, the patient in Dark Passage *(Humphrey Bogart) tries to focus on his beautiful saviour (Lauren Bacall).*

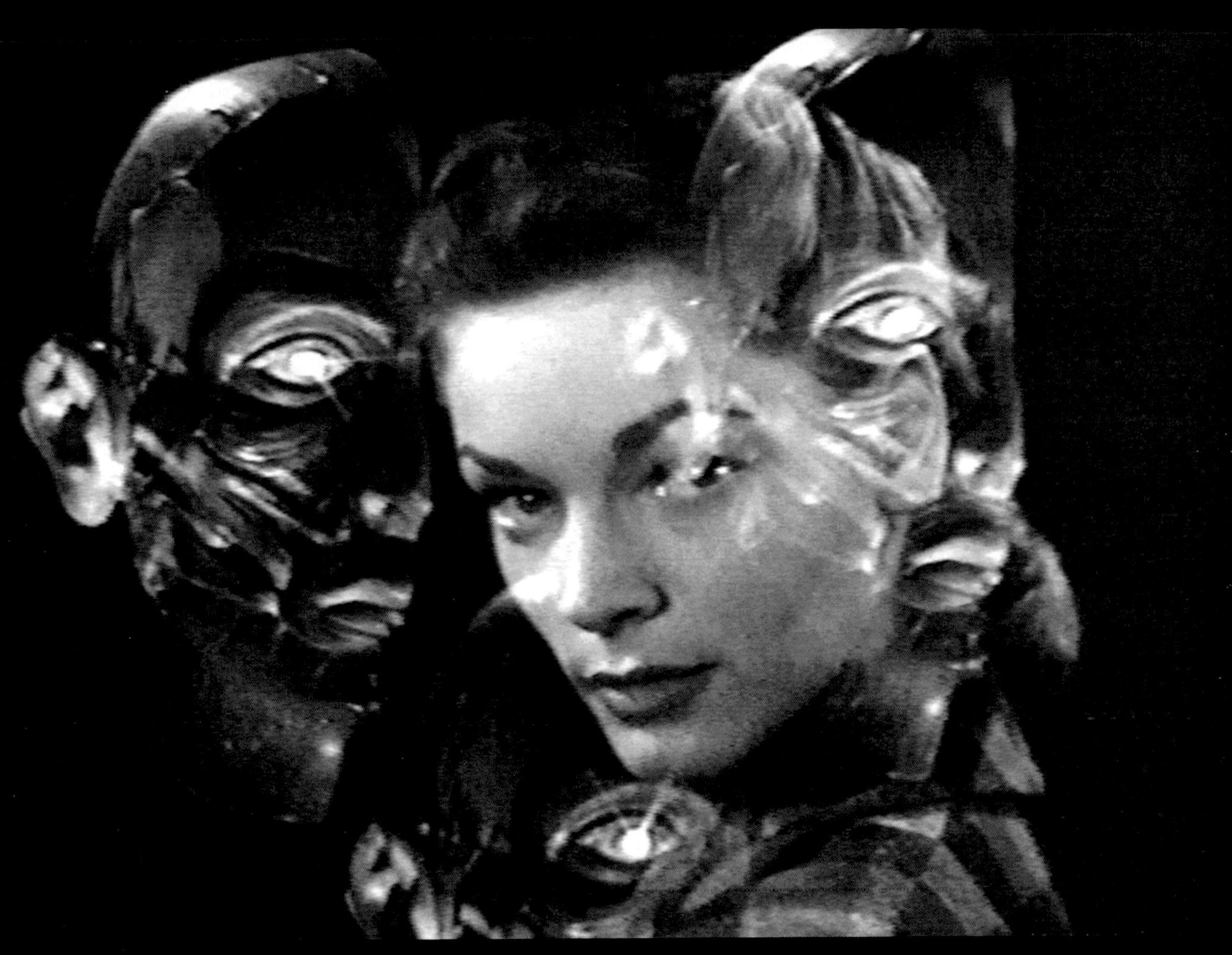

fig. 14

ish images Franju has composed. The cursed, labyrinthine world the disfigured girl has to live in and her cruel destiny, which excludes her from all social contacts, make the operation seem like the only solution — instead, it turns out to be a nightmare far worse. When the victims' faces are peeled off by the surgeon, Franju's imagery is excruciatingly explicit. The tender faces are brutally juxtaposed with the torture instruments used for the surgery — scalpels and pins to dismember the faces and lift off the skin with a sadistically meticulous slowness. The viewer is spared no detail of the gory procedure.

While the facial skin initially promises to be an exchangeable mask, it soon becomes apparent that this inhumane procedure is rejected both by the bodies of the victims and that of the unfortunate daughter. After each operation, the girl's new face gradually mottles, loses its contours and dies off as her flesh rejects the transplant.

Though the film cries out for a psychoanalytical interpretation, we can also just let the images — reminiscent of Cocteau and displaying an undeniable Surrealist influence — speak for themselves. We see the young woman walking around in her white mask, a human being condemned to live in some ghastly limbo. Not even the most qualified surgeon is able to restore his own daughter's beauty, a curse so powerful that even science cannot break it.

In some respects, this film is a variation on the Frankenstein theme. Like Frankenstein, the father character attempts to play God, in this instance to rescue his daughter from the

fig. 15–18

In Georges Franju's Eyes Without a Face *(1959), a deranged cosmetic surgeon attempts to restore his daughter's face, which was disfigured in a car accident. He uses the facial skin of other young and beautiful women for his transplants...*

fig. 19

.... but the operations always fail. The patient's face rejects the foreign tissue.

fig. 20

The moment of horror: The facial skin is lifted off and before the flesh beneath is seen, the camera pans to the perspective of the victim.

realm of facelessness and return her to a life worth living. He is willing to resort to the utmost cruelty if only he can save his daughter. In this context, plastic surgery is presented as a criminal act of hubris; the failed transplants suggesting that a human being only exists as a whole. It is simply not possible to "add" skin to a person to make him or her more complete.

Another vivid portrayal of the figure of the plastic surgeon is presented by Sydney Hayers' *Circus of Horrors* (1960). This film tells the story of Dr. Rossiter (Anton Diffring), who is forced to leave England shortly after the Second World War. After his operation on a young woman, Evelyn Morley (Colette Wilde), has gone wrong, he flees to France to escape arrest. Here, he assumes a new identity as Dr. Bernhard Schueler and takes over a run-down travelling circus. He uses his surgical abilities to attract new additions to his entourage — petty female criminals with disfigured faces, thieves and prostitutes. His operations turn them all into beautiful women. However, as Schueler does not want to rely on the women's gratitude alone to keep them in his ring, he also keeps a file on the criminal past of each of his patients.

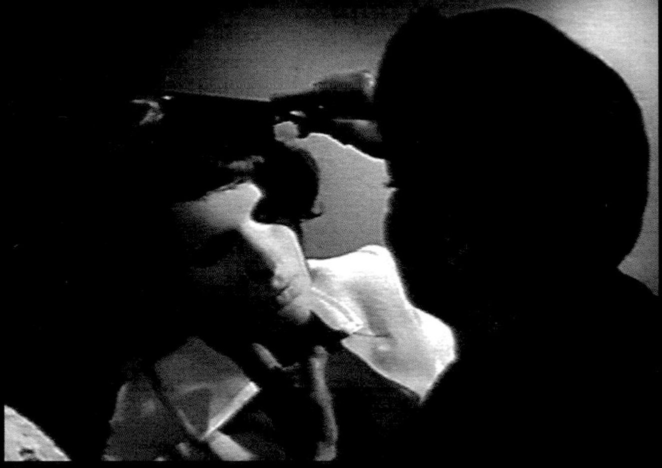

fig. 15

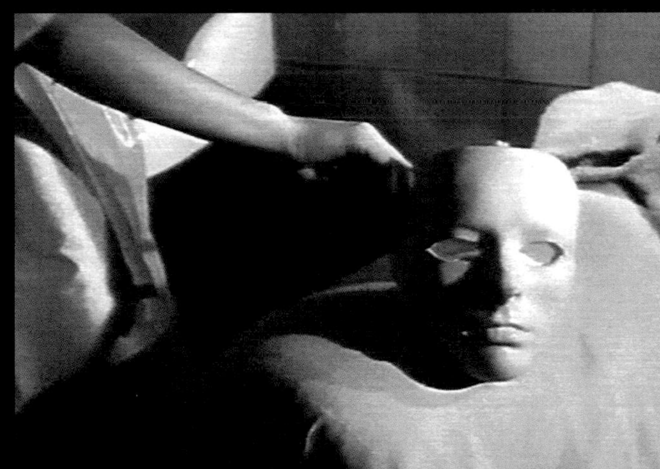

fig. 16

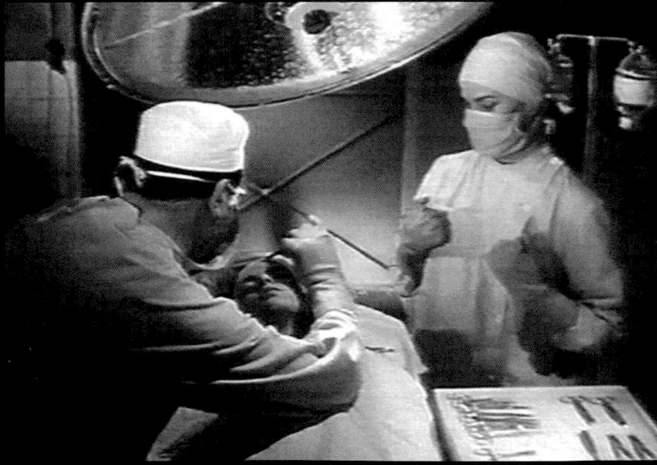

fig. 17

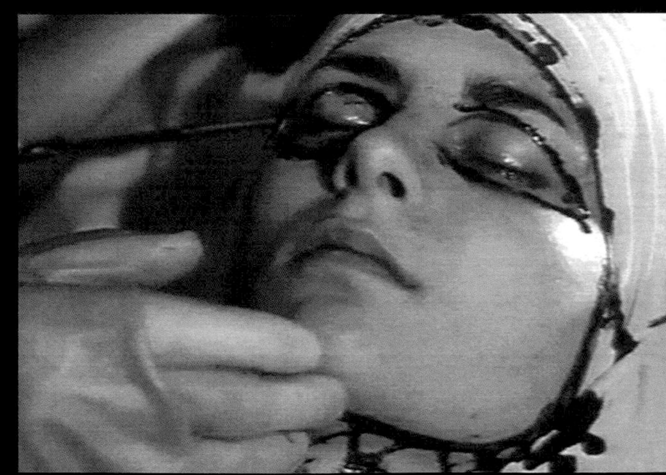

fig. 18

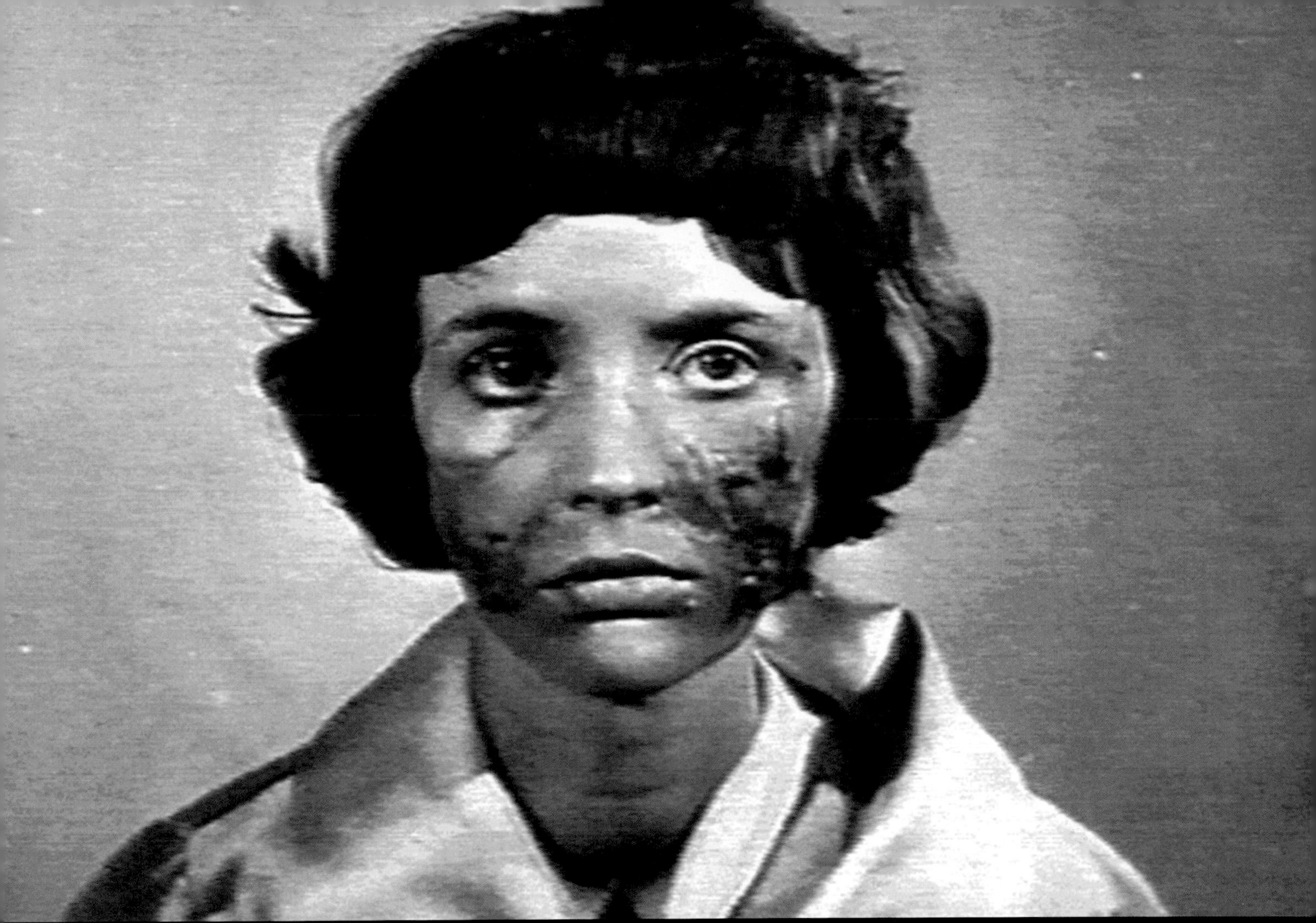

fig. 19 / fig. 20

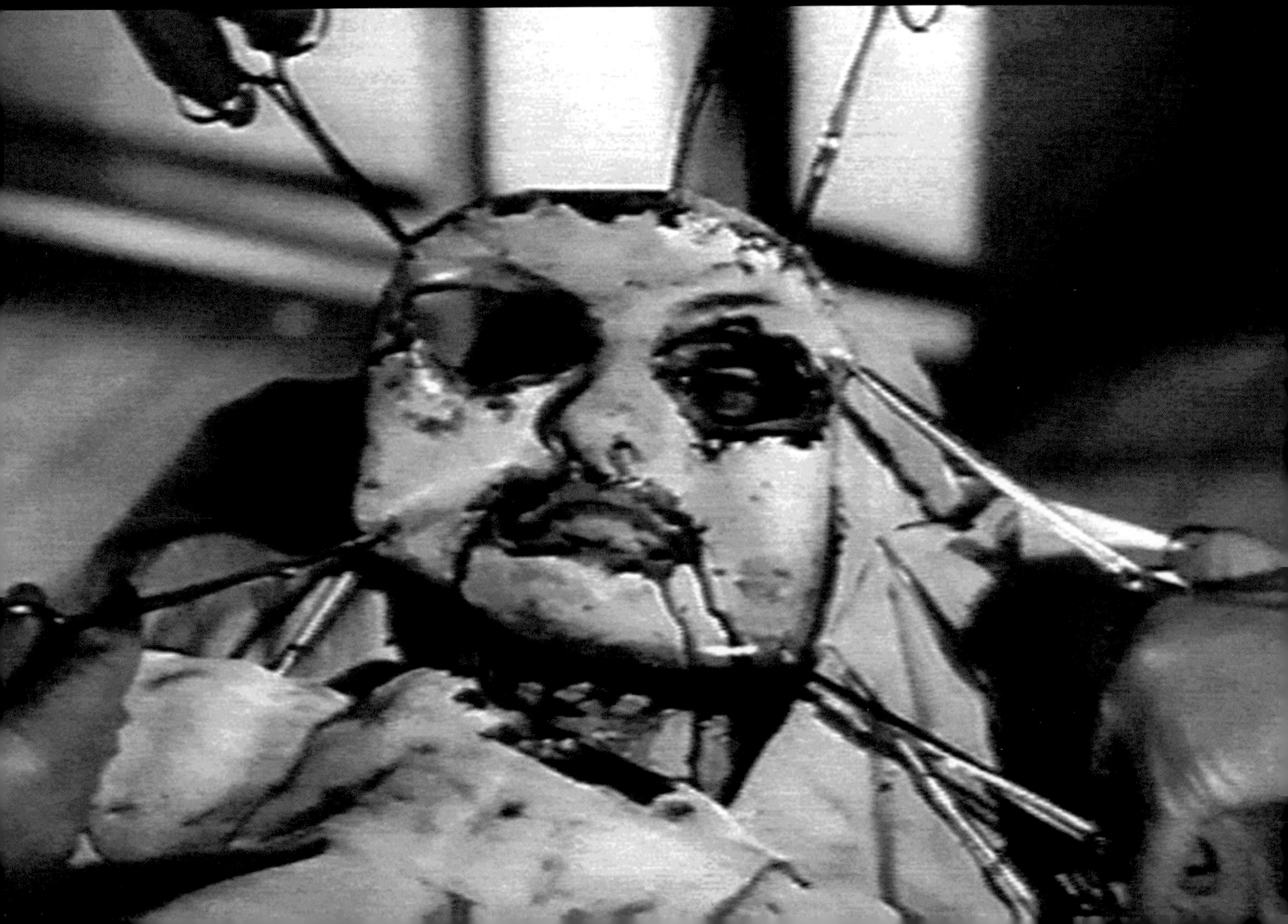

fig. 21–24

*Hubris of the cosmetic surgeon: Dr. Rossiter gets his kicks from turning female petty criminals with disfigured faces into stunning beauties, and then taking them as his lovers. (*Circus of Horrors*, 1960, directed by Sidney Hayers).*

fig. 25

This shot shows us the ambiguity of ugliness: Despite her disfigured face, the woman is depicted as being attractive. We are simultaneously drawn to and repulsed by her.

The circus, as the successor to the freakshow of old, to satisfies the public urge for spectacle and is used as a metaphor for society. All that counts here is outward appearance. The clowns are defined by their make-up as unmistakably as the trapeze artists are by their splendid costumes. This is in stark contrast to the instinctual desire exuded by the caged circus animals. When the character Nicole (Carla Challoner), for whom the surgeon has just removed a scar, runs to the animals to show them her new face, she ecstatically keeps repeating "I am beautiful!" Her entire existence and future have been saved, it would seem. This turns out to be a false promise for most of Schueler's other patients. Although the doctor rids them of their old identities, he refuses to give them their much-hoped-for freedom, instead exploiting them sexually and for his own material wealth. These beautified women have been reduced to mere objects, the "works" of an unscrupulous surgeon who would sooner murder them than set them free. Schueler has one driving ambition, which is to showcase his creations to his old colleagues at the tour's final performance in England. As the highlight of the show, his latest masterpiece Melina (Yvonne Romain) is to tame a sedated lion. As Schueler's helpers rebel against him, Melina is killed by the lions in the ring — only her face remains unscathed.

In Hayers' film, cosmetic surgery is portrayed as an achievement of civilisation that can provide its patients with a better quality of life. In the context of this discussion, however, the figure of the surgeon is of particular interest. Rossiter is initially a surgeon to the richest families of England but falls from grace when one of his operations results in disfigurement. Demoted to the lowest echelons of society, he keeps perfecting his professional skills, but completely abandons his ethical code of practice. Seduced by the powerful possibilities of plastic surgery, he becomes corrupt. It comes as no surprise that his just punishment at the end of the film is to lose his own face.

Like Franju in *Eyes Without a Face*, John Frankenheimer juxtaposes aesthetic surgery with the completeness of the human being in his thriller *Seconds* (1966). In this film, top-level bank clerk Arthur Hamilton (John Randolph) is mysteriously contacted by a secret company offering him a new identity. The company would wrap up his existing life, providing a dead body that would be buried in place of Hamilton. "The question of death decision," company head Ruby (Jeff Corey) explains to him, "may be the most important of your life." After some initial hesitation, Hamilton accepts (and picks death by fire). His marriage had been dysfunctional for some time, and he has long lost all personal motivation and ambition.

The operation is planned with the precision of a military strike; a team of professional cosmetic surgeons is employed to operate on Hamilton. The operation is set in a clinical environment that was convincingly realistic to audiences at the time. We see how a chin inlay is inserted and how the nose is remodelled as if it were a sculpture. When Hamilton's bandages are finally removed a few weeks later, he cannot believe his eyes — the facial operation has not only provided him with a new identity but also replaced the worn-out forty-something's face with a youthful and attractive visage (Rock Hudson). A "masterpiece," as Ruby claims.

After completing a fitness training course, Hamilton is given his new persona: He now is the painter Antiochus Wilson, Tony for short, who lives in a charming beach house on the outskirts of town. Here, he is to get used to his new role as an artist and playboy. The enticing Nora (Salome Jens), who soon begins an affair with him, is there to help him along the way and demonstrate his unfettered freedom to him: "You don't have to prove anything." Despite, or possibly because of this, he fails to slot into his new life. At a party, he almost gives away his secret, and eventually decides to visit his old wife (Frances Reid) in his new guise as the painter Wilson. He is determined to find out what went wrong in the life of Arthur Hamilton.

Back at his old house, he comes across a photo of his former self, and holds it up against his reflection in the living room mirror. Again, the look into the mirror is the film's key scene, its most symbolic moment. More than anything, the mirror reflects the self-image of the character that was thrown into chaos by the operation. By looking into the mirror, the patient is attempting to reconcile his appearance with his self-perception, to re-integrate his consciousness with his identity. It is impossible to tell at this point which will come out on top, the old or the new; fittingly, the mirror image in *Seconds* only serves to show that

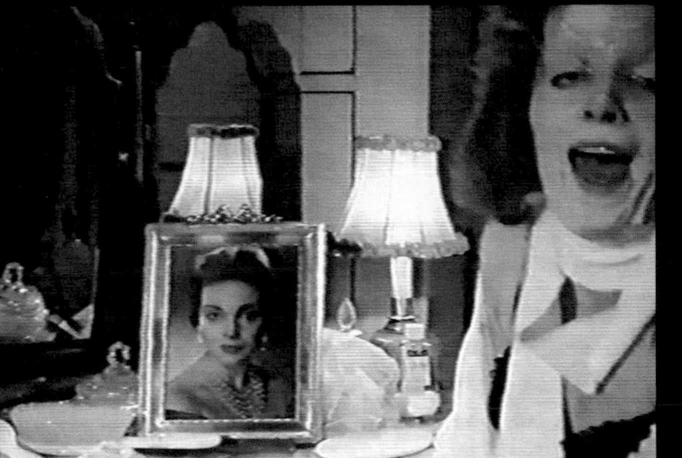
fig. 21

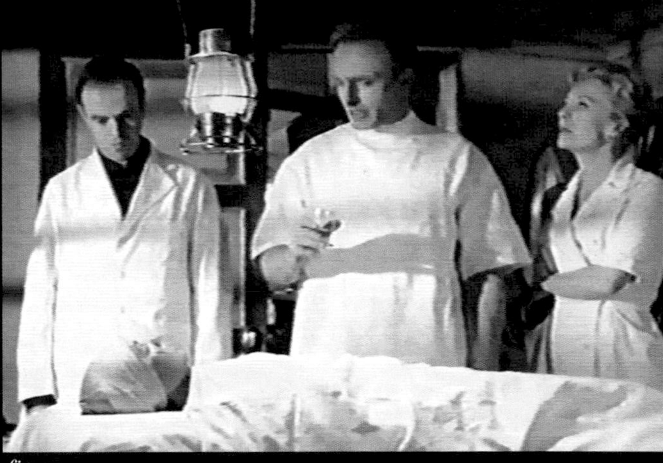
fig. 22

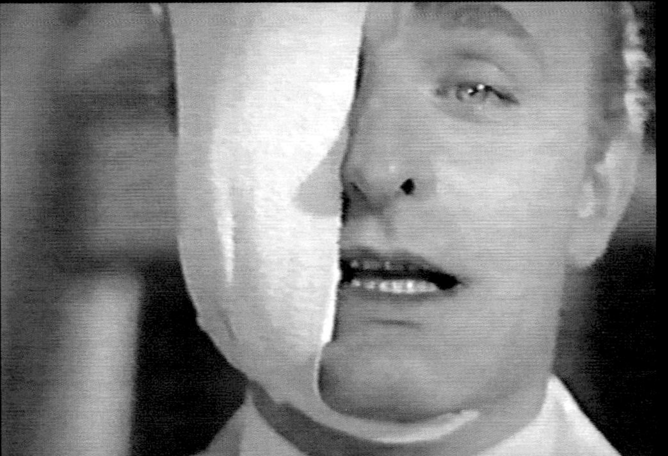
fig. 23

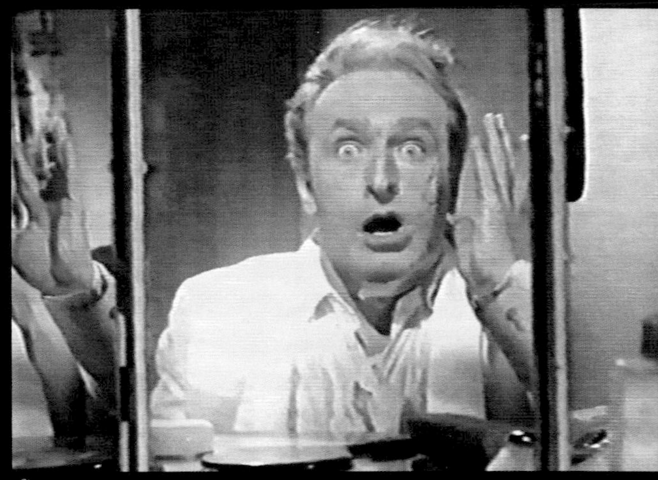
fig. 24

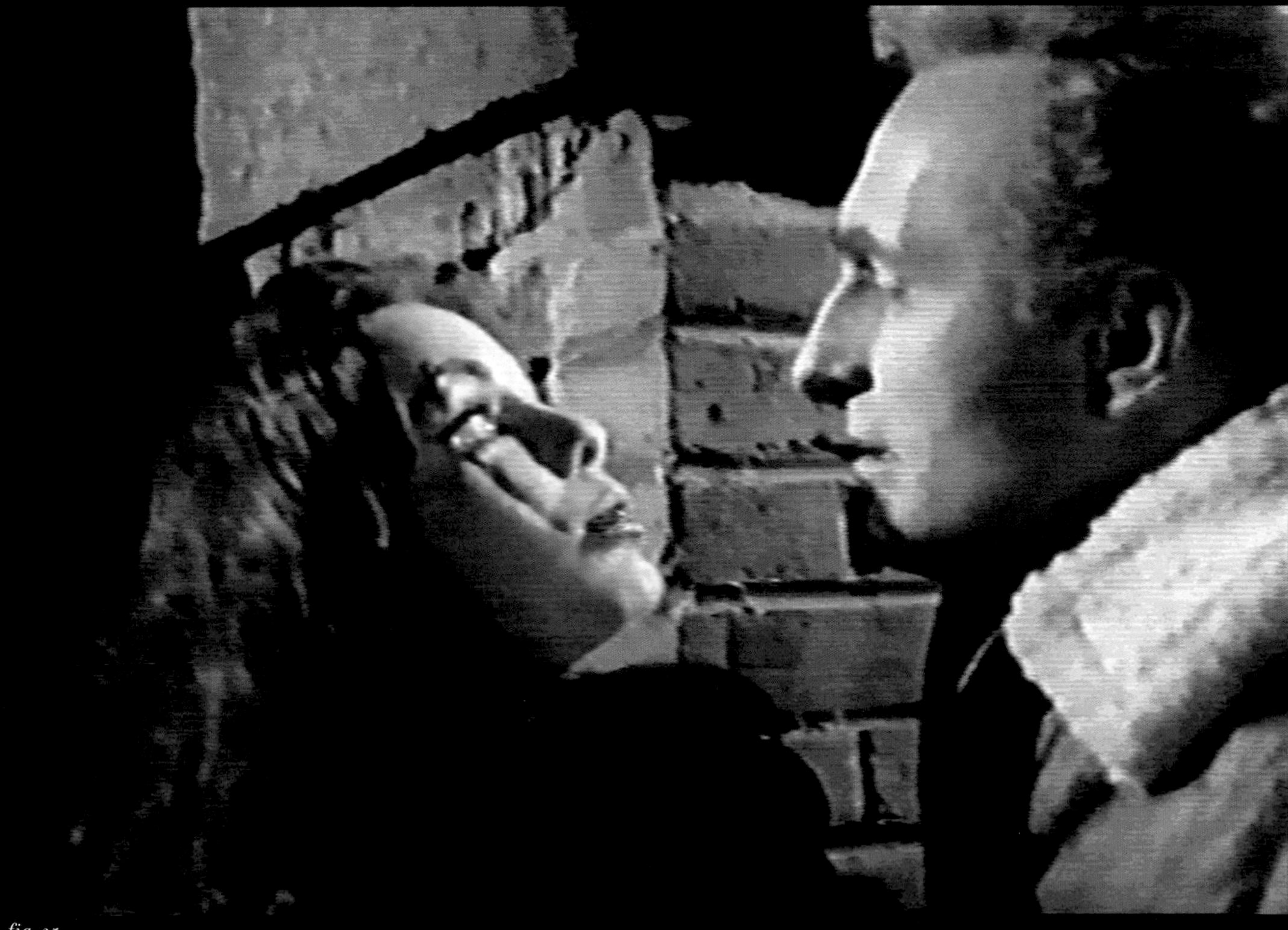

fig. 25

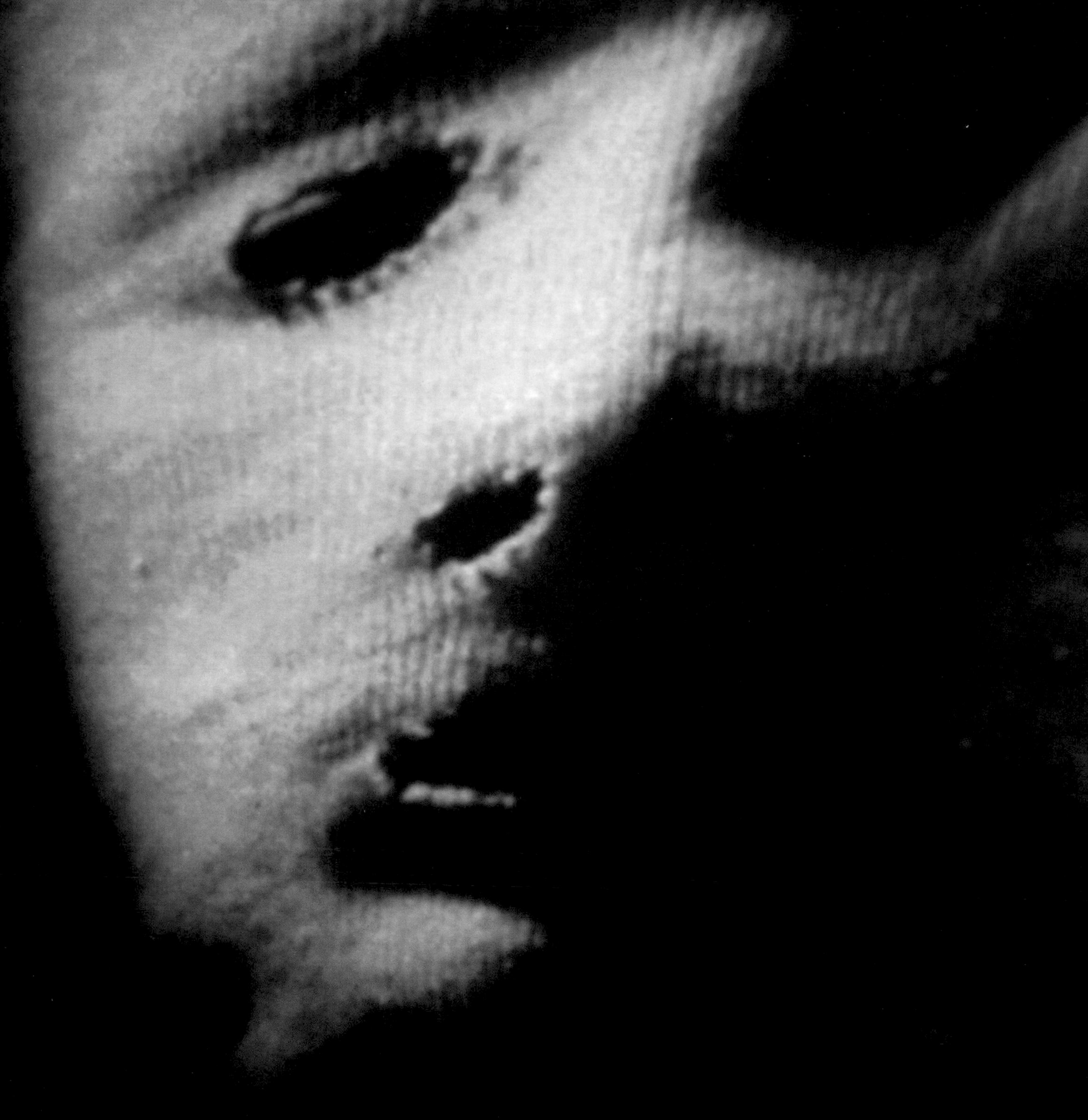

fig. 26

fig. 26

An image of somnambulistic time: In John Frankenheimer's Seconds *(1966), the world no longer conforms to the conventional coordinates of time and space.*

fig. 27 & 28

Just before the operation: The new face already exists on paper as a precisely-measured design.

fig. 29 & 30

Initially, the new face is still obscured by the bandage mask. Then, a new person appears!

fig. 31 & 32

Not only does the mirror multiply the face, it also casts doubt on the identity of the person reflected.

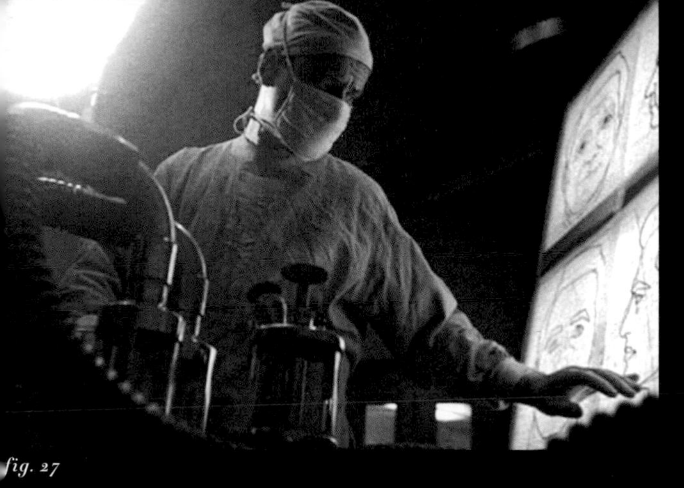

fig. 27

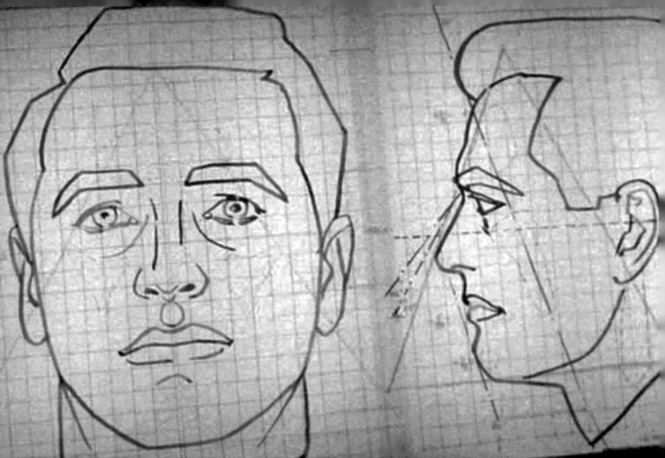

fig. 28

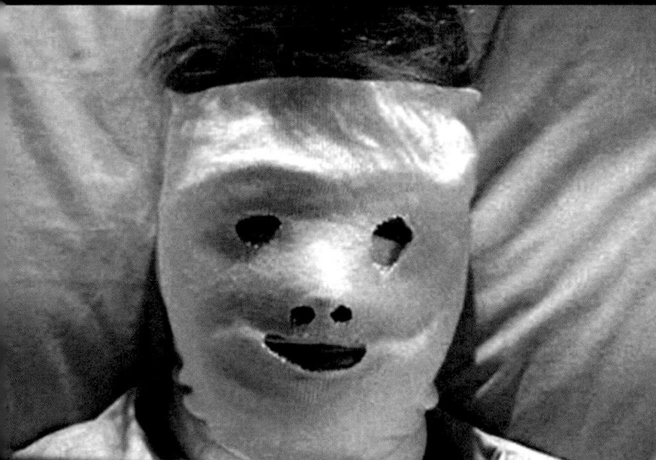

fig. 29

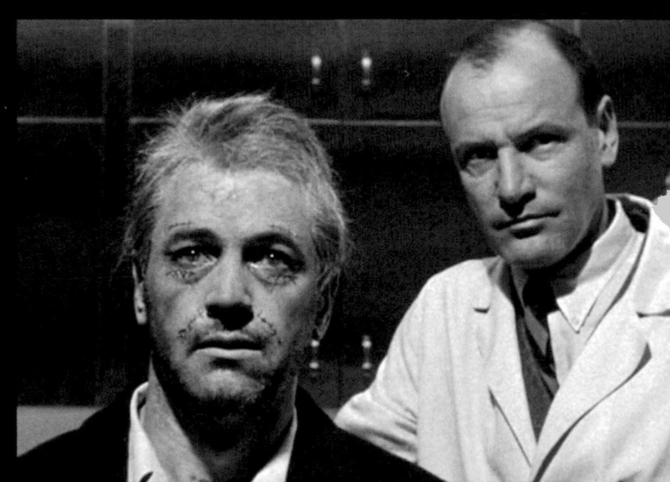

fig. 30

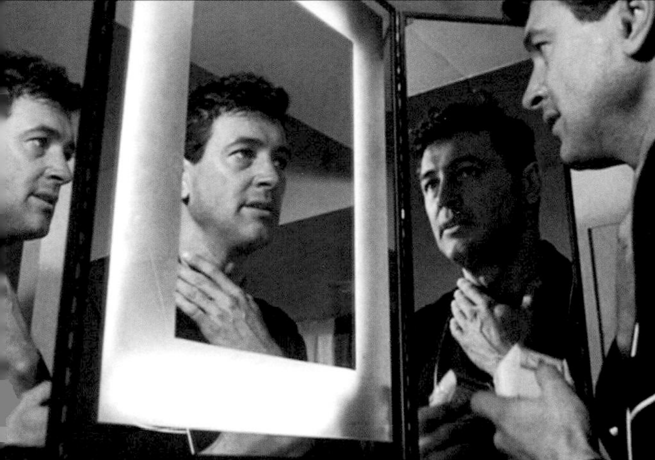

fig. 31

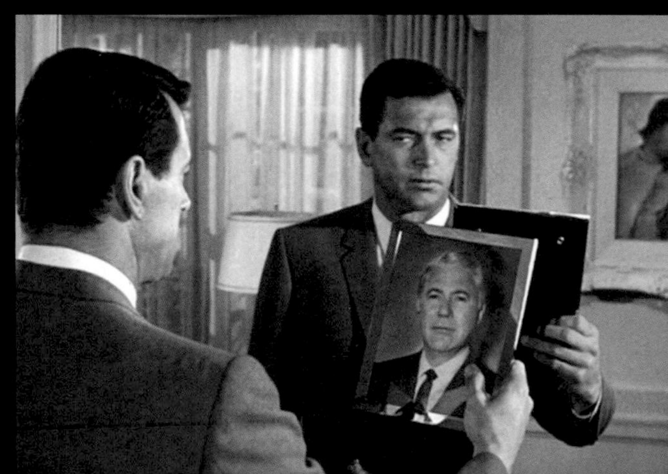

fig. 32

t can give no answer — neither about Wilson nor about Hamilton. Again, the characters are a more reliable source of reflection — it is Hamilton's wife who has the answer the protagonist was looking for. "See, Arthur had been dead a long long time before they found him in that hotel room," she tells him and also explains the reasons behind this. Hamilton simply never knew what he really wanted, it seems, and every time one of his wishes was fulfilled, he would only become more depressed.

For Wilson, i. e. Hamilton, the Gordian knot has suddenly been cut; now that he can see where he failed, he wants a new chance at his old life. But when he confronts the daunting company about wanting to be re-operated, he is told that he will first need to supply the name of a potential new client. However, Wilson / Hamilton simply cannot think of anyone, and dismisses the request. In his enthusiasm about his belated self-revelation, he fails to recognise the gravity of this situation, which catches up with him only when it is too late — on the operating table. This time, the surgeon turns out to be not the giver of another life but the giver of death. His task for this operation is to remodel Wilson into a dead body — which is to be used as the mortal remains for the discarded identity of another client. As the doctor puts the electric chisel to his victim's face to disfigure it, he seems regretful about having to destroy his beautiful work.

fig. 33 & 34

The future is already here: In Logan's Run *(1976, directed by Michael Anderson), the youth craze is elevated to a cultural law.*

fig. 35 & 36

Cosmetic surgery is an established part of everyday life. In this beautiful but not brave new world, an old man is a sensation.

fig. 37

The surgical machine reveals its true nature: Like a menacing spider, it tries to subdue its human victim with a web of laser beams.

The Cult of Youth

In the 1970s, discussions of the role of plastic surgery in the real world were still rare in film. The subject largely remained a theme for escapist fantasies. Michael Anderson's 1976 science-fiction classic *Logan's Run* proposes a society where youthfulness has been elevated to a social norm.

Survivors of a natural disaster, the people of 2274 live in a gigantic underground city, fashioned as a recreational paradise. The only social restriction in this free-spirited world is age. After thirty years, the life clock installed in the palms of the inhabitants' hands runs out, and the affected citizens are required to enter the so-called Carousel — where they are renewed, i. e. executed, in a "rebirthing" ritual. Those who refuse, the "runners," are hunted down and killed by the age police, also known as the "sandmen." The 26-year-old Logan 5 (Michael York) is a sandman, an assassin whose job it is to enforce the youth-based state system. But when the mainframe computer erroneously advances his time clock by four years, the hunter becomes a hunted runner

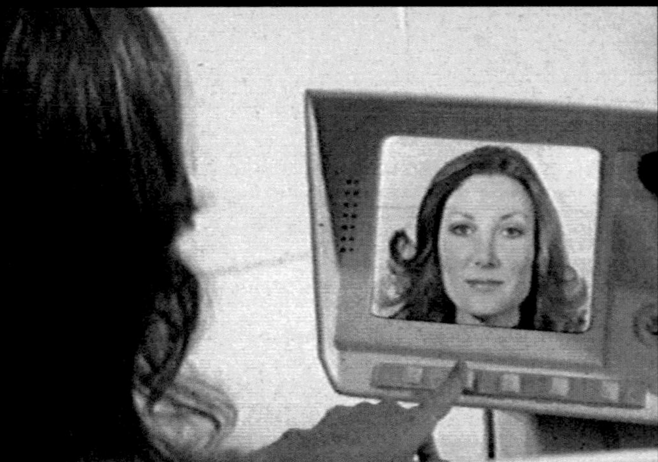

fig. 33

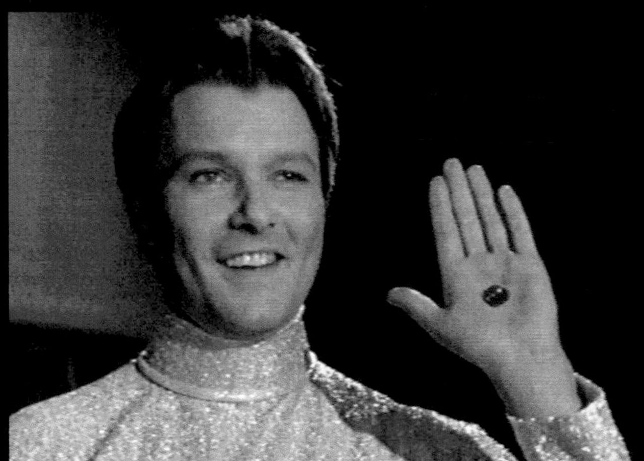

fig. 34

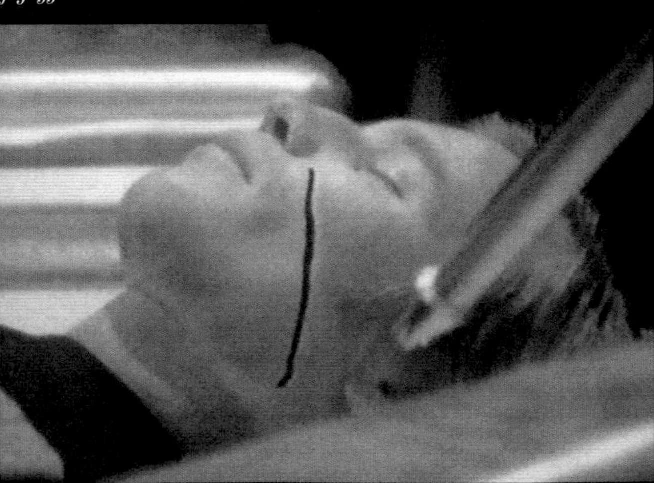

fig. 35

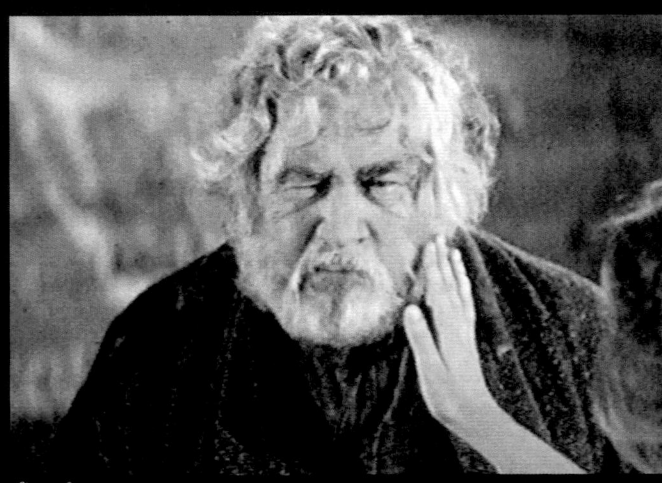

fig. 36

fig. 37

Fedora *(1978) is an allegory for Hollywood's glamour. The film diva has lost control over both her appearance and her life; in the end, she is transformed into an ageless, ideal figure.*

see only the mould, we can already envisage the scalpel incisions that will happen during the operation — and recognise the vulnerability of the face.

The patient's eyes reflect pure terror.

himself. To aid his escape from the city, Logan seeks out a surgeon to provide him with a new face.

The society proposed here is astounding: Although none of the city's subterranean citizens is older than thirty, facial surgery is a common lifestyle choice. A visit to the so-called "New You" centre is no more remarkable than a visit to the hairdresser. (The word combination "New You" further emphasises the equivalence of youth and identity suggested here.) In keeping with sci-fi conventions, the patient uses a computer catalogue to select his or her new facial features, and walks out of the store with a new face half an hour later.

The operating theatre is depicted in an aptly futuristic fashion — an oval glass room with a swivelling chair at the centre (not unlike today's dentist chairs) featuring a number of spider-like metal arms. With a slight whirr, a red laser beam from one of the metal tentacles cuts into Logan's arm; before any blood appears, another laser seals the wound — "instantly, before you feel a thing," as the surgeon explains. In this future, the surgeon-artist has evolved into a precision technician who is "proud of [his] machine."

The highly technical environment — the surgeon performs the operation from a control panel — conveys a sense of

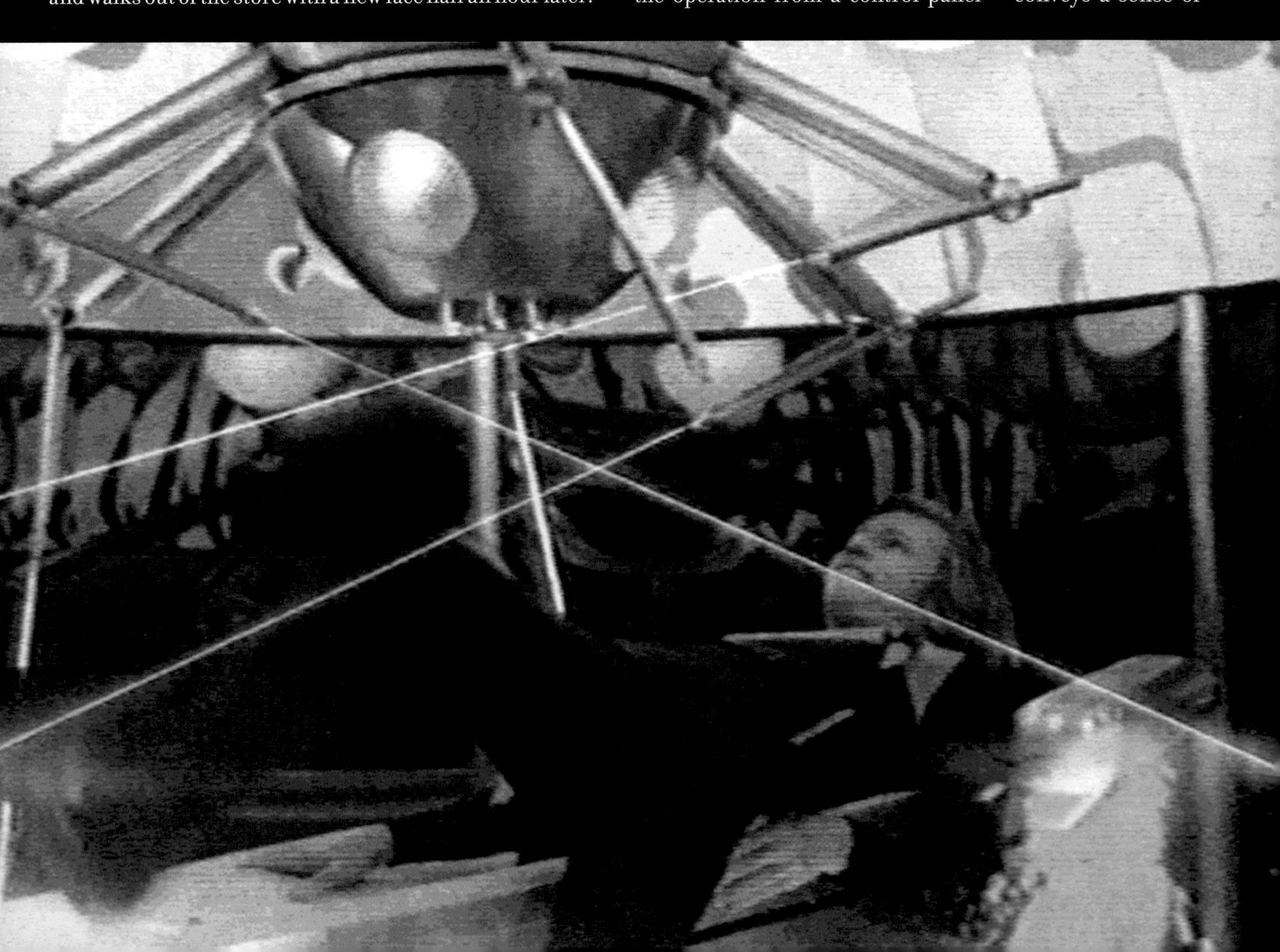

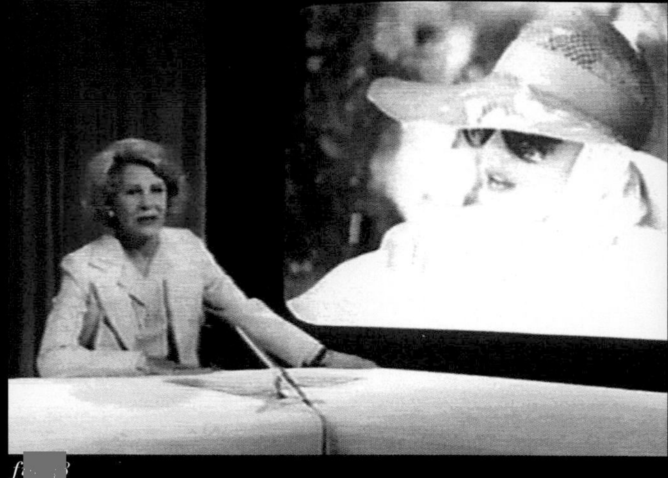

fig. 38

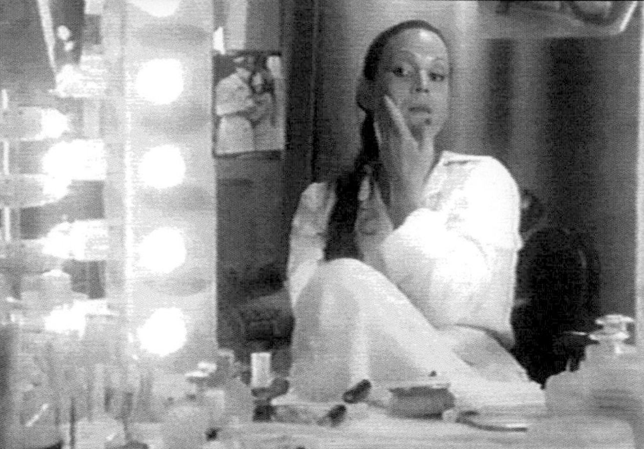

fig. 39

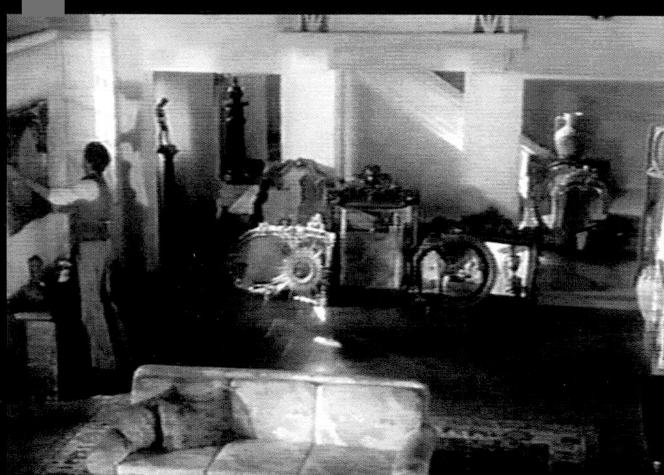

fig. 40

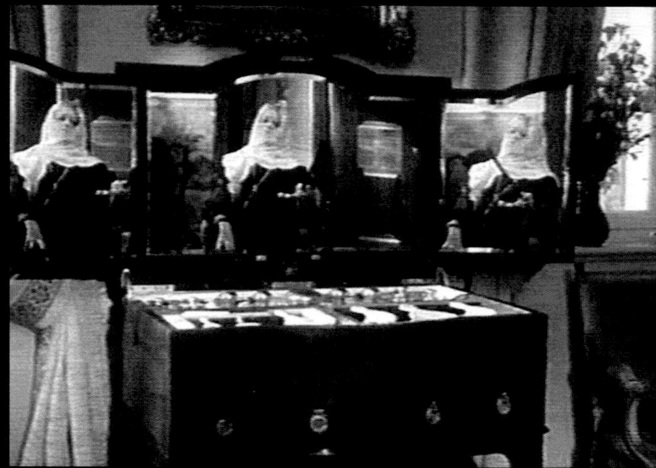

fig. 41

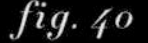

security to the character (and viewer) that soon turns out to be false when the surgeon attempts to kill Logan with his laser apparatus. Before long, the operating table is the scene of a struggle, and amid red and green laser beams and the steam generated by their incisions, the doctor becomes a victim of his own machine.

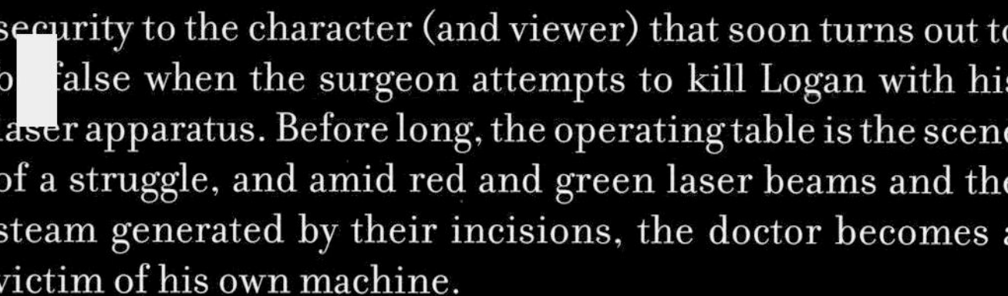

In this instance, aesthetic surgery serves to illustrate the condition of a society that has reached a highly sophisticated level of technical proficiency but lacks the moral foundation to apply it adequately. The citizens go to the aesthetic surgeon as they would go to the hairdresser, simply because they are bored with their current look. "A sandman can get as sick of his face as anybody else," Logan tells the doctor when questioned on his reasons for wanting surgery — a perfectly satisfactory reply. Just as society has found a seemingly ideal form, every person has become an architect of his or her own appearance. Substance and values have become irrelevant in this superficial world. Both on the operating table and in society's beauty image, the person has become a malleable object without a definite identity — perfection has become uniform. A society like this creates suitable myths for itself and it is easy to see the dream factory of Hollywood as the real-world inspiration for this utopian people-making factory.

The subject's potential for self-reference, as discussed earlier, is exemplified by Billy Wilder's *Fedora* (1978). This drama looks closely at the relationship between aesthetic surgery and the world of cinema. At the start of the film, a newsreader announces the death of the actress Fedora: "This world-famous face, shining on the screen for over forty years, is with us no longer." Fedora's radiant looks were attributed to the skill of her surgeon, Dr. Vando (José Ferrer). The following dialogue between Vando and the film producer Barry Detweiler (William Holden) gives a revealing insight into Vando's character:

Detweiler: "You must be a magician. How do you do it?"
Vando: "It's no big secret, you can read up on it in any Sunday paper. Apparently I put them (my patients, that is) on ice for a couple of months, exchange their blood and then pump them full of hormones. I use sheep embryos and baboon sperm. I perform surgery with laser beams and tissue transplants, a little acupressure here, a little skin tightening there, and naturally, plenty of mental and dietary discipline. Yoga and yoghurt, if you like."
Detweiler: "And how much of it is true?"
Vando: "Every single word. Nothing at all. Depends who you ask. To my patients, I'm a genius — to my esteemed colleagues, a quack, a fraud. "

Looking at his nonsensical methods, Vando would indeed seem to be a cynical charlatan. However, he may also be an egocentric genius, it is impossible to tell. His last sentence certainly implies that the patients need to believe in his methods if they are to work.

Her eternal youth and beauty have brought Fedora not only admirers but also much envy, as is evident from the malicious insinuations voiced by the Countess Sobryanski

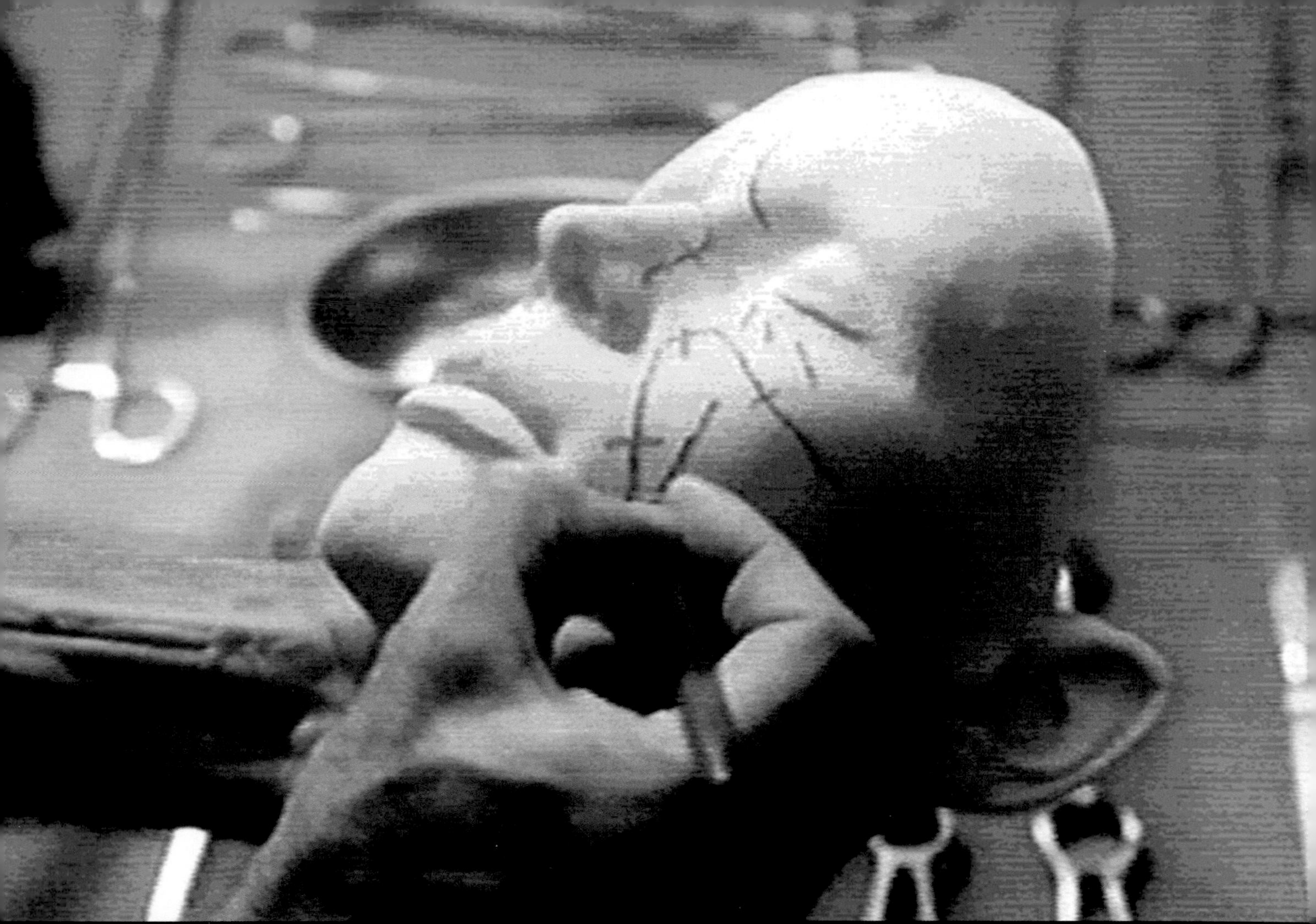

fig. 42 / fig. 43

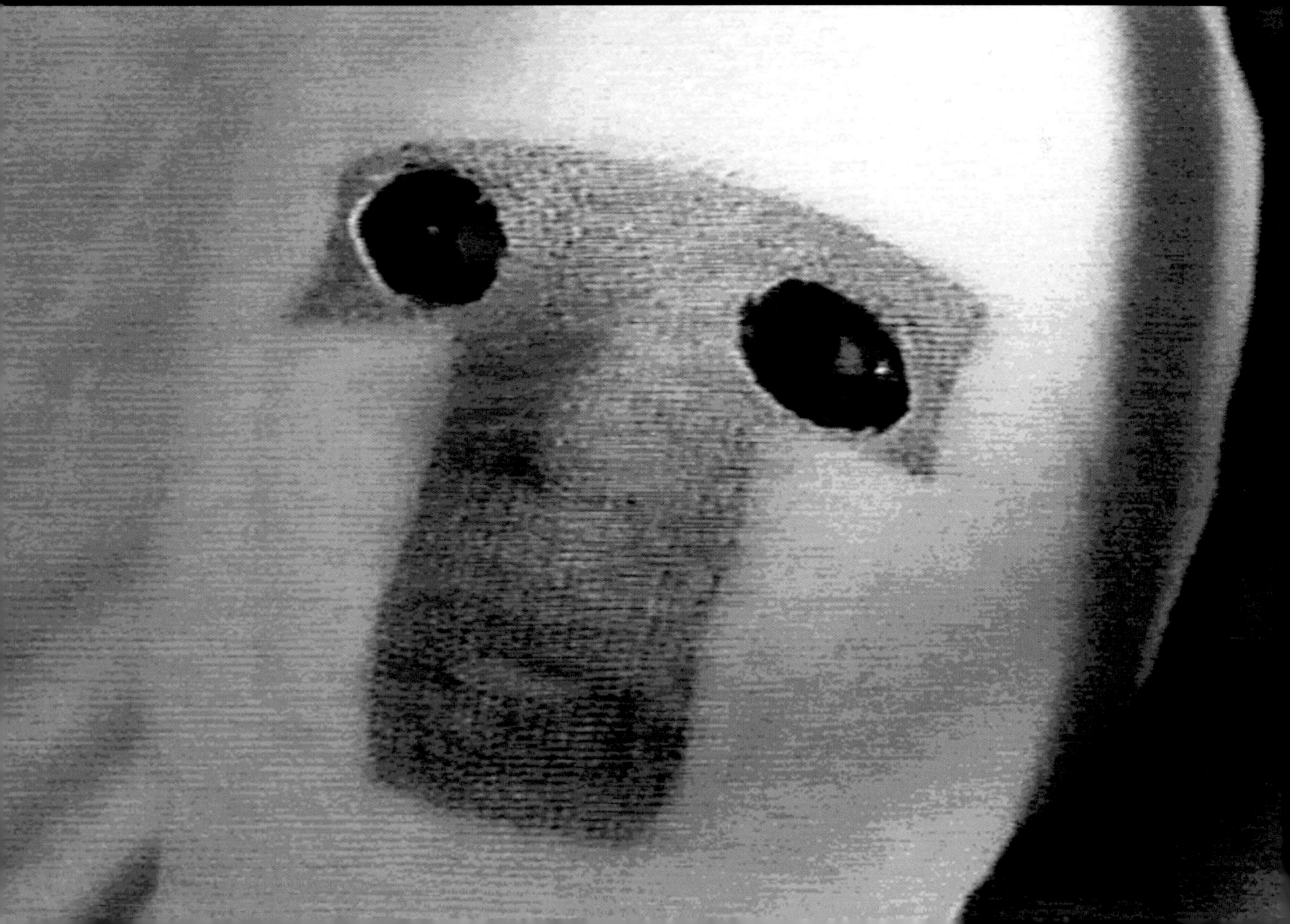

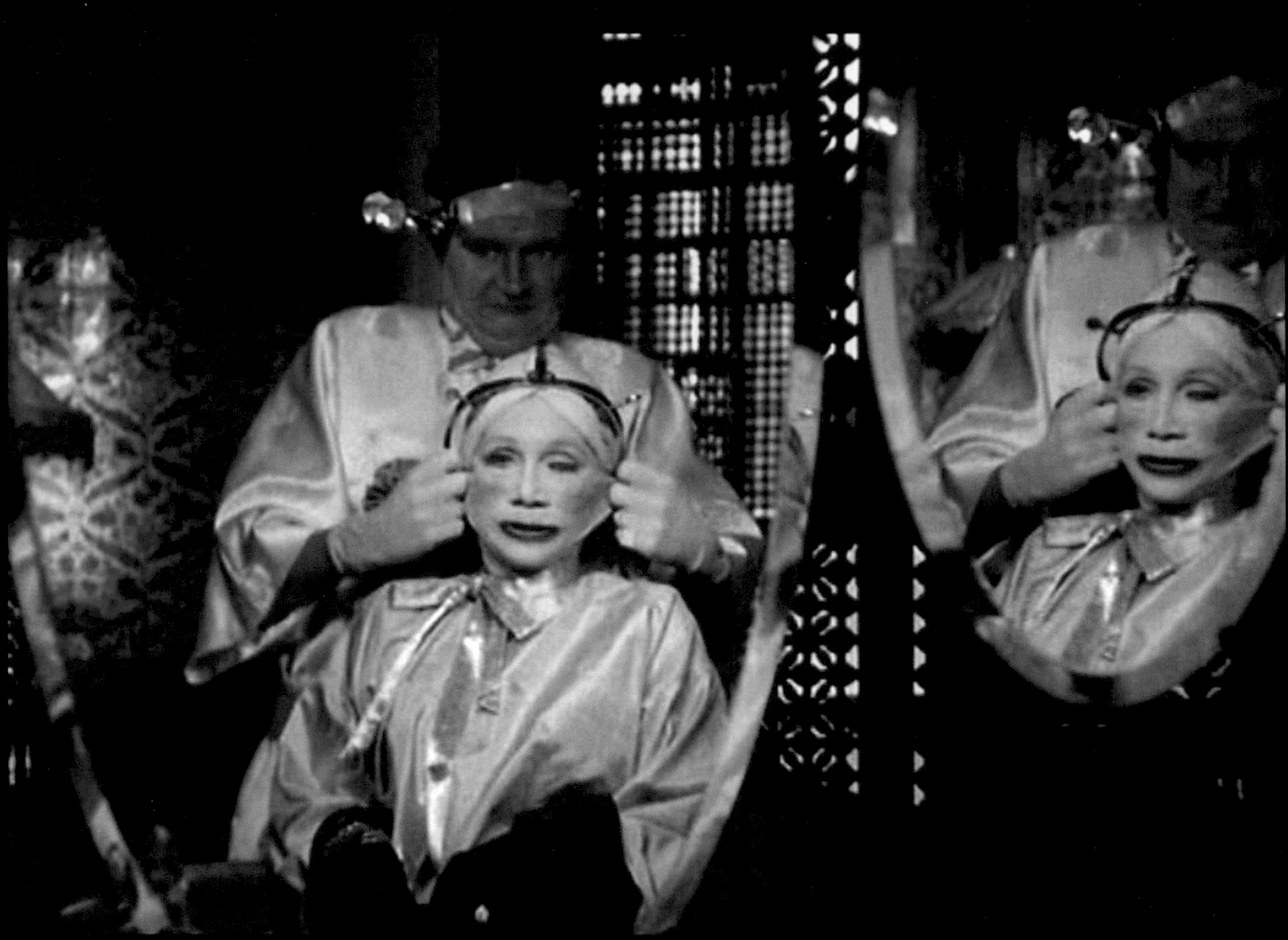

fig. 44

(Hildegard Knef): "A woman considering suicide has only one worry remaining: 'What will I look like when they find me?' She would take pills, slit her wrists, drown herself, even shoot herself — but never would she throw herself under a train. She wants to be remembered as beautiful and elegant, not as disfigured and mutilated." In fact, however, the audience has been aware from the start of the film that this is exactly how the actress took her life.

In *Fedora*, the secret of beauty is also the key to identity. The real Fedora is not the dead woman, we learn, but this very Countess Sobryanski, disfigured by a failed cosmetic operation and bound to a wheelchair. The supposed Fedora was in fact her daughter, who took over the role to continue the glamorous life of the film star and perpetuate her fame.

While the mother was unable to cope with the loss of her beauty, the daughter could no longer cope with the loss of her own identity. The mother could not stand being robbed of her publicity, while the daughter was robbed of her privacy. Both lives failed because of an incongruence of interior and exterior reality. Wilder presents aesthetic surgery as a tragic masquerade, a process of self-denial in the service of show business. Condemned to flawless beauty, the stars are unable to escape its inhumane clutches even in their death: After the eternally beautiful Fedora is disfigured by her grisly suicide, cosmetic surgery is used once more to give her the face she was known for.

It is deeply sarcastic when Wilder presents the old, blemished Fedora as an advocate of the Hollywood glamour aesthetic. In her view, the illusion of beauty is the only reason why Hollywood exists: "Audiences were sick of what they were being offered in the name of entertainment — cinema verité, the naked truth, the uglier the better? No, they wanted glamour."

Hubris and Decadence

As the general public has become increasingly familiar with the practice of plastic surgery, the cinematic treatment of the subject has become less sinister. Instead, surgeons and patients alike are being used as welcome targets for social satire and wholesale ridicule. Consistent with older cinematic approaches are the image of the surgeon as an artist caught between genius and insanity, and the issue of personal identity.

In Terry Gilliam's *Brazil*, aesthetic surgery is elevated to a status symbol for the decadent society depicted. In this futurist fantasy, the rich don't collect art — instead, the ladies of society have turned themselves into art objects, human canvases for competing surgeon-artists to wage their bizarre discourse on. Acid or scalpel — this "scientific" debate of diverging surgical approaches uses live "objects" to prove its points. While one of the patients may be transformed into an attractive young woman, another may end up as an amorphous blob. It is made painfully obvious that the transgression of life's natural order can only end in extreme grotesque, heralding the decay of this society.

A similar perspective, albeit presented not nearly as drasti-

fig. 44

Oh, mother! — Terry Gilliam's Brazil *(1984) uses garish colours to portray an unfettered cosmetic surgery that severs all natural, biological ties between parents and children.*

fig. 45–47

The operation as a farce, the surgeon as a stylist: Facelifting as an artistic performance!

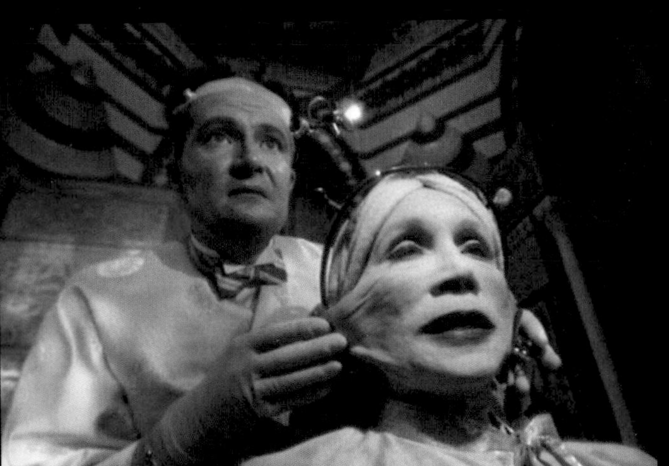

fig. 45

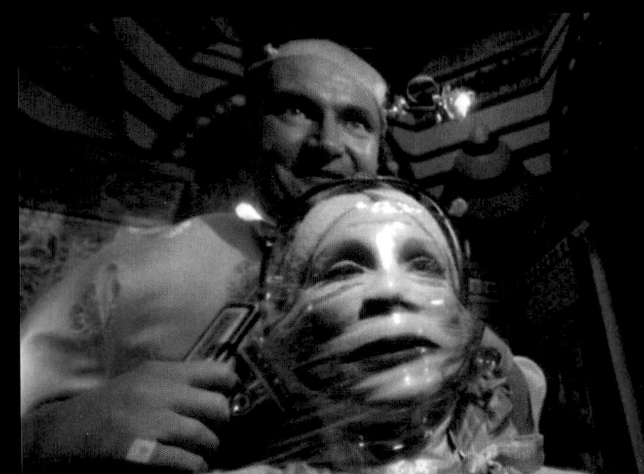

fig. 46

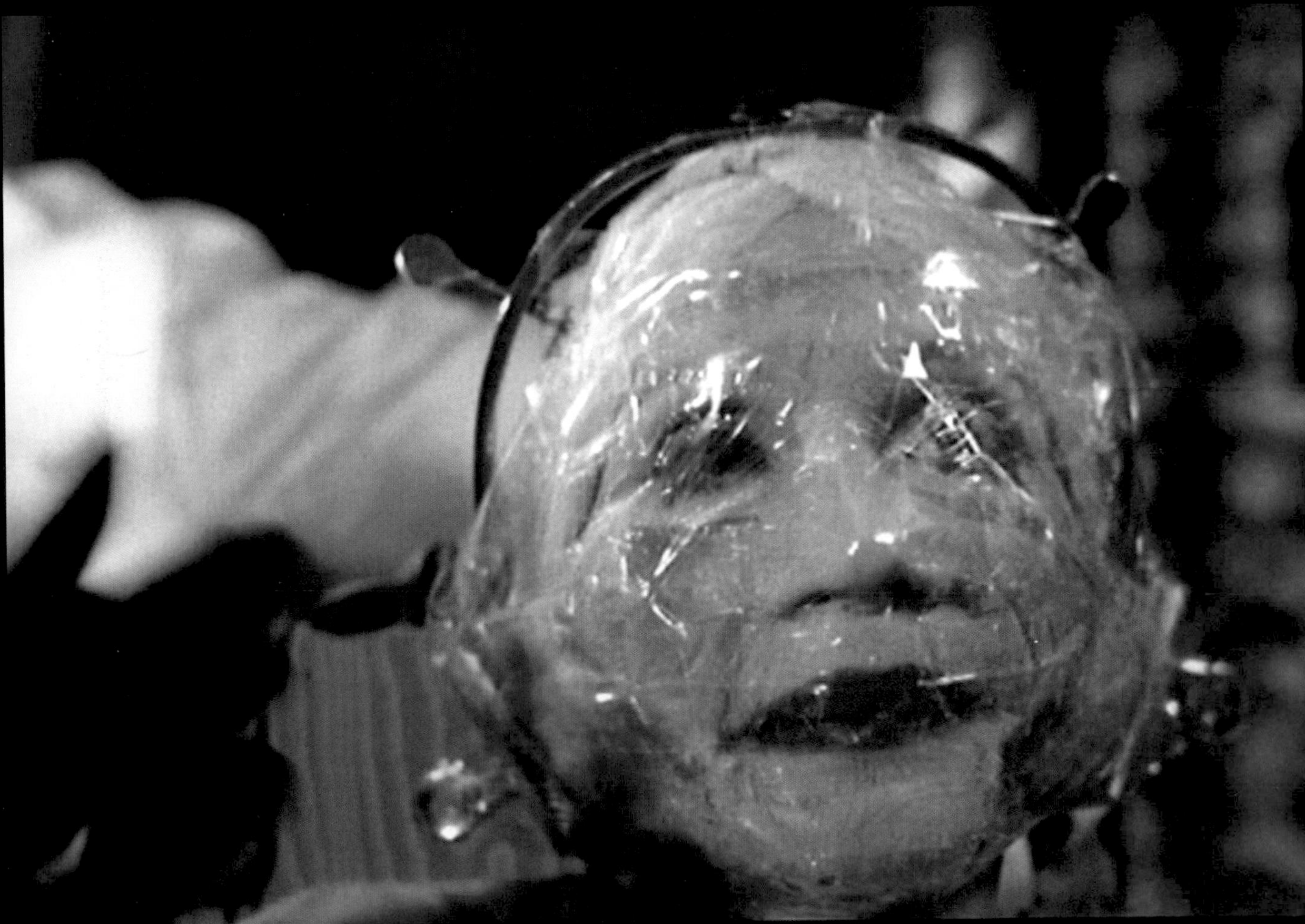

fig. 47

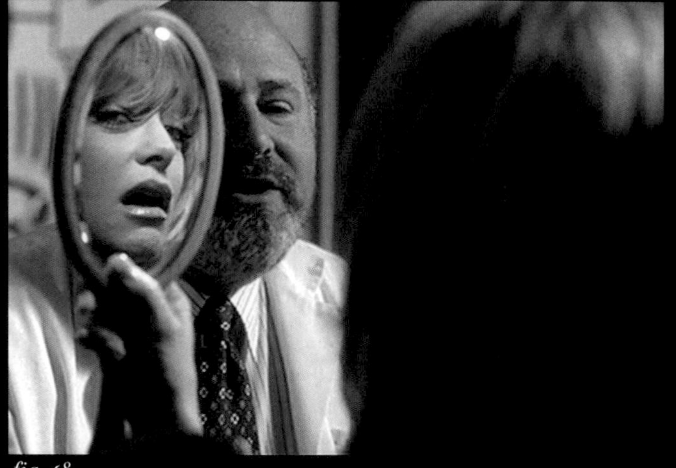

fig. 48

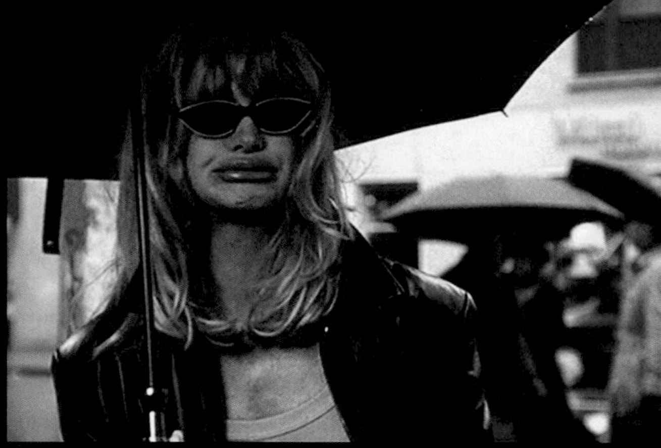

fig. 49

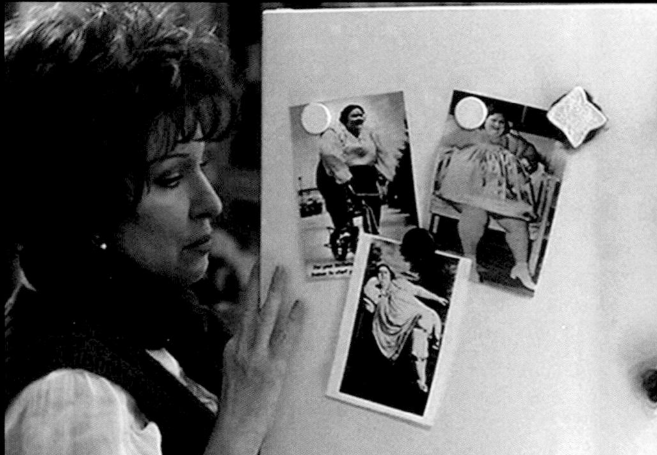

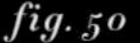

fig. 50

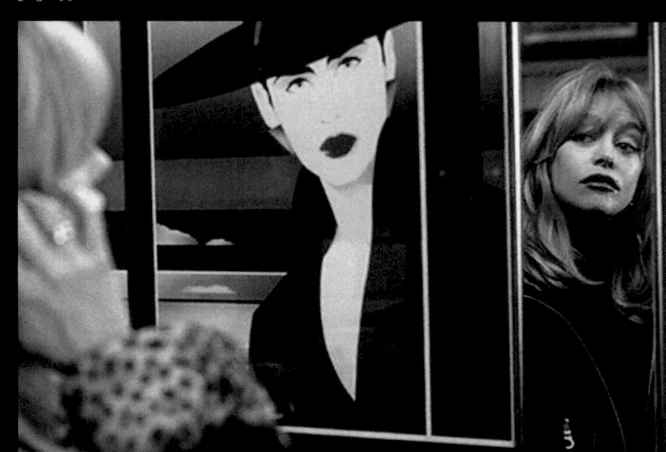

fig. 51

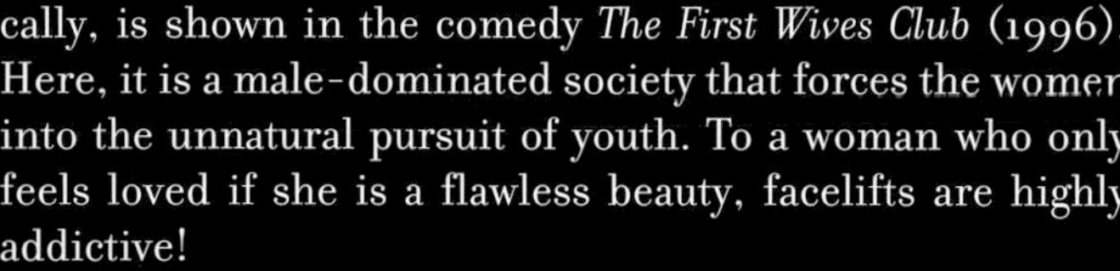

cally, is shown in the comedy *The First Wives Club* (1996). Here, it is a male-dominated society that forces the women into the unnatural pursuit of youth. To a woman who only feels loved if she is a flawless beauty, facelifts are highly addictive!

A notable development in this film is the surgeon's role as a rational, sensible doctor, who warns his patients against crossing the boundaries of reasonability. At the same time, he is still an artist – "You are my masterpiece!" – who will ultimately submit to his client's wishes and chequebook.

One of the characters is presented alternatively as a victim to be pitied – at the end, this patient cannot even smoke a cigarette as her lips have become too puffy – and a figure of fun. Behind her back, rumour is rife that "some parts of her" are indeed fifty years old … Still, there is enough self-awareness here to realise that this desperate search for youthfulness is part of the career-oriented woman's battle to gain power in a male-dominated society, and that the market forces of showbiz demand it. Again, we remember that identity is largely constructed – a construct more than ever based on individual ambition. A beautiful body seems to put every goal within reach. Ultimately, this is a phenomenon for which Hollywood was only a precursor.

When dealing with plastic surgery, it is also one of cinema's repeated aims to present an idealist approach to identity, to show that identity is not anchored in outward appearance. In Walter Hill's *Johnny Handsome* (1989), a criminal who has been disfigured from birth (Mickey Rourk) is transformed into a virtuous beau. In this film, the plastic surgeon (Forest Whitaker) appears as a miracle worker, softly proclaiming the good news that every human being can become a different person if given the chance. The only one not to believe in Johnny's miraculous transformation is the cynical inspector (Morgan Freeman), who, in the end, is proven right. Still, the film declines to resolve the question if "handsome Johnny" was simply unable to beat his old habits or if it was his social environment that brought the ugly side of his personality to the fore again.

Masquerades of the Self

The question remains – *are* we simply who we are, or are we *made* into that which we are? Just as importantly, are we really who we *think* we are? Seeing that outward appearance has become such an important part of our self-definition, and that our physical exterior is becoming [illegible] less predetermined but a ductile expression of our wishes and ambitions, we cannot even trust our mirror image anymore.

In Wolfgang Petersen's *Shattered* (1991), a man (Tom Berenger)is involved in a car accident that he survives with severe amnesia and a disfigured face which is reconstructed in a lengthy series of operations. As he is recuperating, doubts begin to surface: The few fragmentary memories left to him are difficult to reconcile with the details offered by his wife to reintegrate him into his old life. At the end, all initial viewer assumptions of who is the good and who the bad guy in this film are knocked on the head – the sup-

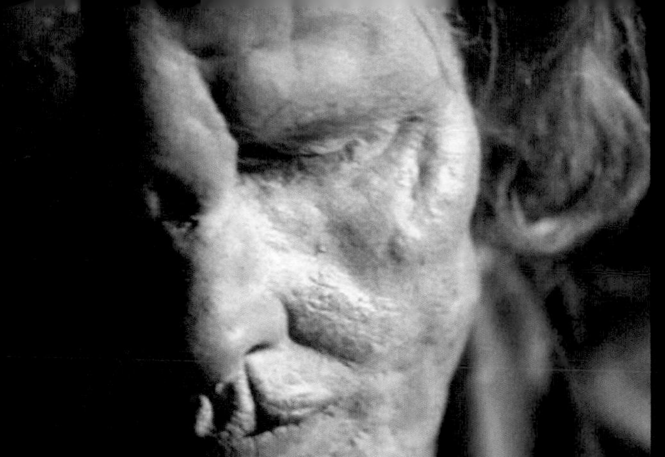

fig. 52

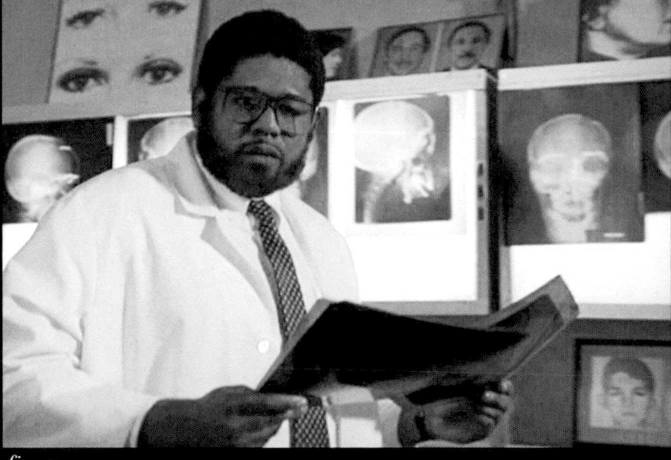

fig. 53

fig. 48–51

The pressures of conformity women are subjected to only make plastic surgeons more powerful. Hugh Wilson's comedy First Wives Club *(1996) portrays facelifting as an addiction.*

fig. 52 & 53

Is it possible to create a new personality together with a new appearance? In Walter Hill's Johnny Handsome *(1989), the cosmetic surgeon seems to affect a change that a social worker could only dream of: A disfigured criminal (Mickey Rourke) is converted into a reformed citizen.*

fig. 54

A world turned upside down: For a moment, reality has lost both direction and scale.

fig. 54

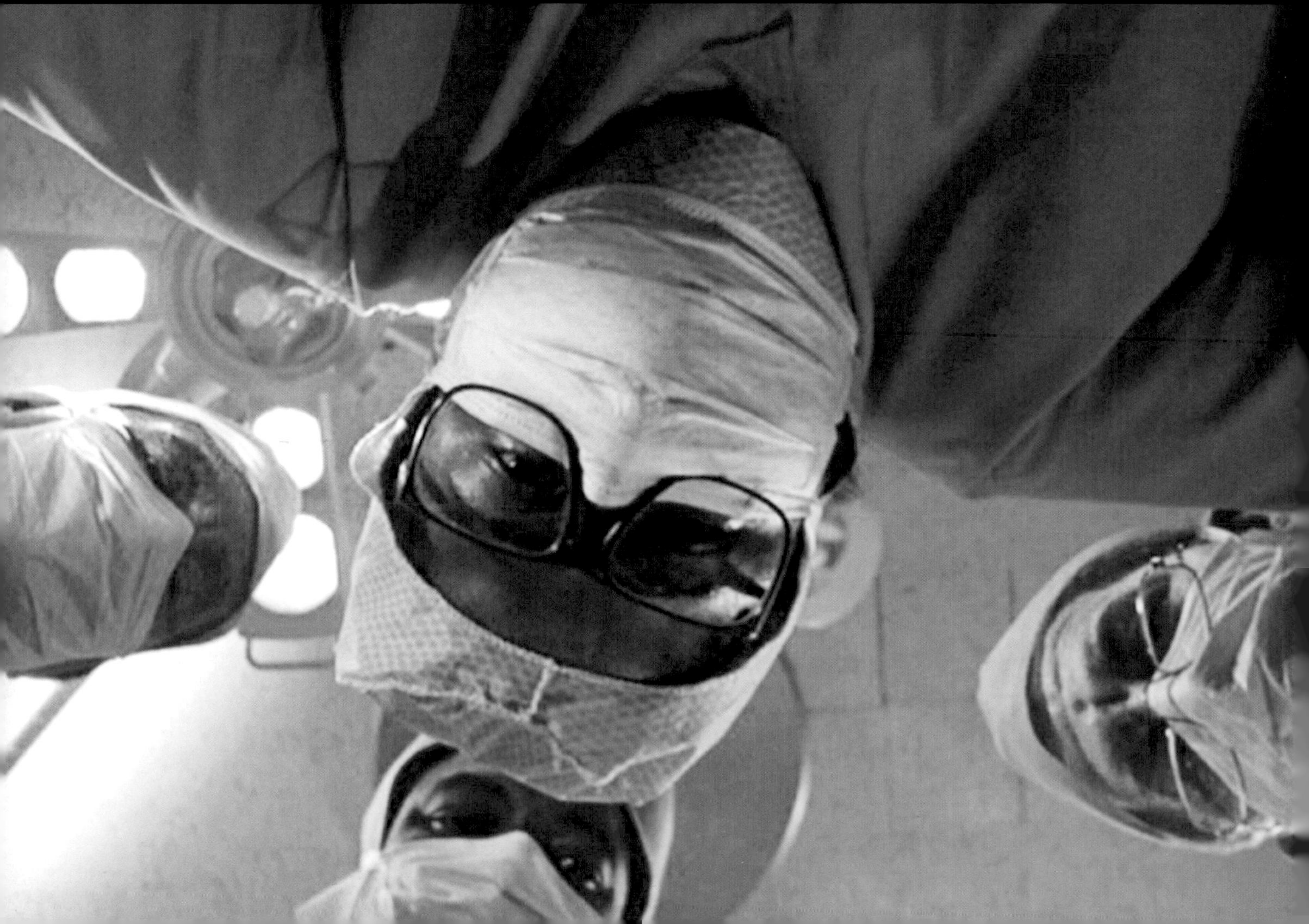

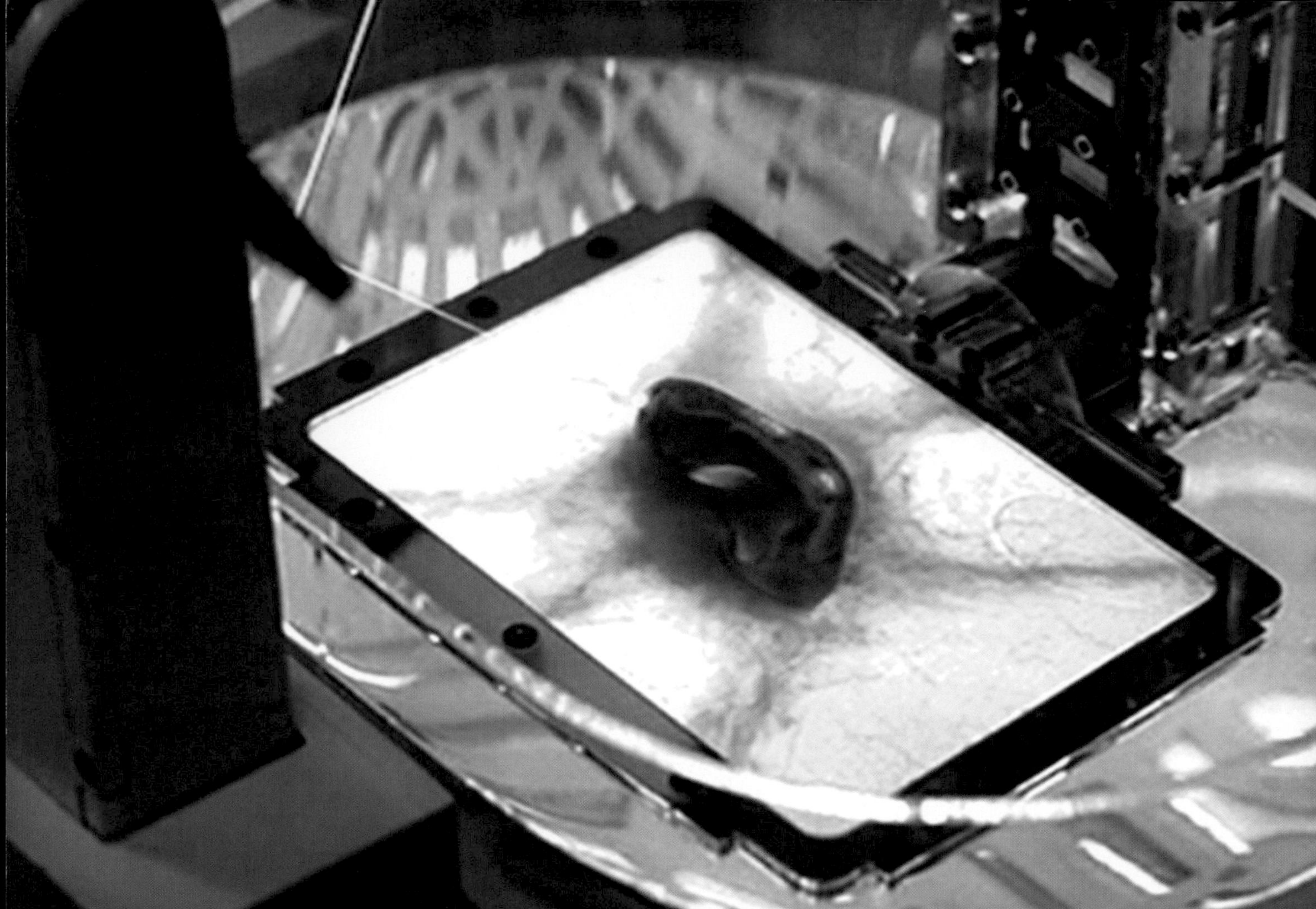

fig. 55

posed wife used her lover to get rid of her husband and then forces the lover to take on her husband's identity to cover up the murder.

More significant than the theme of exchanged identity, which is the key plot element in this thriller, is the realism with which Petersen depicts the operation. Our first image of the protagonist is his totally disfigured face right after the accident. In a dream sequence shown later on, splinters of glass assume the shape of a face, only to shatter again — a metaphor for the shattering of an identity, providing a clue for later plot developments but also implying that the upcoming metamorphosis will be a painful one. Next, a shattering windscreen is superimposed over images of the disfigured face, and finally, the operation itself is recapitulated. The viewer is mercilessly confronted with all the bloody details, from the sanding down of the scars to the slow surgical process of restoring the face.

In retrospect, the viewer knows that the surgeons, having been tricked by the wife, sculpted an entirely new face from the facial "material" remaining after the accident. When the patient finally recovers, he attacks his mirror image in helpless rage. We now know that he had recognised the face of his adversary in the mirror — his own new face. His instinctual response was to destroy the identity that had been cast onto him, and, as in the other films discussed, the inner self ultimately triumphs over the exterior mask.

In his action thriller *Face/Off* (1997), John Woo demonstrates how deeply we rely on facial traits to recognise and trust those close to us. High-tech surgery, presented in this film as a fusion of the classic operating theatre, an alchemist's lab and the Star Trek command bridge, makes it possible for faces to be treated as exchangeable masks. Sean Archer (John Travolta), a policeman, is thus able to assume the identity of his most hated enemy, the terrorist Castor Troy (Nicolas Cage), who previously murdered Archer's son. Archer's aim is to gather information about a bomb strike on L. A. by gaining the confidence of Troy's brother, who is held at a maximum-security prison. Meanwhile Troy manages to take control of the surgeons and forces them to graft Archer's face onto his own faceless head, thereafter effectively assuming control of Archer's life. This exchange is only reversed temporarily in a later scene when the two characters stand on opposite sides of a double-sided mirror.

It may come as a surprise that film distrusts outward appearances so vehemently, seeing that it is a predominantly visual medium itself. Examining this more closely, it makes perfect sense; cinema, after all, is the home to illusion and illustrates the precarious balance of interior and exterior reality better than any other medium.

"Is this your daughter, Mrs. Lefferts?" — "I don't know," answers the old woman, obviously unable to tell. Only a mole on the dead body's hip finally makes it possible for her to identify her murdered daughter. Officer Bud White (Russell Crowe) can understand the confusion. "You're wrong, Officer," the red-haired beauty now lying dead at

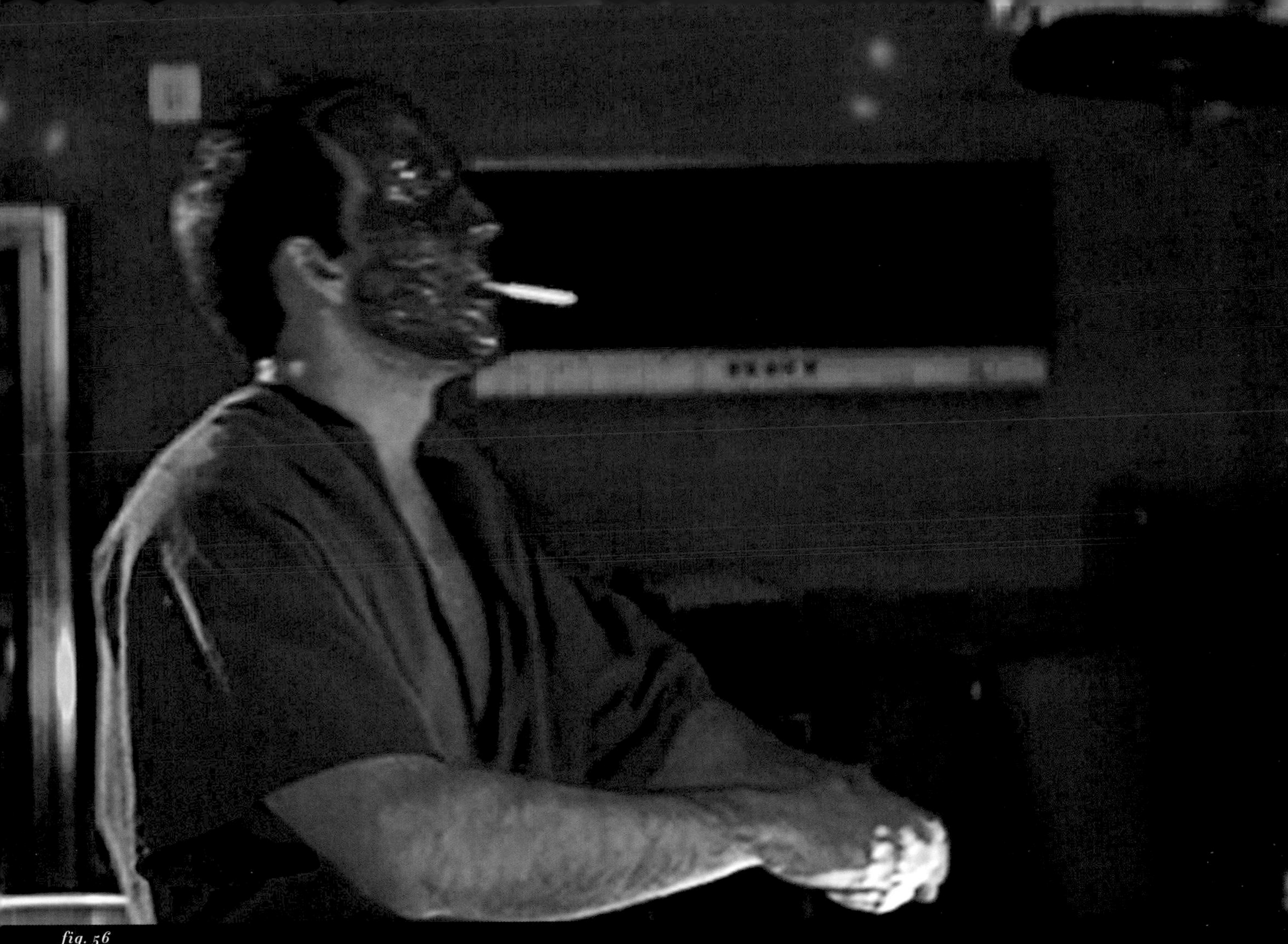

fig. 56

fig. 55

In Face / Off *(1997, directed by John Woo) the possibilities of manipulating human appearance seem to be boundless.*

fig. 56

Stay cool: The terrorist Castor Troy (Nicolas Cage) relaxes with a cigarette while waiting for his new face.

fig. 57–59

John Woo's film presents a high-tech vision of plastic surgery where outward appearance can be transformed flawlessly and permanently.

fig. 60

The face as a membrane between interior and exterior reality: A dormant identity?

the morgue had said to him not long before. Then, the girl's nose was in bandages — not because of an attack or an accident, but because Susan Lefferts was in the process of turning herself into Rita Hayworth.

In this film, *L. A. Confidential* (1997), director Curtis Hanson dramatically shows us an embittered battle for identity — in a world where ideals have become an unaffordable luxury, and self-presentation and prostitution of all kinds are the only effective means of survival. In this man's world, women have been degraded to mere objects of fantasy. The prostitutes depicted here, who slip into the roles and appearances of film stars for the pleasure of their clients, are ultimately more consequent and maybe also more honest than the others. After all, who really is everything they pretend to be? Beauty can't exist without displaying an element of truthfulness. But what is beauty? *L. A. Confidential* reminds us that the value of beauty lies in its recognisability. In the glamorous world of Hollywood, it is not an individual, personal trait, but a look to be marketed. This is the flipside of the beauty concept presented here — one where women are never allowed just to be themselves. In this world, beauty is not a value but a function.

In *L. A. Confidential*, the theme of cosmetic surgery symbolises the illusion and an overwhelming need to conform which people in the media world are confronted with every day. Hollywood is a place where beauty is turned into a sellable commodity, and one could even see it as a metaphor of the Western world and its values: a select few have to be beautiful, happy and eternally young for the rest of us to look up to.

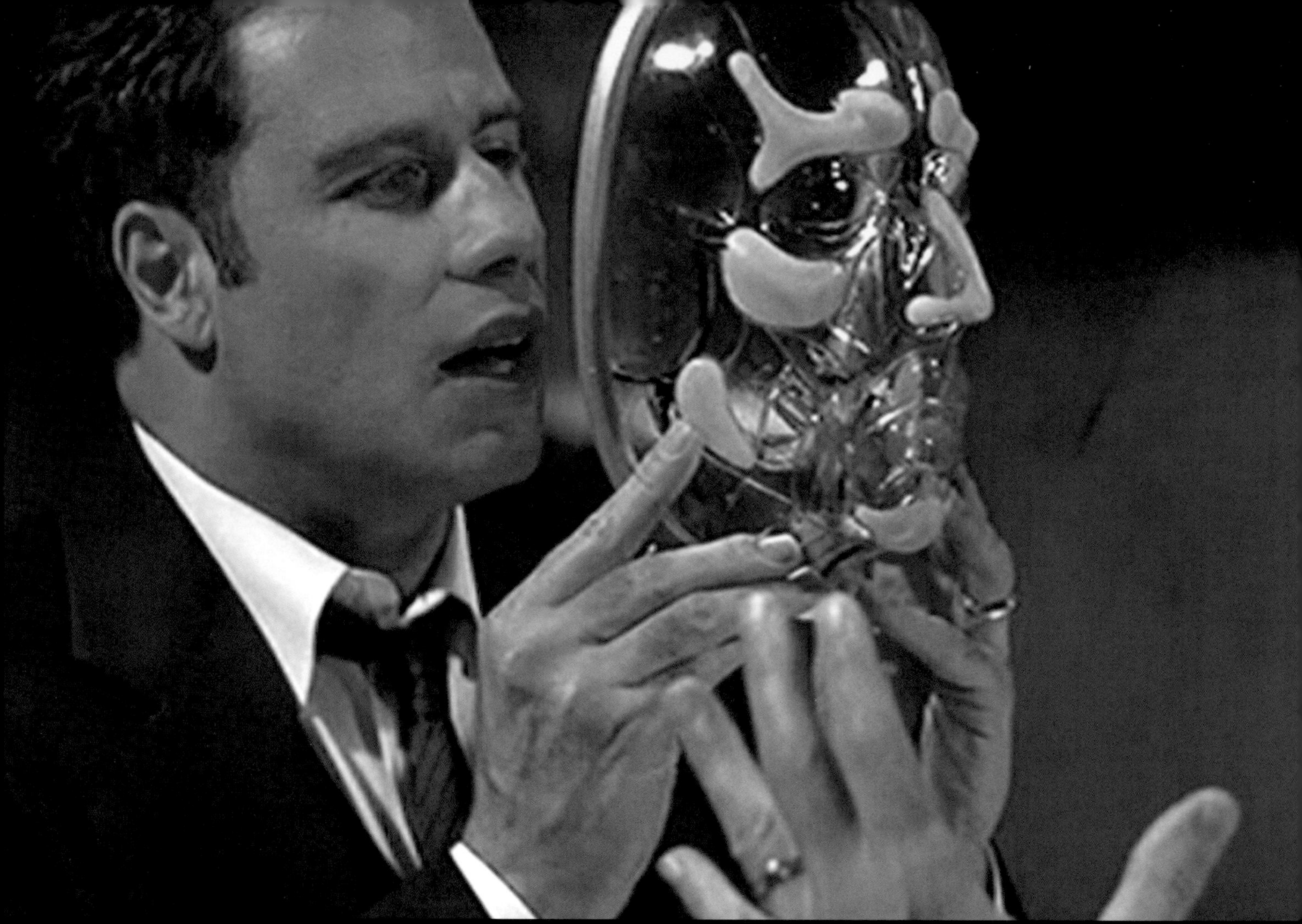

fig. 57 / fig. 58

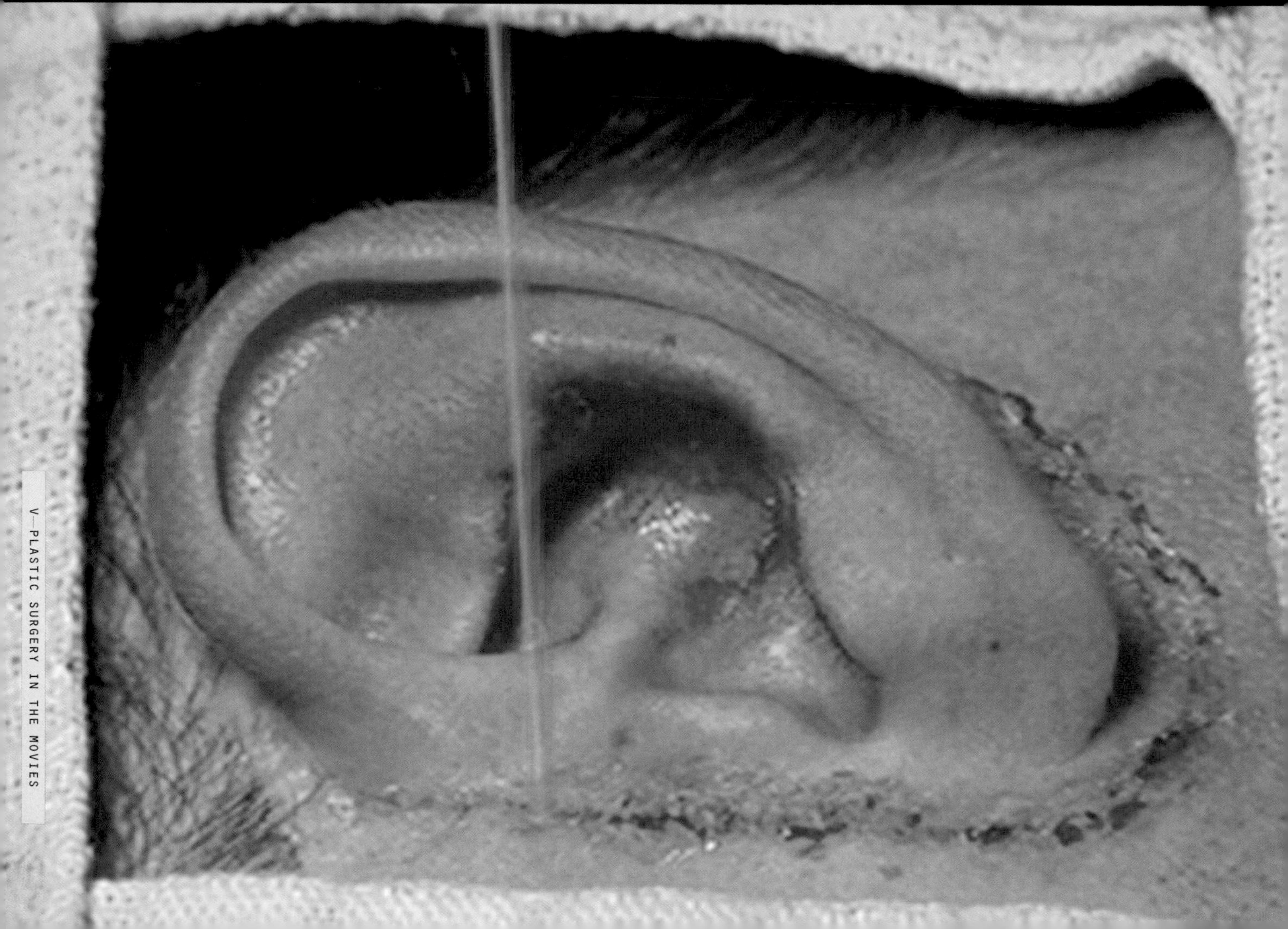

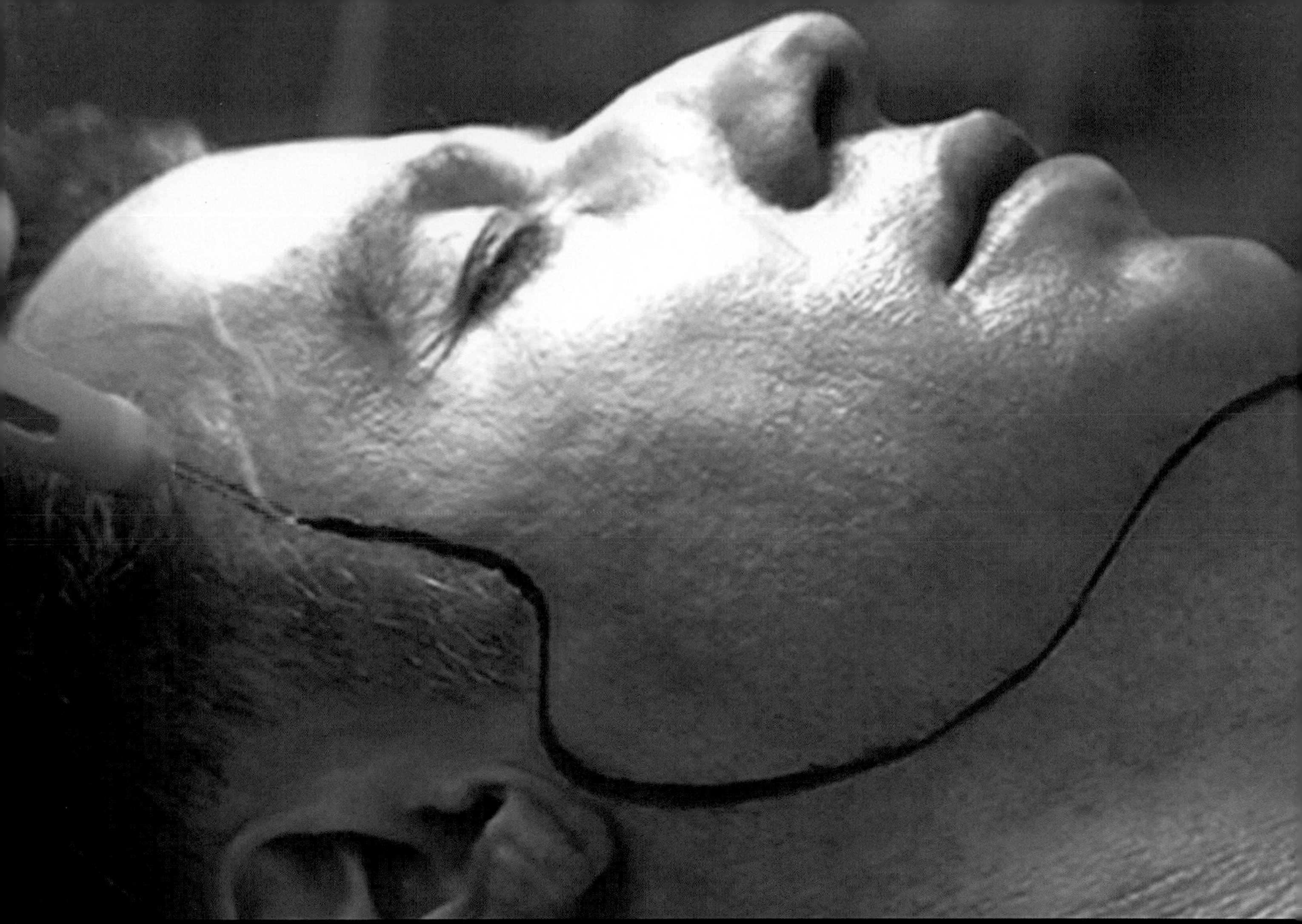

fig. 59 / fig. 60

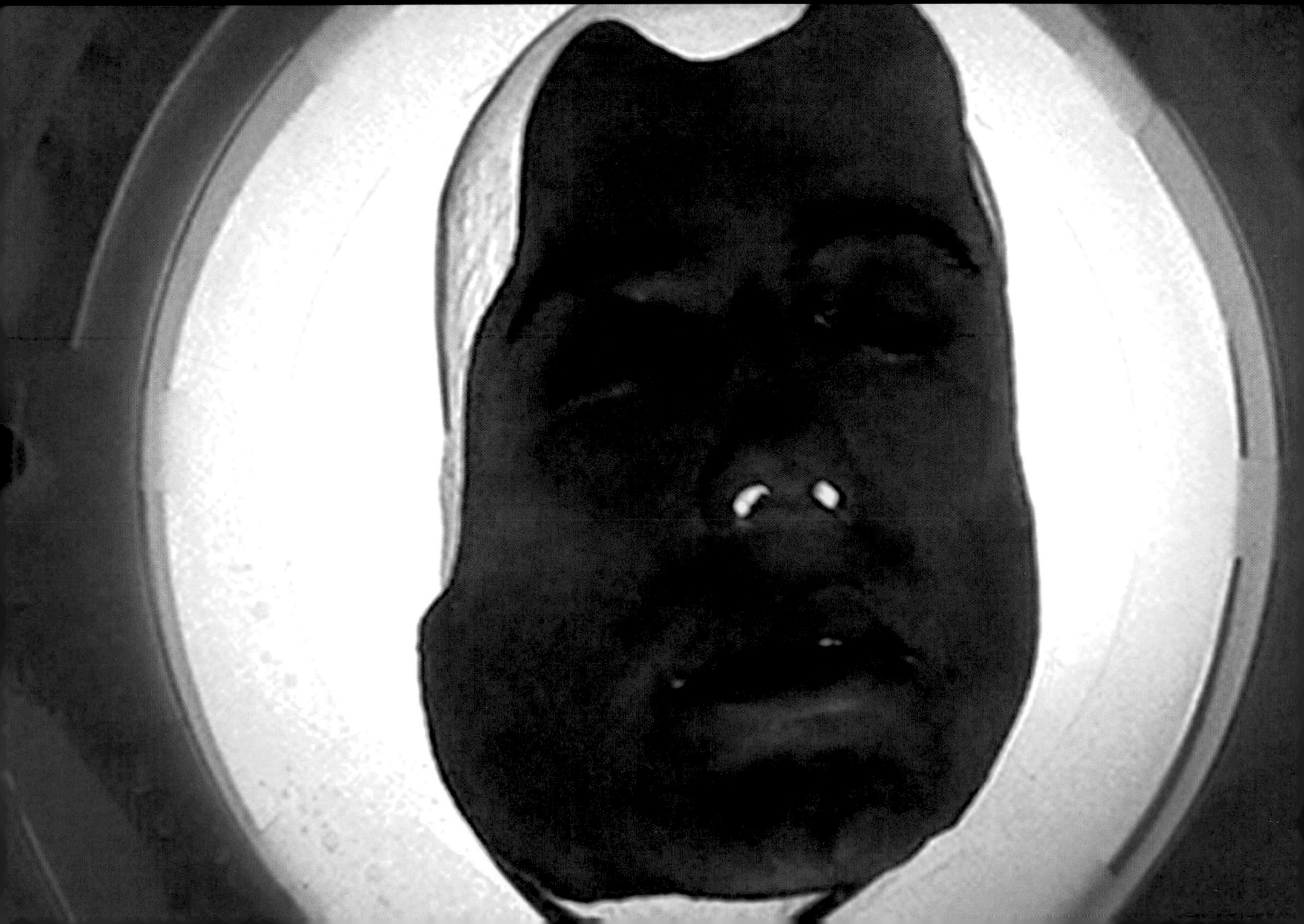

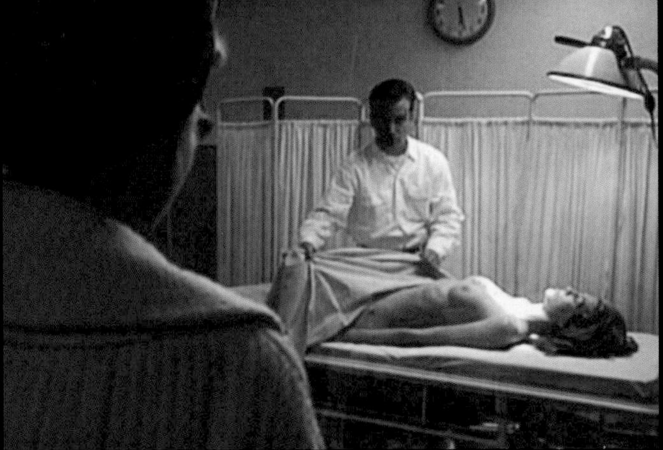

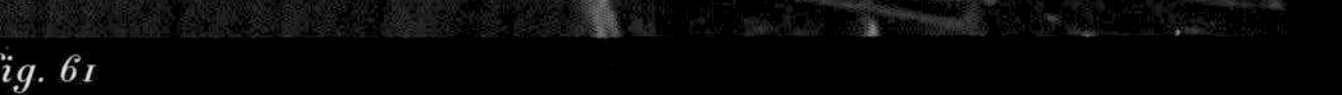

fig. 61

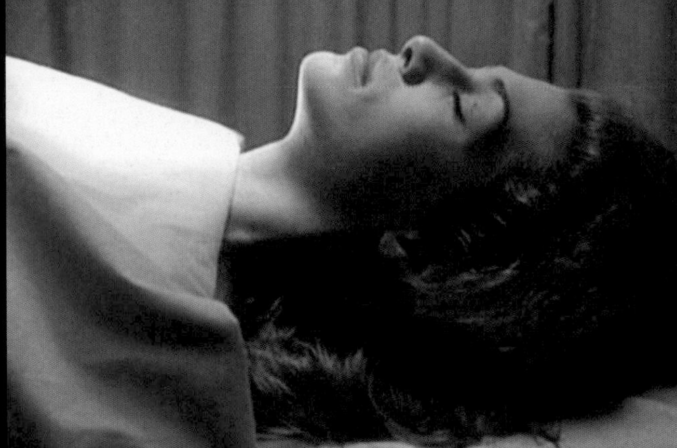

fig. 62

Beautiful Illusion

The object of Cameron Crowe's *Vanilla Sky* (2001), a remake of the Spanish film *Abre los Ojos* (1997) by Alejandro Amenábar, is to present beauty as the fragile foundation of self-worth. David Aames (Tom Cruise), a 33-year-old millionaire heir, has been arrested on suspicion of murder. Together with the psychologist Curtis McCabe (Kurt Russell), he attempts to make sense of the past weeks (and indeed years) of his life. David's privileged life had changed drastically after meeting the beautiful dancer Sofia Serrano (Penélope Cruz). Soon after starting a relationship with her, he becomes the victim of a car accident caused by his disappointed ex-lover. David's face ends up disfigured and the right half of his body is almost paralysed. His perfect world, largely based on superficialities, collapses.

Although his face is soon restored, David refuses to take off his protective mask (made especially to speed up his recovery), and the psychologist does not get to see his face. To David, the loss of his looks is synonymous with a loss of self-worth. The repercussions of this borderline experi-

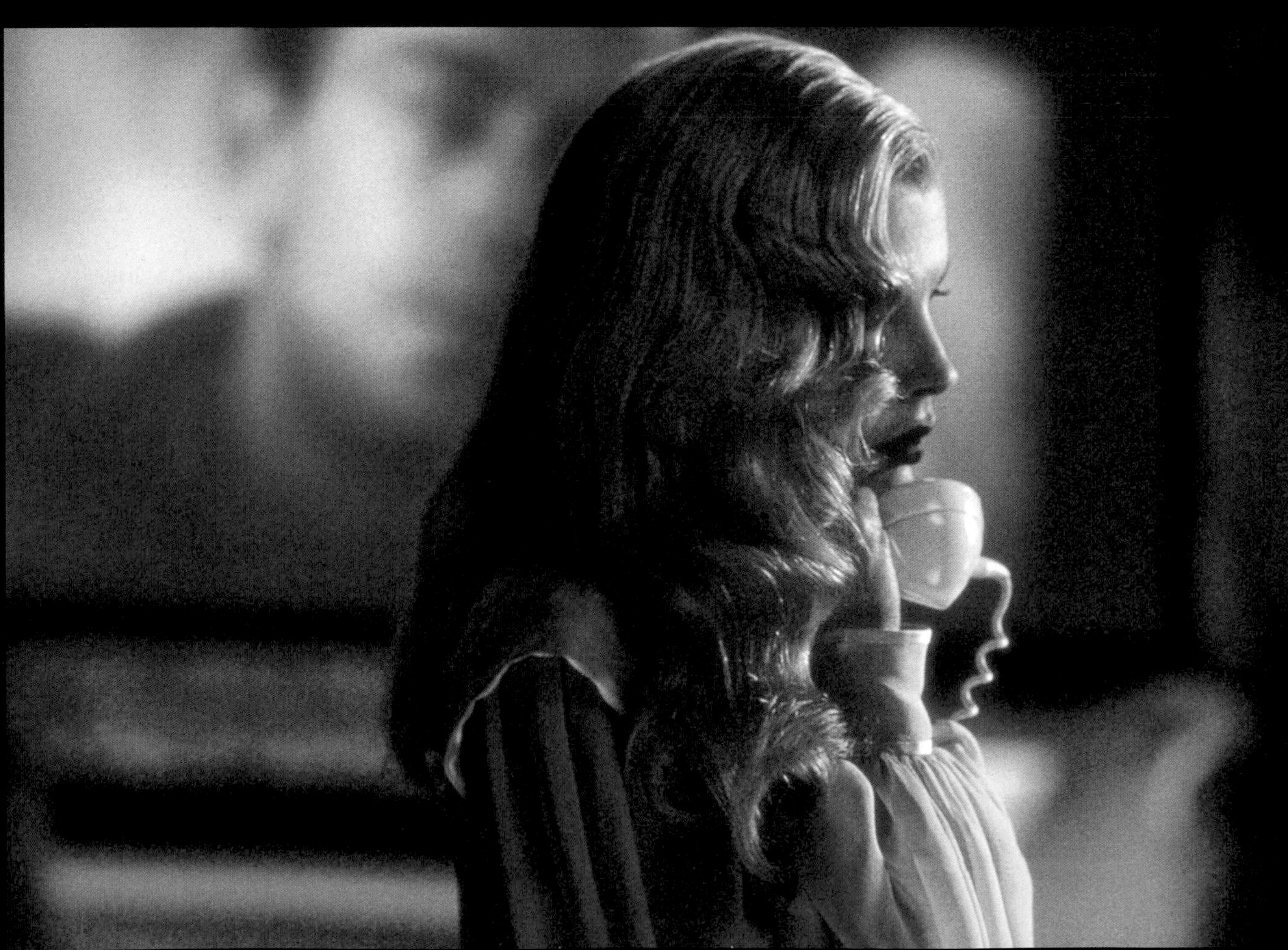

fig. 63

fig. 61

The horror of a mother...

fig. 62

... who is unable to identify her dead daughter: In Curtis Hanson's L. A. Confidential *(1997), young prostitutes are remodelled to look like famous film stars.*

fig. 63

Model and clone: The call girl Lynn (Kim Basinger) gives her clients the illusion of going to bed with Veronica Lake (who is displayed on the poster in the background).

fig. 64

A white hair! Paradise is flawed, a dream catches up with reality. Tom Cruise as David Aames has to face the fact that his world is but a figment of his imagination. (Vanilla Sky, *2001, directed by Cameron Crowe).*

fig. 65

The all-powerful vs. the disempowered: David Aames (Tom Cruise) faces his medical team like a man defending himself.

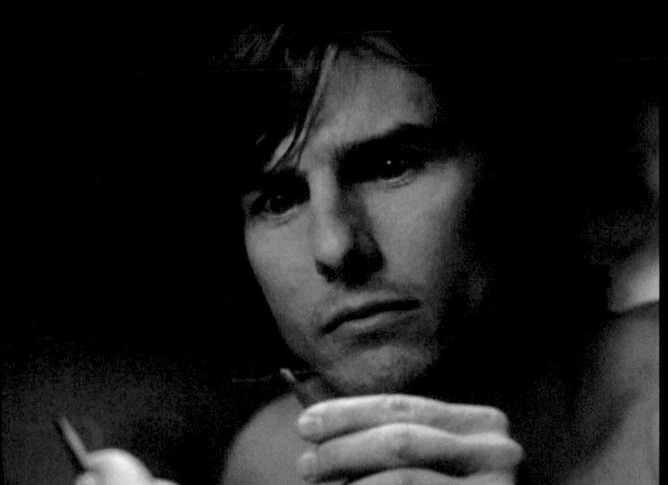

fig. 64

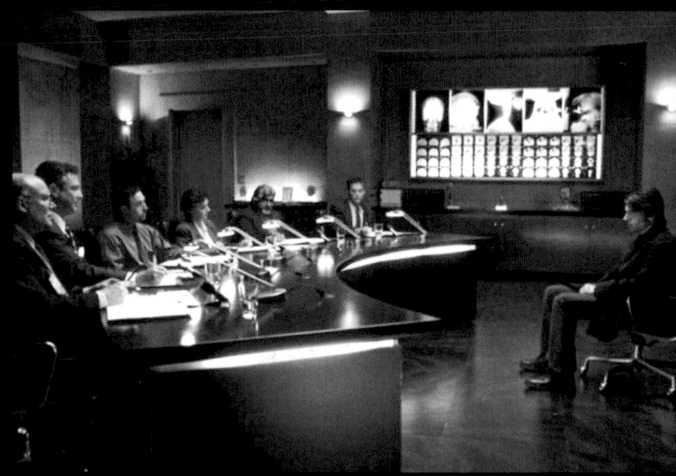

fig. 65

ence, gradually revealed to the viewer in a series of flashbacks, cannot be reversed by surgery alone, as successful as it may be. When treatment starts to look unpromising, Aames challenges his doctors to be more experimental, willing to take any risk to get back his old life. Dr. Pomerantz, a surgeon who does without the white coat usually associated with cinema's "doctor" stereotype, appearing more like a top-level manager instead, appeals to his patient's common sense: "We're not cowboys here who can chop and change you at wish!" Instead of a new surgical strategy, Aames' six-strong medical team presents him with a specially developed facial mask made of latex to aid the regeneration of his skin.

On his first public excursion, the desperate man is unable to cope and runs wild. He wears the hated mask on the back of his head — a macabre symbol of his inner turmoil, and also a symbol for the interchangeability of dreams and nightmarish reality. As David finds out in one of the film's more surreal turns, he is in fact living in an artificial dream state — a dream that is going wrong because of a technical defect. When finally given the choice, he decides to wake up and lead a life beyond the illusion of beauty.

In doing so, he rejects society's pressure to comply with certain standards of appearance. In one of the key lines of the film, David explains to his aesthetic surgeon before operating that "It's not about vanity. Vanity is not the issue here but how I function in the world. It is my job to function out there." Now that this premise has proven to be a fragile illusion and his unconditional belief in the union of beauty and truth has been broken, he is willing to again engage in the adventure of reality.

The Mirror never Lies

The initial apprehensiveness plastic surgery was met with in film, and its relegation to the realm of horror, has largely subsided. Complex views of the subject are evident in films that explore the relationship between a person's identity and their outward appearance, or in films that take a satirical view of plastic surgery. Satire often focuses on the figure of the client or patient, who feels the need to comply with society's conception of beauty — an aspect the viewer is made to both question and identify with.

Similarly, the figure of the surgeon has also grown in complexity. The old clichés are still quoted in some instances, such as Steven Spielberg's *Minority Report* (2002), but usually these are deliberate references to film history. When the surgical operation itself is shown in graphic detail, this is usually for the purpose of drawing attention to technological or medical progress, not to elicit a negative emotional response. The characters' face-swap in *Face/Off*, for example, is an indication that we live in a world that has become so complex and technologically advanced that nothing should be taken at face value — an old topic in a new guise.

Most films involving plastic surgery focus on society's obsession with youthfulness and its superficial approach to

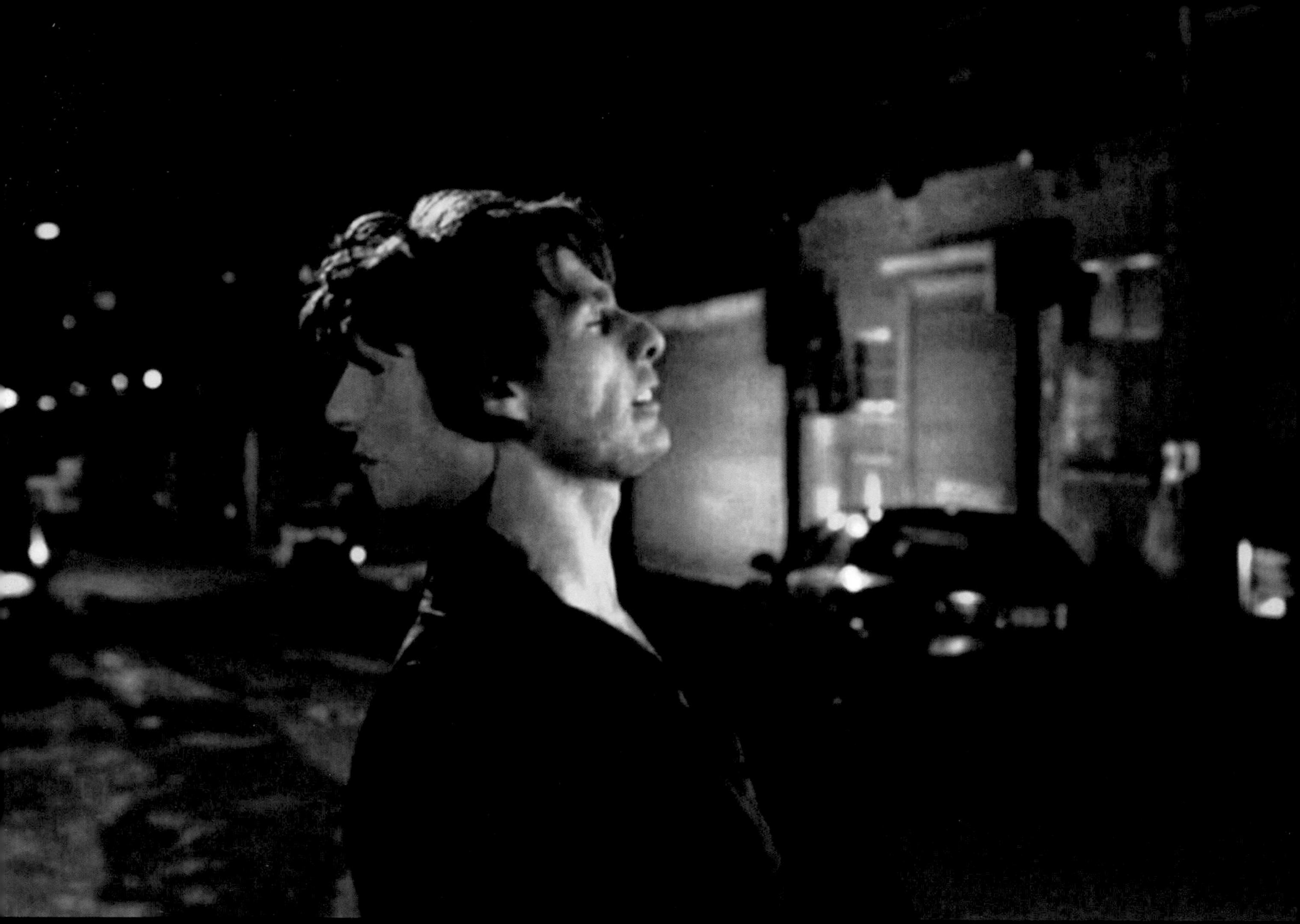

fig. 66 / fig. 67

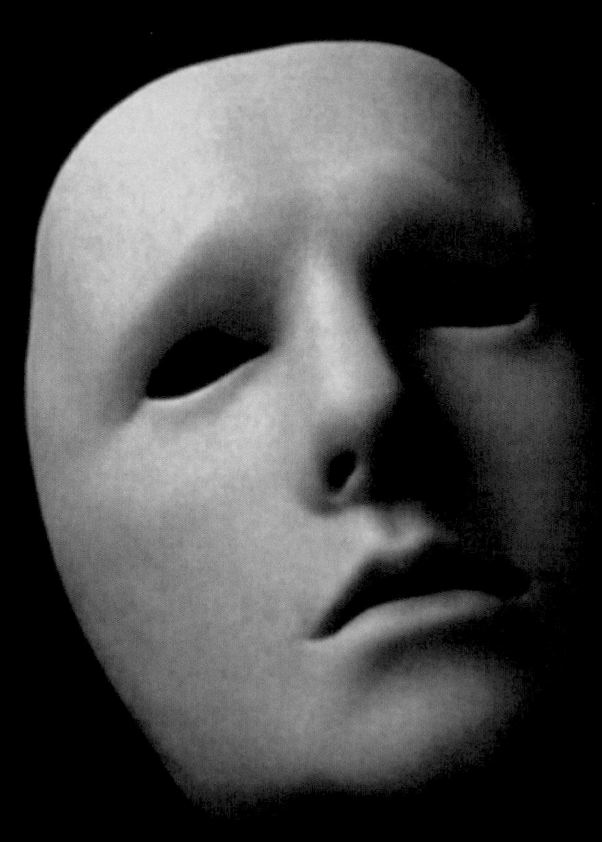

fig. 66

Split identity: David Aames (Tom Cruise) has lost control of his life.

fig. 67

The mask is no less enigmatic than the mirror. What if identity was but a mask with nothing behind it?

fig. 68

We design our "adventure," and our destiny.

human identity and appearance. A new level of filmic reflection quite beyond this is reached in Crowe's *Vanilla Sky*. The film discusses a question that easily transcends the established context of plastic surgery: Once you become aware of the constructed nature of perceived concepts such as beauty, truth, love etc., what relevance does the artificial manipulation of a person's *outward* appearance still have? Film makers from all eras have been thoroughly sceptical towards the practice of plastic surgery. Being at the mercy of your own body, e. g. suffering from disfigurement, is projected onto the helplessness of the patient towards the surgeon. This is presented in a number of contexts:

The treatment of aesthetic surgery is fairly non-specific when used to symbolise the decadence of society. In this instance, the real theme is vanity — of both the patients and the surgeons. This context is predominantly addressed by comedies.

Another means of using the theme is to present the problem of hubris. In this case, the medical professional is seduced into doing evil, deluded by the manipulative possibilities of plastic surgery. This is really part of the much larger 'mad scientist' context, which can also be found in many different genres.

But undoubtedly, the primary filmic context for the subject of aesthetic surgery is the issue of identity. Again, this has been addressed in a wide variety of genres. Aesthetic surgery is a very apt metaphor for the issue of identity vs. illusion, as it so neatly juxtaposes interior and exterior realities. In terms of film aesthetics, the extent of its importance is often underestimated. For as we have seen, it often determines not only the "what" but the "how" of the narrative. Cosmetic and facial surgery offer a number of narrative possibilities that are specific to the medium of film. Only the cinema can really tell us how difficult it is to look in the mirror after a facial operation. Only film can show us images that alternately make us the subject and the object of perception. Only film can depict the uncertainty and doubt a person experiences when their feelings of false superiority give way to feelings of guilt. In this context, the act of stepping in front of the mirror and looking into it is the defining moment; as viewers, we observe (or believe we are observing) a human being's estrangement from him or herself. It is no coincidence that as a filmic device, the mirror is so often used to symbolise loss of identity.

When it comes to identity, film narrative can let us slip into the skin of the character presented, and show us the discrepancies between inner and outer reality. In such instances, the contrast between inside and outside is a visualised reflection of human identity. Again, the mirror serves as a symbol for the issue of personal identity. Not only can it suggest the integrity of outward appearance and inner character; more importantly, it can also emphasise the dissociation and growing polarisation of the two. Yet the mirror remains the placeholder of identity — an identity that is not a state but a vital necessity.

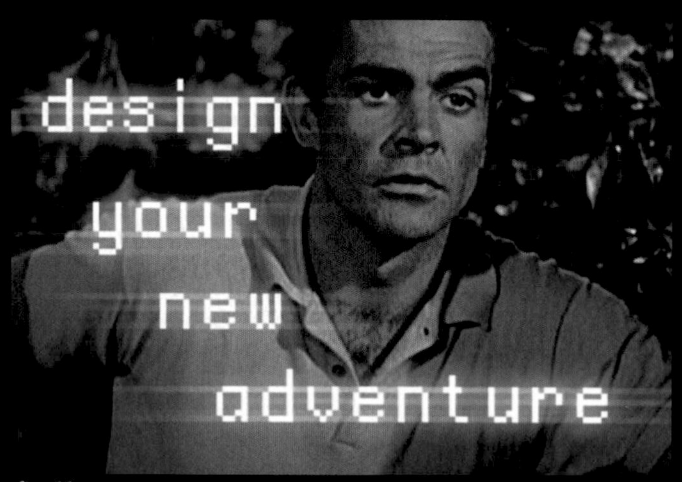

fig. 68

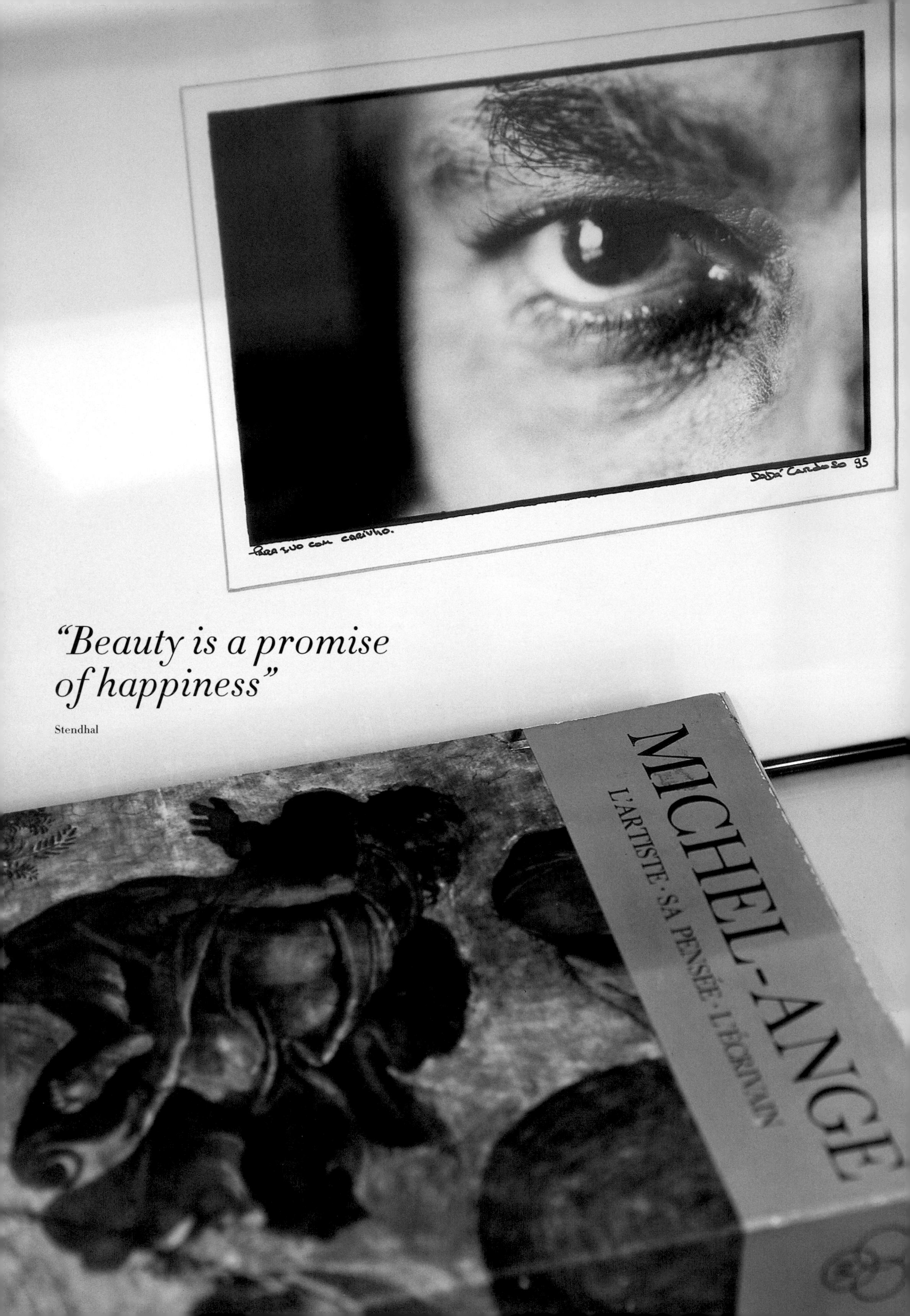

"Beauty is a promise of happiness"

Stendhal

VI.

THE MICHELANGELO OF THE SCALPEL: IVO PITANGUY

Text by

EVA KARCHER

VI.

The Michelangelo of the Scalpel: Ivo Pitanguy

EVA KARCHER, Munich

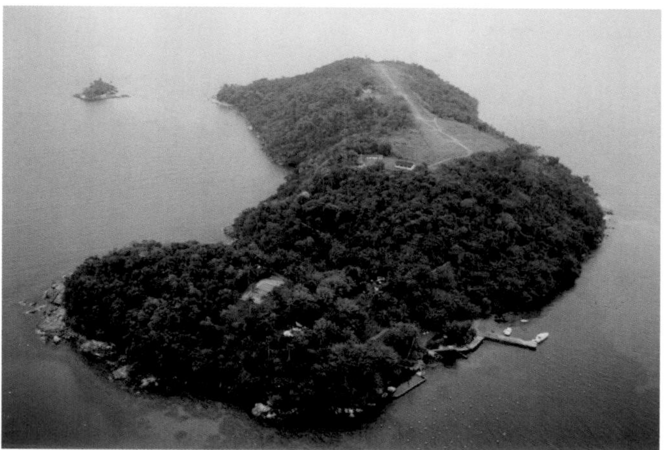

fig. 1

Flying towards her in his helicopter, he feels like her lover. 160 kilometres or 20 minutes' flight time south of Rio de Janeiro, she appears below him — voluptuous and well-rounded, nestling in the emerald-green and azure-blue waves of the Atlantic. "She has the shape of a woman," Ivo Pitanguy enthuses — "she" being his very own island, the three-km-long Ilha dos Porcos Grande (Big Pigs Island). He found this treasure three years ago in the "Angra dos Reis", the Bay of Kings — a haven of the rich and super-rich of Brazil.

The most famous of all living cosmetic surgeons, Pitanguy selected this island from more than 350 others in the bay because "like a siren," it enchanted him. "I conquered her, sculpted her and trimmed her curves," he tells us with a smile, "but I've always respected her wild, primeval nature." Is this the language of an "homme à femmes"?

In his occupation at least, the 79-year-old Brazilian known as the godfather of plastic and aesthetic surgery has proven to be an expert on feminine beauty like no other. Having performed more than 40,000 operations over four decades, Ivo Hélcio Jardim de Campos Pitanguy is the much-lauded guru of a profession still on the rise. Pitanguy's colleagues have the greatest respect for their most prominent public advocate. He tells us that he has trained 500 doctors from 40 countries, and twice as many again — including some of the world's most renowned surgeons — are proud to have been his students, even if only for brief stints of work experience. Student surgeons are literally begging for internships at Pitanguy's clinic.

Ivo Pitanguy's vivid life is the stuff of legend, and it is difficult to distinguish between fact and fiction in the swathes of Hollywood myths surrounding him. Numerous articles and reports describe his prestigious clientele of film stars, ranging from Joan Crawford to Raquel Welch, from Zsa Zsa Gabor to Brigitte Bardot. To thank the maestro for a successful restoration, Gina Lollobrigida reportedly sculpted him a little boy's bust. Marisa Berenson, to whom Pitanguy returned her former beauty following an accident, praises him as a "genius." Fara Diba, the former Empress of Persia, repaid his services with an antique Persian rug and a 1,700-year-old ring. Purportedly.

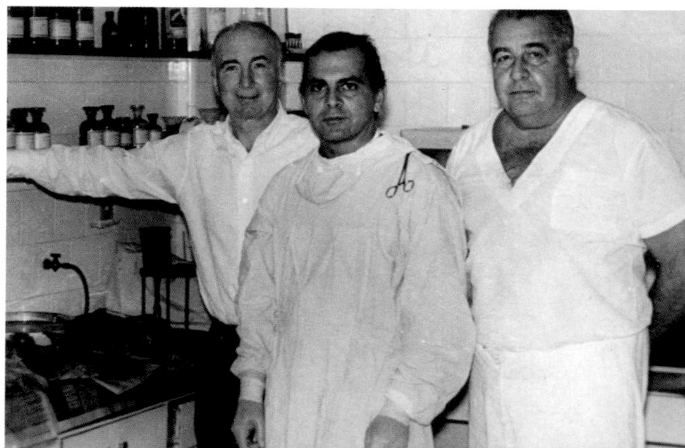

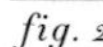

fig. 2

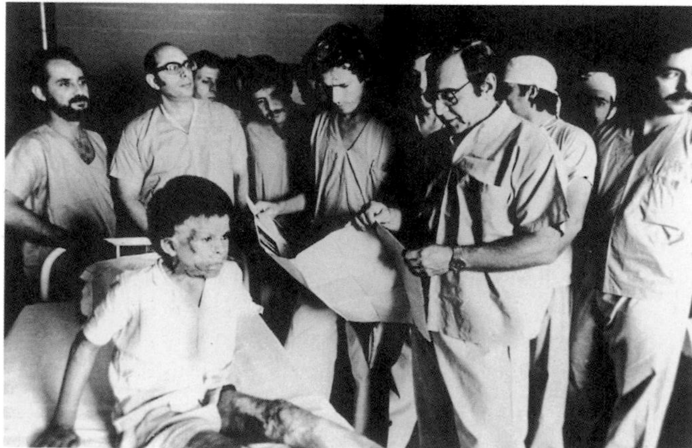

fig. 3

fig. previous pages

Dadá Cardoso photographed Ivo Pitanguy's right eye in 1995. The photograph, signed and dedicated, was a gift to the surgeon. Underneath the photo lies the book on Michelangelo "L'artiste — Sa pensée — L'écrivain." © Tuca Reinés

fig. 1

Ivo Pitanguy's very own slice of paradise — the Ilha dos Porcos Grande — lies in the Atlantic Ocean, just a 20-minute flight from Rio. As he once put it, the island enchanted him like a siren.

fig. 3

Worlds apart from Pitanguy's prestigious private clinic: At Rio de Janeiro's charity hospital Santa Casa de Misericórdia, the surgeon operates on impoverished patients free of charge — such as this boy who suffered facial burns. Source: Private archive Pitanguy

fig. 2

In the course of his career, Ivo Pitanguy (centre) has performed more than 40,000 operations and trained approx. 500 doctors from 42 countries. Even those who have just had stints of work experience under Pitanguy proudly refer to themselves as his "students." © Reuter Raymond / CORBIS Sygma

fig. 4

After his horrific accident on the Nürburgring in 1976, Niki Lauda sought out Ivo Pitanguy for treatment. The cosmetic surgeon completely restored the racing driver's burnt face. © Reuter Raymond / CORBIS Sygma

fig. 5

It is a rare occurrence to see Brazil's most famous doctor sitting at his desk. The list of patients is long and includes international celebrities such as Farah Diba, Leni Riefenstahl, the Duchess of Windsor, François Mitterand and the King of Jordan. © Tuca Reinés

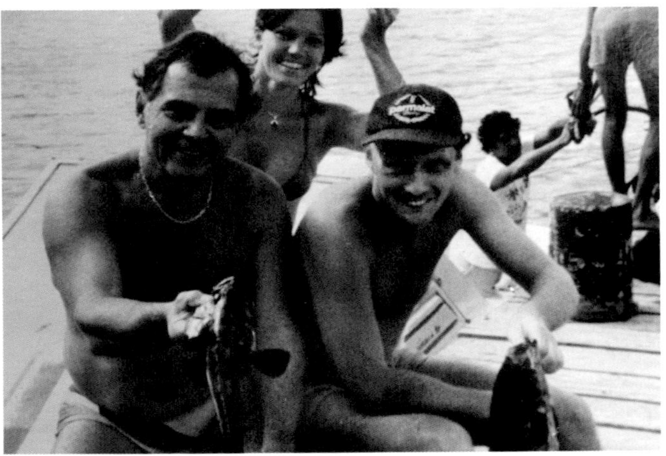

fig. 4

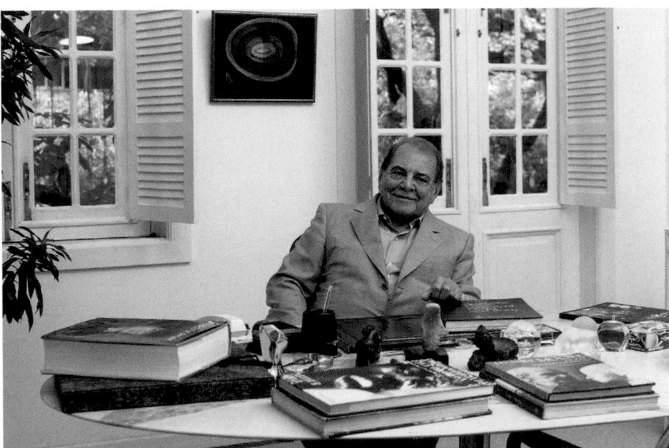

fig. 5

Other celebrities whom Pitanguy did cosmetic repairs for and returned their youthful looks to include Helmut Berger, Candice Bergen, the Princesses Anne and Ira of Fürstenberg, Melina Mercouri, Betty Ford, the Duchess of Windsor, Leni Riefenstahl, François Mitterand, the Kings of Morocco and Jordan — and of course Niki Lauda, whose face Pitanguy reconstructed after his terrible accident on the Nürburgring in 1976. How did they, one wonders, express their gratitude?

In response to this question, the "Michelangelo of the scalpel," as German magazine "Der Spiegel" once described him, seals his lips with his left index finger and smoothly skirts the subject: "All my patients are famous." Never does he reveal the identity of any patient, "jamais!!!" — you can literally hear the three exclamation marks in his impeccable French. As well as French and his native Portuguese, the multi-talented Pitanguy is fully fluent in English, Spanish and Italian, and has a good grasp of German. Almost all of the celebrities who have visited his clinic villa in the Rua Dona Mariana in Rio's uptown suburb Botafogo have left him a personal souvenir. Pitanguy points to a photo of himself having lunch with Paul Bocuse: "As a gift, he presented me with one of his secret recipes. Not as a patient, but as a friend." Naturally.

Another old friend, Salvador Dalí, immortalised Pitanguy with a bronze. The Spanish genius known for his melting clocks, lobster phones and lip couches boldly mounted a model of Pitanguy's head onto the body of a horse, symbolically transforming him into a centaur. Pitanguy is very proud of his sculptural metamorphosis, and his reverence for Dalí is boundless. "I have an incredible admiration for Dalí," he says, "as well as many other Surrealists." Without a hint of irony, he adds: "My entire life has been surreal." The professor's taste in art is not limited to the boundless delirium of the Surrealist virtuoso, but encompasses a wide range of modern styles. He has acquired numerous modernist masterpieces over the last ten years, as well as notable contemporary works when they catch his eye. Pitanguy is no amateur art enthusiast — for a decade, he was the president of Rio de Janeiro's Museum of Modern Art. As a collector, too, this diminutive, stormy man with the olive skin, black hair and bushy eyebrows is setting new standards. Although most cosmetic surgeons appreciate art, few can claim to own works by Pablo Picasso, Henri Matisse, René Magritte, Marc Chagall, Joan Miró or Balthus, or a sculpture by Henry Moore. Nor do they have mobiles by Alexander Calder and paintings by Pierre Soulages or Yves Tanguy hanging on their walls. Pitanguy also likes to support contemporary local artists like his son Bernardo: "Anita Malfatti, Manabu Mabe and Cândido Portinari," he lists his current favourites. "Paintings are my passion," he adds pensively, "because they are akin to poetry."

As Pitanguy sees it, poets — French poets especially — are more intimately aware of the ideal of beauty than others. As

fig. 6

Ivo and Marilu Pitanguy have been married for over 45 years. They share a passion for modern art; their villa in Rio de Janeiro's uptown suburb Gávea is home to a world-class collection including original works by Magritte, Chagall and Picasso.
© Reuter Raymond / CORBIS Sygma

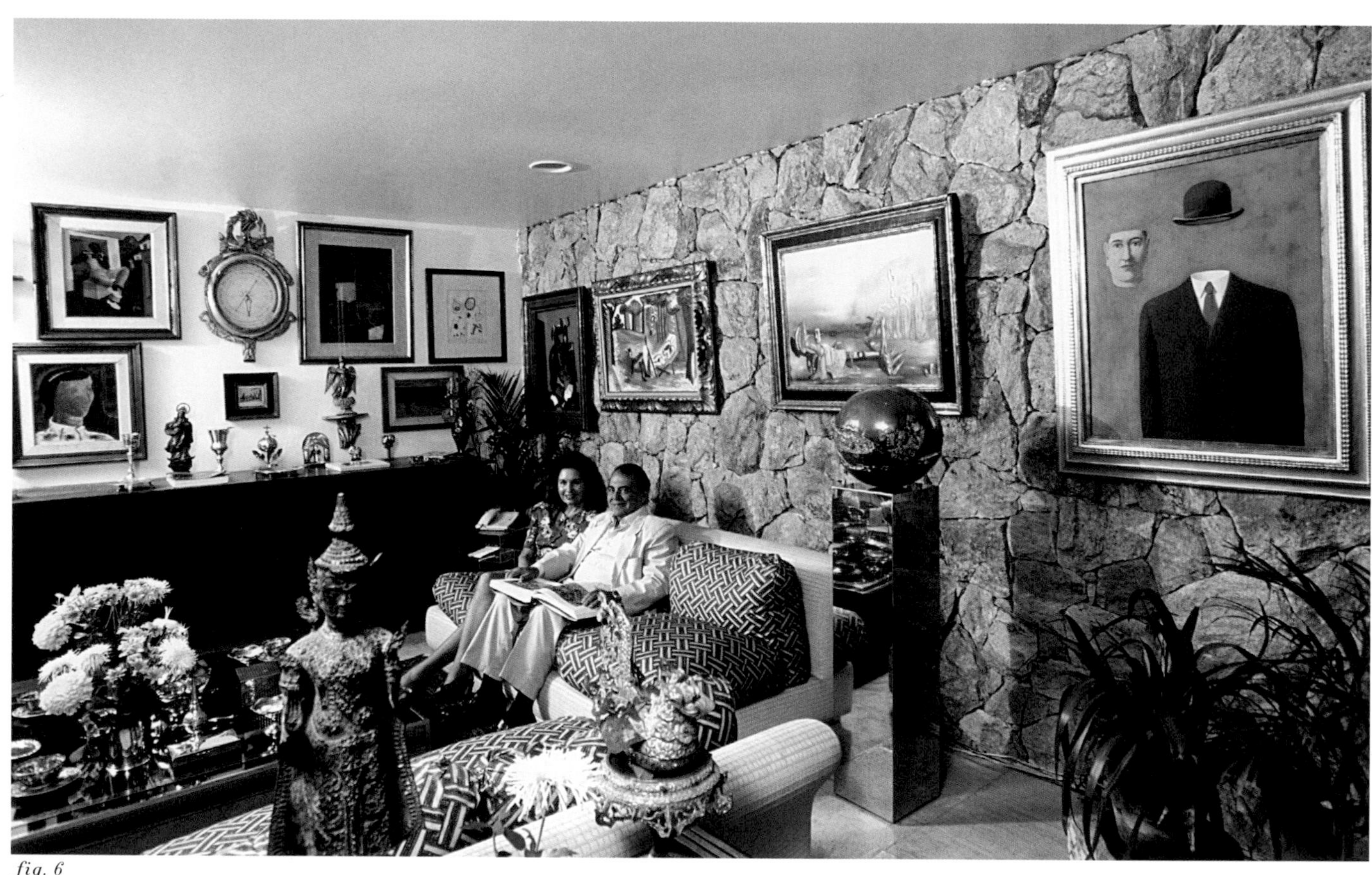

fig. 6

a craftsman, he is envious of the "boundless freedom" artists enjoy. "They are permitted to create new works, whereas we need to work within the limitations of nature."
With a passion as if he himself had helped the poets to compose their verses, he recites lines by Stendhal and Honoré de Balzac. "Beauty is a promise of happiness," hopes the former, and "Beauty is a necessity; it grants peace to the soul," claims the latter. To Ivo Pitanguy, such sentences are the tenets of his personal beliefs. He is obsessed with the concept of beauty, a beauty that has to exist beyond the "stereotypes of fashion." "It's not about perfect proportions or regular features," he explains. "A face that is completely symmetrical is monotonous." When it comes to this subject, Pitanguy is unable to restrain himself — he jumps out of his chair and gesticulates wildly, his speech getting faster, his voice straining. "The media always focus on a statuesque form of beauty. This beauty is like the mask of death, it is the opposite of being alive! Time and again I explain to my patients that beauty is always a happy coincidence, a coincidence of minute deviations from the norm — not an arbitrary combination of classic Greek noses, almond eyes and pouting lips. True beauty radiates from the inside, it is an expression of personal qualities." To perceive this inner beauty, explains the expert surgeon, you need "a feel for aesthetics. This is the most important prerequisite for success in a profession like mine."
A feel for luxury also seems to help. Pitanguy has plenty of it and is not ashamed to show it, for example in his private residences — the chalet in the Swiss Alps, the apartment in Paris, his island and of course his home address in Rio. To-

fig. 7

Ivo Pitanguy's private clinic, founded in 1963. Here, the surgeon maintains a team of 70 professionals. The clinic director is Pitanguy's own daughter, Gisela. © Tuca Reinés

fig. 8

The waiting rooms in Pitanguy's clinic confirm his reputation as "the world's most expensive cosmetic surgeon." Designed as glamorous salons, they are adorned with works by Brazilian and French artists. © Tuca Reinés

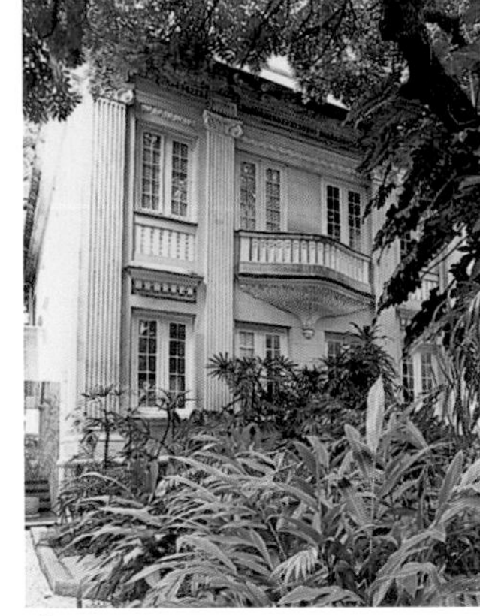
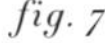

fig. 7

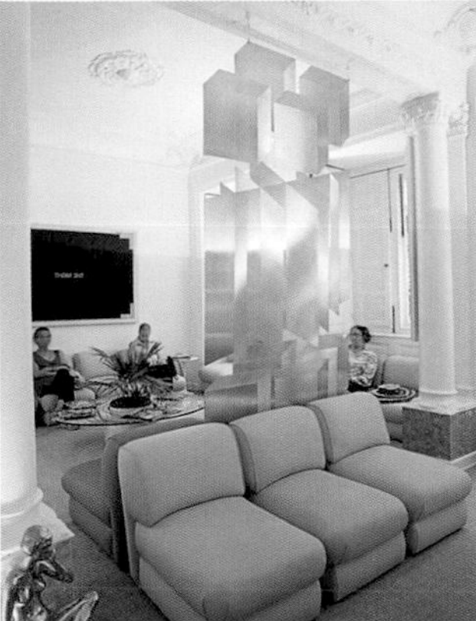

fig. 8

fig. 9

Evidence of skill and renown: Ivo Pitanguy has been honoured with countless awards, diplomas, prizes and medals. He is widely regarded as the prime "global player" in his profession. © Tuca Reinés

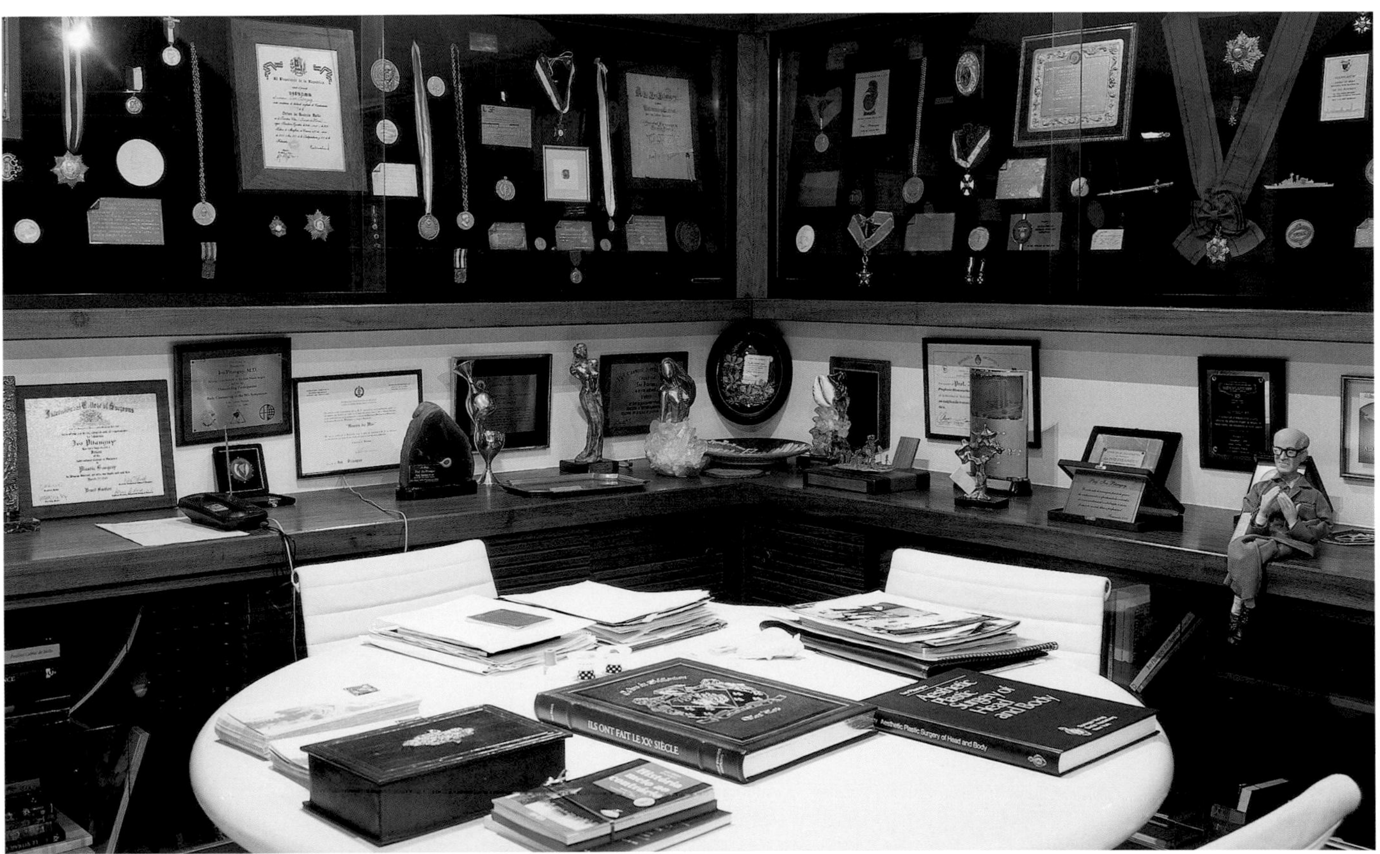

fig. 9

gether with his wife Marilu, to whom he has been married for more than 45 years, he lives in Gávea, one of the city's rich suburbs among the hills. The puritan design of his house, built in the 1960s, is clearly influenced by Japanese architecture. The minimalist cube is surrounded by palm trees, acacias, hibiscus and orchids, a cocoon of leaves, flowers and tropical scents. Heavily armed bodyguards constantly patrol the premises with five dogs, growling rather fiercely. Pitanguy bred the dogs himself: "They are Great Danes crossed with Weimaraners." An effective artillery indeed. Pitanguy's security team is on duty around the clock, guarding the people, furniture, paintings, sculptures and antiques, as well as the swimming pool and the tennis court. By way of a wooden bridge that could come straight out of a Monet, the doctor and his wife visit their small garden pavilion three times a week. Here, they practice karate. Sport is the secret to Pitanguy's physical vitality and unbridled energy. He has been a swimmer since childhood; for six years, he played competitively for the Minas Tennis Club, the team that produced Brazil's champion tennis player. Pitanguy's tennis successes are demonstrated by his collection of trophies, which visitors can admire in the fitness compound. The doctor also likes scuba-diving, fishing and skiing. "Keeping fit is the foundation of your health and good looks," he declares, and with a humorous wink, he flexes his muscles: "I believe in *preparing* the body as well as *repairing* it." His credo may be light-hearted, but it requires a lot of discipline and stamina to keep his body constantly fit. As the professor explains, he gets up at 6 a. m. every morning. He then reads several international newspapers and eats a

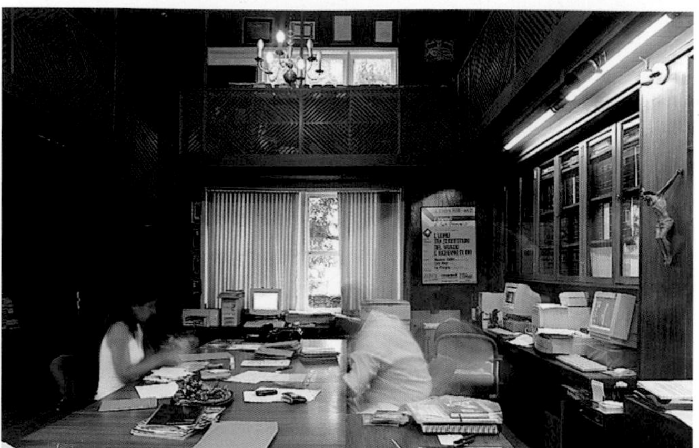

fig. 10

fig. 11 & 12

Ivo Pitanguy in the operating theatre. He treats more than 1500 patients every year, and refuses to distinguish between medical and aesthetic indications. "My operations are not just for my patients bodies, they are also for their souls" he is convinced. © *Ricardo Azoury / CORBIS*

fig. 10

The library of Pitanguy's private clinic. The surgeon has also established an in-house study centre for his students and assistants to pursue their reading and research in peace and quiet. © *Tuca Reinés*

"très petit déjeuner." This is followed by a one-hour body workout with exercises that vary according to season. Later, his chauffeur drives Pitanguy to the clinic; on the way, the surgeon reads his emails, makes telephone calls, dictates letters or memos and simply enjoys the fresh sea breeze blowing from the beaches of Ipanema, Copacabana and Leblon.

The most expensive cosmetic surgeon in the world, as the tabloids sometimes label him, also likes to display an abundance of luxury and glamour at his workplace. The waiting lounges and consultation rooms of the clinic, founded by Pitanguy in 1963, are designed as comfortable salons. They are adorned with art objects and paintings by local, French and anonymous artists, including works by the Brazilian painter Antônio Dias, prints by the French artist Pierre Doutreleau and a tapestry by Jean Lurçat, to name but a few examples. Most of the artworks displayed here revel in a dynamic, cheerfully decorative aesthetic and feature feminine curves aplenty — Pitanguy's tribute to his feminine ideal of "the harmonious proportions and graceful movements of a dancer."

At every turn, there is evidence of Pitanguy's role as a well-liked "global player" — in his field as well as in the international jet-set society. We see awards, honorary diplomas and dozens of snapshots of Pitanguy meeting great artists and scientists such as Marc Chagall, the writer Jorge Amado, the cardiac specialist Christiaan Barnard or Sir Harold Gillies, one of the pioneers of cosmetic surgery in the United Kingdom.

Around 70 doctors, assistants, surgical nurses, lab technicians, administrative staff and other professionals are employed at Pitanguy's clinic. One of these is his daughter Gisela, the clinic's director and a trained psychotherapist. His sons have followed different callings. Together with his team, Pitanguy effortlessly masters a considerable mountain of work every day. As well as his sophisticated clinic featuring three operating theatres, fifteen patient suites and a study centre for trainee research, Ivo Pitanguy has been running a department for reconstructive and aesthetic plastic surgery at Rio's charity hospital Santa Casa de Misericórdia since 1982. The towering Baroque building, which dates back to the 16th century, was financed and renovated entirely by Pitanguy.

The master surgeon and his medical team come here once a week, usually Wednesdays, to operate on injuries, burns and malformations such as harelips and tumours. They also perform cosmetic work on eyes, breasts and noses, and carry out routine facelifts and liposuction. Despite the 1,500 operations performed every year, the waiting list of men and women wanting free cosmetic surgery is always a long one — much to the satisfaction of the many student surgeons that have an invaluable opportunity here: to practice, practice and practice again.

How does Pitanguy bridge the gap between the elementary suffering encountered at the hospital and the vanity-based needs of most of his private clinic's patients? Is it not a cynical, almost obscene contrast? "No," counters Pitanguy, "in both instances I perceive human pain. I don't draw a line between medical and aesthetical indications of suffering. To be happy with yourself is by no means a superficial desire. My operations are not just for my patients' bodies, they are also for their souls."

Although Pitanguy is sometimes accused of playing the role of the Samaritan for purely tactical reasons, the vast majority of Rio's and indeed Brazil's population celebrates Pitanguy like a national hero at every festive occasion. The only Brazilian arguably more popular than Pitanguy is soccer legend Pelé, but the gap between the two is fast closing. In 1999, the surgeon was the guest of honour on the carnival float of *Caprichosos de Pilares*, one of Rio's biggest samba schools, at the celebrated *Carnaval do Brasil*. Feted like a hero, his white dinner jacket was covered in flower wreaths and his face was one huge, radiant smile. It may have been then that the word "pitanguiser" was coined to describe the aura surrounding this man — a mix of charisma, intelligence and compassion.

Little did Pitanguy know as a youth that one day he was to be such a celebrity. Born on July 5, 1926, he grew up far from any glamour in Belo Horizonte in the state of Minas Gerais. His father was a general surgeon, his mother came from a family of Portuguese diamond traders. Between his older brother and three younger sisters, Ivo was regarded as a dreamer, a child who liked to read lots or roam around the neighbourhood — "timid and wild," as he likes to describe himself as a child. "When I was 13, my dearest toy

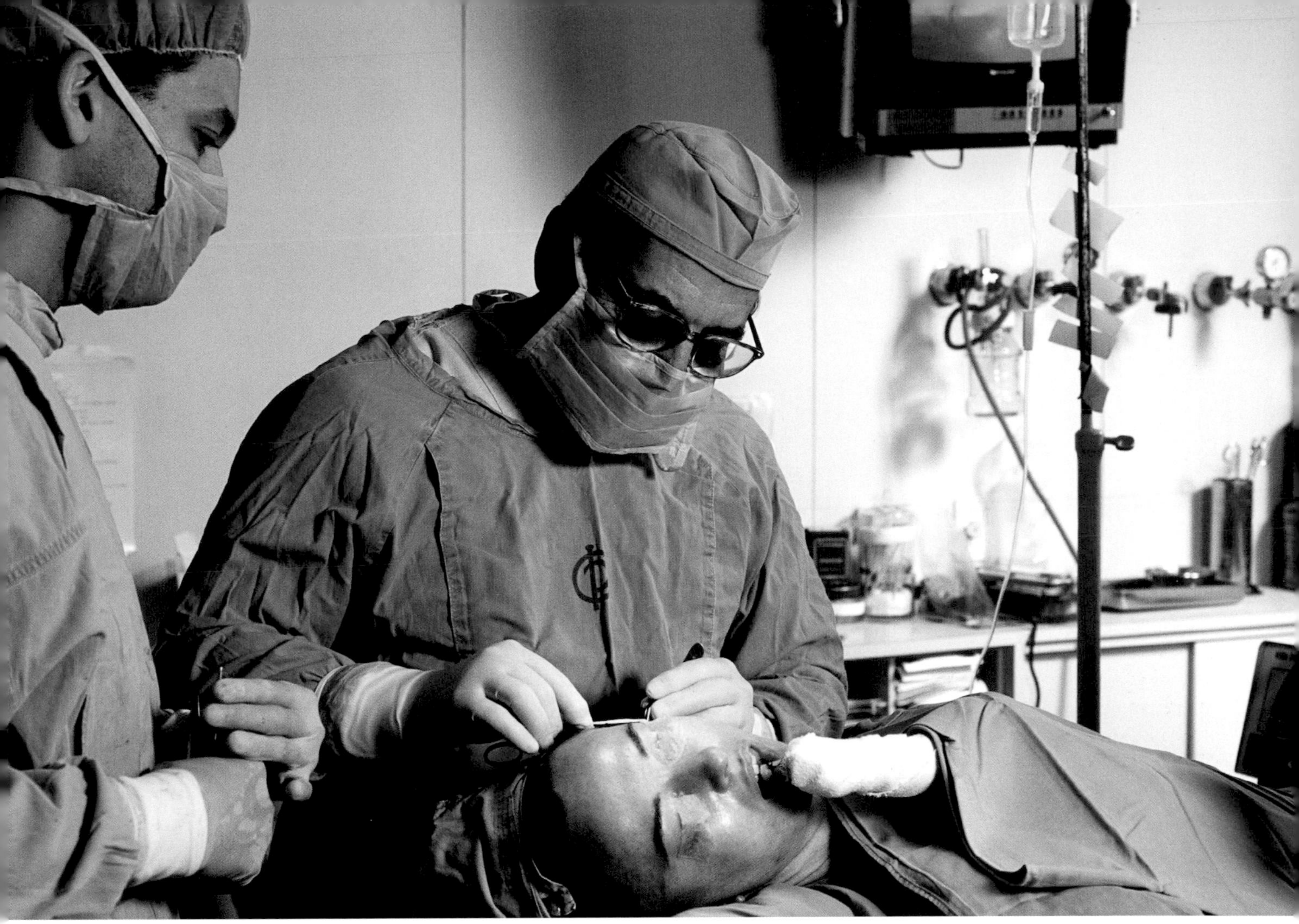

fig. 11 / fig. 12

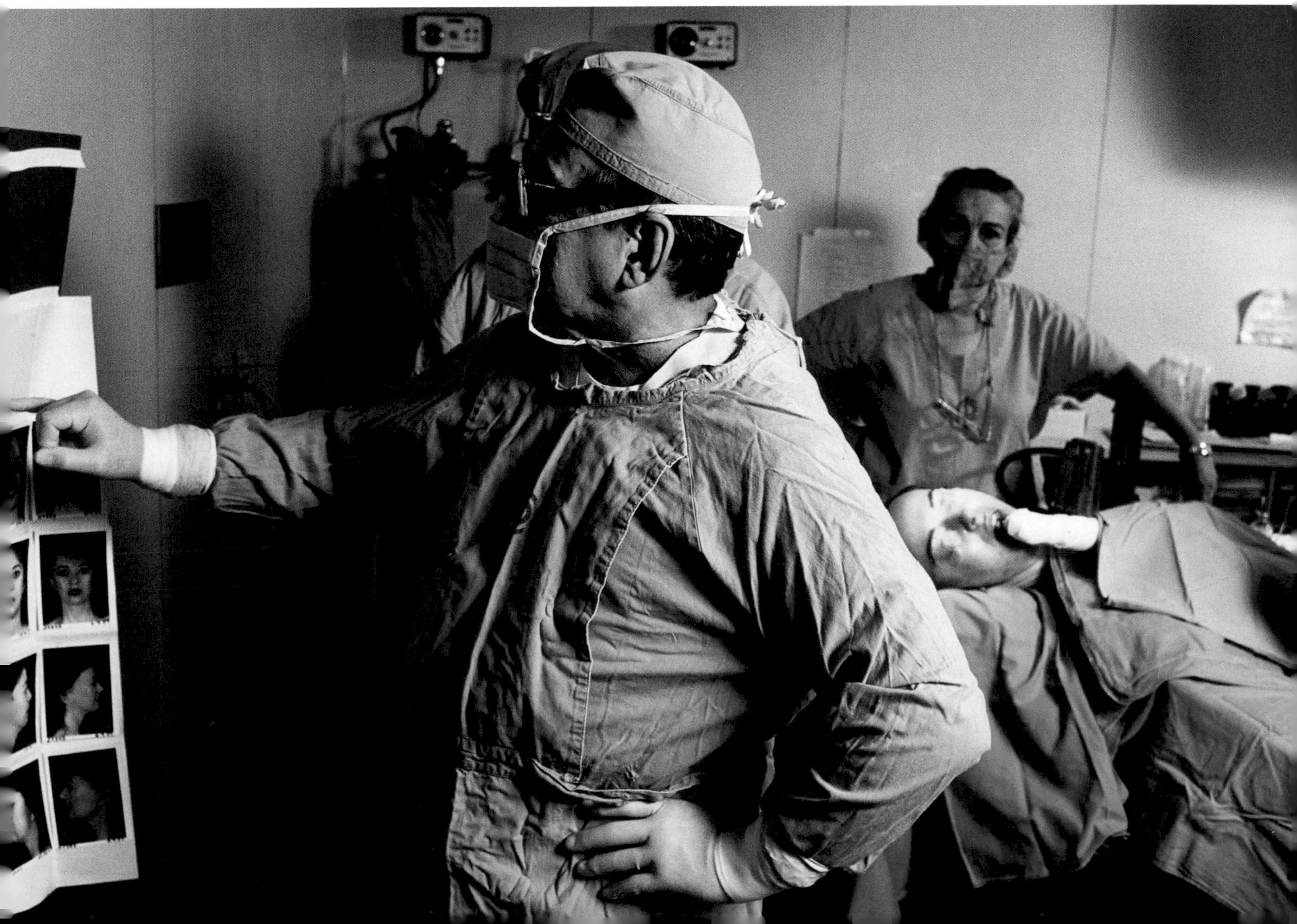

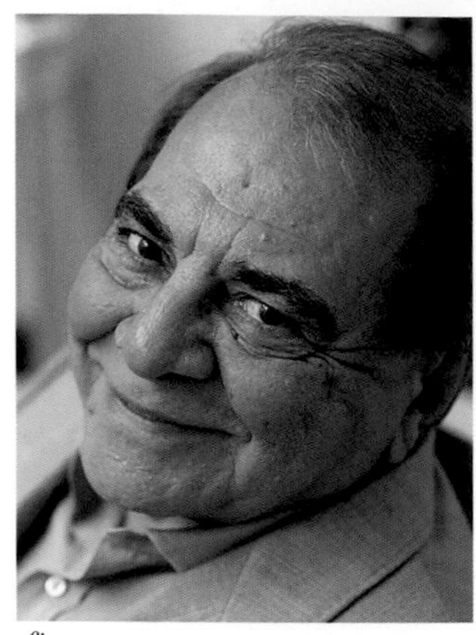
fig. 13

fig. 13

Ivo Pitanguy was born in 1926 in Belo Horizonte. He commenced his medical studies at the University of Minas Gerais at the age of 14, having stated his age as three years older on the enrolment form. Thanks to Pitanguy, Brazil has become the Silicon Valley of cosmetic surgery. © *Tuca Reinés*

fig. 14

Ivo Pitanguy points out a page in his book "Aesthetic Plastic Surgery of Head and Body"*. The book was published in 1981 by Springer Verlag, a standard reference work used by most of today's cosmetic surgeons.* © *Tuca Reinés*

was a boa constrictor. It had suddenly appeared in front of me on one of my many forest walks. Much to the distress of my parents, I took it back home." And much to the relief of his parents, the reptile disappeared just as suddenly only a few days later.

Still, this loss signified the end of childhood for young Ivo. Growing up was a competitive process, he now understood, and the introverted thinker turned into an ambitious fighter. He decided to follow in his father's footsteps and study medicine. With the help of his father, he successfully exaggerated his age by three years on the enrolment application and was thus able to commence studies at the medical faculty of the Minas Gerais University at the tender age of 14.

In Rio, he completed his training to become a general surgeon and was soon operating on accident and emergency cases. Next, he travelled to Europe and the US to specialise in the field of plastic surgery. At 22, he was an intern at the Bethesda Hospital in Cincinnati, immediately moving on to train under luminaries such as Marc Iselin in Paris and Sir Harold Gillies as well as Sir Archibald McIndoe in London. With all of his teachers, he communicated exclusively in their local language. When he returned to his home country, he was like a matador certain of victory.

At Rio's charity hospital, the Santa Casa de Misericórdia, Ivo Pitanguy founded the hospital's department for hand surgery. It would have been entirely possible for him to still be working as a reconstructive surgeon today, and an excellent one at that, had it not been for that terrible night of December 17, 1961. "I will never forget the inferno," he recounts quietly, "when the Gran Circo Norte Americano in Niteroi was on fire. 2,500 people were consumed by the flames; 300 children were brought to my clinic, many of them with extremely severe burns. Our team was working non-stop for three days and three nights." The tragedies encountered here, particularly the pain suffered by the children and the cruel deformations many of them were subjected to, determined the future course of Pitanguy's career. "I suffered immensely with these children. When they saw their destroyed faces, they would rather have been dead. At this point I vowed to dedicate my life to one cause: to unite reconstructive and aesthetic surgery."

Pitanguy fulfilled his pledge. In the process of doing so, he achieved much more: he has developed and established many important surgery techniques, such as the one where the abdominal wall is tightened with a low-down incision. And thanks to Pitanguy's efforts, Brazil has become the Silicon Valley of cosmetic surgery. Generations of cosmetic and other plastic surgeons have worked on the international clientele Pitanguy brought to them. When Rio became a capital of glamour in the 1950s, Pitanguy was kissing the hands of divas such as the heavenly Liz Taylor or the spirited Queen Elizabeth II. Many of the ladies were to return – but not just for the magnificent beaches. With them they brought a jet set hungry for cosmetic surgery, and before long, Brazil had established its reputation as a body-shaping Mecca.

The Brazilian Society of Plastic Surgery has more than a thousand members, making it the world's largest association of plastic surgeons outside of the US. In 2002, its members performed a total of 370,000 operations – a world record. As in the US and Europe, breast enlargements and reductions, facelifts and liposuction enjoy the greatest popularity. The number of male clients is growing steadily – currently, men make up 30% of the patients. The Brazilian cosmetic surgery market is thriving not only because of the consistently high standard of operations and surgeons; compared to the US, the operations are also significantly cheaper. Among other factors, this is due to patients being able to leave the clinics sooner than in the US.

What is the future of Pitanguy's profession? "Today, beauty is marketed as youth," the master says. "The benefits of age, such as maturity, are neglected. This is a terrible oversight." Pitanguy has five grandchildren by now, but assures us that he himself has never had a facelift. "I feel young because I have held on to my passion," he beams. If the field of cosmetic surgery "remains the dominion of professionally-trained specialists," Pitanguy believes it will continue to flourish.

Increasingly, he is withdrawing from his surgical activities, focusing on his properties and island instead. "I am thoroughly familiar with death," Ivo Pitanguy claims, and once again shows us his sphinx-like smile. "I'm not at all afraid of it. As Marc Aurel once described it – when it is time for me to go, I want to fall like a ripened olive and give thanks to the tree that has borne me and the earth that has nourished me."

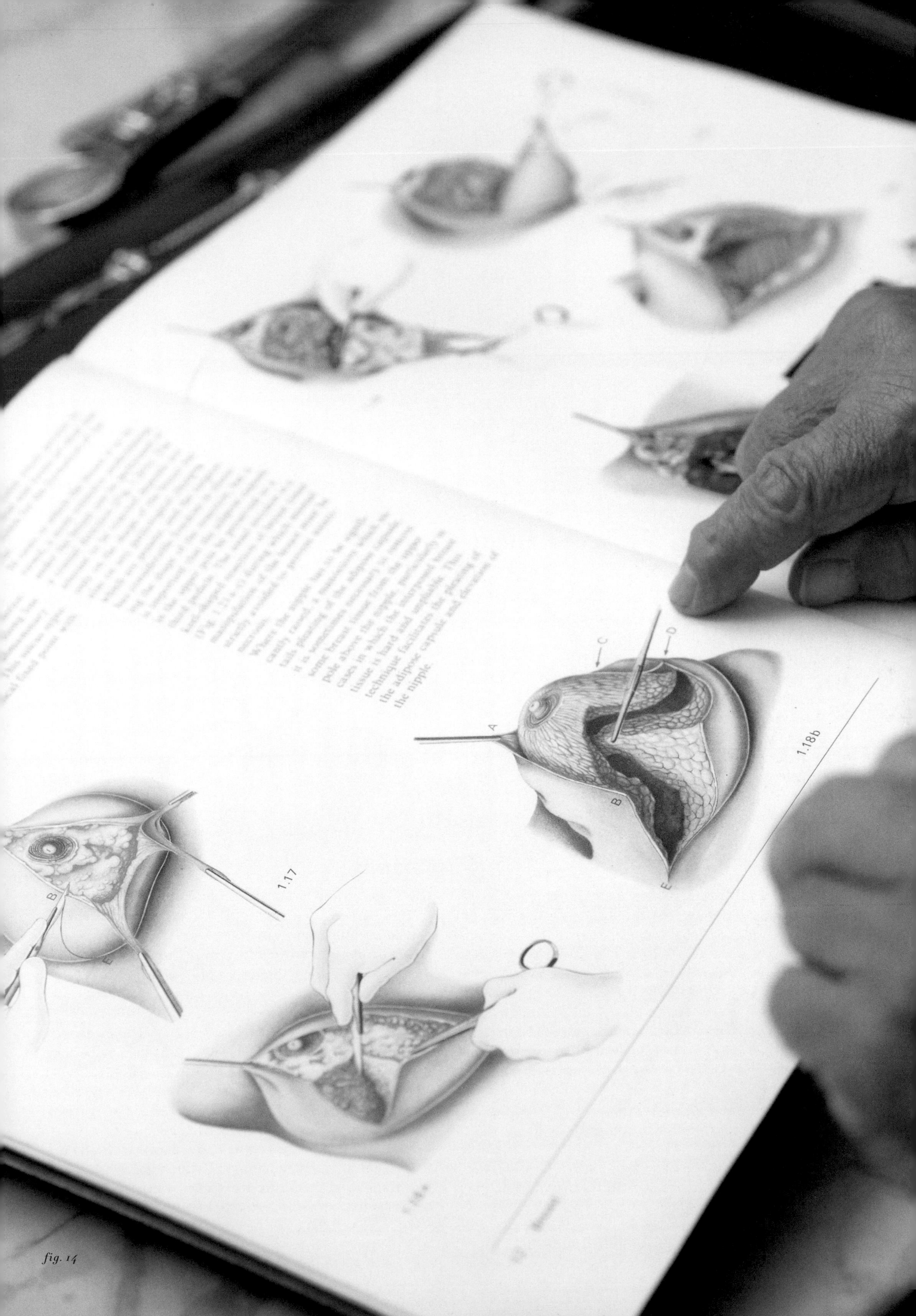

fig. 14

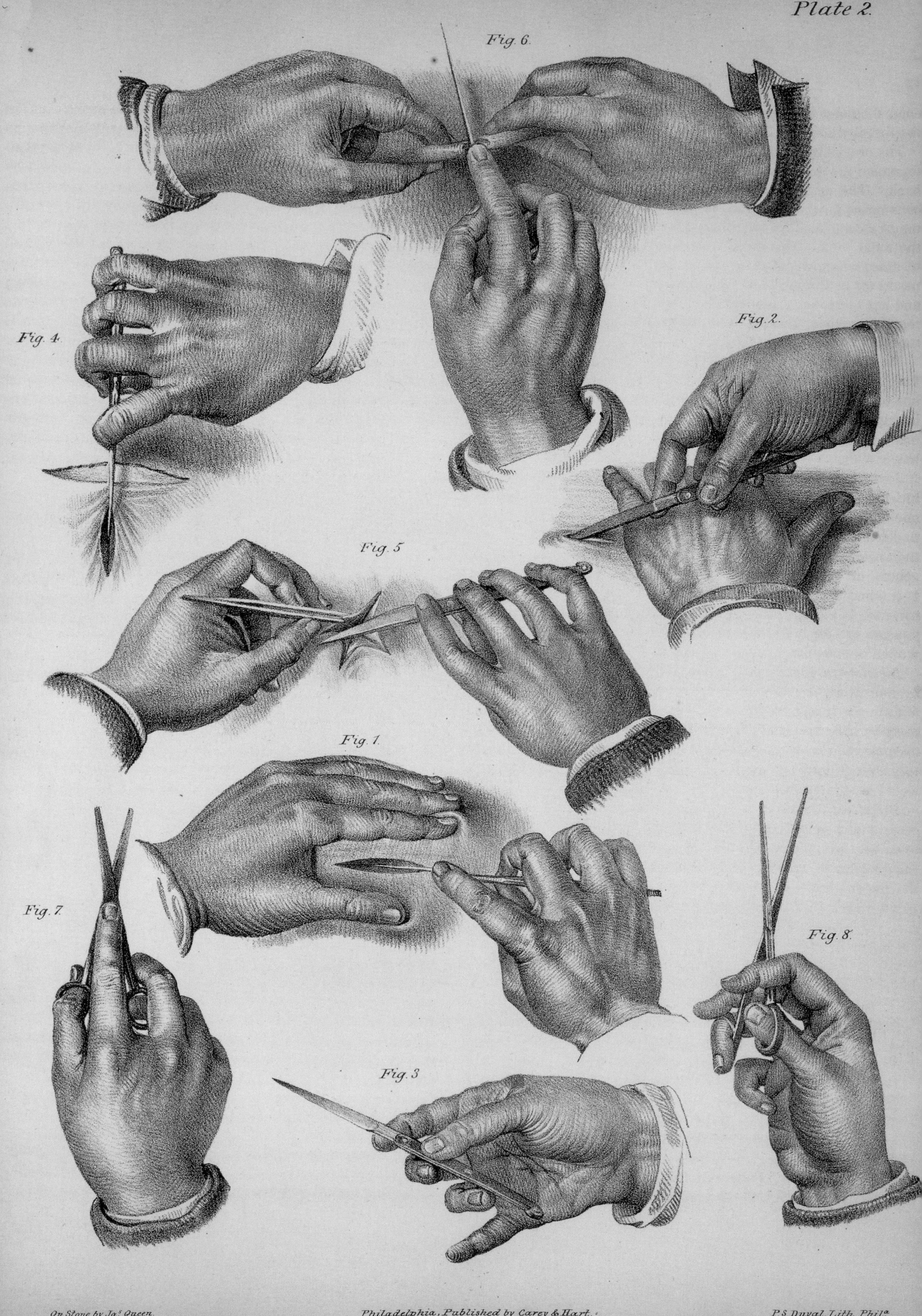

On Stone by Jas. Queen.   Philadelphia, Published by Carey & Hart,   P.S. Duval, Lith. Phila.

VII.

THE WORLD'S MOST FAMOUS AESTHETIC SURGEONS

Interviews by

EVA KARCHER

and

RICHARD RUSHFIELD

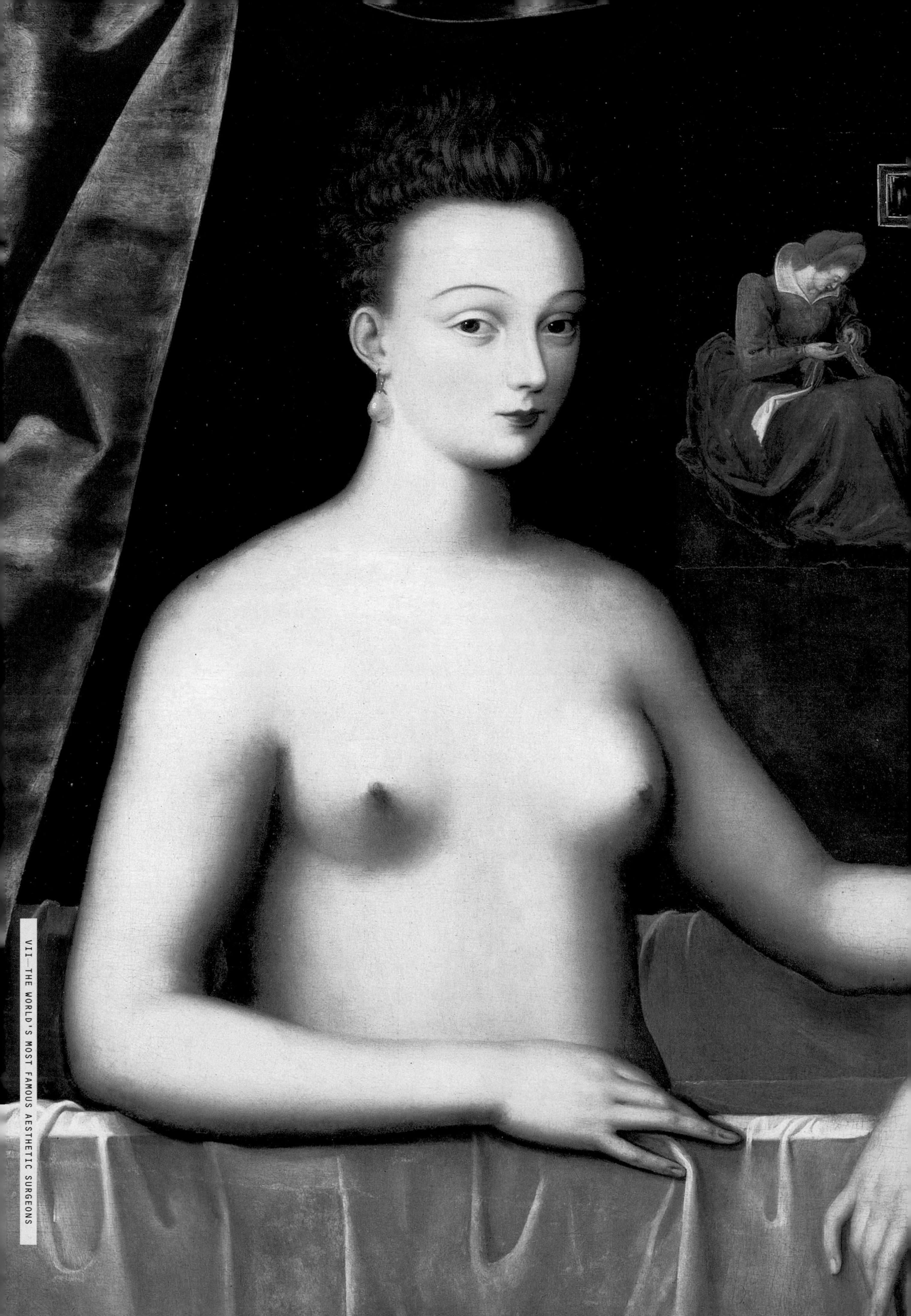

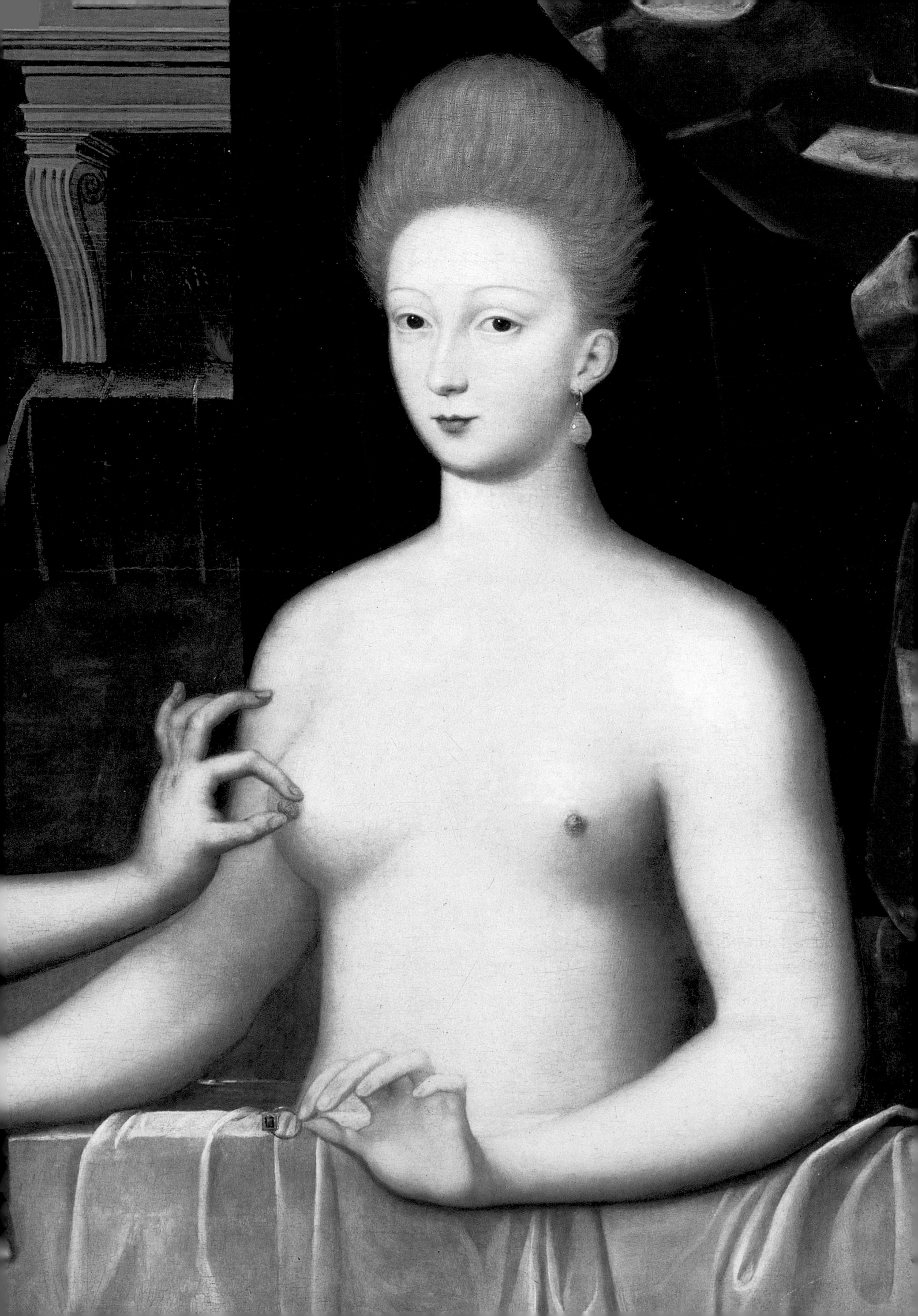

"My aim is not to create beauty but normality"

DAI M. DAVIES, London

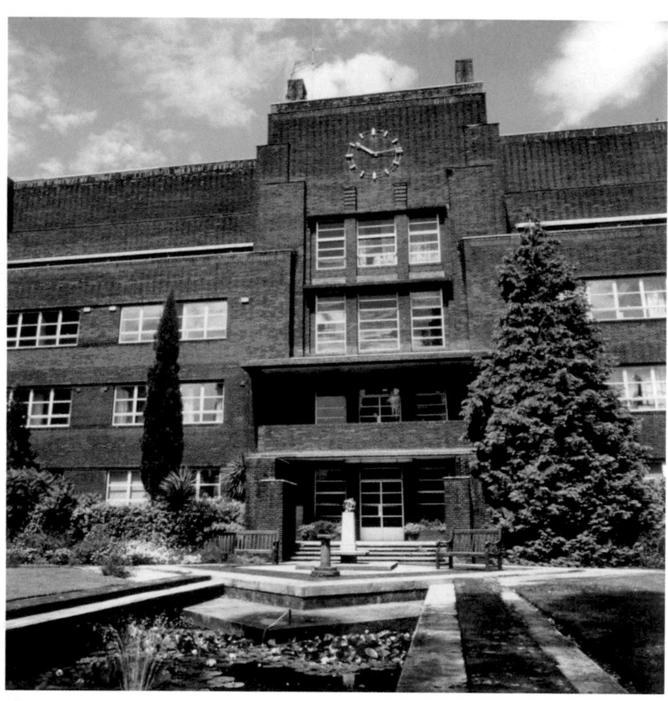

fig. 1

1. WHAT FASCINATES YOU MOST ABOUT BEING AN AESTHETIC SURGEON?

There are several aspects that fascinate me. On the one hand, it demands a very high level of professional skill, where accuracy is a matter of millimetres. On the other hand, it is very satisfying to be able to see the results of my work. But the greatest privilege to me is that many of the patients I work on have thought very carefully about their decision to undergo a life-changing operation, a decision not made quickly or lightly. It is a great honour and responsibility for me to take part in this with them.

2. WHICH AREAS DO YOU SPECIALISE IN?

I concentrate on breast reductions, facelifts and other facial operations, especially corrective surgery on eyes, noses and chins.

3. DO YOU REGARD YOURSELF AS AN ARTIST?

Not really. Obviously, I need to have a sense for aesthetics and be able to imagine, for example, how a certain nose fits a certain face. But unlike an artist sitting in front of a blank canvas and interpreting his subject, the surgeon has a finished "work" in front of him and needs to carry out the patient's interpretation, not his own. That's the difference, really. We don't necessarily make our patients more beautiful; we just tighten their skin and remove some of the wrinkles.

4. WHAT IS YOUR CONCEPT OF BEAUTY?

Beauty is fleeting. I don't have a set concept of beauty. With my work, my aim is not to create beauty but normality. For example by reducing an overly large breast to a normal size, i. e. a size that is proportionate to the body. Looking at the changing views of beauty over the centuries, beauty has a number of constants — but also a near-infinite number of variations that depend on the fashion of the time.

5. IN ART HISTORY, WHAT IS YOUR FAVOURITE NOTION OF BEAUTY?

I don't have a specific one. As I hold lectures on the historical development of the ideal of female beauty, I have researched art history. In the middle ages, for example, the significance of the female breast was to symbolise nourishment and also spirituality. Only later did it become an erotic or sexual symbol.

6. TO YOU, WHO ARE THE MOST BEAUTIFUL WOMAN AND MOST BEAUTIFUL MAN ALIVE?

Most definitely my wife.

7. DO YOU REGARD YOURSELF AS ATTRACTIVE?

Well, I don't think I'm unattractive.

8. WHAT DOES AGING MEAN TO YOU?

Body and mind weaken, the mind especially in terms of short-term memory performance. At the same time, we become enriched by experience; but this also makes us less tolerant.

9. ARE YOU AFRAID OF GETTING OLDER?

No — it's inevitable. Sure I'd like to be ten years younger, but it's an irreversible process. That's why I compensate

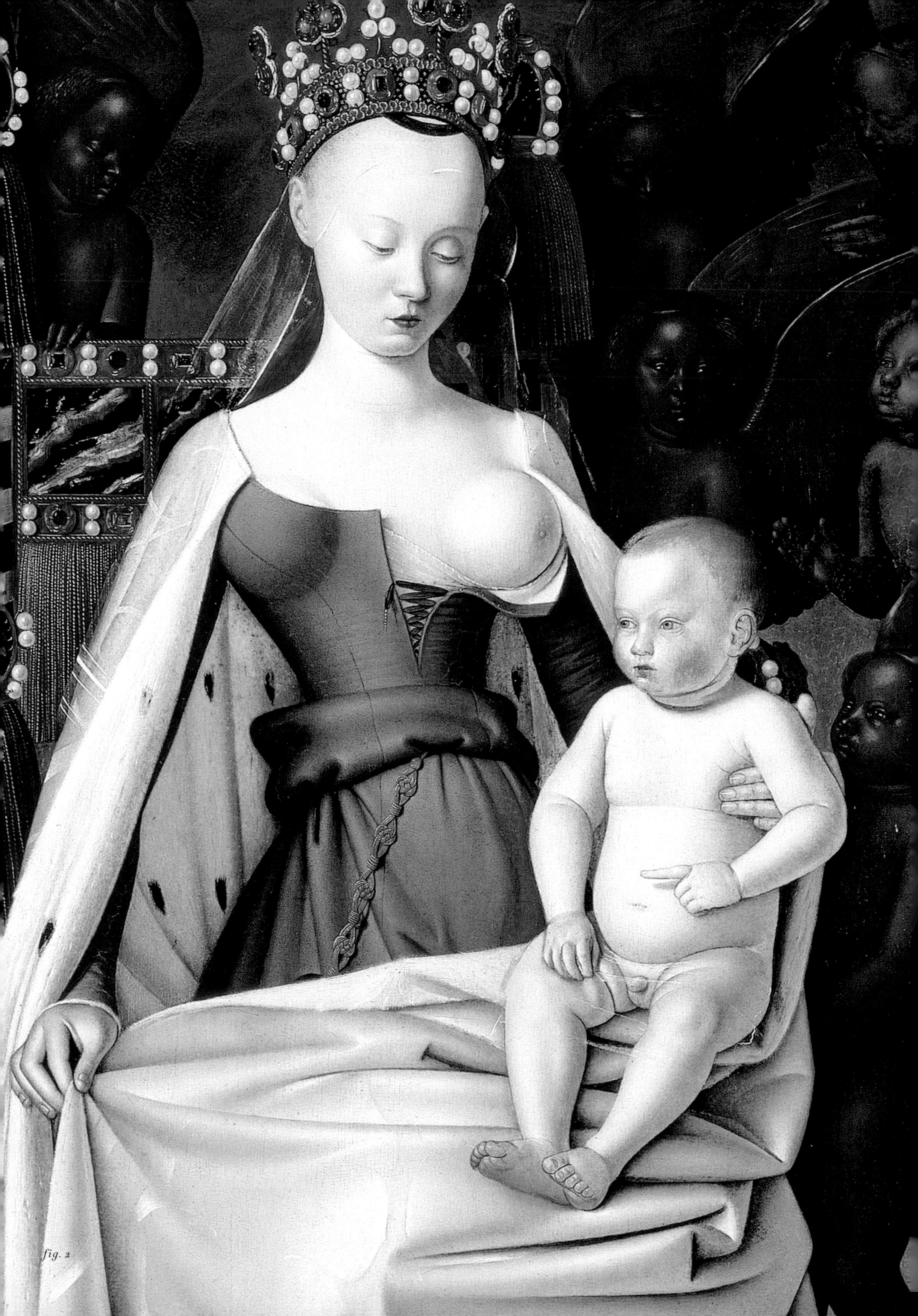

fig. 2

fig. previous pages

Plastic surgery has always demanded great skill: These instructions on how to use surgical implements are taken from the seminal reference work "A Treatise on Operative Surgery" by Joseph Pancoast (1805–1882). © Columbia University Health Science Library. Photo: Dwight Primiano

"Gabrielle d'Estrées and one of her sisters" was painted around 1600 by an artist from the School of Fontainebleau. © Paris, Réunion des Musées Nationaux; Photo: G. Blot

fig. 1

The London practice of Dai Davies. In contrast to many of his colleagues, the surgeon doesn't see himself as an artist. © Private archive Dr. Davies

fig. 2

For much of art history, the female breast symbolised nourishment and spirituality. Only later did it become a symbol for sexuality. This is a close-up from Jean Fouquet's "Melun Diptych" (1456). Koninklijk Museum voor Schone Kunst, Antwerp

in other areas. For example, I enjoy observing my children growing up, seeing how they themselves are getting older and more mature. Nobody can live forever — I'm happy with my life as it is, and I enjoy my existence as much as I can.

10. HAVE YOU EVER UNDERGONE AESTHETIC SURGERY YOURSELF? IF SO, WHAT WAS IT FOR?

No, and I can't see myself wanting it. Maybe the eyelids one day ...

11. HAVE YOU EVER OPERATED ON YOUR WIFE/PARTNER AND/OR CHILDREN? IF SO, WHY?

I would never operate on my wife or on one of my children. It just seems too arrogant. Also, it would be too emotional. Looking at the many cosmetic surgeons whose wives and girlfriends have had facelifts, especially those in the US, you start asking yourself who's really doing who the favour! Does the partner really want to meet her man's expectations by being a walking business card for his work?

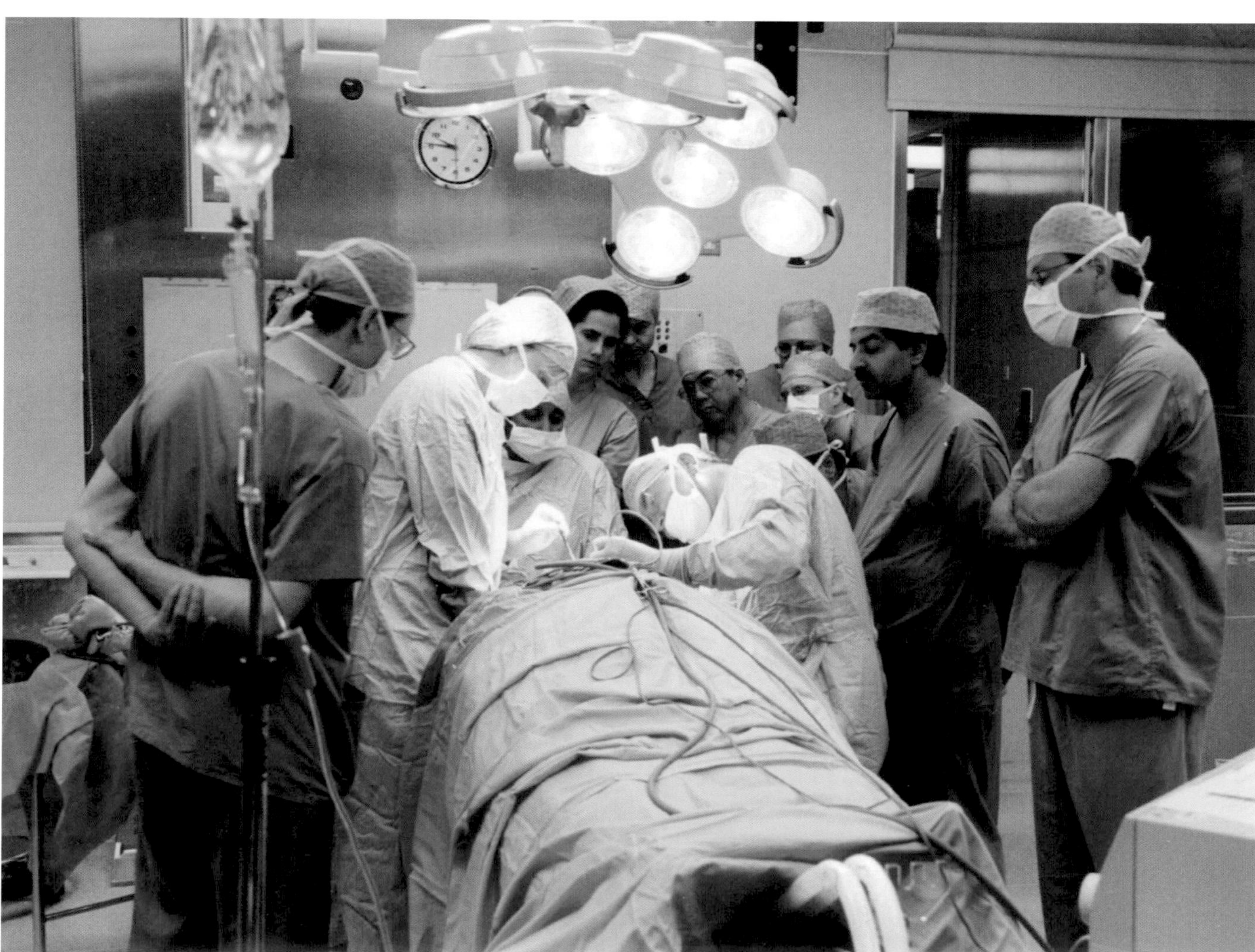

fig. 3

fig. 3

As a surgeon, Dai Davies specialises on the breast and the face. He thrives on the technical challenges of his work and the trust his patients place in him. © Private archive Dr. Davies

fig. 4

The surgeon and his wife. "I would never operate on my wife or on one of my children," he states. "It just seems too arrogant." © Private archive Dr. Davies

12. CAN YOU JUSTIFY EVERY OPERATION AND PATIENT REQUEST, OR IS THERE A POINT WHEN YOU REFUSE TO DO AN OPERATION?

If patients have unrealistic expectations concerning the outcomes of an operation, I decline their request. Luckily, most of my patients have very pragmatic ideas. It's crucial for the surgeon and the patient to spend time discussing the outcomes they expect in detail.

13. WHAT IS THE MOST UNUSUAL REQUEST FOR SURGERY YOU HAVE ENCOUNTERED IN YOUR CAREER?

One of my patients was a young girl at the onset of puberty; her breasts had grown quite dramatically within a few months. When I operated on her, I removed approximately eight kilograms of breast tissue. That was my most extreme case, an emergency scenario really.

14. WHAT ARE YOUR PATIENTS' REACTIONS FOLLOWING SURGERY?

It varies from procedure to procedure. Female patients often get depressed and tearful when coming out of a facelift. They suffer from swollen skin, pain and tension. It usually takes a few weeks before they can appreciate the changes, but when they finally do, they are always very happy. Patients that I've corrected the breasts or noses for are normally satisfied and pleased straight away.

15. COULD YOU NAME SOME OF YOUR MORE WELL-KNOWN PATIENTS?

I don't do so as a matter of principle.

16. DO YOU BELIEVE THAT BEAUTY LARGELY EMANATES FROM WITHIN?

That depends on how you define beauty. To me, beauty is more than physical attractiveness, it also encompasses personality and aura. I would say that beauty is equally internal and external.

17. DO YOU THINK THAT BEAUTIFUL PEOPLE ARE HAPPIER AND LEAD MORE FULFILLED LIVES?

No. In many ways, beauty is a form of tyranny. If you are a beauty icon, you need to conform to an image dictated by

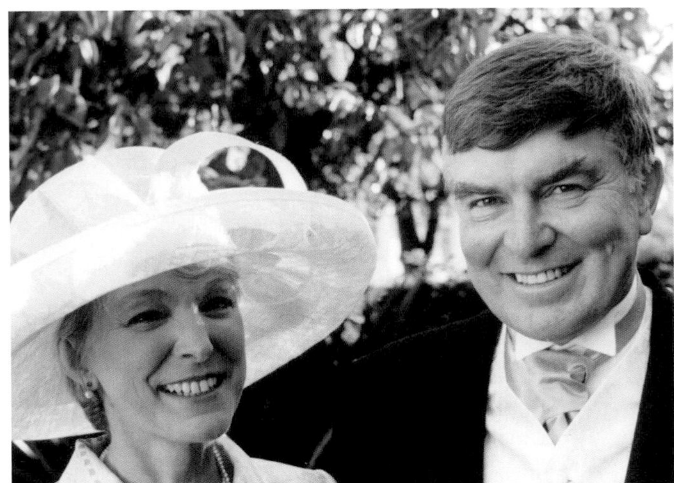

fig. 4

the media. You can't ever relax. Beauty can also cause uncertainty. I think that being normal is highly preferable to being beautiful; the price of beauty is very high. Unfortunately, society places far too much importance on beauty.

18. DO BEAUTIFUL PEOPLE HAVE BETTER SEX?

No, to the contrary! I think they can't enjoy it as much because they constantly have high expectations projected onto them, and fulfilling these expectations can be very stressful.

19. WHAT DOES THE FUTURE HOLD FOR AESTHETIC SURGERY?

Very soon, procedures will have become much less invasive. The scars will be smaller or gone altogether, the procedures will increasingly take place outside of the theatre and also become more affordable. Anti-aging treatments such as injections, laser therapy and drugs will become more important — not for rhinoplasty etc. but for typical symptoms of aging such as loose skin, drooping faces and sagging breasts. Genetic research will also introduce innovative new forms of treatment. Who knows, maybe someone will soon discover the anti-aging gene.

Interview: Eva Karcher, Munich

"I may be the only surgeon to have done psychoanalysis"

SERDAR EREN, Cologne

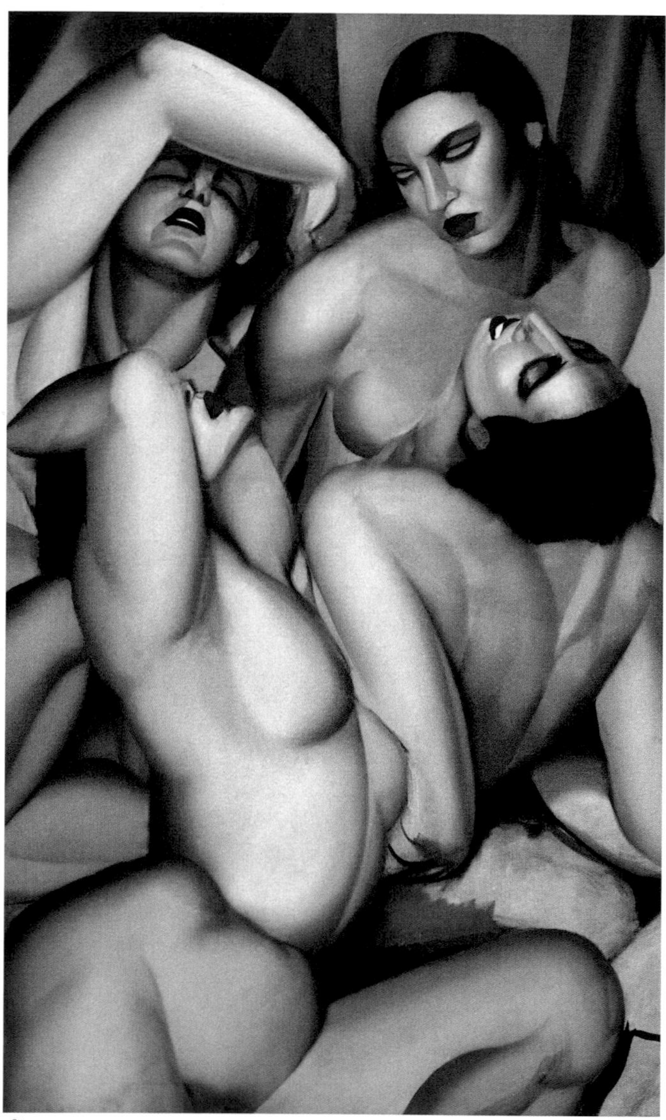

fig. 1

1. WHAT FASCINATES YOU MOST ABOUT BEING AN AESTHETIC SURGEON?

The essential prerequisite of my work is a keen eye for detail. Almost as important as this are a perfectionist attitude and a high level of manual proficiency. These are characteristics I have displayed from an early age. I grew up in Turkey. We often did sewing work, and I soon noticed that I was working much faster and much better than my brothers and sisters, sometimes even faster than my mother. I had already decided to become a surgeon when I was at school. 27 years ago, I first got in contact with traumatology. Accident-related surgery is often very messy, so my professional interests shifted to plastic surgery. This is an area where I feel I can truly improve my patients' quality of life.

2. WHICH AREAS DO YOU SPECIALISE IN?

Actually, I would describe myself as one of the few all-round surgeons in Germany. I am well known for my combination operations, for example performing a facelift, breast correction and liposuction in a single session. The area I am most demanded in is breast enlargement. I have developed my own method for this type of surgery, which I describe as an "interior bra." Aside from this — well, I believe I may be the only plastic surgeon to have done psychoanalysis. This has contributed very much to my ability to recognise the psychological structures and motivations of my patients. In plastic surgery, it is crucial to understand the psychological subtleties displayed by your patients. Ideally, every cosmetic surgeon should also have experience in psychotherapy and should have done psychoanalysis. You see, surgery is an aggressive profession — an aspect that should not be played down. Of course the surgeon's main role is to master his or her skills and functions, but 30 to 40 percent of the occupation rely on psychology and aesthetics.

3. DO YOU REGARD YOURSELF AS AN ARTIST?

In a manner of speaking, yes. When I operate on birth malformations, I am creating something new. As a cosmetic surgeon, I re-create something that has already existed before. I don't change, I restore. As I mentioned before, I regard a substantial part of my role as a surgeon to be psychological. This is also the angle I take, for example, when explaining to patients the relationship between muscular activity and appearance. If somebody always frowns with worry, worry lines will eventually appear on their forehead. Somebody who laughs a lot keeps his or her lips trained in doing so, and consequently, the corners of

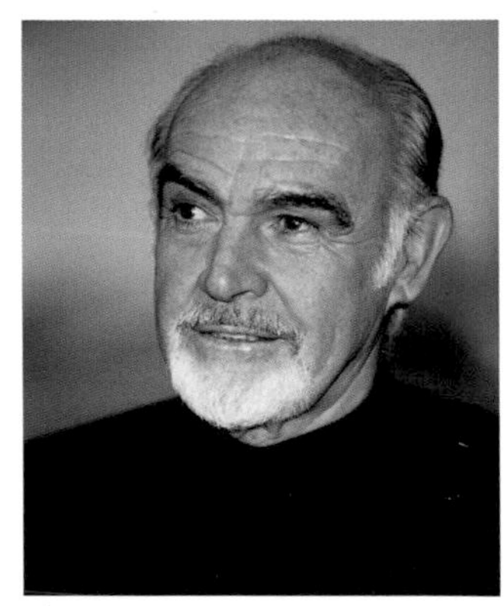
fig. 2

fig. 1

Serdar Eren is fascinated by Art Deco. This oil painting from 1925, "Groupe de quatre nus," is by Tamara de Lempicka (1898–1980). *© akg-images*

fig. 2

To Serdar Eren, Sean Connery is living proof that a balding man with wrinkles can also be attractive. *© Rufus F. Folkks / CORBIS*

fig. 3

Serdar Eren and his wife. "She is a natural beauty," believes the surgeon – and has never needed cosmetic surgery. *© Private archive Dr. Eren*

their mouth won't droop! Personal character is displayed in a person's face just like their emotions — the transitions are seamless. Looking at it from this angle, you could say that I am a psychologist with an artistic perspective.

4. WHAT IS YOUR CONCEPT OF BEAUTY?

I reject standards and guidelines. To me, attractiveness consists of harmony. That's why I think liveliness and vitality are sexy. The question is, can these qualities be physically enhanced? I believe they can. One of my favourites is eyelid surgery. Correcting the upper or lower eyelid has a positive effect regardless of age, it simply helps patients to feel more secure about themselves and their age.

5. IN ART HISTORY, WHAT IS YOUR FAVOURITE NOTION OF BEAUTY?

I love Art Deco and Turkish antiques — tapestries, furniture, accessories. I have recently discovered contemporary art for myself, maybe it's the beginning of a collection.

6. TO YOU, WHO ARE THE MOST BEAUTIFUL WOMAN AND MOST BEAUTIFUL MAN ALIVE?

That would be my wife; to me, she has a perfect face. Of men, I think Sean Connery is a particularly beautiful example.

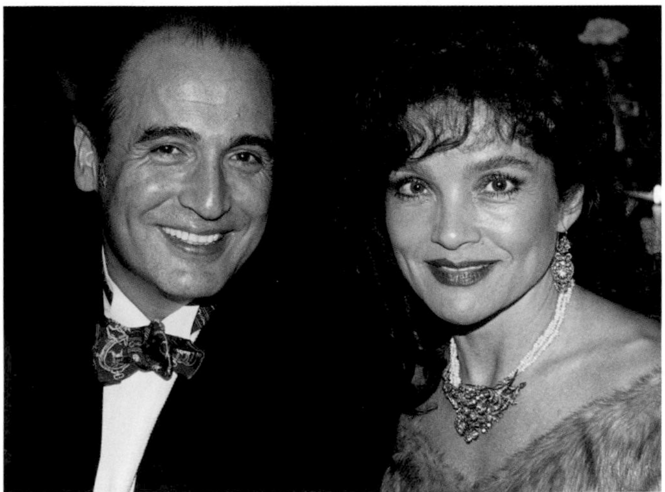
fig. 3

7. DO YOU REGARD YOURSELF AS ATTRACTIVE?

Yes. However, I'm not just talking about external attractiveness, but also about self-confidence. My self-confidence comes from my experience and from my work. I often try to convey to my colleagues and patients that it's not just shapes that make a person beautiful, but also the dynamics displayed by the person.

8. WHAT DOES AGING MEAN TO YOU?

I'm very curious. I can't wait to see what will happen in ten years' time! My priorities used to be to have a well-trained body, plenty of hair and enough virility. I was a competitive sportsman and quite narcissistic, but I never had much confidence in myself. Looking back, I can see how my values have shifted. I consider myself lucky for having changed for the better.

9. ARE YOU AFRAID OF GETTING OLDER?

Not at all. I try to live the present as vividly as possible. My life is so exciting that I experience the aging process as something positive, not something negative.

10. HAVE YOU EVER UNDERGONE AESTHETIC SURGERY YOURSELF? IF SO, WHAT WAS IT FOR?

No, and I'm not planning on having any.

11. HAVE YOU EVER OPERATED ON YOUR WIFE/PARTNER AND/OR CHILDREN? IF SO, WHY?

No, my wife is beautiful by nature, see question number six!

12. CAN YOU JUSTIFY EVERY OPERATION AND PATIENT REQUEST, OR IS THERE A POINT WHEN YOU REFUSE TO DO AN OPERATION?

Complications only ever happen before a procedure. On several occasions, I have operated on patients at the wrong point in time. This doesn't happen anymore because I can anticipate it now. I have also stopped operating on patients that want to drastically change their appearance. I can smoothen faces and make them appear younger, but I cannot recreate them. My favourite patients are women who are psychologically very stable.

fig. 5 a+b & 6 a+b

Serdar Eren's business is to remodel bodies, as shown by this tummy tuck and upper thigh/hip contouring procedure. This is as far as the Cologne-based surgeon goes. "I've stopped operating on patients who want to radically change their appearance," he explains. © Private archive Dr. Eren

fig. 4

Serdar Eren in the operating theatre. He is one of the few all-round surgeons in Germany, known for his multiple procedures. © Private archive Dr. Eren

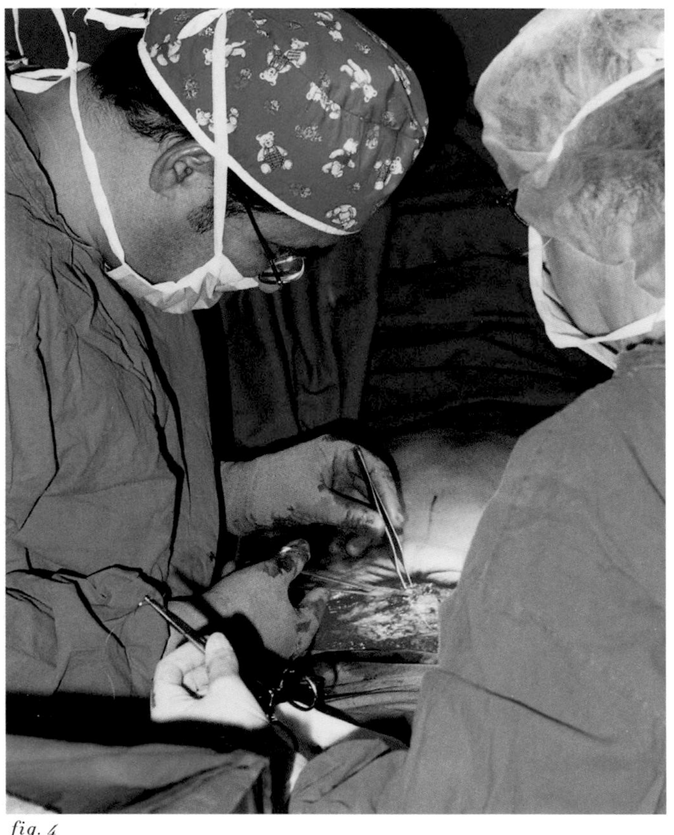

fig. 4

13. WHAT IS THE MOST UNUSUAL REQUEST FOR SURGERY YOU HAVE ENCOUNTERED IN YOUR CAREER?

20 years ago, I transplanted a toe onto a thumb! I performed a sex change once, turning a woman into a man. That was the biggest challenge of my career. I wouldn't do it again; we cannot heal these people of their problems. They always have to repress the fact that they used be of the opposite sex.

14. WHAT ARE YOUR PATIENTS' REACTIONS FOLLOWING SURGERY?

Once they realise that their improved looks register positively with the people around them, my patients are happy and full of thanks. When they start getting compliments, they feel desirable and start to enjoy their lives again. They often send me letters and thank-you presents.

15. COULD YOU NAME SOME OF YOUR MORE WELL-KNOWN PATIENTS?

No, I always maintain professional discretion.

16. DO YOU BELIEVE THAT BEAUTY LARGELY EMANATES FROM WITHIN?

Yes. A person who feels wanted, desired — in whatever way — also feels more self-confident and more beautiful. A woman who isn't considered good-looking will still feel beautiful when she is wanted. Those feelings definitely radiate from within.

17. DO YOU THINK THAT BEAUTIFUL PEOPLE ARE HAPPIER AND LEAD MORE FULFILLED LIVES?

Not at all. Many beautiful people are entirely preoccupied with themselves.

As a result, they focus on their appearance and come to expect a high standard of living. This, however, requires more than just looks! Still — society is more accepting towards beautiful people, provided they present themselves well.

18. DO BEAUTIFUL PEOPLE HAVE BETTER SEX?

No. Appearance has no effect on the production of pheromones.

19. WHAT DOES THE FUTURE HOLD FOR AESTHETIC SURGERY?

I'm not as optimistic as many of my colleagues. Not much has changed over the last 20 years in aesthetic surgery. Facelifts have basically remained the same. Cosmetic surgery has become an industry, and more and more people have operations. They will increasingly invest in their appearance instead of their emotional well-being, which is an unfortunate development. On the other hand, aesthetic surgery has the power to make people more attractive and bolster their self-esteem. For this reason, it will remain indispensable.

Interview: Eva Karcher, Munich

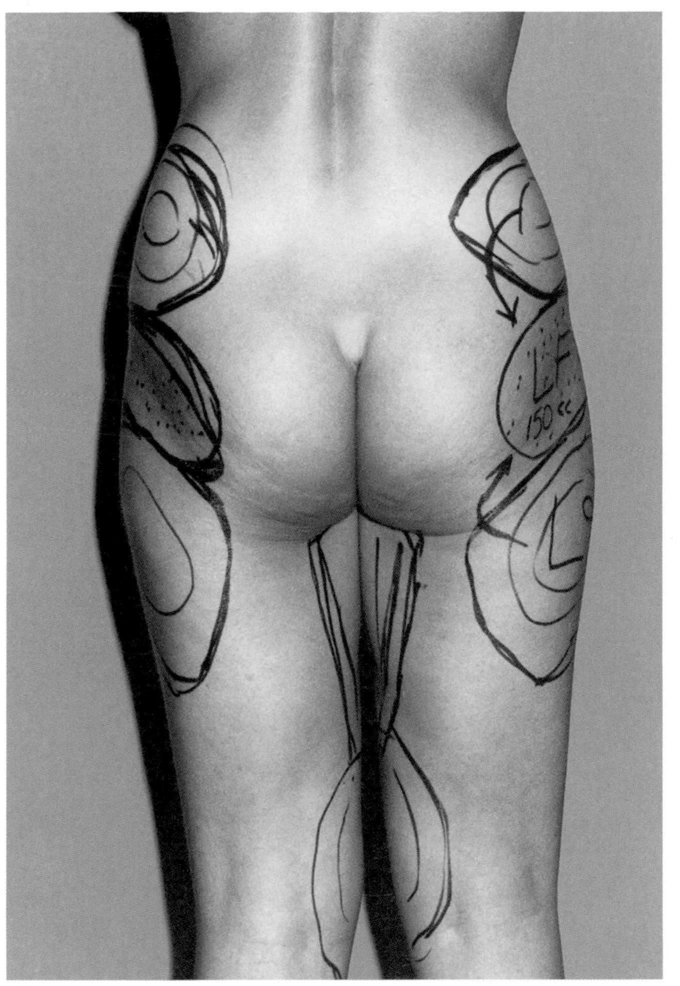

fig. 5 a

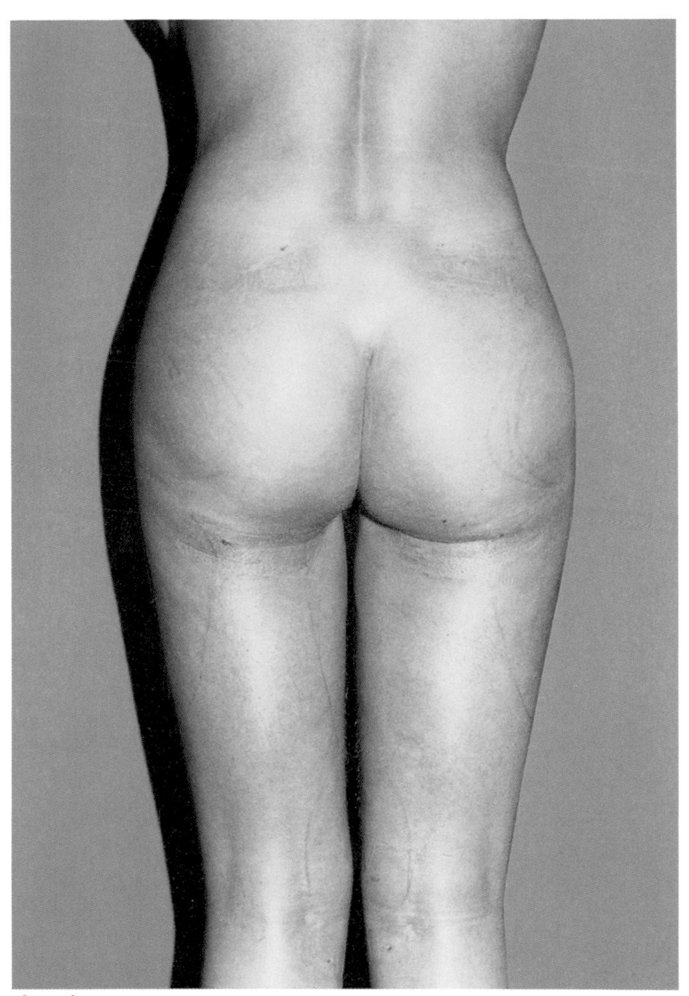

fig. 5 b

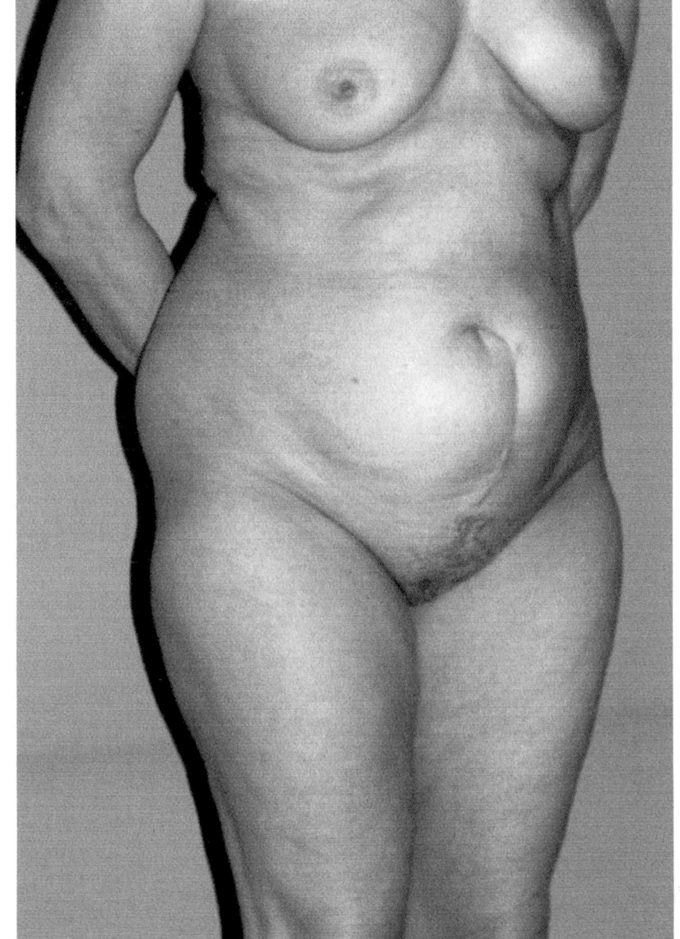

fig 6 a

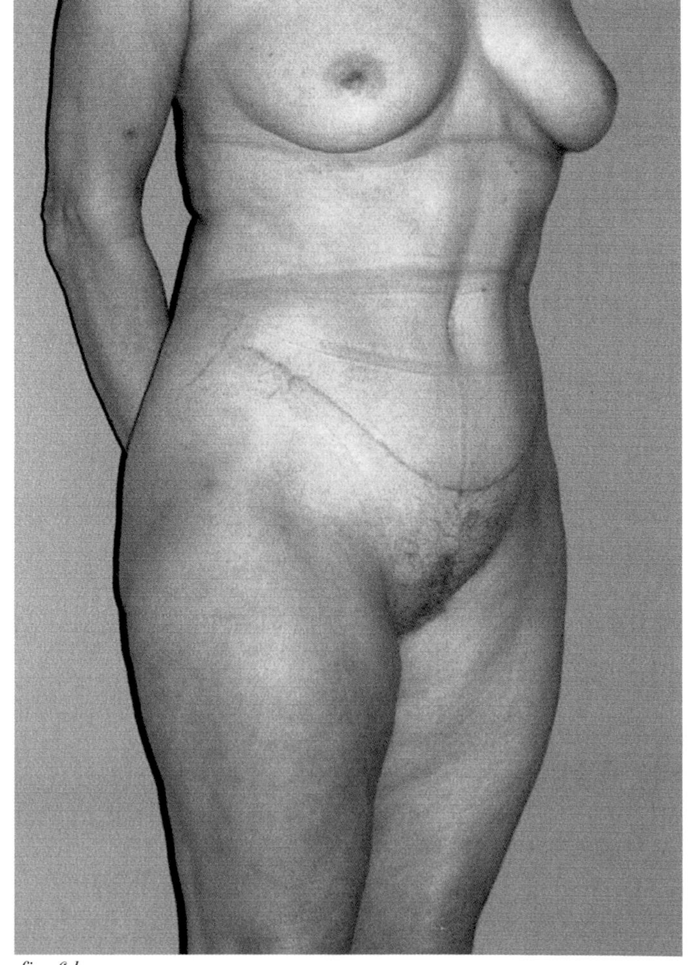

fig. 6 b

fig. 7

Dr. Eren's centrally pedunculated reduction mammaplasty and "interior bra" technique. Two de-epithelised lateral corium flaps are created to sculpt the reduced mammary gland. © Private archive Dr. Eren

fig. 8

The corium flap envelops the lower parts of the centrally pedunculated gland like an interior bra. It is fastened to the rib periosteum and the pectoral muscle – and suspends the reshaped mammary gland. © Private archive Dr. Eren

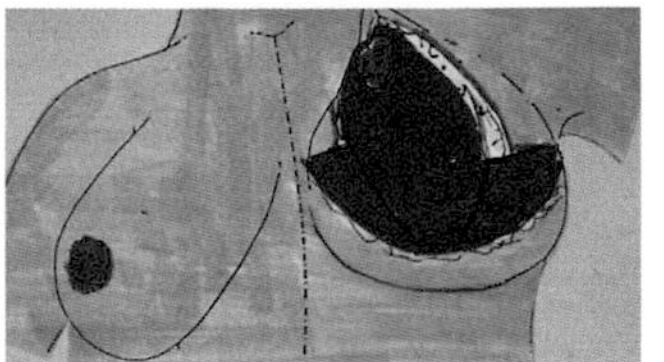

fig. 7

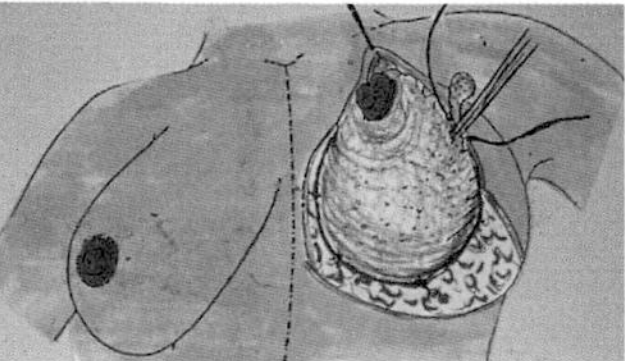

fig. 8

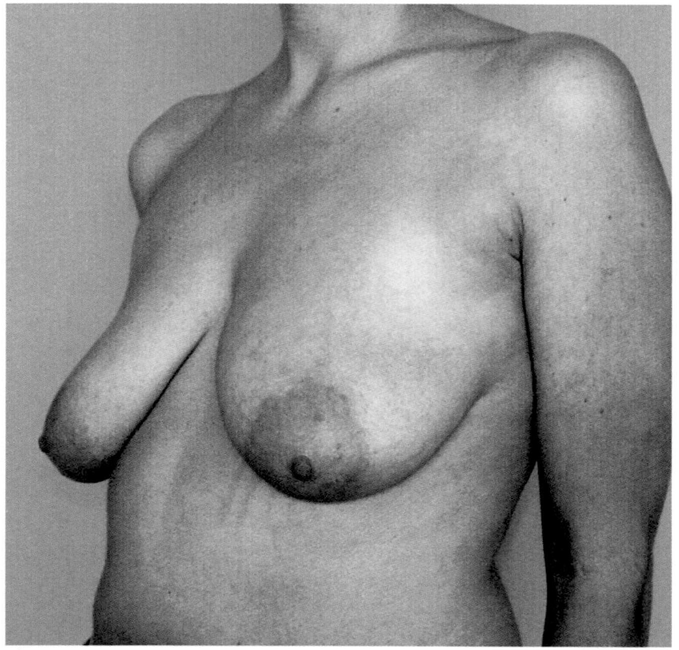

fig. 9 a

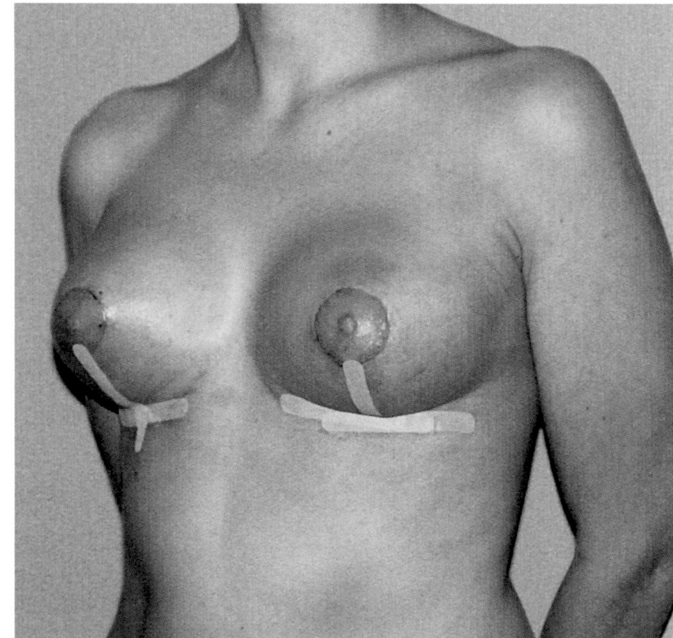

fig. 9 b

fig. 10 a

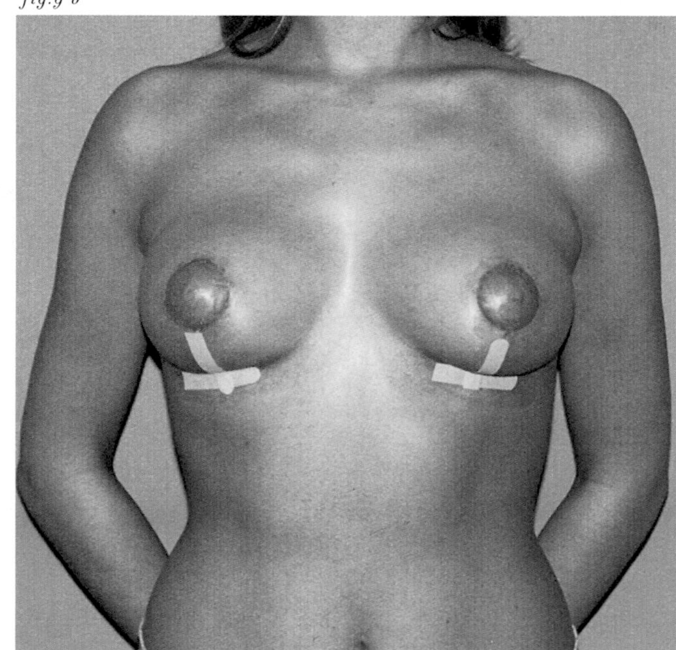

fig. 10 b

fig. 9 a+b

A 52-year-old patient. The breasts are lifted and contoured using the interior bra technique – without any implants. © Private archive Dr. Eren

fig. 10 a+b

A 20-year-old patient who had suffered from sagging breasts. The sutures were removed two weeks after the operation. © Private archive Dr. Eren

fig. 11 a+b

A 28-year-old patient with heavily deformed and sagging breasts; three years after the operation. © Private archive Dr. Eren

fig. 12 a+b

A 32-year-old patient with sagging breasts; four years after the operation. © Private archive Dr. Eren

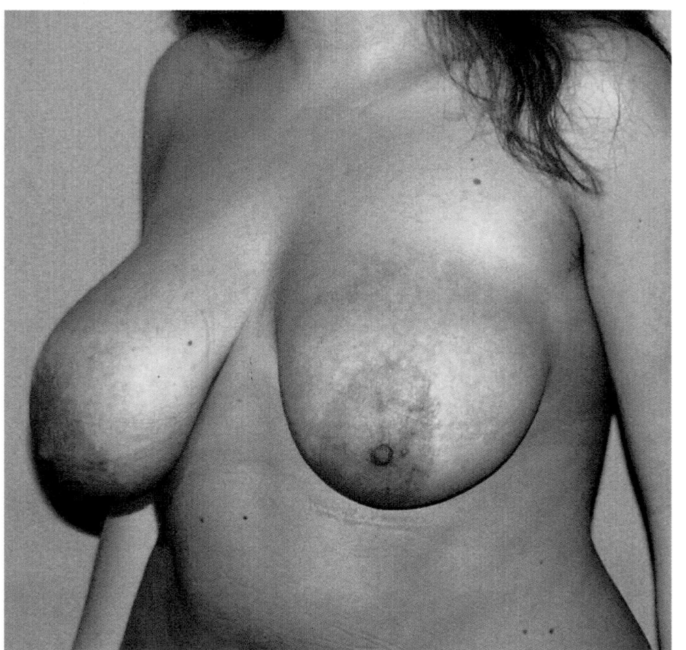

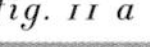

fig. 11 a

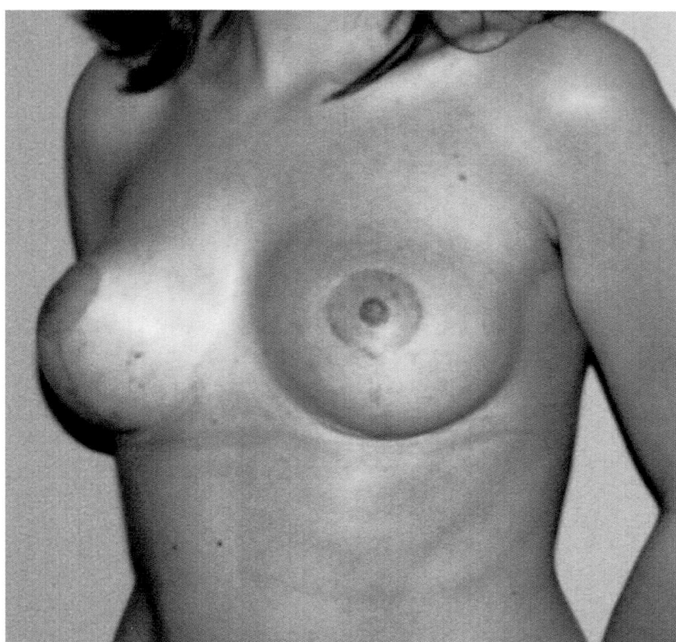

fig. 11 b

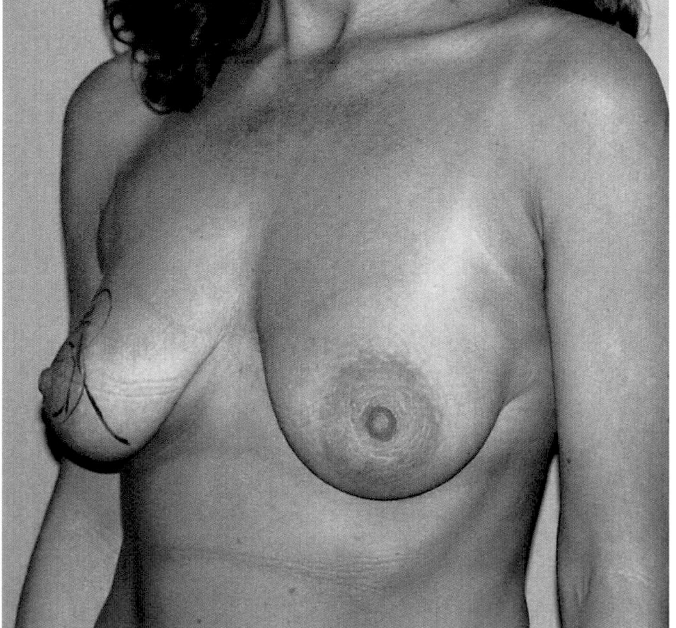

fig. 12 a

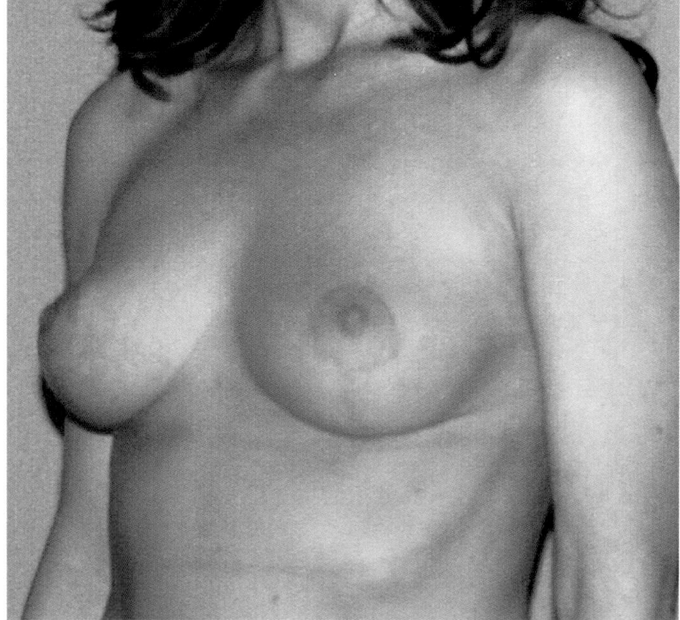

fig.12 b

"My operations are very relaxed"

WERNER L. MANG, Lindau/Munich

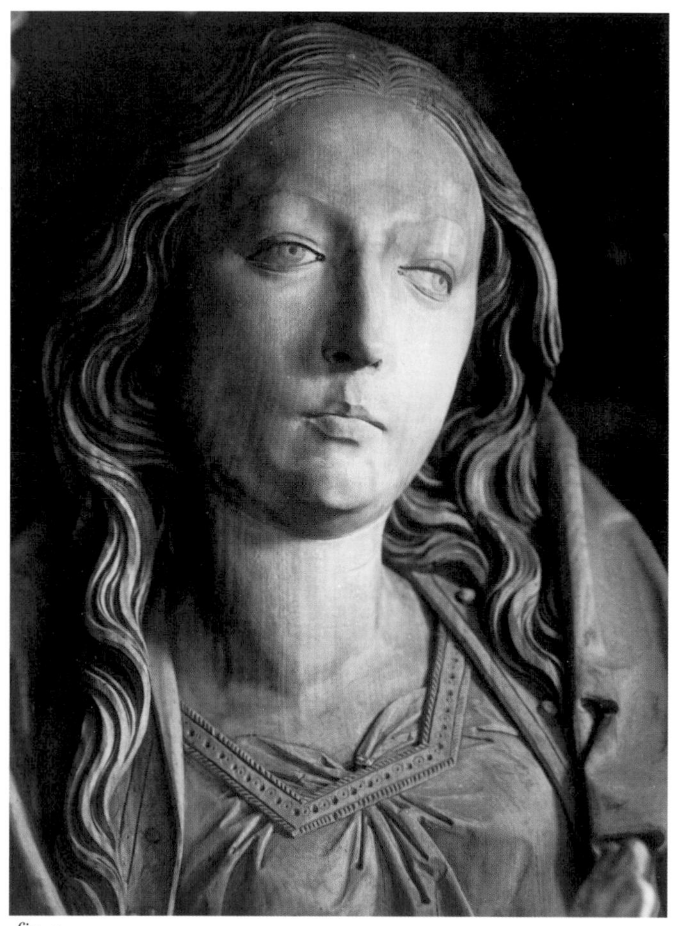

fig. 1

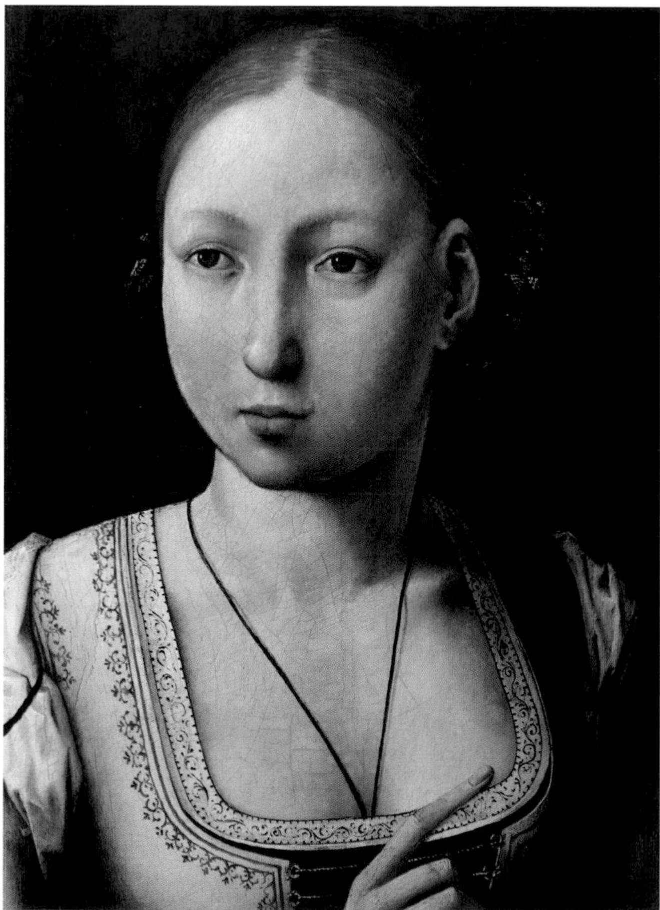

fig. 2

1. WHAT FASCINATES YOU MOST ABOUT BEING AN AESTHETIC SURGEON?

Aesthetic surgery is my passion since I was 14 years old. I was constantly drawing noses and sculpting faces. My aim was to make the faces look more harmonious — pinning back the ears and smoothing out the bumpy noses. I think I only did well at school because I had this single-minded ambition. As soon as I finished school at the age of 18, I used all my savings — 320 Deutschmarks were not to be sneezed at then! — and bought a plane ticket from Amsterdam to Rio de Janeiro. I wanted to learn from Ivo Pitanguy directly. When I arrived at his clinic, I had to wait from 8am until 8pm before he would finally see me! Today, we are good friends. I perform around 2,000 surgical procedures every year; my operations have become very relaxed. Aesthetic surgery is still my first and foremost passion, as it is so demanding. Not only do you need faultless technique, you also need to be a psychologist and have the aesthetic sensibilities of an artist.

2. WHICH AREAS DO YOU SPECIALISE IN?

After completing my studies as a general surgeon, I specialised in otolaryngology (ENT). In plastic surgery, rhinoplasty is my speciality (nasal corrections) — the most demanding procedure in the field of cosmetic surgery. This is my foremost passion, my obsession; I have developed my

fig. 1

Tilman Riemenschneider (1455 / 60–1531) carved this head of the Virgin Mary. The figure is part of the central shrine of the Altar of the Virgin Mary in Creglingen, titled the "Ascension of Mary." © akg-images

fig. 2

Joan "the Mad," Queen of Castile and Aragon (1479–1555), wife of Philip "the Fair" and mother of Emperor Charles V. This portrait was painted by Juan de Flandes around 1496. © akg-images / Erich Lessing

fig. 3 & 4

In a study conducted in cooperation with the University of Paris, Werner L. Mang discovered that the modern ideal of masculine beauty still corresponds to the Ancient Greek profile. Hollywood star Richard Gere, whom the surgeon regards as one of the world's most attractive men, is one of best examples to prove this theory. © akg-images / John Hios (36), Robert Eric / CORBIS SYGMA

fig. 5

To Werner L. Mang, film diva Sophia Loren (pictured in 1965) is one of the most beautiful women alive. Despite her age, he explains, she still has an erotic aura. © Getty Images

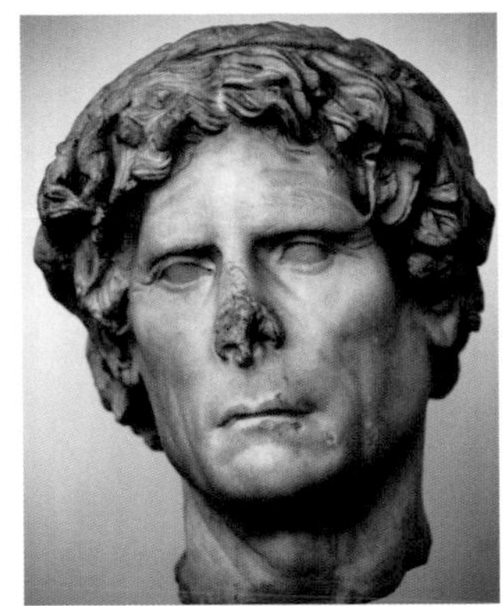

fig. 3

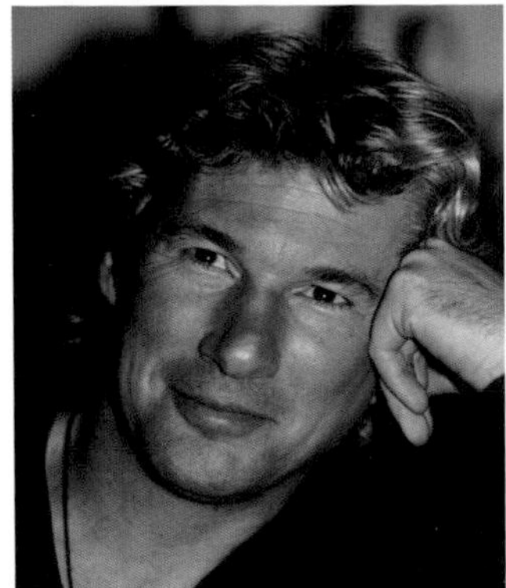

fig. 4

own special techniques for it, referred to as the Mang-nose. With my team, I also daily perform facelifts, breast enlargements, liposuction and general body contouring.

3. DO YOU REGARD YOURSELF AS AN ARTIST?

If anything, I regard myself as an athlete — a marathon man or a decathlete who needs to be fit and ready at all times. In my occupation, there is plenty of physical and psychological stress to deal with. I do regard myself as an artist, but only in that I view every facelift or nasal correction as an aesthetic decision. To make this decision, I work as closely with the patient as possible.

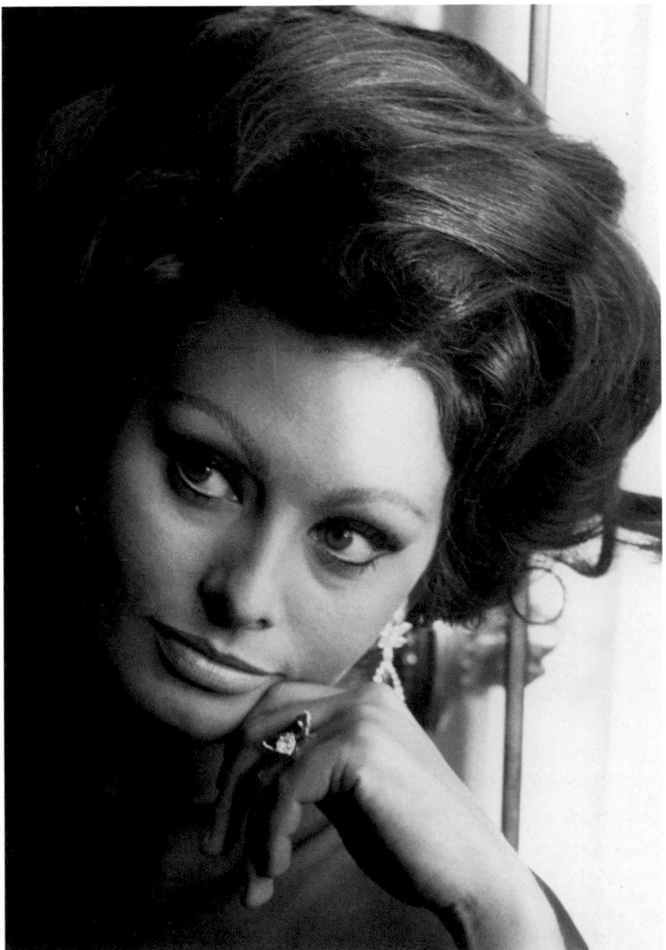

fig. 5

4. WHAT IS YOUR CONCEPT OF BEAUTY?

That is a difficult one. Ten years ago, we conducted a study into beauty concepts together with the University of Paris. Our findings led to the conclusion that Gothic portrayals of the face tend towards a feminine idea of beauty, whereas the Early Greek faces reflect a more masculine aesthetic. To me, beauty needs to be timeless and radiant. It does not need traits such as regularity or symmetry; on the contrary, these can quickly get boring and even mar beauty. By no means does our work aim to force aesthetic standards onto people — the objective is to increase our patients' well-being. Doll noses, gigantic breasts and inflated lips are quirks of fashion that are either outdated already or will soon be on their way out.

5. IN ART HISTORY, WHAT IS YOUR FAVOURITE NOTION OF BEAUTY?

I love the German Expressionists, especially the artists of Dresden's "Brücke" group. I'm also interested in contemporary art. I collect works by artists of my age, such as Georg Baselitz, Jörg Immendorf and Gerhard Richter, as well as works by young artists from southern Germany. In my new clinic in Lindau, I regulary present art by young painters from around the world whose works deal with the subject of beauty. I also enjoy painting creatively myself. Once I have retired from my career, I want to study art history and live in the south of France.

6. TO YOU, WHO ARE THE MOST BEAUTIFUL WOMAN AND MOST BEAUTIFUL MAN ALIVE?

My wife. Among the more well-known film stars, Sophia Loren is one of the most attractive women, still very sexy despite her age. Of the men, Richard Gere is very attractive, both in terms of his looks and his personality. But I don't have any real idols. My father was my only role model.

7. DO YOU REGARD YOURSELF AS ATTRACTIVE?

Someone else will have to be the judge of that! Personally, I regard myself as honest, undiplomatic and highly ambitious. In my horoscope, I attribute this to my ascendant,

fig. 6

In the operating theatre, Prof. Mang is at ease and able to relax. He does approx. 2000 operations per year, and has done a total of 30,000 in the course of his career, which makes him one of the world's top ten. Here, he is demonstrating new operating techniques to plastic surgeons at the University clinic of St. Petersburg. He is a reowned visiting operator throughout the world. © Private archive Prof. Mang

fig. 7

After his wife had a skiing accident, Werner Mang operated on her nose; after she gave birth, he remodelled her lower abdomen. © Private archive Prof. Mang

fig. 8

The lobby of the new clinic in Lindau at Lake Constance, Europe's largest clinic for aesthetic surgery. Werner L. Mang, a keen collector of contemporary art, aims to bring together medicine and culture at his clinic by exhibiting works of contemporary artists from around the world. © Private archive Prof. Mang

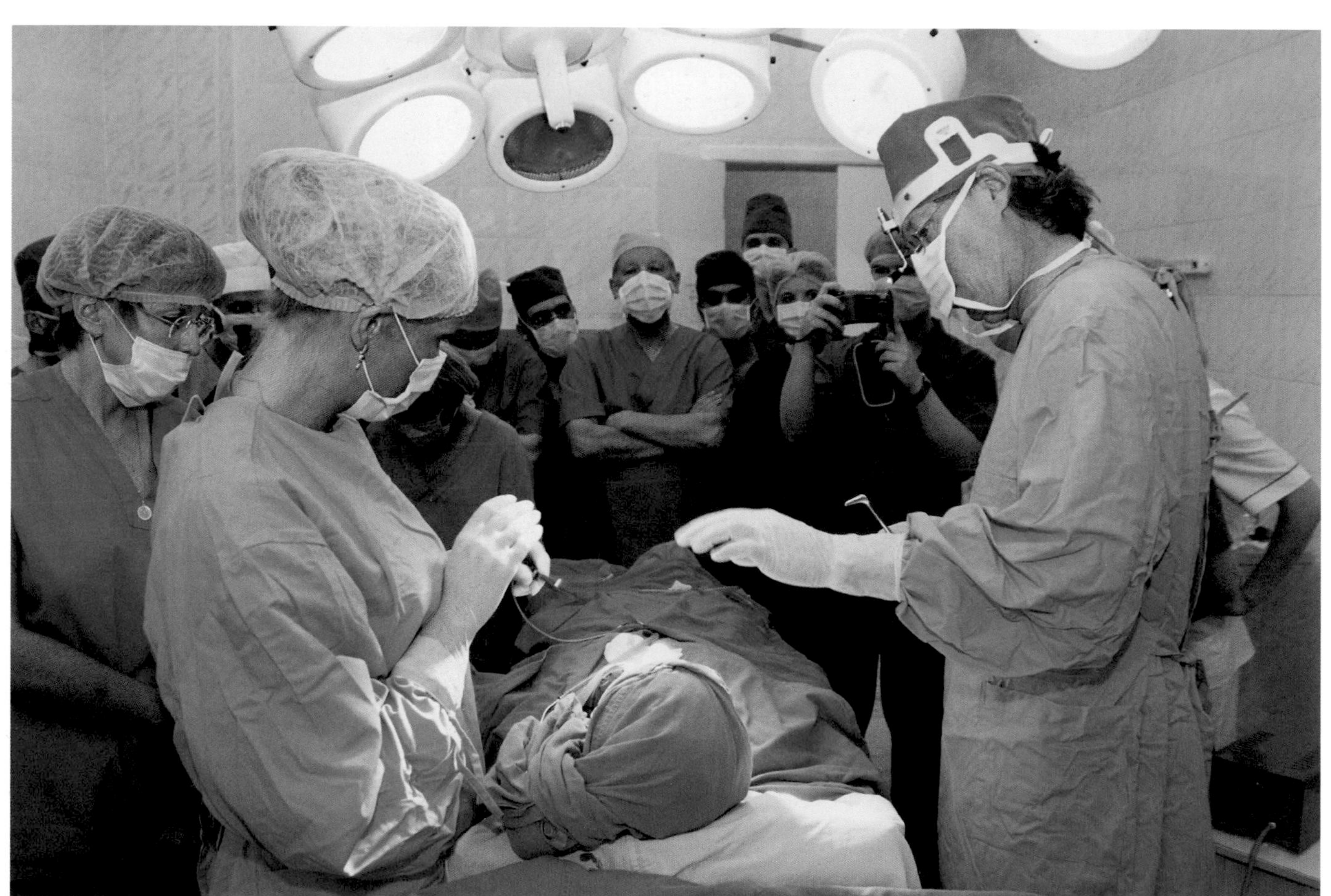

fig. 6

Virgo, whereas my star sign, Leo, explains my preference for glamour, high society and parties. I think I'm a highly interesting person with two different souls. People tell me that I have a strong aura, that they can sense my presence when I enter a room.

8. WHAT DOES AGING MEAN TO YOU?

My greatest treasure is my health. Unfortunately, aging means that you become more susceptible to diseases and ailments. I take preventive measures against this by having a healthy lifestyle — I play several sports, I go jogging, play tennis and enjoy sailing.

9. ARE YOU AFRAID OF GETTING OLDER?

Yes. I cannot see anything positive about death. Maybe I will be able to confront my mortality once I have reached a certain age. At the moment however, I try not to think about it.

10. HAVE YOU EVER UNDERGONE AESTHETIC SURGERY YOURSELF? IF SO, WHAT WAS IT FOR?

No, and I'm not planning on it. My vitality is more important to me. I could get the bags under my eyes removed, but I don't really want to be operated on unless there is a medical necessity.

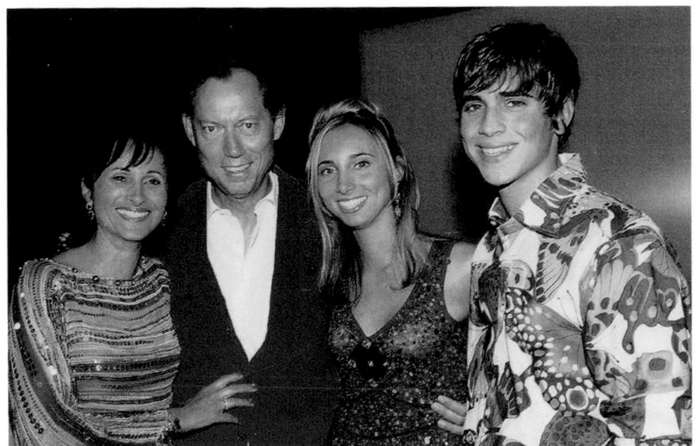
fig. 7

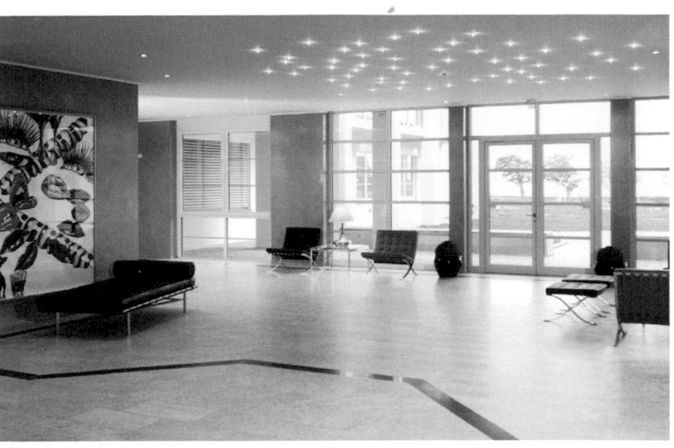
fig. 8

11. HAVE YOU EVER OPERATED ON YOUR WIFE/PARTNER AND/OR CHILDREN? IF SO, WHY?

My wife had a skiing accident once, and I operated on her nose. And after the birth of our children, I operated on her lower abdomen. Apart from instances such as these, I don't advocate operations within the family.

12. CAN YOU JUSTIFY EVERY OPERATION AND PATIENT REQUEST, OR IS THERE A POINT WHEN YOU REFUSE TO DO AN OPERATION?

To approximately ten percent of my patients, I recommend the services of a psychologist. If people approach me wanting an operation to save their marriage or to look like Claudia Schiffer, I send them away — similarly if they feel ugly and "just want to be beautiful." These people are so unstable psychologically that I refuse to take responsibility for operating on them. Also, they would never be satisfied with the results, as their problems are not of a cosmetic but psychological nature. Because of this, I work very closely with psychologists.

13. WHAT IS THE MOST UNUSUAL REQUEST FOR SURGERY YOU HAVE ENCOUNTERED IN YOUR CAREER?

One time I was approached by a young business manager who wanted me to transform him into Brad Pitt. After he came back year after year, I finally did an operation for him. He was the only extreme case I caved in to. Today he looks exactly like Brad Pitt and he feels great.

14. WHAT ARE YOUR PATIENTS' REACTIONS FOLLOWING SURGERY?

Even when procedures are objectively successful, some patients, approximately three percent, are not satisfied — sometimes they even sue me! Everything worked out as planned, but they project their personal issues onto me, the surgeon. This can make my work very difficult at times.

15. COULD YOU NAME SOME OF YOUR MORE WELL-KNOWN PATIENTS?

No. All I can tell you is that I've made friends with many celebrities I have operated on.

16. DO YOU BELIEVE THAT BEAUTY LARGELY EMANATES FROM WITHIN?

Yes and no. The inside and the outside need to be in harmony with each other. To me, beauty needs to have an erotic aspect to it. Enlarged breasts or a face with even features are not enough; outside of the context of a person's sexual energy, they are boring.

17. DO YOU THINK THAT BEAUTIFUL PEOPLE ARE HAPPIER AND LEAD MORE FULFILLED LIVES?

No. When beauty is coupled with vanity, the results can be hideous. I don't believe happiness relies on appearance — or on money. You can't buy happiness. I experience moments of happiness when I ride my bicycle to the clinic. Or when my daughter arrives from her studies in England.

18. DO BEAUTIFUL PEOPLE HAVE BETTER SEX?

No. That's rubbish.

19. WHAT DOES THE FUTURE HOLD FOR AESTHETIC SURGERY?

The field will continue to become more popular, it will become a mainstream industry with discount prices and mass-produced products. Housewives will be able to afford operations that used to be the prerogative of film stars. That's where the problems will start; we need to ensure that professional training is strictly enforced. In fact, I have recently founded an International Academy for Aesthetic Surgery as part of my new clinic at Lake Constance. Our board, made up of ten well-respected professors, is lobbying to legally regulate usage of the professional title of the "aesthetic surgeon." The second problem that aesthetic surgery is and will be facing is of a more philosophical nature. Our culture is increasingly focusing on external aspects. As a result, people's emotional well-being is becoming too reliant on their appearance. People are losing their personal values and integrity because the predominant face of culture does not care for such private qualities. I find this very depressing. You cannot use a scalpel to create a meaningful existence.

Interview: Eva Karcher, Munich

"Beauty consists of subtle asymmetries, not flawlessness"

HANS-LEO NATHRATH, Munich

1. WHAT FASCINATES YOU MOST ABOUT BEING AN AESTHETIC SURGEON?

I enjoy working with my hands and I like helping people, even if they are challenging. My occupation allows me to engage in aesthetics – especially feminine aesthetics. Women fascinate me. I try to put myself in the woman's position to find out how she perceives herself. Naturally, I also enjoy operating on men. In either case, my work entails considerable responsibilities; every surgical procedure has potential risks associated with it. I make myself aware of this every morning – by asking myself if I would be willing to have the operation I'm about to perform done on me.

2. WHICH AREAS DO YOU SPECIALISE IN?

Facial surgery, especially facelifts. Also liposuction. I also do breast corrections frequently – mostly enlargements, but also reductions and contouring. However, I refuse to enlarge breasts to disproportionate sizes. This can lead to health risks or complications.

3. DO YOU REGARD YOURSELF AS AN ARTIST?

The ideal scenario is for my aesthetics to be congruent with the patient's aesthetics. When this happens, it makes me happy – but does it make me an artist? On the other hand, I do shape and sculpt, and that requires a certain amount of aesthetic sensibility.

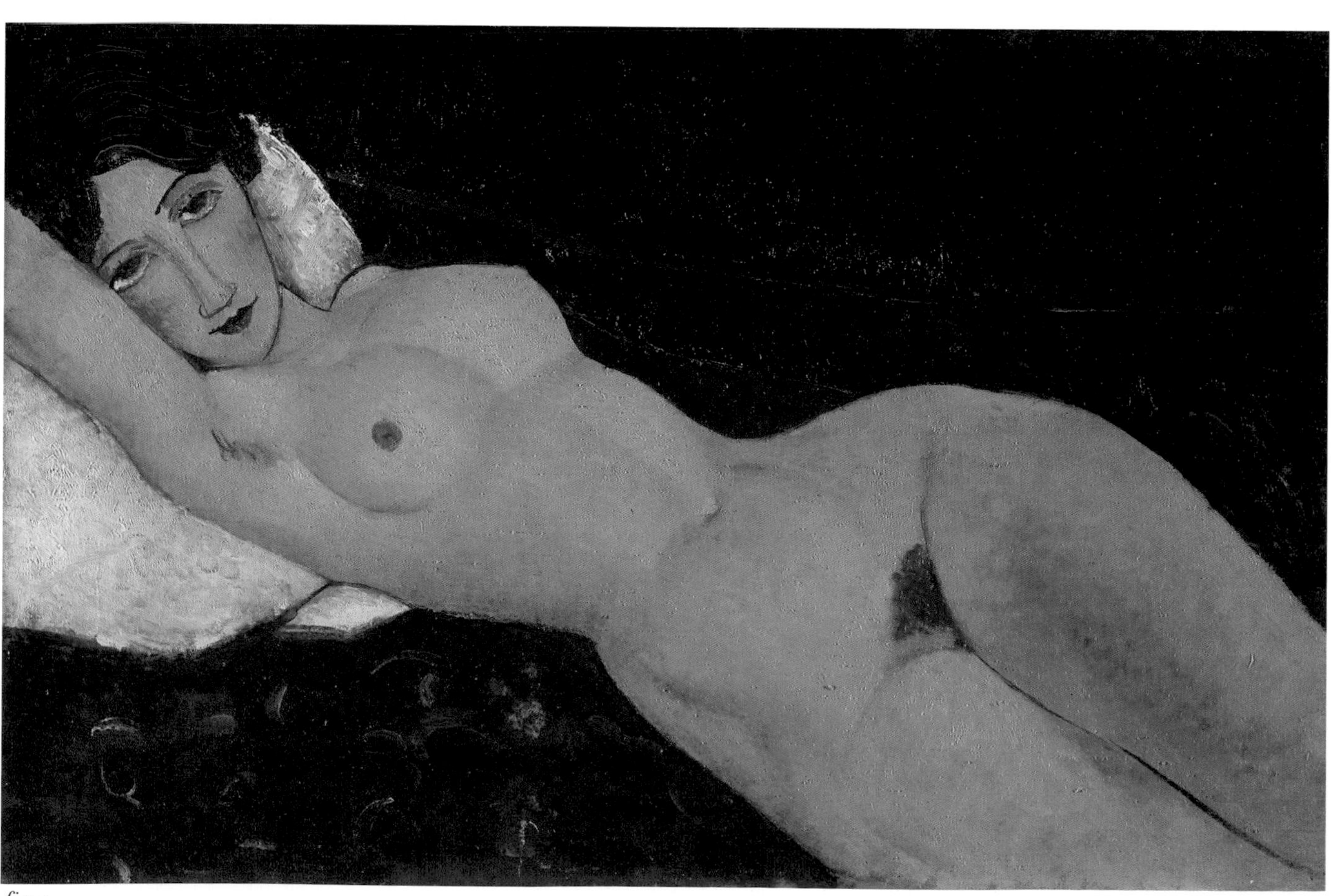

fig. 1

fig. 1

"Reclining Nude' by Amadeo Modigliani (1884–1920) is simply stunning," enthuses Hans-Leo Nathrath about his favourite example of beauty in art. © Staatsgalerie Stuttgart

fig. 2

Hans-Leo Nathrath (Shown with his family in front of the opera house) could imagine having cosmetic surgery done on himself – for example corrections on the lachrymal sacs. © Private archive Dr. Nathrath

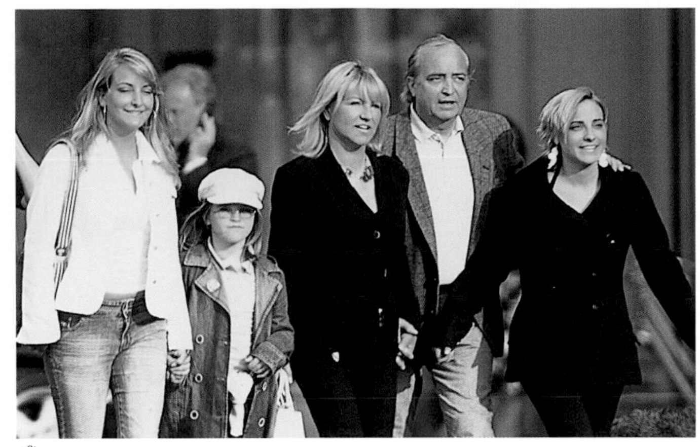

fig. 2

4. WHAT IS YOUR CONCEPT OF BEAUTY?

My personal concept of beauty doesn't necessarily have to match the patient's. However, I wouldn't perform an operation if I considered it aesthetically wrong. There is a good catchphrase in my profession — "don't do what you don't like." I stick with this as much as I can. Regarding my personal concept of beauty — I believe in the harmony of proportions suggested by the classical Greek ideal of beauty.

5. IN ART HISTORY, WHAT IS YOUR FAVOURITE NOTION OF BEAUTY?

Modigliani's "Reclining Nude" is simply stunning. In contemporary art, I enjoy artists who present the subjects of beauty and youth, i. e. the subjects most relevant to my work, in subtle and ironic ways. My favourites include the photographic artists Mette Tronvoll and Rineke Dijkstra.

6. TO YOU, WHO ARE THE MOST BEAUTIFUL WOMAN AND MOST BEAUTIFUL MAN ALIVE?

Catherine Deneuve and Romy Schneider. Sean Connery.

7. DO YOU REGARD YOURSELF AS ATTRACTIVE?

I never think about it. However, it would be a lie to tell you that I've never looked at myself critically in the mirror. I think I'm a good type of person. By this I mean that I'm somebody who is secure and confident about himself. I also see this as a key criterion for success in a profession like the one I practice.

8. WHAT DOES AGING MEAN TO YOU?

Most of all, it means maturity, the ability to approach life in a more relaxed manner. For me personally, this may well mean that I shall need to temper my craving for adventure. A point will come when my body simply won't be able to cope with my extensive skiing tours, mountain hikes and kayak trips on the ocean.

9. ARE YOU AFRAID OF GETTING OLDER?

No. I think I'll be able to deal with the age-related restrictions on physical activities such as sports. Of course I'm scared of diseases and afflictions, and also of physical, psychological and mental decay. And like everybody else, I am scared of dying. The benefits of age, on the other hand, are that you don't have to search anymore, that you no longer need to fight for love, recognition and power. Also, my occupation is one where experience is crucial, where you get better over the years and receive more recognition.

10. HAVE YOU EVER UNDERGONE AESTHETIC SURGERY YOURSELF? IF SO, WHAT WAS IT FOR?

Not yet. If I had the time for it, I probably would! For example, I would like to get rid of the bags under my eyes. That'll have to happen sometime soon.

11. HAVE YOU EVER OPERATED ON YOUR WIFE/PARTNER AND/OR CHILDREN? IF SO, WHY?

I have done aesthetic surgery for members of my family, including my wife. Taking this question to mean whether it is possible to operate on people you are intimate and familiar with — I believe yes. Regardless of this, I find my wife as appealing as ever. And although looking at plastic surgery from the outside may not suggest it, operations can in fact be very aesthetic.

12. CAN YOU JUSTIFY EVERY OPERATION AND PATIENT REQUEST, OR IS THERE A POINT WHEN YOU REFUSE TO DO AN OPERATION?

If a 30-year-old woman comes to my practice and wants me to do a facelift on her, I tell her "sure, come back in ten years' time." A different example: An actress approached me for facial surgery once, and brought along lots of photos and detailed ideas. She wanted me to change her face so that her likeness to a well-known international film star would be even more obvious. I thought about it very carefully and decided to go ahead with it. The result is actually very convincing.

13. WHAT IS THE MOST UNUSUAL REQUEST FOR SURGERY YOU HAVE ENCOUNTERED IN YOUR CAREER?

A 40-year-old man approached me with his childhood photos and wanted me to make him look like he was twelve years old again. I tried to persuade him to seek psychological help. Another case: An Ethiopian patient came to me for a facelift. The woman also had a torn earlobe because of an

fig. 3

In this room, Hans-Leo Nathrath undertakes minor operations, mostly eye lid corrections. Operations such as face-lifts and liposuction procedures are taken care of in the operating theatres of the clinic. To him, surgical success is measured in the harmony of proportions. © Private archive Dr. Nathrath

fig. 4 a–d & 5 a–d

An example of a breast reduction (4 a–d), before and five years after the surgery, and a breast enlargement (5a–d), before and three years after the operation. According to Hans-Leo Nathrath, these are not the only procedures becoming increasingly common. The surgeon fears that aesthetic surgery will soon turn into a popular sport – with possibly very negative results. © Private archive Dr. Nathrath

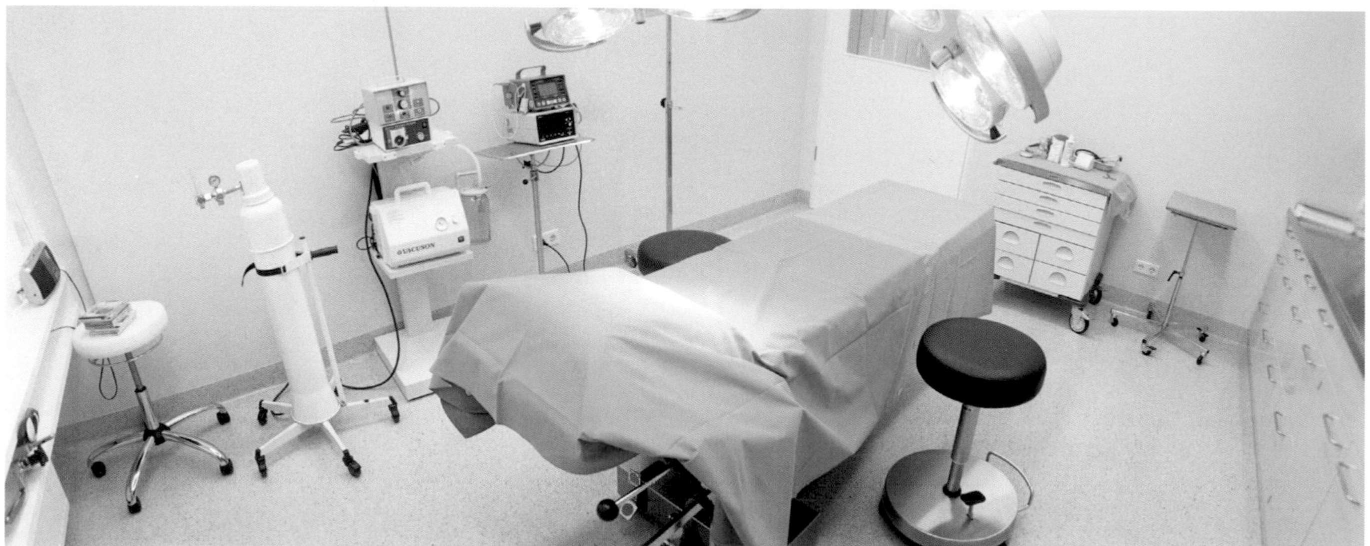

fig. 3

earring. When I asked her if I should fix this for her as part of the operation, she asked me instead to tear the other ear-lobe as well!

14. WHAT ARE YOUR PATIENTS' REACTIONS FOLLOWING SURGERY?

They are usually very realistic because I brief them about the procedure in great detail. Swellings and other typical healing reactions don't come as a shock to them. My patients generally feel better and happier than before once they see the final result.

15. COULD YOU NAME SOME OF YOUR MORE WELL-KNOWN PATIENTS?

No.

16. DO YOU BELIEVE THAT BEAUTY LARGELY EMANATES FROM WITHIN?

Yes. Although my job is to harmonise contours and proportions, I am quite aware that beauty is more than skin-deep. Older faces are often the most beautiful! Beauty consists of subtle asymmetries, not the flawlessness suggested by the media. The illusions propagated by the media can be dangerously misleading.

17. DO YOU THINK THAT BEAUTIFUL PEOPLE ARE HAPPIER AND LEAD MORE FULFILLED LIVES?

No. It may well be that they lead more luxurious lives, as high society requires people to be attractive. But people aren't happy simply because they are beautiful. However, people can conversely be beautiful as a result of their happiness and inner peace.

18. DO BEAUTIFUL PEOPLE HAVE BETTER SEX?

No, because eroticism is a mental phenomenon. Beauty can be a starting point, but desire and passion are triggered by other things.

19. WHAT DOES THE FUTURE HOLD FOR AESTHETIC SURGERY?

In 20 or 30 years, many operations will be performed much faster. Aesthetic surgery will become like a popular sport — which will also have negative repercussions. The gap between the rich and the poor will continue to widen, and medical ethics will need to address this. I sincerely hope that the elites of Europe will continue to favour a natural concept of beauty.

Interview: Eva Karcher, Munich

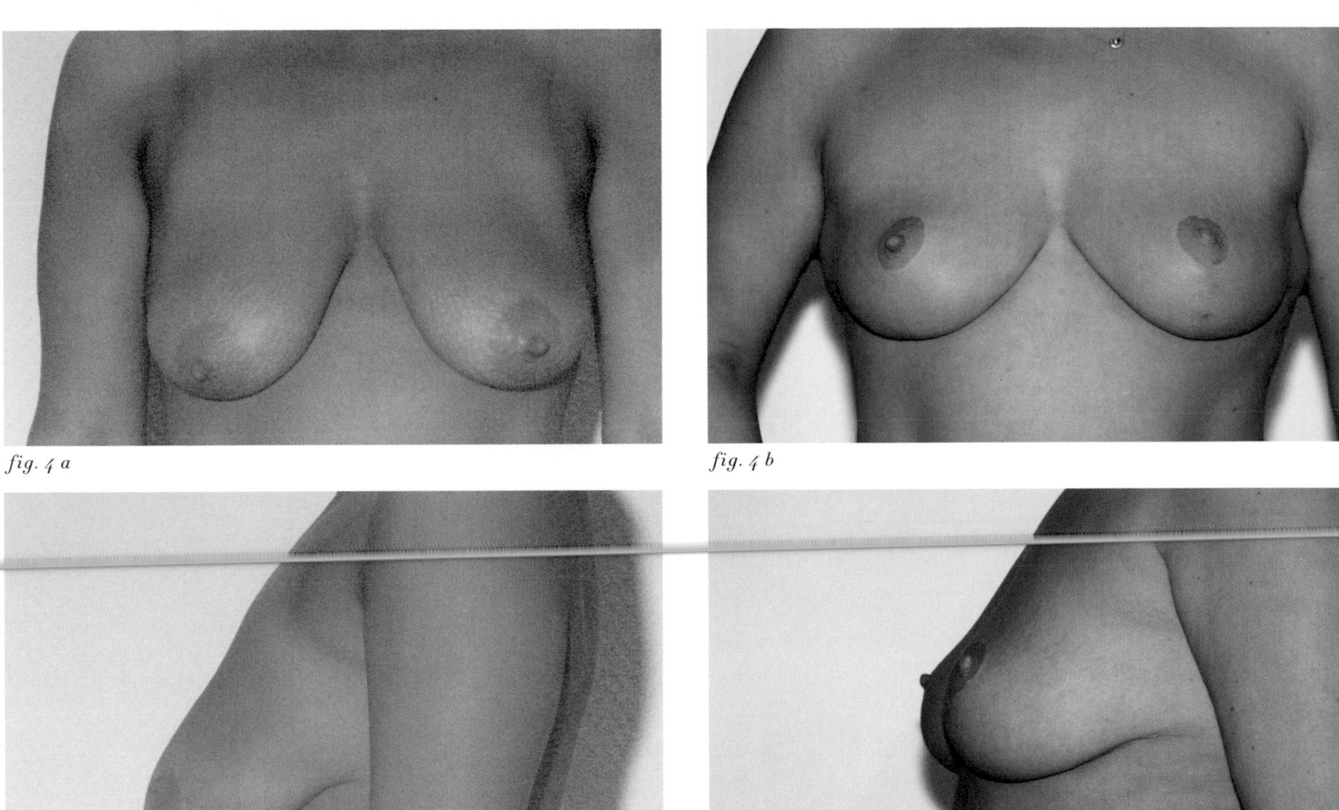

fig. 4 a

fig. 4 b

fig. 4 c

fig. 4 d

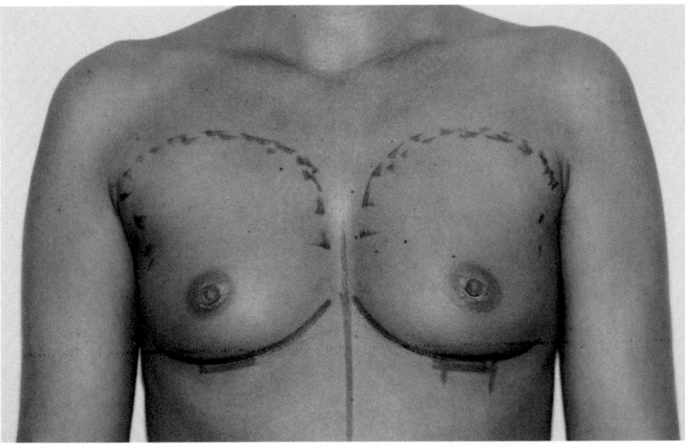

fig. 5 a

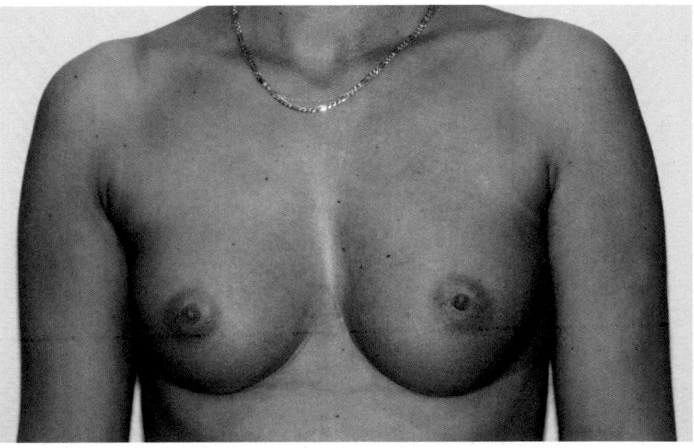

fig. 5 b

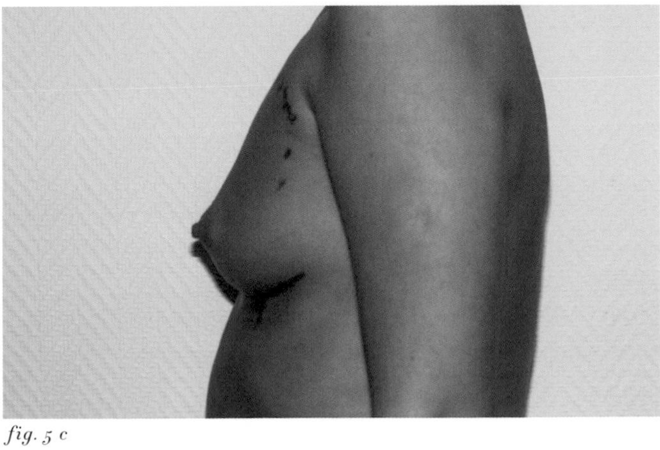

fig. 5 c

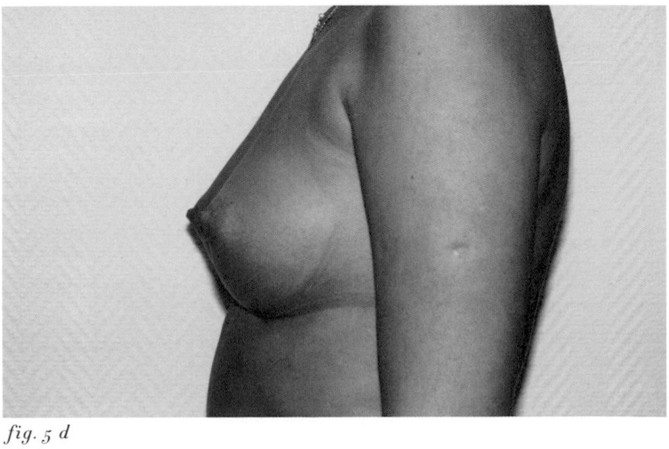

fig. 5 d

"I love women – J'aime la femme"

BERNARD CORNETTE DE SAINT CYR, Paris

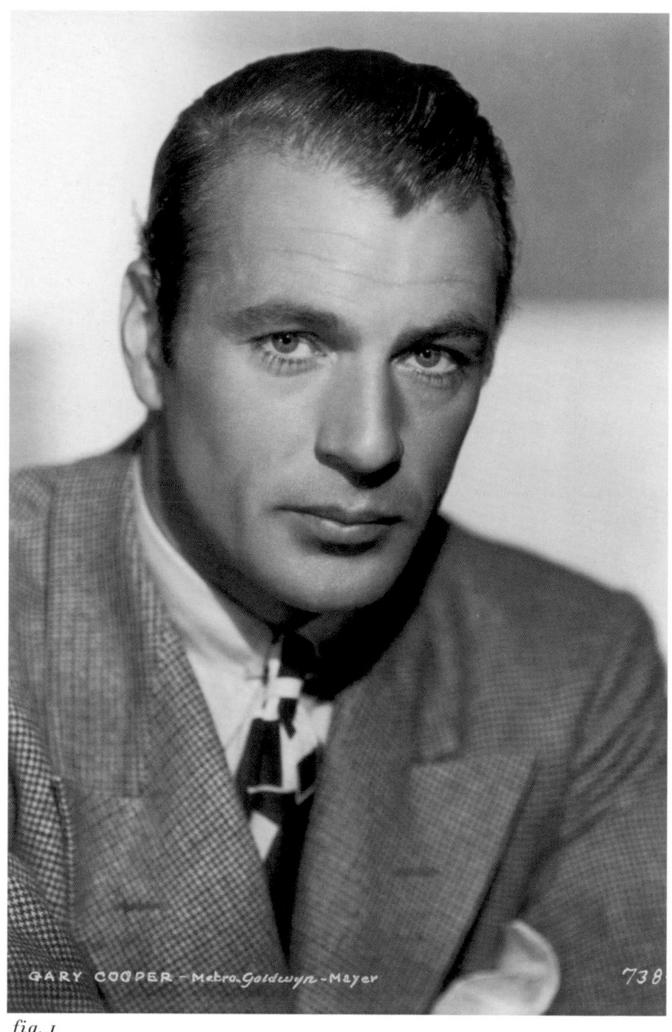

fig. 1

1. WHAT FASCINATES YOU MOST ABOUT BEING AN AESTHETIC SURGEON?

First of all, this would be the technical skill required of me as a surgeon. My work furthermore requires an ability to empathise with people, as well as a certain degree of artistry. In a way, I regard myself as a sculptor because I work on the body. But the most important aspect may well be the human dimension. I am a doctor with all my heart and soul. When I see how my patients are transformed after a successful operation, how they suddenly radiate more self-esteem, I am truly happy. Because I have brought happiness to others.

2. WHICH AREAS DO YOU SPECIALISE IN?

Facelifts, breast operations – enlargements, reductions and contouring – and rhinoplasty. These are areas requiring a great deal of creativity. Like most surgeons in my field, I have taken established surgical methods and developed them to suit my areas. I also perform liposuction and tummy tucks.

3. DO YOU REGARD YOURSELF AS AN ARTIST?

One should be modest about one's own achievements. This is for someone else to decide. I would never describe myself as an artist, but ...

4. WHAT IS YOUR CONCEPT OF BEAUTY?

I love women – J'aime la femme. I don't have one single, stereotypical concept of beauty. Of course there are universal criteria of beauty, but they can appear in so many different ways. Two women can look completely different, yet both can be beautiful. I find all kinds of standardising and cloning despicable. Beauty is individual.

5. IN ART HISTORY, WHAT IS YOUR FAVOURITE NOTION OF BEAUTY?

I enjoy and collect contemporary art. Artists like Jan Saudeck and Frank Stella, but also many pop artists, like Andy Warhol, Robert Rauschenberg, Yves Klein, César, Arman and Antoni Tàpies. My brother is one of the world's most renowned experts on modern and contemporary art. He is an art auctioneer. Our entire family consists of art lovers; another one of my brothers collects pottery, for example. I regard my exposure to art as an important prerequisite for my work. In art, you learn to discover the nature of beauty.

6. TO YOU, WHO ARE THE MOST BEAUTIFUL WOMAN AND MOST BEAUTIFUL MAN ALIVE?

There are so many. Queen Rania of Jordania is one of my favorites. But any day at the corner of the street, I can have an emotional aesthetic shock catching sight of the most

fig. 1

To Bernard Cornette de Saint Cyr, Gary Cooper is one of the most handsome men of the 20th century: "He was masculine and gallant, grown-up but still full of dreams." © Getty Images

fig. 2

The distinguished architecture of Bernard Cornette de Saint Cyr's practice in Paris is evidence of his family's deep appreciation of art. One of his brothers is a renowned international authority on modern and contemporary art. © Private archive Dr. de Saint Cyr

fig. 3

Bernard Cornette de Saint Cyr's personal Top Ten: Jennifer Lopez is a prime example of feminine beauty, and Sophia Loren is another main contender. © Frank Trapper / CORBIS

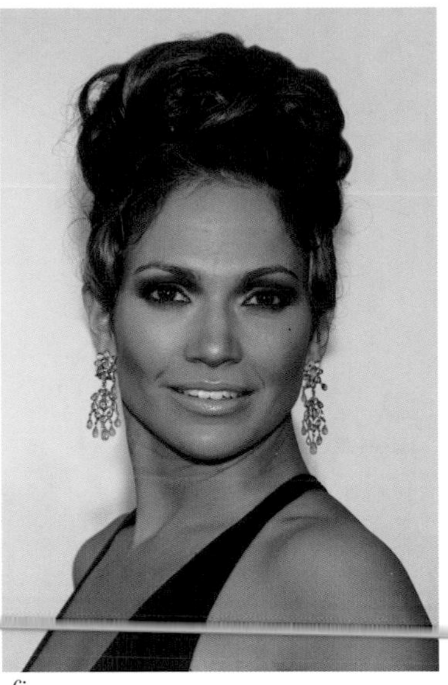

fig. 3

beautiful woman for this short instant. All men know this feeling which increases the hormones. To me, the most beautiful man of the 20th century was Gary Cooper. He was masculine and gallant, grown-up but still full of dreams.

7. DO YOU REGARD YOURSELF AS ATTRACTIVE?

On the occasions when beautiful women tell me they think I'm attractive, I tend to believe them. It probably helps that I don't have any hang-ups.

8. WHAT DOES AGING MEAN TO YOU?

Aging depends on genetic factors and on attitude. Externally we eventually lose the fullness and smoothness of our youth — depending on our genes and our lifestyle: eating and drinking too much, smoking and sun-tanning all accelerate the aging process. But in complete disregard of these factors, there are 25-year-olds who look frighteningly old and 55-year-olds who are bursting with energy and vitality. Some people become more beautiful with age, others become less attractive. I think that people have a lot of control over how they age.

9. ARE YOU AFRAID OF GETTING OLDER?

Yes. I do whatever I can to slow down the aging process. I do physical exercise every day, I watch my nutrition, I don't drink or smoke. I feel so young, and time is moving so quickly. What scares me the most is that I may not have enough time for all my plans and ideas.

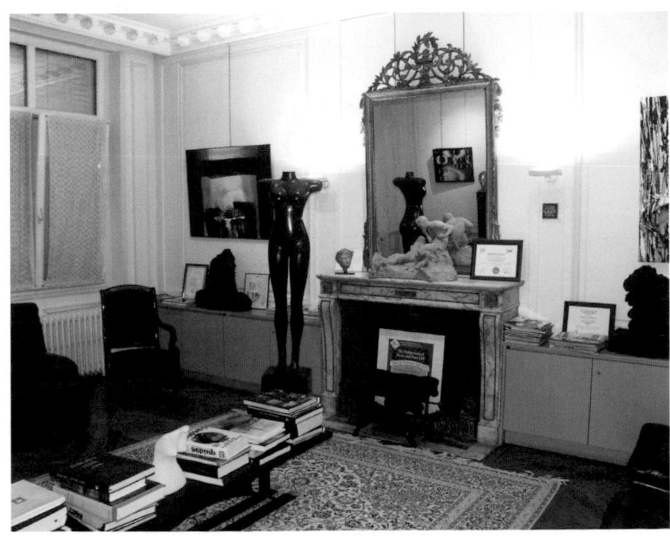

fig. 2

10. HAVE YOU EVER UNDERGONE COSMETIC SURGERY YOURSELF? IF SO, WHAT WAS IT FOR?

I've had a facelift and had my eyelids tightened. It's becoming more acceptable for men to have cosmetic surgery now. Most popular among men are corrections on the neck and the eyelids, tummy tucks and liposuction, and among younger men also nasal corrections. Interestingly, men from the Arab world are more open to cosmetic surgery than their European counterparts.

11. HAVE YOU EVER OPERATED ON YOUR WIFE/PARTNER AND/OR CHILDREN? IF SO, WHY?

Yes, I've worked on my wife's face. Also on the faces of my mother, my father, my sister and my cousins — almost my entire family, in fact.

12. CAN YOU JUSTIFY EVERY OPERATION AND PATIENT REQUEST, OR IS THERE A POINT WHEN YOU REFUSE TO DO AN OPERATION?

Most of my patients are sensible. Only around five percent demand procedures that are too extensive or too extreme. That's the point when I refuse.

13. WHAT IS THE MOST UNUSUAL REQUEST FOR SURGERY YOU HAVE ENCOUNTERED IN YOUR CAREER?

The most reckless patient I've had to operate on was a female artist called Orlan. She wanted a facelift, lip injections and liposuction all at the same time, as an artistic concept and performance. I did this only once, a second time would have been unethical.

14. WHAT ARE YOUR PATIENTS' REACTIONS FOLLOWING SURGERY?

My patients are often overjoyed and tell me: "You've changed my life!" This sentence is the biggest reward for my work. Sometimes there are complaints about complications, and sometimes there are petty gripes. My motto

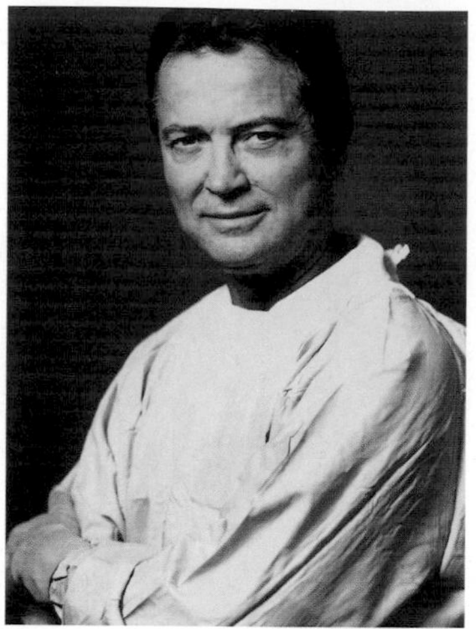

fig. 4

fig. 4

Bernard Cornette de Saint Cyr does not have a stereotypical concept of beauty. He despises nothing more than uniformity. © Private archive Dr. de Saint Cyr

fig. 5

Beauty and egocentricity can be close companions, as demonstrated by the "Narcissist" (1987), a work by the Czech photographer Jan Saudek. © Jan Saudek, Prague

fig. 6

For his sculpture "Blue Venus," Yves Klein applied colour pigments and a synthetic binder to a plaster cast of the famous "Venus de Milo." © 1994 Image of Yves Klein: Daniel Moquay, Paradise Valley, AZ

is: "The patient is always right." After I've operated on them, I tell my patients to return regularly for one or two years; if there are any minor corrections they would like me to see to, I perform these at no additional charge. 98 percent of my patients are happy with the surgical results.

15. COULD YOU NAME SOME OF YOUR MORE WELL-KNOWN PATIENTS?

Obviously, I won't reveal any names. I can, however, tell you that many of my high-ranking patients come from the Middle East — from Saudi Arabia, Kuwait, Ghana, Dubai, and also from the royal families of these countries. Still, most of my patients are from Europe; some also come from the United States.

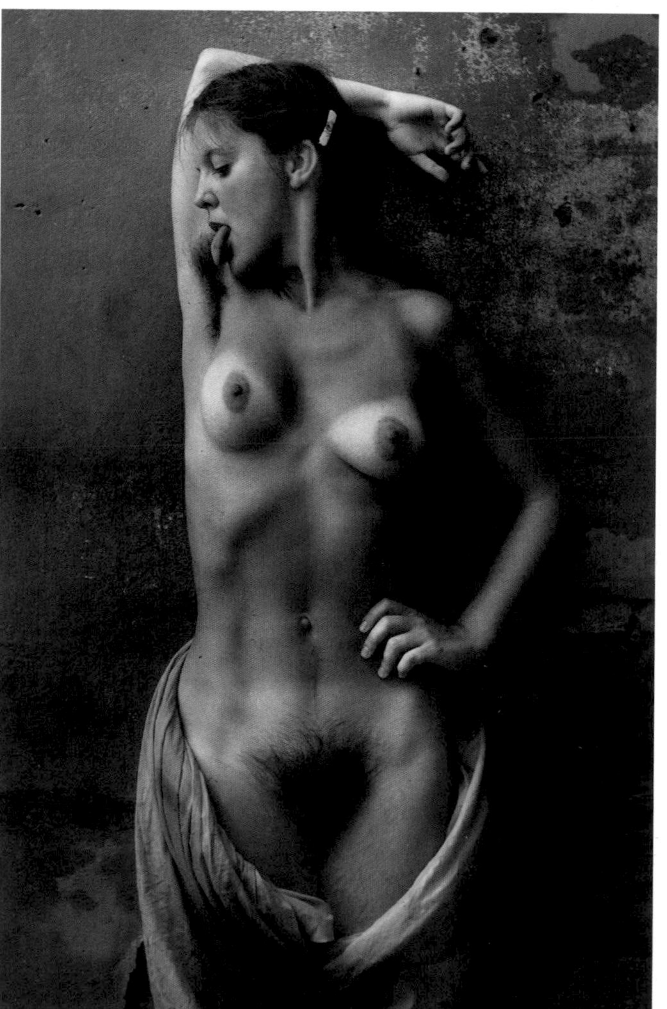

fig. 5

16. DO YOU BELIEVE THAT BEAUTY LARGELY EMANATES FROM WITHIN?

Let me tell you a joke. In a TV talkshow, a young woman is surrounded by cosmetic surgeons, psychologists and journalists. She is really overweight and ugly, and very unhappy with her appearance. The host tries to comfort her: "Mademoiselle, it is much more important that you have an inner beauty." The girl's answer — "Every time I take my inner beauty out on the town, I end up going home alone." It may not be very fair, but beauty — female beauty — is the most important asset in the world. The continued existence of mankind relies on it!

17. DO YOU THINK THAT BEAUTIFUL PEOPLE ARE HAPPIER AND LEAD MORE FULFILLED LIVES?

Yes. People who aren't attractive may be able to compensate for this disadvantage with charisma and intelligence. But they need a lot more energy. And for women, it's twice as hard as for men.

18. DO BEAUTIFUL PEOPLE HAVE BETTER SEX?

Yes. For the same reason as described in Question 17.

19. WHAT DOES THE FUTURE HOLD FOR COSMETIC SURGERY?

More and more people will seek out the help of cosmetic surgeons. The taboos that have been established by Jewish-Christian culture and education are fast disappearing. People are free to have operations to increase their attractiveness. Our objective is to give people more self-esteem. That's why we make them more beautiful. It's very important that aesthetic plastic surgeons communicate on an international level and exchange ideas and knowledge. The more transparency there is within the profession, the better the procedures will become.

Interview: Eva Karcher, Munich

fig. 6

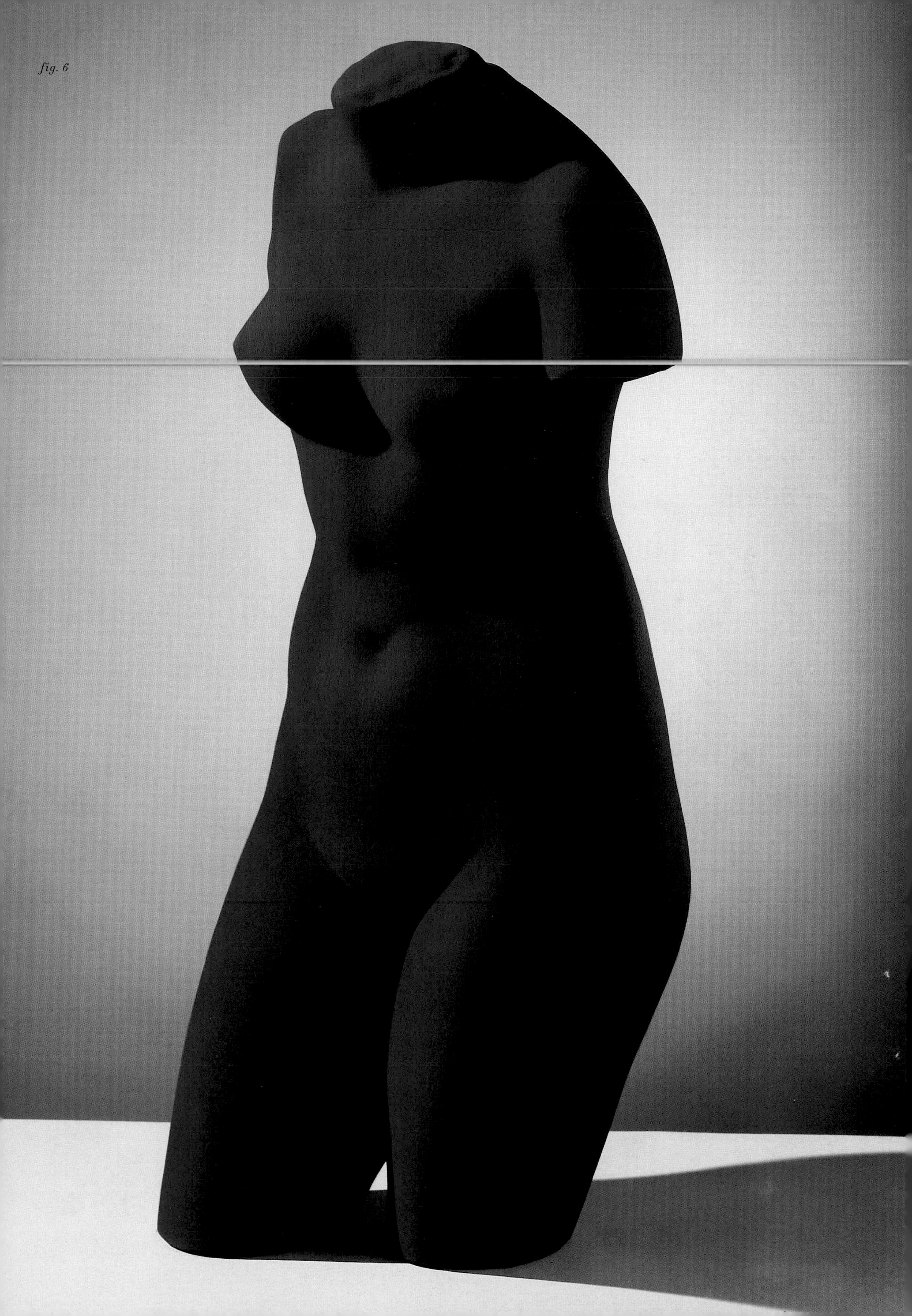

"I am a surgeon of emotions"

CHRISTOPH WOLFENSBERGER, Zurich

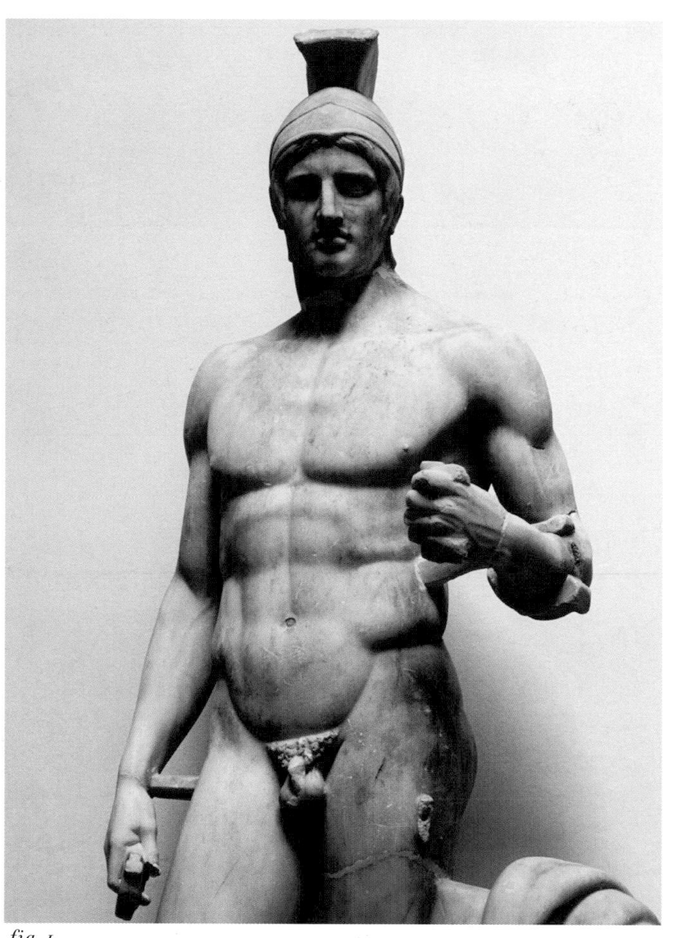

fig. 1

1. WHAT FASCINATES YOU MOST ABOUT BEING AN AESTHETIC SURGEON?

We create, or try to create, works of art using a medium that is as fascinating as it is challenging — the human body and the human face. There is no duty more noble than this. In contrast to other fields of medicine that also shape and create, everything we sculpt is immediately transparent and visible to the patient and his or her family. We perform a surgery of emotions!

Our work is a continual balancing act, without routines but full of unpredictable factors: wound healing, psychological acceptance, reasons behind the operation and the patient's social environment. Last but not least, aesthetic surgery is the last remaining medical profession that permits freelance work. There simply isn't the level of state control and overbearing financing regulation that other fields of professional medicine are burdened by. The importance of this cannot be overestimated.

2. WHICH AREAS DO YOU SPECIALISE IN?

Aesthetic plastic surgery on the face and body. This includes both invasive and non-invasive procedures — face, brow and neck lifting, liposuction, breast contouring and implants, breast reduction and laser treatment, chemical peelings, injection wrinkle treatment with fillers such as Botox (Botulinum-Toxin-A) and collagen, Restylane and Perlane.

Our surgical department is complemented by an Institute for Anti-Aging Medicine (age prevention), where comprehensive individual diagnoses, consultation and support are provided by experienced endocrinologists. We also have our own wellness day spa for consultation and treatment sessions, offering medical skin care, general cosmetics, laser hair removal and "Endermology," which is cellulite treatment with a computer-controlled lymph drainage massage unit by LPG.

3. DO YOU REGARD YOURSELF AS AN ARTIST?

Yes. I don't, however, regard myself as a genius, like for example my favourite composer, Wolfgang Amadeus Mozart. Nor do I attempt to reflect society in the manner of a writer or poet. I regard myself as a down-to-earth, technically highly-skilled craftsman — akin to the traditional goldsmith or sculptor. In a way, my profession is a craft based on science. These two elements, the creative and the scientific, keep each other in balance. However, I do not have the artist's whim or freedom in my work; a surgeon has to deliver a consistently high level of service and display a consistently professional and constructive attitude. This requires a lot of discipline.

Personally, I have a very close relationship to art. Since the days of my youth, I have been producing pencil-drawings, sketches, collages and design drawings. Calligraphy is another one of my passions. A beautiful, hand-written letter is so much more appealing than an e-mail! My wife

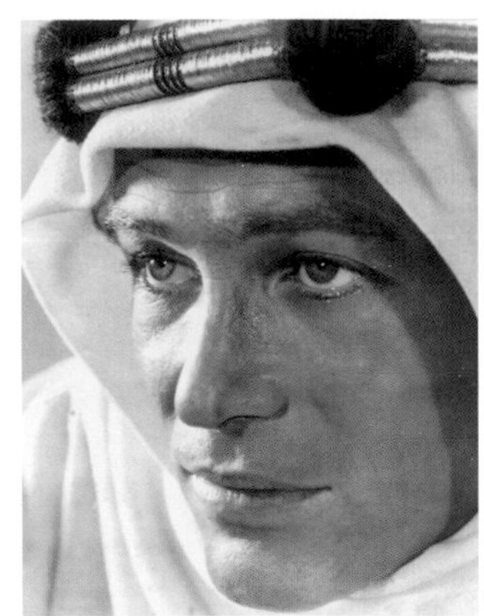

fig. 3

fig. 1

Mars, the Roman god of war, complete with muscular torso and classical profile. © Roger Wood / CORBIS

fig. 2

Egyptian, Greek and Roman culture are of seminal importance to his work, says Christoph Wolfensberger. This photo shows part of a Greek sculpture of a sleeping hermaphrodite. © Araldo de Luca / CORBIS

fig. 3

Christoph Wolfensberger ascribes an expressive beauty to Peter O'Toole. Here, the British actor is pictured in his most famous role, Lawrence of Arabia. © picture-alliance

and myself regularly attend concerts and opera performances; we are acquainted with renowned musicians and also host concerts at our home. I also play the piano myself, actually a Bechstein grand, as well as the trumpet — I have a wonderful instrument by Vincent Bach, one of the best trumpet makers in the United States. When I play music, I can relax and find new inspiration.

4. WHAT IS YOUR CONCEPT OF BEAUTY?

To me, beauty is an experience of the soul. Because it can appear in countless ways, my notion of beauty always comes back to nature. The best example of this is love. It is one of the marvels of nature that women who are in love radiate so much beauty. I revere this primeval, mystical, mysterious force of female beauty, and it still touches me deeply. Style-focused, purely cosmetic and "virtual" beauty and the commercialised, stereotypical beauty propagated by tabloids and magazines mean nothing to me. In my work, it is very important to maintain a strong link to nature. This ensures the results don't derail into

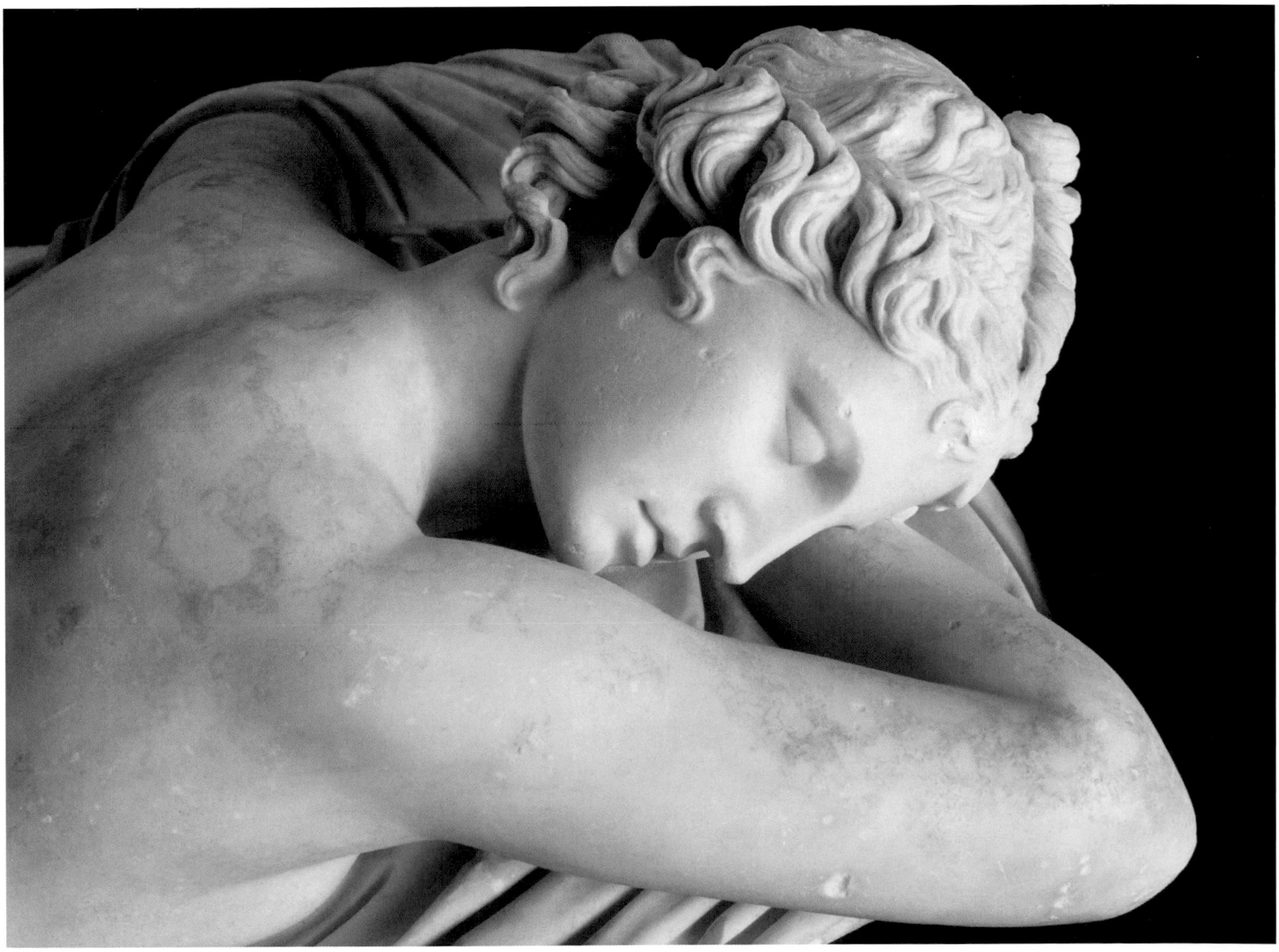

fig. 2

fig. 4

Christoph Wolfensberger (right) as young assistant doctor in the Swiss Alps.
© Private archive Dr. Wolfensberger

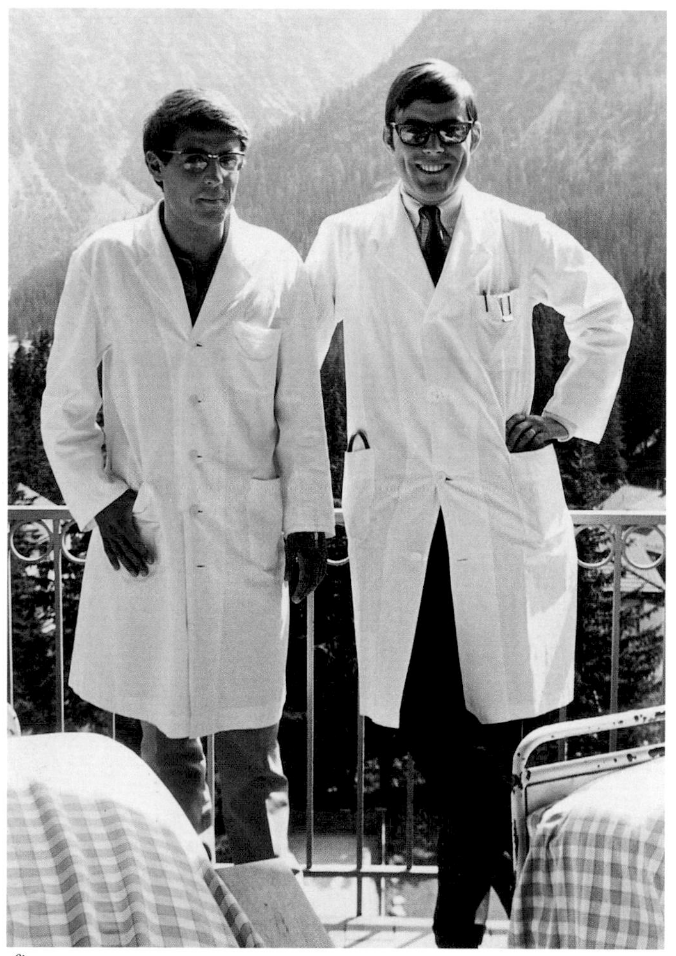

fig. 4

artificiality. Cosmetic surgery is not meant to manipulate — it should only attempt to preserve or restore a person's natural grace.

5. IN ART HISTORY, WHAT IS YOUR FAVOURITE NOTION OF BEAUTY?

As a plastic surgeon, I deal with the harmonies of proportion every day. Essentially, all our insights into these harmonies can be traced back to the Ancient Egyptians, later the Greeks and the Romans, and even later the Renaissance and its timeless art. As the cradle of Western culture, the Mediterranean region and its art are a paramount influence even in my profession.

6. TO YOU, WHO ARE THE MOST BEAUTIFUL WOMAN AND MOST BEAUTIFUL MAN ALIVE?

The most beautiful woman alive in my world is obviously my wife Petra, whom I love and adore. Together with our respect for each other, this adoration has proven to be the most enduring pillar of our 25-year relationship.
If you want me to name film celebrities — with her highly expressive beauty, Sophia Loren has been an idol of mine since my teenage years. Among the male stars, the British actor Peter O'Toole is my ideal of beauty. His "Lawrence of Arabia" was a sensational performance.

14. DO YOU REGARD YOURSELF AS ATTRACTIVE?

I know I have many faults, but nevertheless I have the self-confidence to answer this question with "yes." Why? Well ... I'm tall, slender, dark-haired, an international type of man with Mediterranean blood — sounds like it's straight from the personals! I guess somebody else will need to answer this question. In terms of my work — it is essential to present a healthy ego in the first conversation with the patient so that a foundation of trust is established. All further interaction and work hinges on this.

15. WHAT DOES AGING MEAN TO YOU?

Primarily that it gradually becomes easier to distinguish between the important and less important aspects of life. I can feel it every day how life becomes lighter when unnecessary burdens are jettisoned.

9. ARE YOU AFRAID OF GETTING OLDER?

Yes.

10. HAVE YOU EVER UNDERGONE AESHTETIC SURGERY YOURSELF? IF SO, WHAT WAS IT FOR?

I've had a neck and facelift done — like most men should in their fifties. It just looks neater and makes you feel better.

11. HAVE YOU EVER OPERATED ON YOUR WIFE/PARTNER AND/OR CHILDREN? IF SO, WHY?

fig 5 & 6

Christoph Wolfensberger has performed a facelift on his wife Petra, who also manages his practice. Wolfensberger himself has received a neck lifting. © Private archive Dr. Wolfensberger

fig. 7

In the operating theatre, Christoph Wolfensberger specialises in aesthetic surgery to remodel the face and the body. His holistic approach has inspired him to provide his patients with an Institute for Anti-Aging Medicine and a state-of-the-art day spa. © Private archive Dr. Wolfensberger

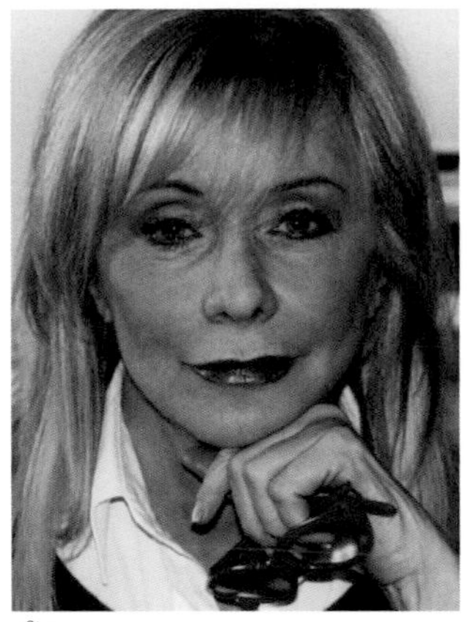

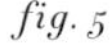

fig. 5

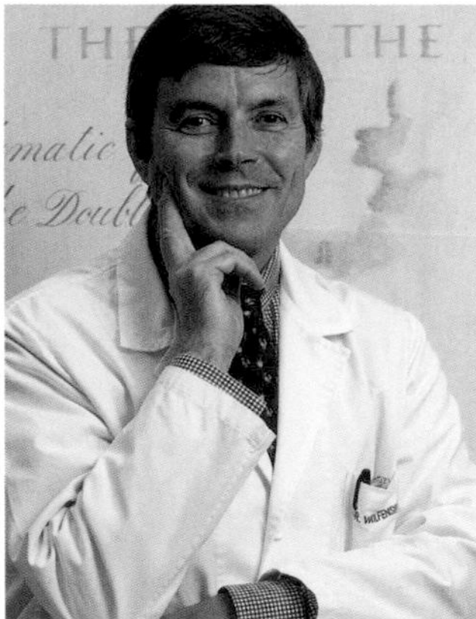

fig. 6

Yes. In January 2000, I did a facelift on my wife Petra. It motivated her greatly. As she is also managing my office, it means that she can give patients advice based on personal experience.

12. CAN YOU JUSTIFY EVERY OPERATION AND PATIENT REQUEST, OR IS THERE A POINT WHEN YOU REFUSE TO DO AN OPERATION?

I regularly decline requests for surgery. For example, a 16-year-old girl from Israel wanted me to do some liposuction on her. Her figure was beautiful, a little voluptuous maybe but not overweight or with much subcutaneous fat. I simply had to say no. She called my office several times to see if I would change my mind, but I had to be firm – I knew she'd regret the operation later.

13. WHAT IS THE MOST UNUSUAL REQUEST FOR SURGERY YOU HAVE ENCOUNTERED IN YOUR CAREER?

One time, a young patient came to an appointment with a Marlboro Cigarettes advertising poster. He wanted to have a nose just like the nose of the cowboy on the poster. I did as he wanted and designed the rhinoplasty around this nose. Although the patient had a different type of face, the reshaped nose fitted perfectly.

I often encourage my patients to bring along pictures of film stars or models and show me exactly what they are imagining. I then try to turn their ideas into reality – of course without ever promising a total match. It makes a lot of sense to integrate these kinds of visual sources into the preoperative plan.

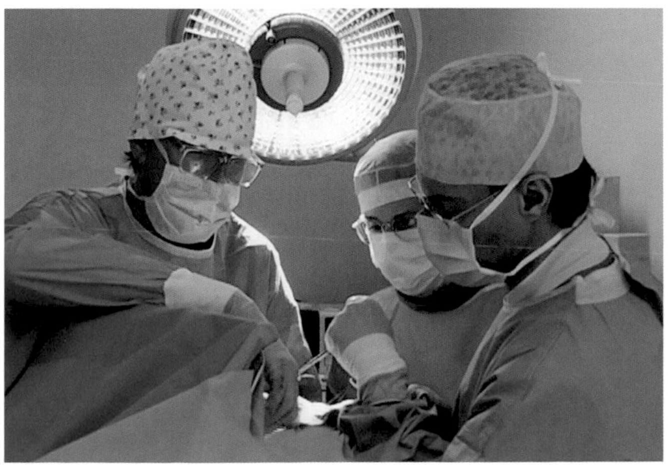

fig. 7

14. WHAT ARE YOUR PATIENTS' REACTIONS FOLLOWING SURGERY?

When patients are pleased with the results, their eyes are much more radiant and their faces more relaxed than before the operation. If their expectations had been causing tension in their faces, it is completely gone after a successful operation. Often, I also hear sentences like "Doctor, you are an artist!" – a compliment I appreciate greatly.

15. COULD YOU NAME SOME OF YOUR MORE WELL-KNOWN PATIENTS?

No. I am fully committed to the utmost discretion. I subscribe to one of the key phrases of Mozart's "Magic Flute" – it's like it was written with cosmetic surgeons in mind: "Be steadfast, patient and discreet."

16. DO YOU BELIEVE THAT BEAUTY LARGELY EMANATES FROM WITHIN?

To me, beauty is always a harmonious balance of the inside and the outside.

17. DO YOU THINK THAT BEAUTIFUL PEOPLE ARE HAPPIER AND LEAD MORE FULFILLED LIVES?

This is often the case, but by no means always. Marilyn Monroe is a tragic example of how beauty can be a burden.

18. DO BEAUTIFUL PEOPLE HAVE BETTER SEX?

No.

19. WHAT DOES THE FUTURE HOLD FOR AESTHETIC SURGERY?

Treatment strategies need to be integrated more productively. The main future concept I can see coming is a healthy lifestyle combined with anti-aging measures, ranging from developments in molecular genetics to the latest innovations of aesthetic surgery. Tissue engineering and stem cell therapy will also be important.

Interview: Eva Karcher, Munich

"As long as mankind has existed, it has worked on its beauty"

JAVIER DE BENITO, Barcelona

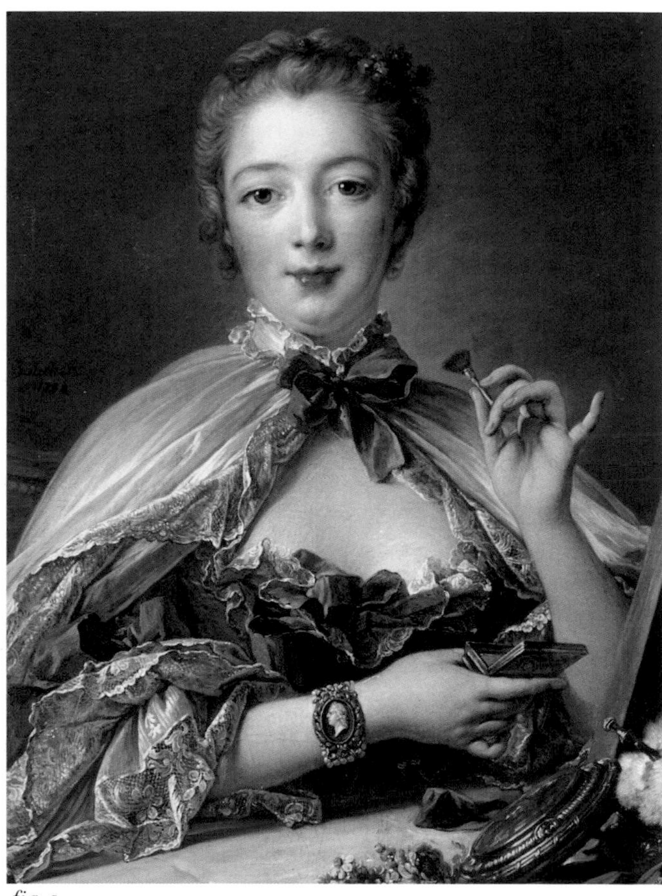
fig. 1

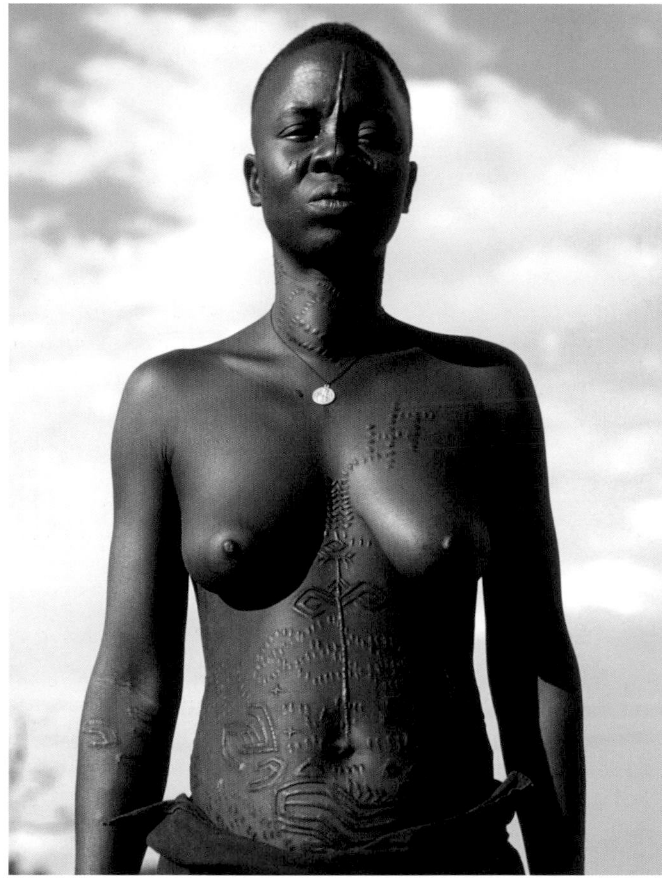
fig. 2

1. WHAT FASCINATES YOU MOST ABOUT BEING AN AESTHETIC SURGEON?

From a very young age, my dream was to become a doctor. I find it satisfying to help people. What fascinates me about my work as a plastic surgeon is that I can endow my patients with a higher quality of life, one they can experience every time they look in the mirror. When they are able to enjoy their appearance, their self-esteem increases and they become more attractive, even seductive. To increase people's overall happiness is the greatest pleasure of my work.

2. WHICH AREAS DO YOU SPECIALISE IN?

Foremostly aesthetic plastic surgery and breast augmentations. I also have extensive experience with endoscopic brow lifting, face and neck lifting, blepharoplasty, which tightens the eyelids, and rhinoplasty, which reshapes the nose.

3. DO YOU REGARD YOURSELF AS AN ARTIST?

Yes. I think that much like an artist, a plastic surgeon needs to have a heightened sensibility for volume, proportions and dimensions. The outcome of an aesthetic surgical procedure is only successful if it is in harmony with the entire body.

4. WHAT IS YOUR CONCEPT OF BEAUTY?

Beauty is something that causes a pleasant sensation when we see or touch it; our tasting, smelling and hearing facul-

fig. 1

In the Rococo period, a powdered white face and skin as delicate as porcelain were considered most attractive. François Boucher (1703–1770) painted this oil portrait, "Madame de Pompadour à sa toilette," in 1758. © akg-images

fig. 2

To a Kuba woman, being beautiful means having as many scars on your face and upper body as possible. The Kuba tribe is based in the Democratic Republic of Kongo. © Otto Lang / CORBIS

fig. 3

In his operations, Javier de Benito concentrates on volume, proportions and dimensions. © Private archive Dr. de Benito

fig. 4 & 5

The Instituto Dr. Javier de Benito is housed in a wing of the Centro Médico Teknon, one of Barcelona's most advanced medical centres. © Private archive Dr. de Benito

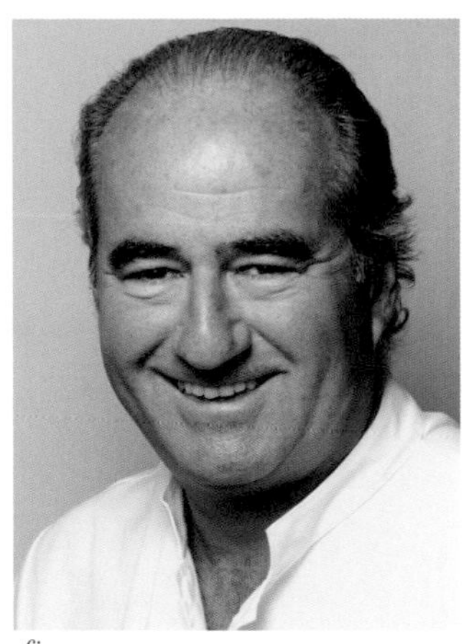

fig. 3

ties may or may not be stimulated. The experience of beauty can be triggered by looking at a painting or a landscape for example, or a face or a body.

5. IN ART HISTORY, WHAT IS YOUR FAVOURITE NOTION OF BEAUTY?

Art history has illustrated that the concept of beauty is an ever-evolving one, depending on time, location and also ethnicity. In the Rococo period, women powdered their faces white and men wore silver-coloured, curly wigs. In Africa, some natives tattoo their bodies with scars, and nomadic tribes artificially enlarge their lips and earlobes. Women in the Western world get silicone injected into their lips. And just like the Masai pierce their noses and tongues with rings and needles, Europeans pierce all kinds of body parts. As long as mankind has existed, it has worked on its beauty — maybe in an effort to forget its mortality …

6. TO YOU, WHO ARE THE MOST BEAUTIFUL WOMAN AND MOST BEAUTIFUL MAN ALIVE?

It's impossible for one single person to encapsulate all the different aspects of human beauty. My personal choice would be to combine the face of Michelle Pfeiffer with the eyes of Kristin Scott Thomas, with the body of Elle McPherson and the legs of Nicole Kidman. This virtual being would be the most beautiful woman in the world to me.

7. DO YOU REGARD YOURSELF AS ATTRACTIVE?

No, I don't think I'm very good-looking. But I'm fairly sophisticated, and I've got plenty of humour. And I've got qualities such as being able to sing and play the guitar. I also much enjoy doing sports. If these characteristics were mixed in a cocktail shaker, the result may well be quite attractive.

8. WHAT DOES AGING MEAN TO YOU?

Aging is a biological process, one where a person ideally becomes more mature, more experienced and more understanding. The person should also develop a greater sense of responsibility and be able to better appreciate the smaller, minor aspects of everyday life. It is very important to anticipate the inevitable process of aging, to prepare for it in advance.

9. ARE YOU AFRAID OF GETTING OLDER?

No. To be honest, I see it as an opportunity to enjoy my life more fully. Of course I will need to maintain the best possible physical condition. At our institute, we have established a department for this very purpose, dedicated exclusively to anti-aging. Thanks to genetic research, we are now able to analyse hereditary factors that influence the aging process. We can then apply specific measures to prevent, delay or altogether avoid weaknesses and ailments.

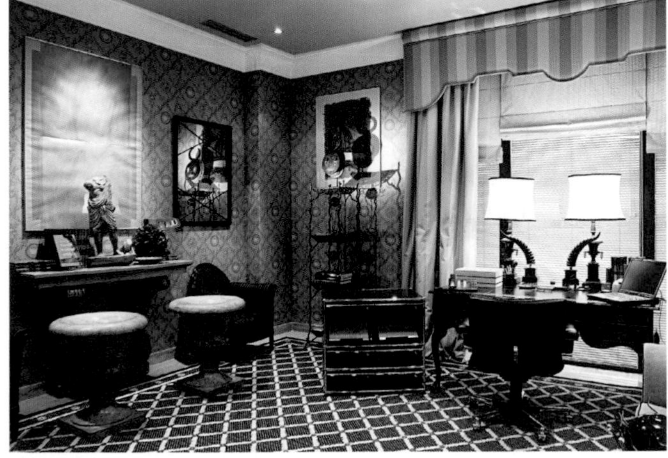

fig. 4

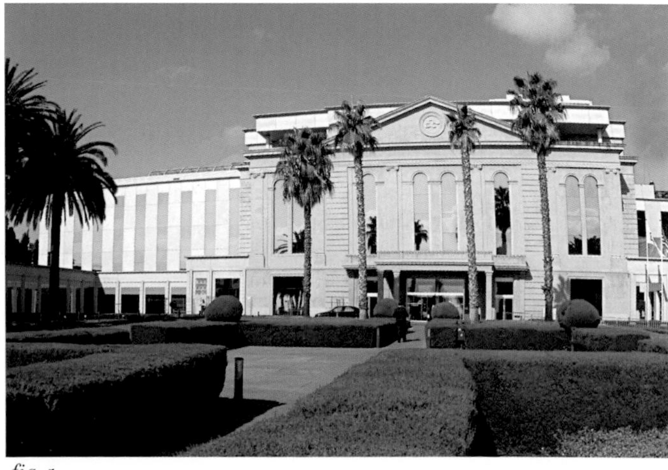

fig. 5

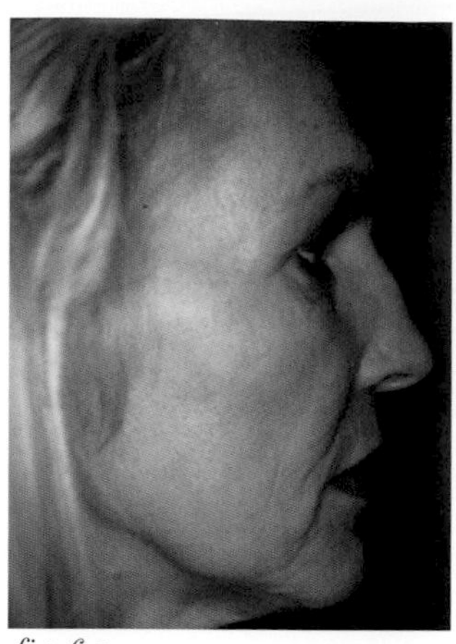

fig. 6 a

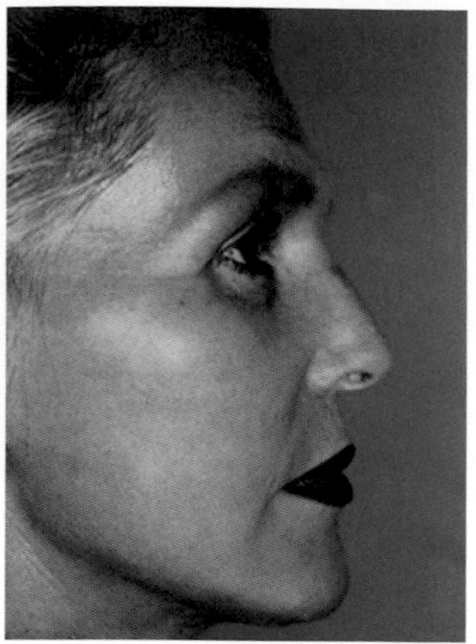

fig. 6 b

fig. 6 a+b

'Before' and 'after' photographs of a patient Javier de Benito performed a facelift on. © Private archive Dr. de Benito

fig. 7 a+b & 8 a+b

These photographs show a female patient before (7 a+b) and after (8 a+b) her buttocks and upper thighs were operated on. © Private archive Dr. de Benito

10. HAVE YOU EVER UNDERGONE AESTHETIC SURGERY YOURSELF? IF SO, WHAT WAS IT FOR?

Yes, I had a hair transplant four years ago. And I think I will get my eyelids worked on one day.

11. HAVE YOU EVER OPERATED ON YOUR WIFE/PARTNER AND/OR CHILDREN? IF SO, WHY?

Both my wife and my daughter have benefited from having a plastic surgeon in the family. I find this perfectly normal.

12. CAN YOU JUSTIFY EVERY OPERATION AND PATIENT REQUEST, OR IS THERE A POINT WHEN YOU REFUSE TO DO AN OPERATION?

No. Some people want the impossible, others want to redefine their personalities and escape reality, and others again want to eradicate flaws that only exist in their imagination. The first interview with the patient is crucial in this respect; as well as arriving at a diagnosis and suggesting a treatment, we also find out what the patient is expecting from the procedure.

13. WHAT IS THE MOST UNUSUAL REQUEST FOR SURGERY YOU HAVE ENCOUNTERED IN YOUR CAREER?

A man once came to me for a nose job. He had already been operated seven times, but none of the surgeons had truly understood what he wanted: to have a nose that looked exactly like the nose of Princess Caroline of Monaco!

14. WHAT ARE YOUR PATIENTS' REACTIONS FOLLOWING SURGERY?

When they look into the mirror a few days after the operation, their reaction is usually quite positive. Sometimes they are a little apprehensive when they realise that their appearance has changed. Ultimately, their reactions depend on how well they understood the information they were given before the operation.

15. COULD YOU NAME SOME OF YOUR MORE WELL-KNOWN PATIENTS?

Certainly not. The vow of Hippocrate includes the vow of secrecy – this is essential to the medical profession. I can only tell you what kinds of celebrities have been treated at our institute: actors, film and TV stars, politicians and famous sporting personalities.

16. DO YOU BELIEVE THAT BEAUTY LARGELY EMANATES FROM WITHIN?

There is an old saying claiming that "beauty is the mirror of the soul," but I don't believe it to be true. A person can be beautiful and at the same time depressed or even psychopathic. If somebody on the other hand is happy and feels good, this will be clearly reflected by the stance and energy displayed. The greatest state of happiness would therefore be reached when beauty and well-being converge.

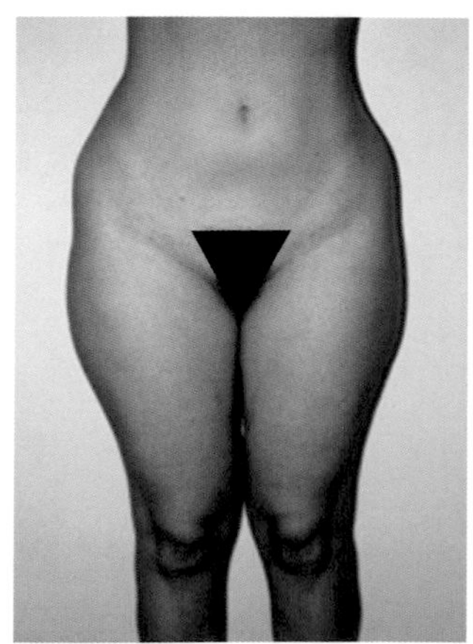

fig. 7 a

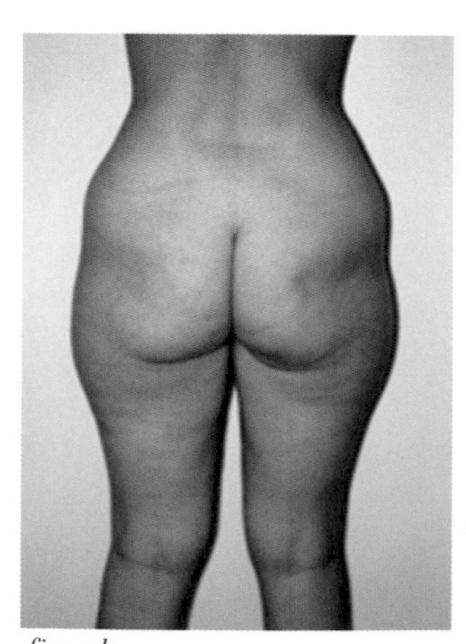

fig. 7 b

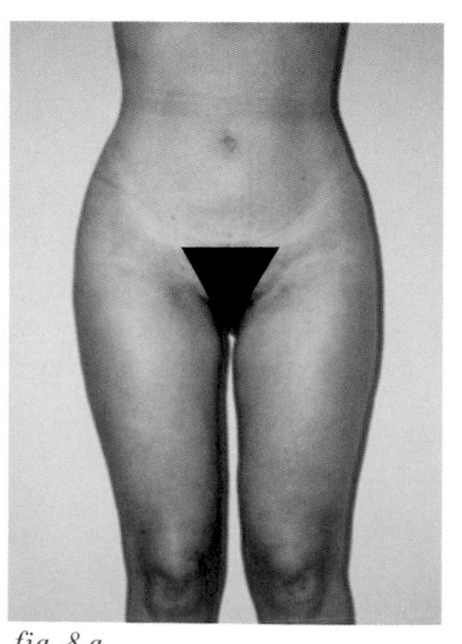

fig. 8 a

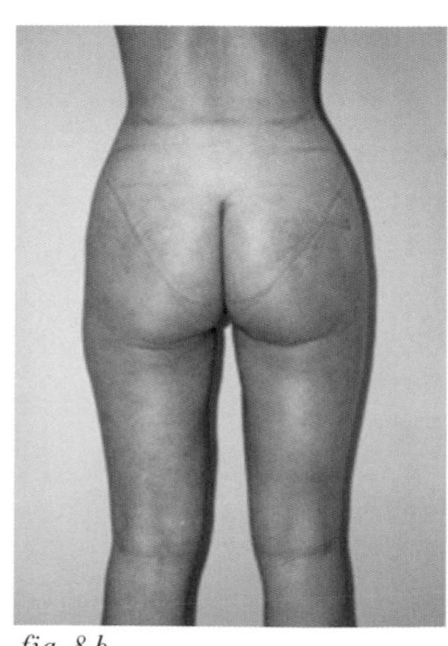

fig. 8 b

fig. 9 a–c & 10 a–c

This patient wanted the contours of her almost boyish body to be rounded – silicon implants have made it possible.

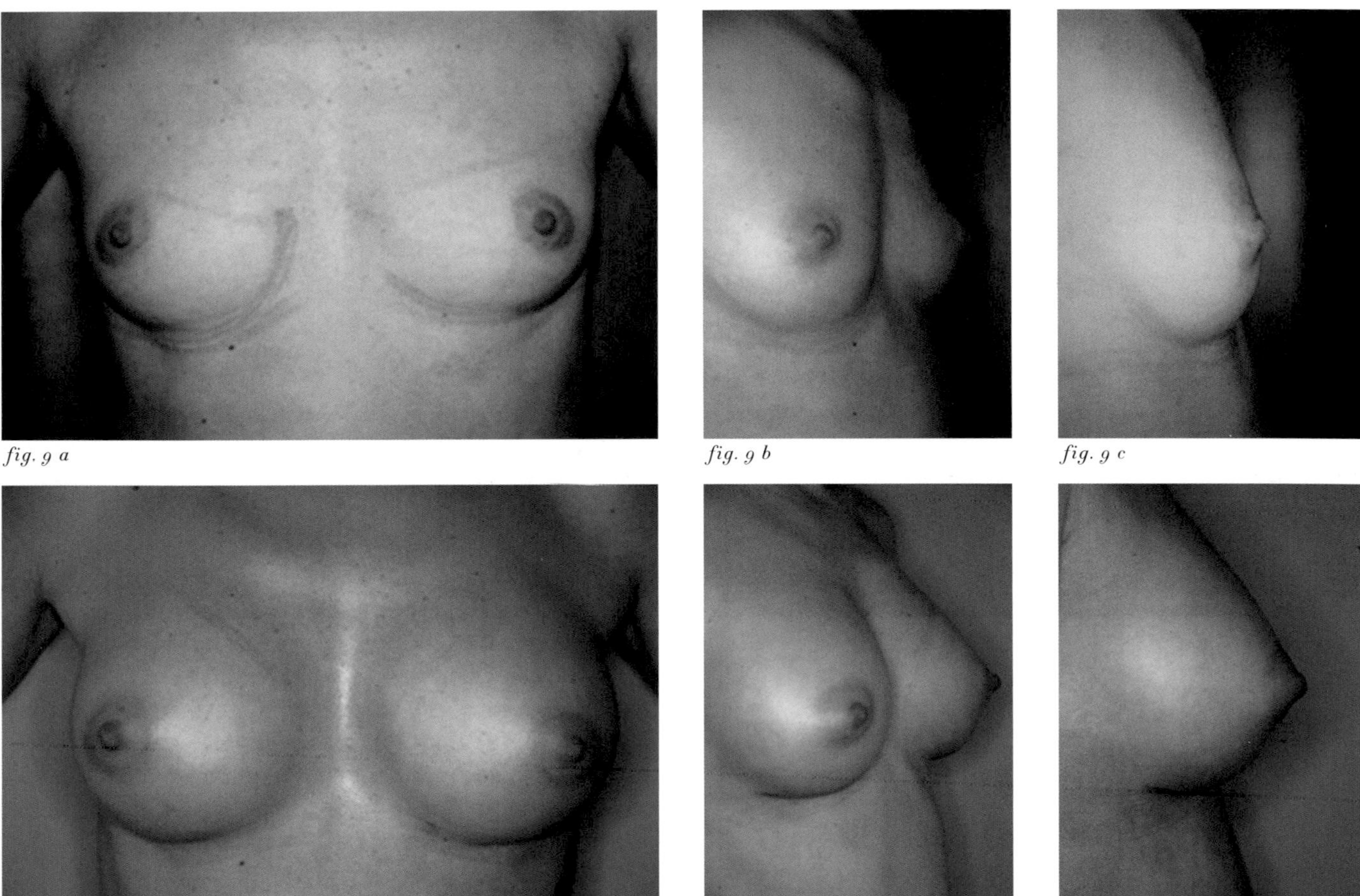

fig. 9 a *fig. 9 b* *fig. 9 c*

fig. 10 a *fig. 10 b* *fig. 10 c*

17. DO YOU THINK THAT BEAUTIFUL PEOPLE ARE HAPPIER AND LEAD MORE FULFILLED LIVES?

Already in the age of classical Antiquity, Socrates noted that beauty was the best letter of recommendation. This suggests that a good-looking person has an advantage when applying for jobs etc., and finds it easier to gain access to many kinds of events than an ugly person would. Lasting success and happiness, however, depend on other qualities and values.

18. DO BEAUTIFUL PEOPLE HAVE BETTER SEX?

See previous answer.

19. WHAT DOES THE FUTURE HOLD FOR AESTHETIC SURGERY?

I believe plastic surgery has a great future ahead of it, especially now that genetic research has opened the doors to a longer life. As our life expectancy is growing, we shouldn't only prepare our organism for a longer lifespan — our appearance should also match our vitality.

Interview: Eva Karcher, Munich

"I see a global trend towards cosmetic surgery"

ISMAIL KURAN, Istanbul

1. WHAT FASCINATES YOU MOST ABOUT BEING AN AESTHETIC SURGEON?

Our work is never based on routine. Every patient is a highly complex individual, a new challenge. Also, we get to operate patients who are usually very happy after surgery.

2. WHICH AREAS DO YOU SPECIALISE IN?

Nasal corrections, breast enlargements and reductions, liposuction. Liposuction is becoming more and more popular, with men as with women. I also perform reconstructive surgery. An interesting fact on the side — in Turkey, facelifts are not as much in demand as they are in Germany. This is because the skin of Turkish men and women is thicker and not as delicate as the skin of fair-haired Europeans; it doesn't age as quickly.

3. DO YOU REGARD YOURSELF AS AN ARTIST?

Yes. Plastic surgery is a combination of art and medicine. You cannot perform it without having some artistic sensibilities. You will find a great many amateur painters and sculptors in our profession.

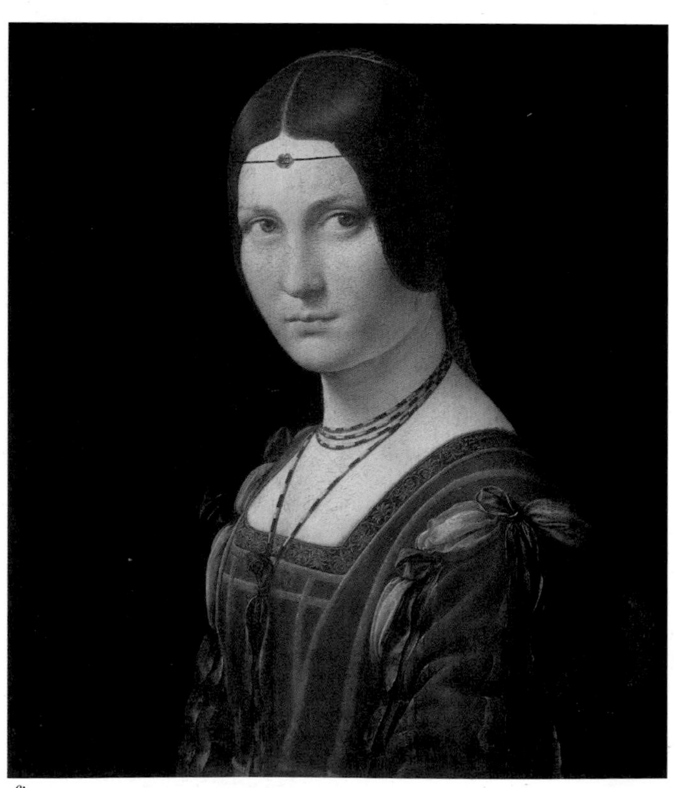

fig. 1

4. WHAT IS YOUR CONCEPT OF BEAUTY?

I like the look cultivated in the 1930s and 1940s. But in my opinion, beauty must always be accompanied by sensitivity. Without a pair of caring eyes, a perfect body means nothing to me.

5. IN ART HISTORY, WHAT IS YOUR FAVOURITE NOTION OF BEAUTY?

I admire the artists of the Renaissance, like Michelangelo and Leonardo da Vinci; they produced works that exhibit ideal proportions as well as an enormous expressivity.

6. TO YOU, WHO ARE THE MOST BEAUTIFUL WOMAN AND MOST BEAUTIFUL MAN ALIVE?

For me, there is no such thing as the single most beautiful woman or man. To me, it is more interesting to look at the differences in beauty, for example between the American and European ideas of beauty. American women want everything to be bigger, bigger breasts, bigger cheekbones. European women, on the other hand, want to look as natural as possible – as do Turkish women. I definitely advocate the European aesthetic.

7. DO YOU REGARD YOURSELF AS ATTRACTIVE?

Sometimes. Especially when an operation was successful and the patient is literally rejoicing. In their gratitude, the patients sometimes worship their surgeon as if he were some kind of god. Obviously, that's good for the ego.

8. WHAT DOES AGING MEAN TO YOU?

I can mainly see benefits. I now look at the world from a lighter perspective; I am more mature, and enjoy the small things in life more – smells, voices, nature.

9. ARE YOU AFRAID OF GETTING OLDER?

I'm only afraid of getting into a situation where I need to rely on other people. A slight feeling of panic stirs in me at the idea of this happening.

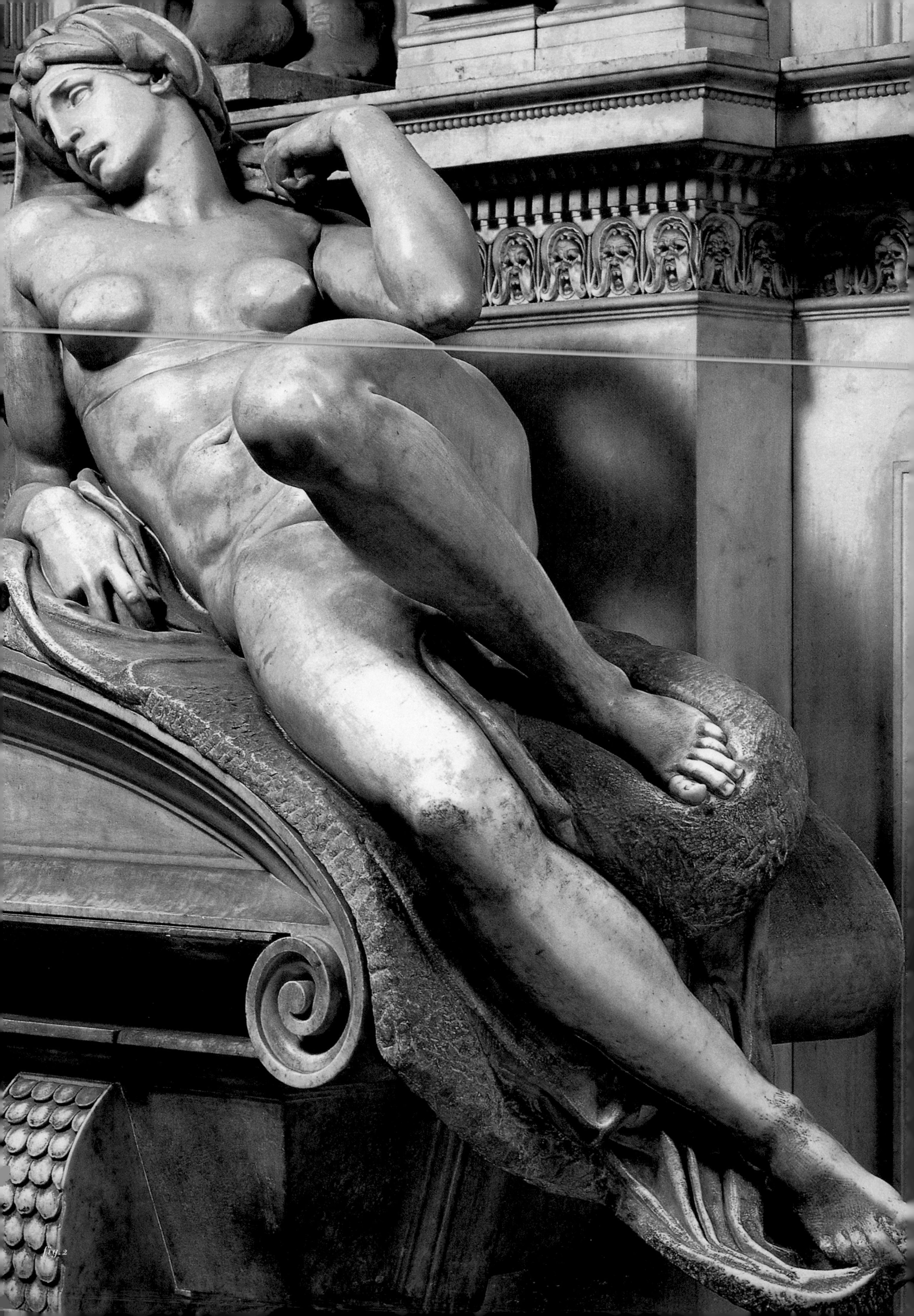

fig. 2

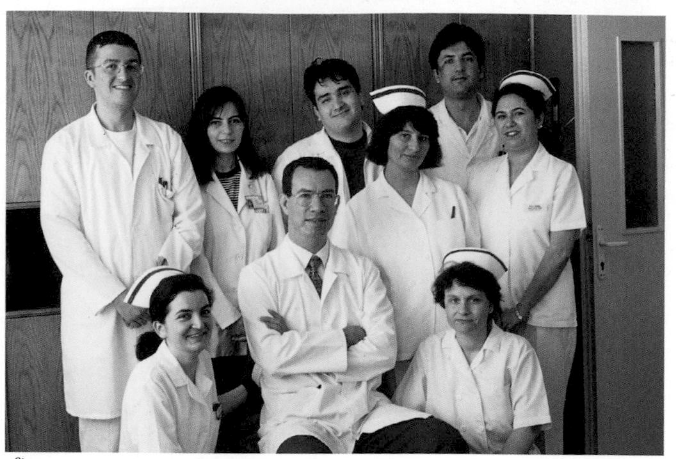

fig. 3

fig. 1

Ismail Kuran appreciates the idealised proportions of Renaissance art. This "Portrait d'une inconnue" (around 1490) is of unknown origin – art experts are still unsure if it was painted by Leonardo da Vinci (1452–1519). © Paris, Musée du Louvre; Photo: RMN – C. Jean

fig. 2

"The morning sun" by Michelangelo (1475–1564). Today, Ismail Kuran distinguishes between two ideals of beauty: the American ideal, which focuses on size and fullness, and the European one, which aims for a more natural look. Florence, Medicichapel San Lorenzo

fig. 3

Ismail Kuran and his team of professionals in Istanbul. They report that demand for aesthetic surgery in Turkey is growing steadily in all sectors of society and across all religious divides, despite the fact that some denominations prohibit cosmetic procedures. © Private archive Dr. Kuran

fig. 4

Michelangelo painted strong, muscular bodies. Modern Turkish patients prefer slender contours – liposuction is their procedure of choice. Facelifts, on the other hand, are much less popular than in Germany, for example, as most Turkish people's skin is tougher and ages less rapidly. © Rome, Photo Vatican Museums

10. HAVE YOU EVER UNDERGONE AESTHETIC SURGERY YOURSELF? IF SO, WHAT WAS IT FOR?

Not yet. I don't really have the time for it. If I did, I would probably get my skin worked on.

11. HAVE YOU EVER OPERATED ON YOUR WIFE/PARTNER AND/OR CHILDREN? IF SO, WHY?

I have operated on benign skin problems for my wife and children. For my aunts and daughter-in-law, I have done liposuction, and I've also given them facelifts.

12. CAN YOU JUSTIFY EVERY OPERATION AND PATIENT REQUEST, OR IS THERE A POINT WHEN YOU REFUSE TO DO AN OPERATION?

If people have unrealistic expectations, for example if they want to look like an existing film star, I decline to work on them. If they are unsure of what they want, I also refuse.

13. WHAT IS THE MOST UNUSUAL REQUEST FOR SURGERY YOU HAVE ENCOUNTERED IN YOUR CAREER?

The most extreme operation I have performed was on a patient who had highly asymmetrical breasts. It was very difficult to correct this imbalance.

14. WHAT ARE YOUR PATIENTS' REACTIONS FOLLOWING SURGERY?

Generally, they are grateful and pleased. The preoperative talks I have with them are so detailed that misunderstandings and surprises are avoided as much as possible.

15. COULD YOU NAME SOME OF YOUR MORE WELL-KNOWN PATIENTS?

No. But I can tell you what areas our patients come from. Most of them are from Turkey, but we are increasingly also getting Turkish people who live in Germany, as well as Germans and Scandinavians. One of the reasons for this may well be that operations are more affordable in Turkey.

16. DO YOU BELIEVE THAT BEAUTY LARGELY EMANATES FROM WITHIN?

Beauty is a combination of interior and exterior characteristics. I notice this especially when performing reconstructive surgery. After a successful operation on a patient with a birth defect or malformation caused by disease, the person not only gains an improved appearance but also looks much more radiant – as if given a new lease on life.

17. DO YOU THINK THAT BEAUTIFUL PEOPLE ARE HAPPIER AND LEAD MORE FULFILLED LIVES?

Yes. They can accept their body more easily, which gives them greater inner harmony. Their life is more enjoyable and carefree. Of course, an operation cannot guarantee happiness.

18. DO BEAUTIFUL PEOPLE HAVE BETTER SEX?

Yes, I believe they do. A person's libido also relies on their self-esteem. A confident person has more fun with everything, including sex.

19. WHAT DOES THE FUTURE HOLD FOR AESTHETIC SURGERY?

In Turkey, the number of patients is growing daily. Aesthetic surgery is no longer restricted to the upper class; today's clients come from all walks of life. More interestingly, they also come from all kinds of religions – even though some of the denominations do not permit them to have these kinds of operations. Hair transplants, rhinoplasty and body-contouring liposuction are the most popular procedures. I see a global trend towards aesthetic surgery. The most important aspect with this is that patients are always informed correctly about the procedures, and that they aren't lured in by larger-than-life promises that will only end in disappointment. Non-invasive techniques will become increasingly important, such as injections with Botox and fillers such as Restylane and Perlane for the lips and nasolabial creases, for example. However, these are only effective for around eight months. Autologous fat works better and lasts longer, and it can also be preserved and reused at a later date. We are increasingly combining surgical and non-invasive procedures – this is one of the great opportunities for aesthetic surgery in the future.

Interview: Eva Karcher, Munich

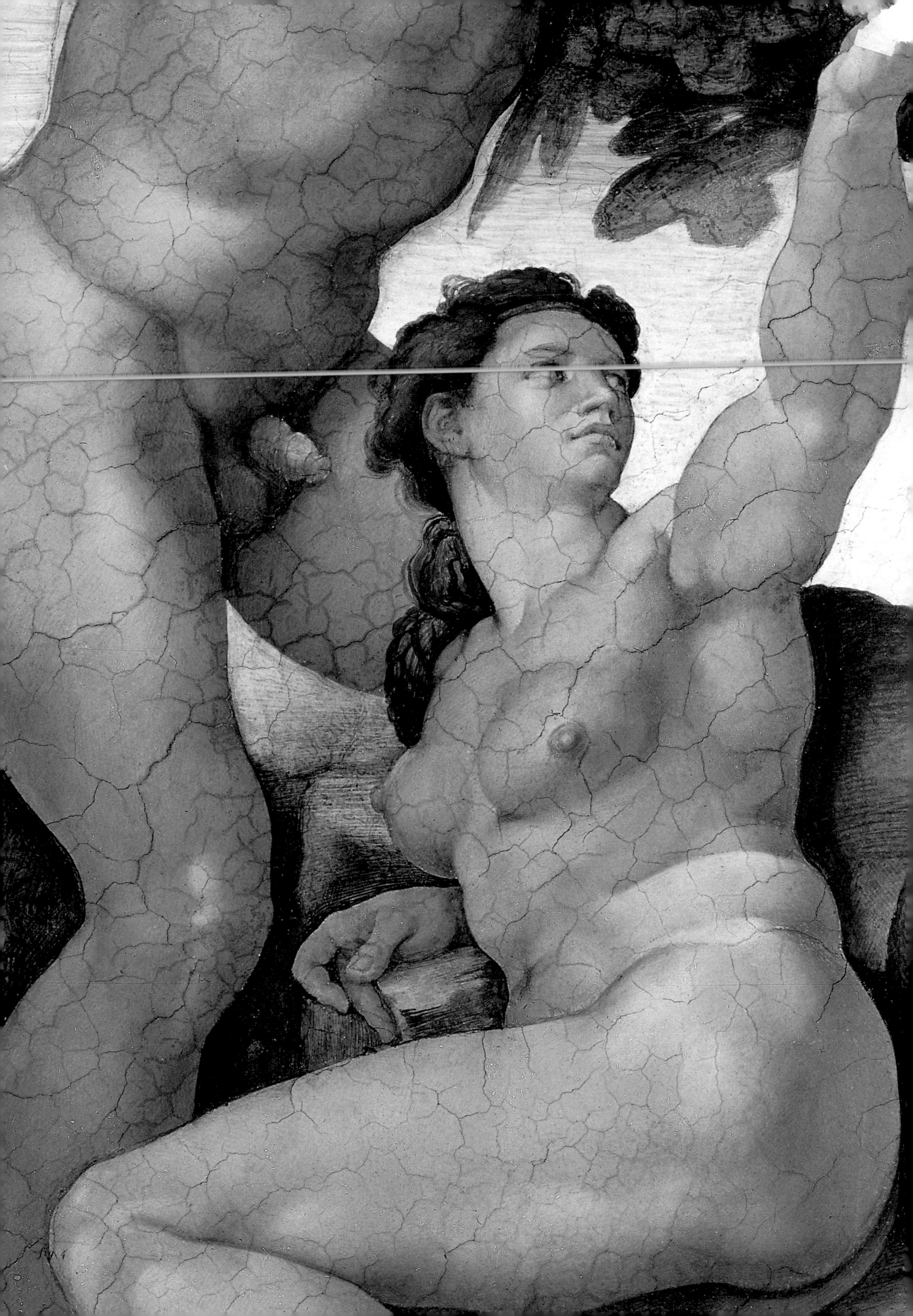

"One can be beautiful at any age"

ALAA EL DIN GHEITA, Cairo

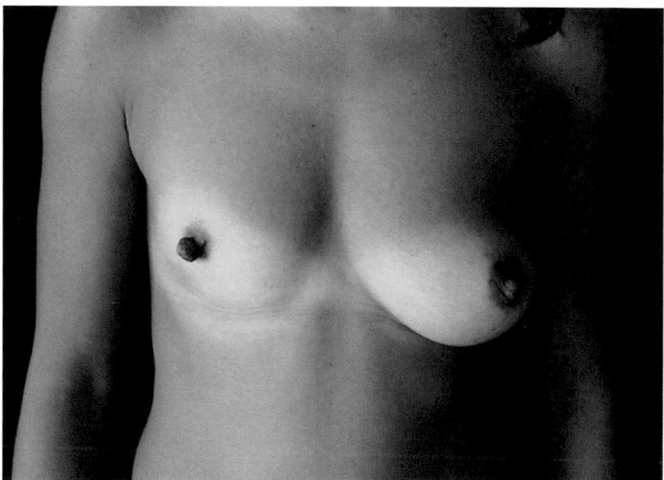

fig. 1 a

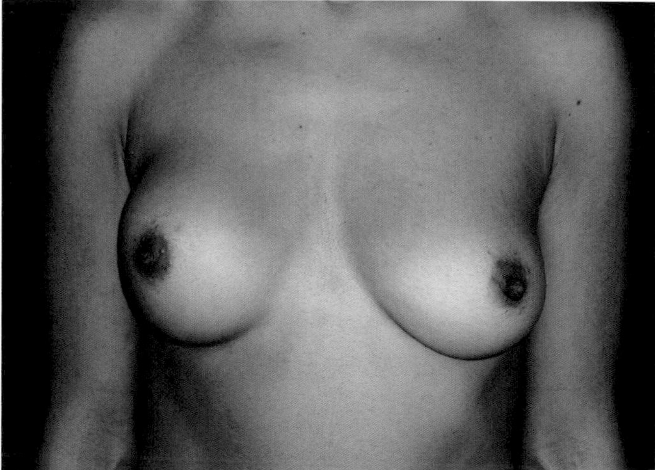

fig. 1 b

1. WHAT FASCINATES YOU MOST ABOUT BEING AN AESTHETIC SURGEON?

I love beauty in all its guises. In the arts, in sports, in fashion. There are 11,000 plastic surgeons in the world, possibly more. To be good, you need excellent training – but also creativity and discerning taste. The complexity of this mix fascinates me the most about my profession.

2. WHICH AREAS DO YOU SPECIALISE IN?

Face and neck lifting. The neck is an integral part of most facelifts. I also specialise in eyelid surgery and breast enlargements and reductions. For non-invasive methods, I reject synthetic fillers and therefore only use autologous fat; this is injected not under the skin, but into the muscle tissue. The lips are the most difficult to shape, and I avoid injections as much as possible.

3. DO YOU REGARD YOURSELF AS AN ARTIST?

Yes. I create, and I have a good eye for the nuances of form and proportion.

4. WHAT IS YOUR CONCEPT OF BEAUTY?

To me, ideal beauty is a sum of three components: the look of the face, the shape of the body and the spirit of the person. In women, I love the harmony that exists between a beautiful face and a beautiful body. It is rare to encounter both at the same time, and even rarer to see beauty coupled with spirit.

5. IN ART HISTORY, WHAT IS YOUR FAVOURITE NOTION OF BEAUTY?

I admire the works of Michelangelo the most.

6. TO YOU, WHO ARE THE MOST BEAUTIFUL WOMAN AND MOST BEAUTIFUL MAN ALIVE?

If we're talking about film stars, there are plenty of beautiful, attractive actresses at the moment, ranging from Catherine Zeta-Jones to Nicole Kidman. Of the male stars, I admire Richard Gere for his looks and Jack Nicholson for his outstanding talent as an actor.

7. DO YOU REGARD YOURSELF AS ATTRACTIVE?

I see myself as normal. I think I have a rather large nose. But many women, as well as men, tell me I'm attractive.

8. WHAT DOES AGING MEAN TO YOU?

Nobody wants to age, let alone die. But everybody knows that both are inevitable. We need to be realistic about this and prepare for our old age. When I was 30, I wanted to be together with a 22-year-old. Now that I'm 57, I prefer a woman who is the same age as me, or no more than 10–15 years younger. She would be able to understand me better

fig. 1 a+b

Right breast congenital hypoplasia. The same patient six months following the implant to achieve symmetry with the opposite breast. © Private archive Dr. Gheita

fig. 2

Alaa El Din Gheita has, apart from a Botox injection into his brow, declined to have any cosmetic surgery performed on his own body. © Private archive Dr. Gheita

fig. 3 & 4

In the eyes of Alaa El Din Gheita, Nicole Kidman has "that certain something." The surgeon also regards Jack Nicholson as beautiful – not for his looks but his outstanding on-screen presence. © Getty Images (4), picture-alliance (3)

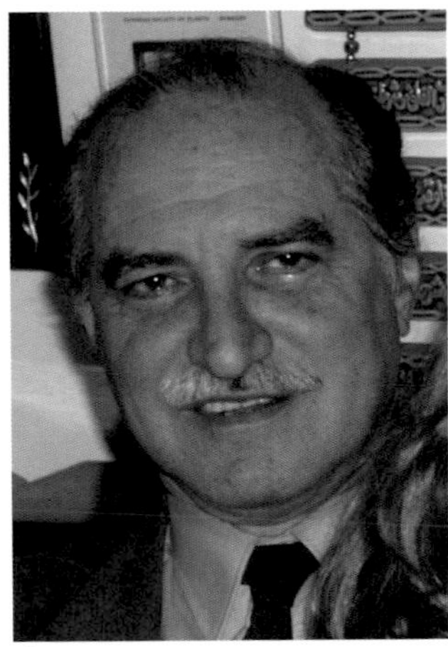

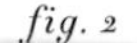

fig. 2

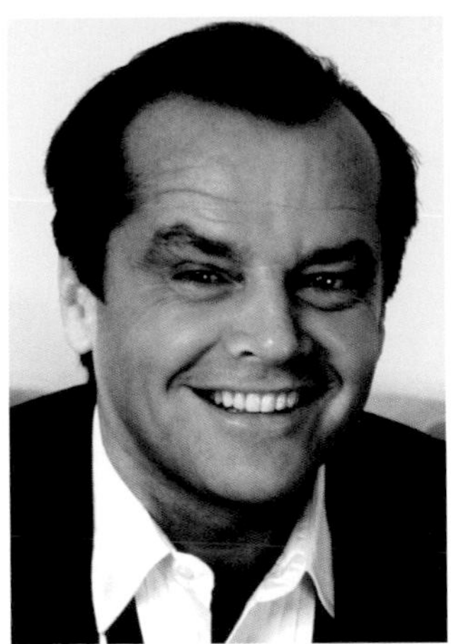

fig. 3

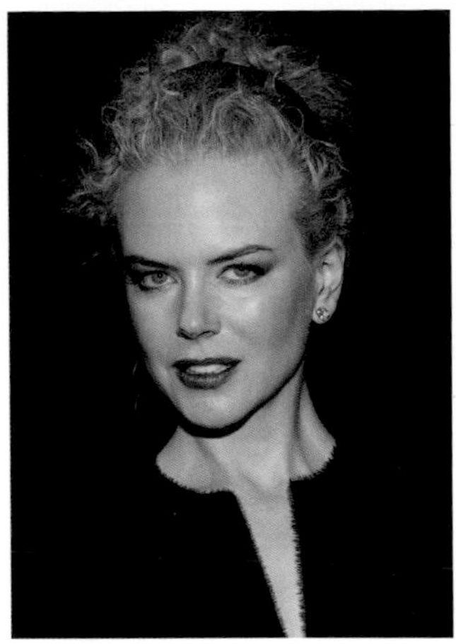

fig. 4

and share my pace of life. I like the classical elegance of women who have arrived at a certain level of maturity. Women with a loud dress sense don't excite me very much anymore. You can be beautiful as well as elegant, at any age in your life.

9. ARE YOU AFRAID OF GETTING OLDER?

No, because I seem to be enjoying life more intensely the older I get. Apart from that, I have two little children who keep me on my toes.

10. HAVE YOU EVER UNDERGONE AESTHETIC SURGERY YOURSELF? IF SO, WHAT WAS IT FOR?

One and a half years ago, I injected Botox into my brow to see how painful it is and how long the effects last. I haven't done anything else, nor have I repeated this procedure. Still, the creases have never been as deep again.

11. HAVE YOU EVER OPERATED ON YOUR WIFE/PARTNER AND/OR CHILDREN? IF SO, WHY?

Yes, I have operated on my wife. I won't tell you where.

12. CAN YOU JUSTIFY EVERY OPERATION AND PATIENT REQUEST, OR IS THERE A POINT WHEN YOU REFUSE TO DO AN OPERATION?

I refuse to do approximately ten percent of the procedures requested, either because they are unrealistic or because the people wanting them are psychologically unstable.

13. WHAT IS THE MOST UNUSUAL REQUEST FOR SURGERY YOU HAVE ENCOUNTERED IN YOUR CAREER?

I regularly operate on children with monstrously malformed faces, for example where the eyes are positioned very oddly. This is a type of reconstructive surgery that couldn't be more extreme.
One of the most demanding aesthetic operations I have performed was on an elderly female patient; despite her age, she was still very attractive. It was a great challenge to restore her exquisite former beauty to her.

14. WHAT ARE YOUR PATIENTS' REACTIONS FOLLOWING SURGERY?

They are usually very pleased, because both parties have kept their side of the agreement. My patients often present me with gifts as a sign of their gratitude. Sometimes, a lasting friendship ensues.

15. COULD YOU NAME SOME OF YOUR MORE WELL-KNOWN PATIENTS?

I have many prominent female patients from the Arab world, well-known actresses for example. But I maintain full discretion for all of my patients, not just the famous ones.

16. DO YOU BELIEVE THAT BEAUTY LARGELY EMANATES FROM WITHIN?

This is essentially a philosophical question. Personally, I believe that a person's inside is responsible for a large part of their beauty. It doesn't create beautiful facial features, but it defines the expression and character of the face.

17. DO YOU THINK THAT BEAUTIFUL PEOPLE ARE HAPPIER AND LEAD MORE FULFILLED LIVES?

No, but beauty can enhance a person's quality of life.

18. DO BEAUTIFUL PEOPLE HAVE BETTER SEX?

No. Why should they? Even if you are very beautiful, it may well be that you are not really sexy at all.

19. WHAT DOES THE FUTURE HOLD FOR AESTHETIC SURGERY?

Aesthetic surgery has only existed for 80 years, so we are still at the beginning. Genetics will contribute significantly to the future of plastic surgery, for example the research conducted into genes that are responsible for the growth of the nose or the shape of the breasts. New and improved types of lasers will also be developed, as well as new injection fillers to better remodel body contours. Surgery will become less and less invasive because we will use new lasers that don't cut the skin. Computers will also become more important in operations. The end of aesthetic surgery will only be reached when we have discovered the aging gene. But that will take some time yet.

Interview: Eva Karcher, Munich

"People's beauty comes from their aura, not their muscle power"

ALI AL-NUMAIRY, Dubai

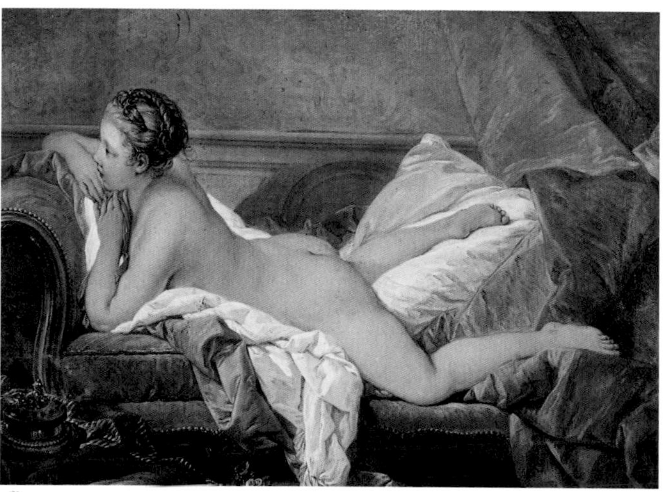

fig.1

1. WHAT FASCINATES YOU MOST ABOUT BEING AN AESTHETIC SURGEON?

The human body is nature's crowning achievement. To be able to work on it is a deeply satisfying joy. An aesthetic surgeon has the unique opportunity of improving the human body as well as making his patients happy. To me, the magnificence of God manifests itself in the beauty of existence. The longer I work in my profession, the more I believe in and love God.

2. WHICH AREAS DO YOU SPECIALISE IN?

I have been working in the field of reconstructive surgery for over 20 years, but my main interest lies in plastic and cosmetic surgery. I specialise in body contouring and lifting as much as I do in breast operation, nose jobs, eyelid surgery, non-invasive injection procedures and surgical laser treatments.

3. DO YOU REGARD YOURSELF AS AN ARTIST?

Yes. Plastic surgery is two thirds science and one-third artistic talent. Aesthetic surgery on the other hand, is two thirds creativity and one third science. A true work of art is but a shadow of divine perfection and we work on getting the perfection with artistic creativity and surgical knowledge.

4. WHAT IS YOUR CONCEPT OF BEAUTY?

In addition to complete harmony and symmetry, which are the universally accepted conditions of beauty, I regard beauty as a spiritual energy rather than a set of measurable proportions. Ideal beauty is a combination of physical attractiveness and the intellectual capacity. Spiritual beauty is the balancing act between seemingly disparate worlds. An erotic tapestry of spirituality over physical and mental harmony is beauty for me.

5. IN ART HISTORY, WHAT IS YOUR FAVOURITE NOTION OF BEAUTY?

As an Arab from the Eastern Arab Peninsula, I look back on a cultural heritage of 8000 years. I believe that past civilizations had ideals of beauty that are still valid today — especially if we place them in the context of contemporary concepts. The woman of Ur, Queen Shabaad of Mesopotamia, or a nude woman from Al-Hadr or a Francois Boucher nude, for example, will always stimulate our aesthetic sensibilities.

6. TO YOU, WHO ARE THE MOST BEAUTIFUL WOMAN AND MOST BEAUTIFUL MAN ALIVE?

Jennifer Lopez and Alain Delon.

7. DO YOU REGARD YOURSELF AS ATTRACTIVE?

Yes — I'm tall, I have an athletic body, I'm educated, I love aesthetics and music, I love riding motorbikes as well as driving fast cars, shooting, painting, flying. I also enjoy hunting and archery.

8. WHAT DOES AGING MEAN TO YOU?

Age is a matter of feeling, not of years. Over the years, men as well as women change physically and psychologically. When we're 50, we simply cannot look like 20. However, we can do a lot to preserve our vitality and vivacity. In my work I help slow down the inevitable loss of youthful elasticity.

9. ARE YOU AFRAID OF GETTING OLDER?

Youth is a gift of nature, but age is a work of art. As we cannot halt the aging process, we should attempt to lead our

fig. 1

To Ali Al-Numairy, the beauty ideals of past ages will always retain their validity – as exemplified by the paintings of François Boucher (1703–1770). Reproduced here is "Girl Resting" (1752). © Munich, Bayerische Staatsgemäldesammlungen Alte Pinakothek

fig. 2

Ali Al-Numairy regards himself as a doctor and an artist. "Aesthetic surgery is two thirds creativity and one third science," he claims. © Private archive Dr. Al-Numairy

fig. 3 & 4

Dr. Al-Numairy's private villa in Dubai. © Private archive Dr. Al-Numairy

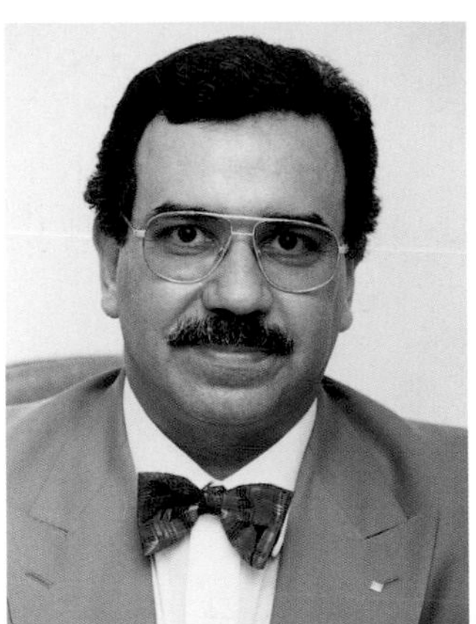

fig. 2

lives in accordance with our age. We will then be able to fully enjoy every stage of our lives. The older the fiddler, the sweeter the tune.

10. HAVE YOU EVER UNDERGONE AESTHETIC SURGERY YOURSELF? IF SO, WHAT WAS IT FOR?

No.

11. HAVE YOU EVER OPERATED ON YOUR WIFE/PARTNER AND/OR CHILDREN? IF SO, WHY?

My profession forbids me to divulge any details about my patients even if these were members of my family.

12. CAN YOU JUSTIFY EVERY OPERATION AND PATIENT REQUEST, OR IS THERE A POINT WHEN YOU REFUSE TO DO AN OPERATION?

I refuse to operate when I am convinced that the outcome will ultimately make the patient unhappy. Sometimes the patient's wishes are too great a risk to his or her health; sometimes I can tell that the results of the operation would be aesthetically dissatisfying to the patient. I also reject patients if they want to have an operation just to please another person, even if there are no medical objections.

13. WHAT IS THE MOST UNUSUAL REQUEST FOR SURGERY YOU HAVE ENCOUNTERED IN YOUR CAREER?

Once, there was a patient who resembled a very famous Arabic singer. He came to me with a major depression and a wish to commit suicide because of his strong resemblance with that Arabic singer. He said that everybody called him with the singer's name and this was eliminating him from his own existence. He told me that unless I did something drastically different, he could live with, he would commit suicide. First of all I had to do his plastic psychology therapy for two to three weeks to change his approach from negative to positive and then I worked on his face. I removed the chin implant and placed it properly to remove the elongated look of his face, then I injected soft tissue filler to lift his cheeks and also performed blepheroplasty on him and a little touch-up work on his nose was done, too. The outcome was very positive. He no more looked like the singer and did not think about ending his life again.

14. WHAT ARE YOUR PATIENTS' REACTIONS FOLLOWING SURGERY?

Because I explain every surgical detail to my patients, frequently even simulating visual outcomes on a computer screen, they see the possible negative outcome. Initially, I

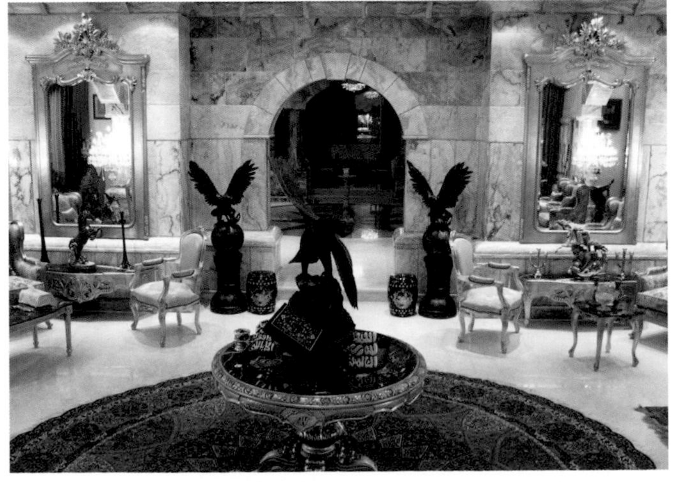

fig. 3

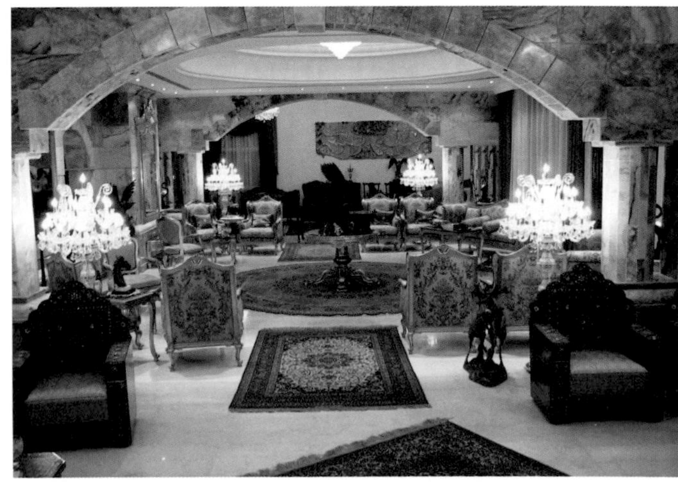

fig. 4

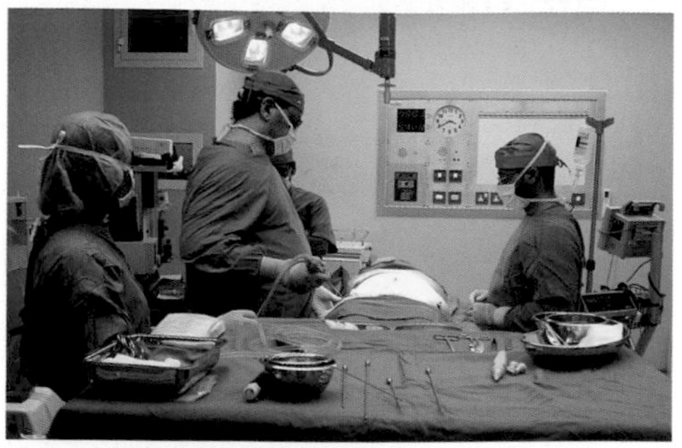

fig. 5

fig. 5

Before an operation, Ali Al-Numairy explains every detail to his patients using digital animations. Because of this thorough preparation, he rarely gets complaints about his work. © Private archive Dr. Al-Numairy

fig. 6 a+b

Body contouring as performed by Ali Al-Numairy. © Private archive Dr. Al-Numairy

fig. 7

A classical beauty: This female torso of Nefertiti is from the period of the 18th dynasty, Ancient Egypt (c. 1350 BC). © akg-images / Erich Lessing

may receive a negative reaction but later it changes. After an operation has succeeded, any initial apprehensiveness and unease soon gives way to palpable relief. Any previously built-up depression is dispelled and the patients' self esteem increases; they display a new-found pride in their enhanced attractiveness.

15. COULD YOU NAME SOME OF YOUR MORE WELL-KNOWN PATIENTS?

For ethical and professional reasons, I never disclose any details about my patients.

16. DO YOU BELIEVE THAT BEAUTY LARGELY EMANATES FROM WITHIN?

Yes, it is a spiritual feeling that permeates the body from within and radiates to the outside. People's beauty comes from their aura, not their muscle power.

17. DO YOU THINK THAT BEAUTIFUL PEOPLE ARE HAPPIER AND LEAD MORE FULFILLED LIVES?

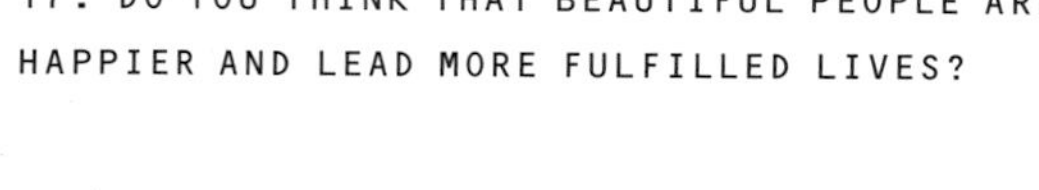

Yes, however, they need to learn to recognize and accept their personal limits.

18. DO BEAUTIFUL PEOPLE HAVE BETTER SEX?

Yes.

19. WHAT DOES THE FUTURE HOLD FOR AESTHETIC SURGERY?

The number of people undergoing cosmetic procedures will continue to rise steadily. The interest displayed by the media will also continue to contribute to this boom. Plastic surgeons themselves will play a crucial role in this global process of popularization, as it is they who develop and refine techniques and discover innovative new methods.

Interview: Eva Karcher, Munich

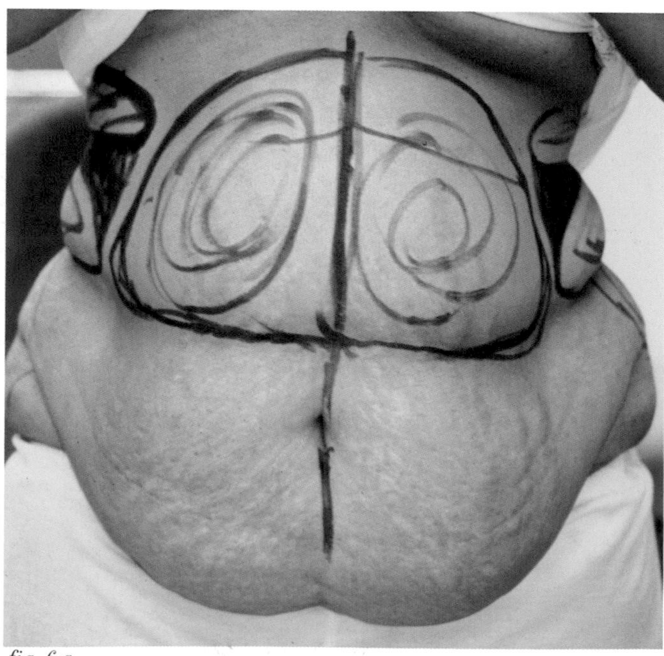

fig. 6 a

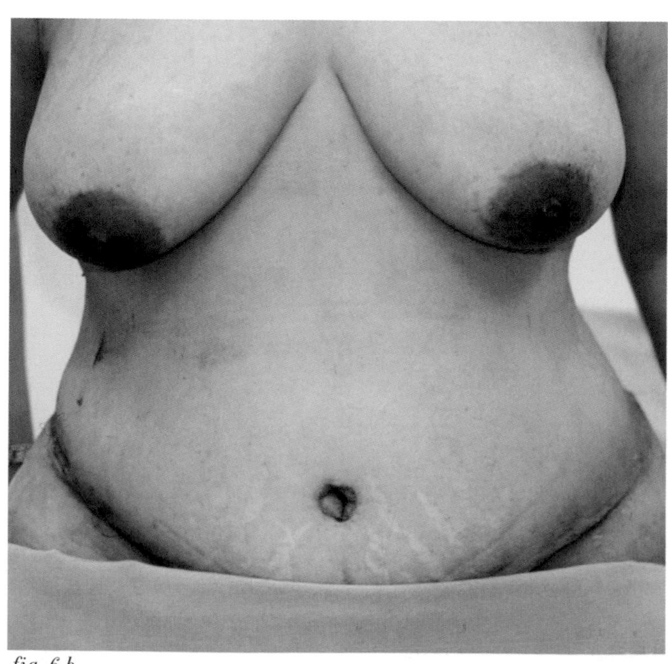

fig. 6 b

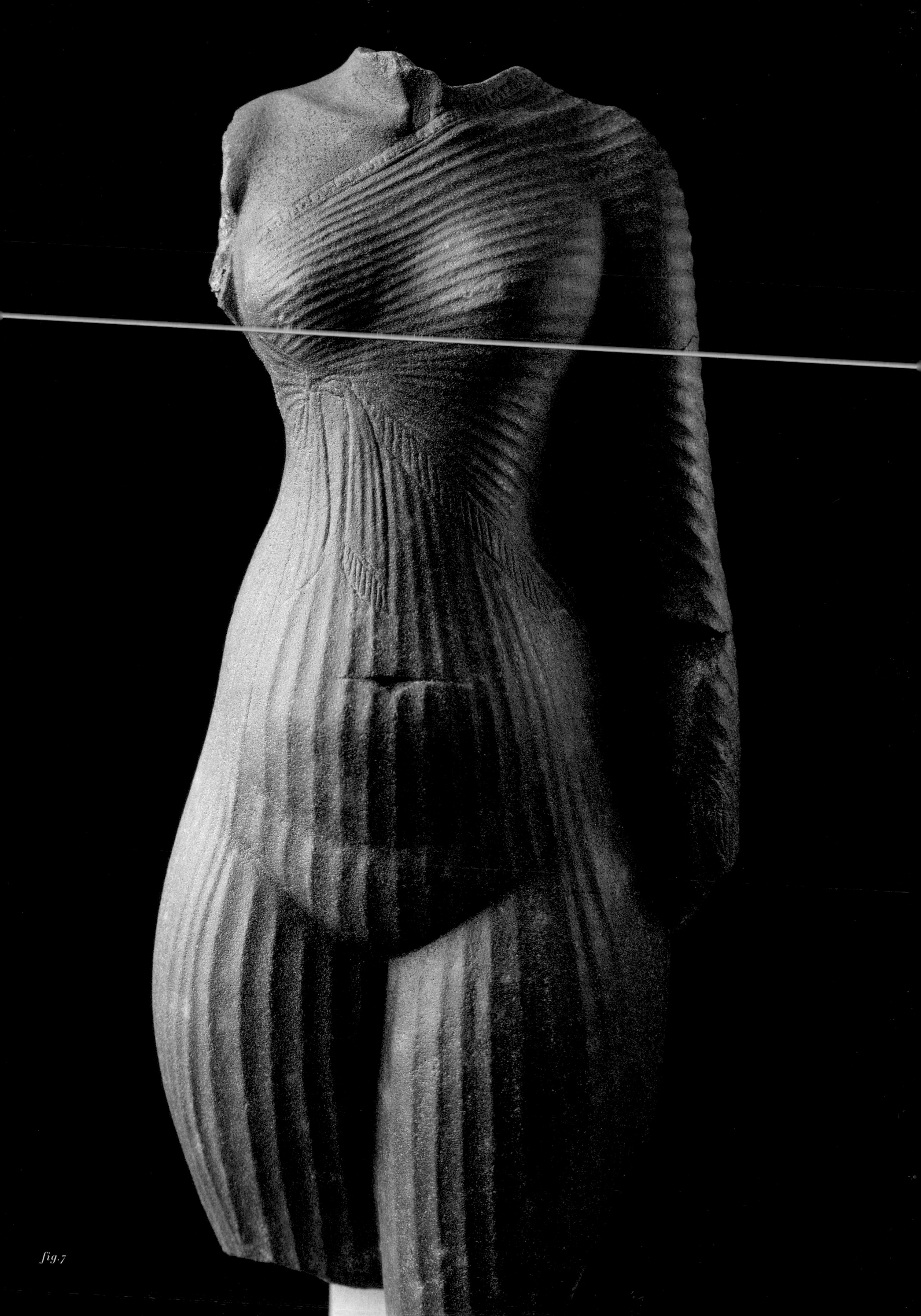

fig.7

"I have created the first mathematical definition of the beautiful face"

STEVEN M. HOEFFLIN, Santa Monica

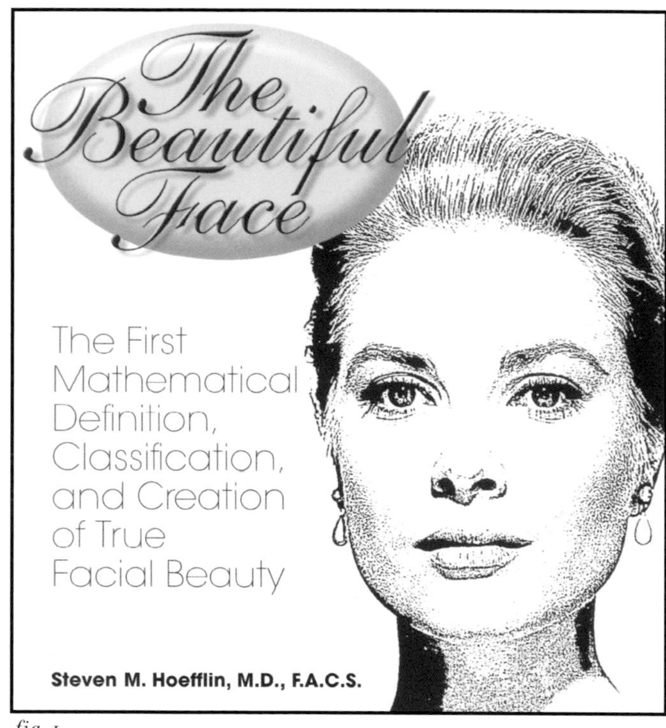

fig. 1

1. WHAT FASCINATES YOU MOST ABOUT BEING AN AESTHETIC SURGEON?

Other than the happiness that I bring to my patients I am invigorated by the continuing challenges. As an example, in my book, I have created the first mathematical definition of the beautiful face. In many aspects of beauty we have exact mathematical measurements. We can take the measurements 34–24–35, for instance, and make beautiful breasts, waists and hips. When somebody has a waist that's a 38 and wants to have a waist that's a 32, we can do liposuction or an abdominoplasty. But until now no one has developed a mathematical formula for the face. So I studied thousands of average, attractive and unattractive faces, computerised all the measurements and developed a formula that enabled me to create very accurate surgical results.

2. WHAT IS YOUR SPECIALISATION?

Starting 30 years ago, I had a busy practice in microsurgery, 20 years ago it was nasal surgery, liposuction and body sculpting, in the last 15 years or so I have been working in face lifts, I have developed a lot of techniques and have written books and numerous scientific articles about it.

3. DO YOU CONSIDER YOURSELF ALSO AN ARTIST?

Yes, I do. I enjoy pencil drawing and sculpting. An artist is somebody who can transfer ideas onto paper, a piece of clay or some other medium. It is a form of communication, which I used to communicate ideas from a patient's to a surgeon's point of view.

4. WHAT IS YOUR IDEAL OF BEAUTY? HOW WOULD YOU SEE THIS IN ART?

Other than my wife, my standard of beauty is someone like Grace Kelly. I have patients from all over the world. Standards of beauty are usually very uniform across the world. The media have dissolved a lot of geographical barriers, and certainly the movie industry and the media have portrayed beautiful faces. I see beautiful faces from China or from Japan, Europe, South America etc. But by and large, if somebody were to judge the world's true standard of beauty, it would be someone like Grace Kelly.

5. WHAT LIVING MAN OR WOMAN FOR YOU IS THE MOST BEAUTIFUL?

My standard of beauty is my wife. In the past it was Grace Kelly. Today, for example, it is Rebecca Romijn-Stamos.

6. DO YOU BELIEVE YOURSELF TO BE ATTRACTIVE AND WHY?

I think I'm average to a little bit above average. Most men inherit their health and looks from their mothers' side of the family, especially their maternal grandfathers.

7. WHAT DOES AGING MEAN TO YOU?

For some, the mind and body slow down with age, others say they feel younger than they look, and they would like to re-adjust this as time goes on. The other day I did a facelift on an 82-year-old woman who is active, has a social life and had a 50-year-old boyfriend after she had lost her husband. She didn't want to look 82, she wanted to

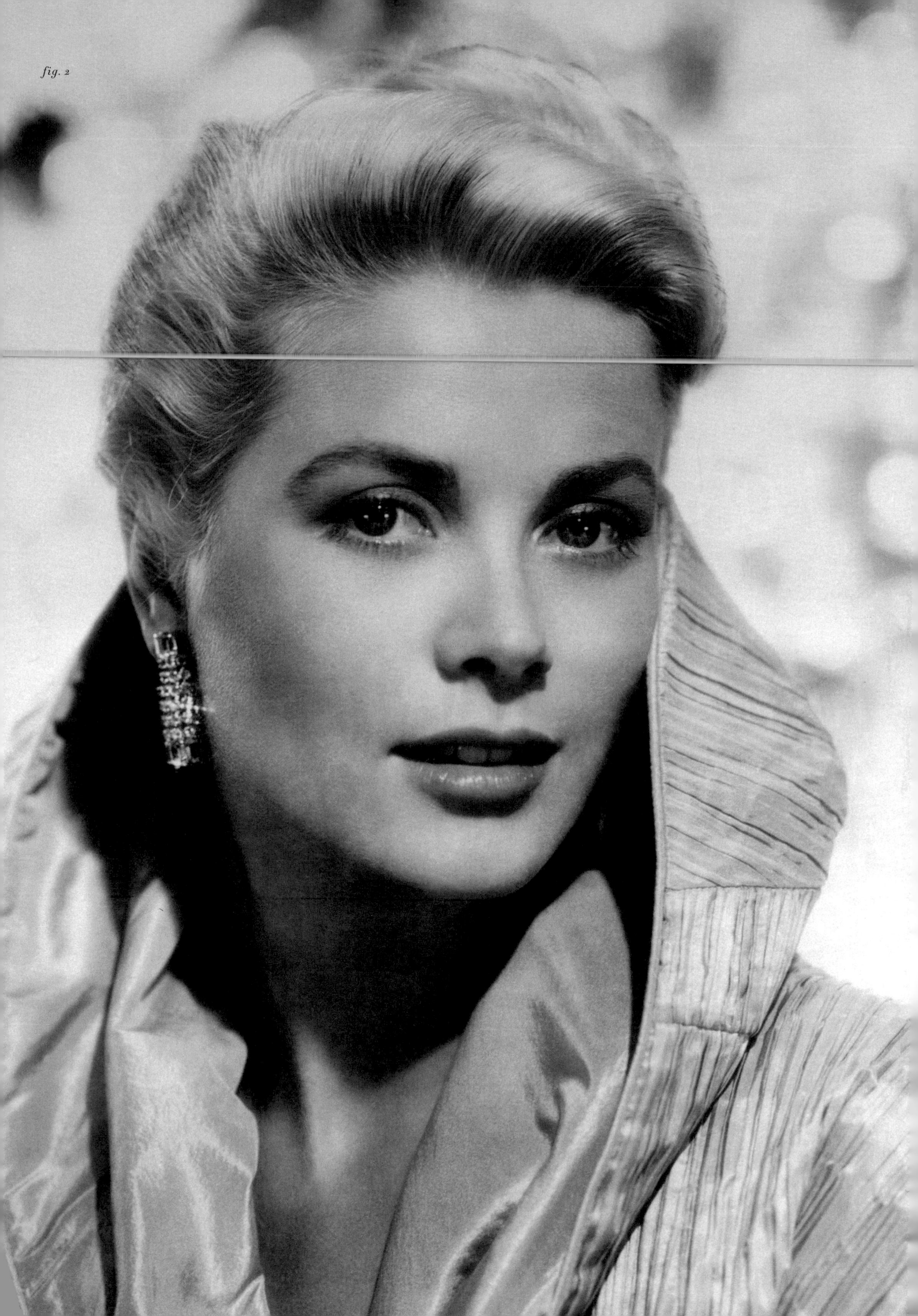

fig. 2

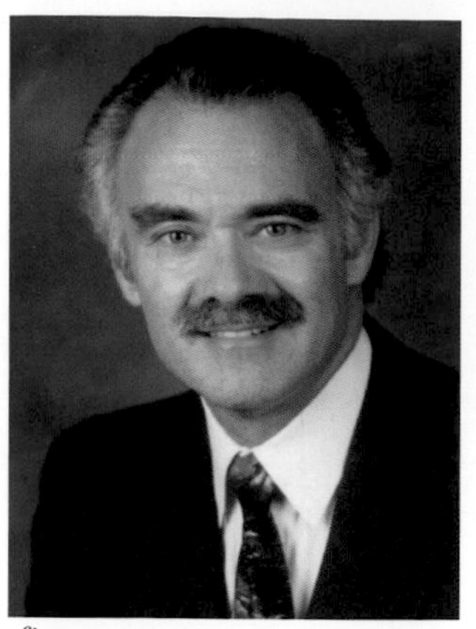

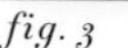

fig. 3

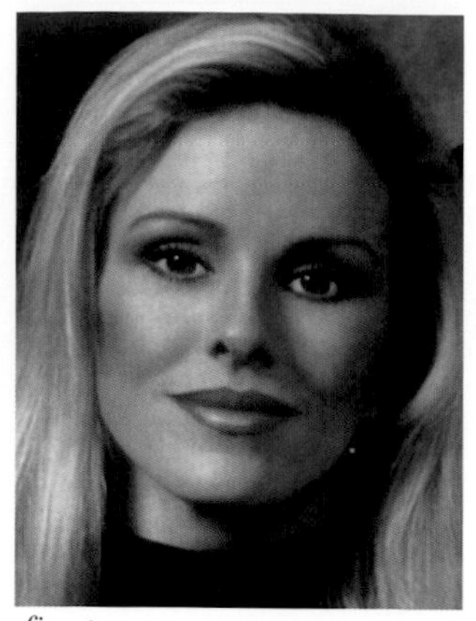

fig. 4

fig. 1

Cracking the beauty code: The president of the Los Angeles Society of Plastic Surgeons, Steven M. Hoefflin M. D., FACS, has measured and analysed thousands of faces. Based on his studies, he published the first mathematical definition of beauty. © Private archive Steven M. Hoefflin M. D.

fig. 2

Made to measure: According to Dr. Steven M. Hoefflin's calculations, Grace Kelly had a perfect face. His entire work is based on these standards. © Bettmann / CORBIS

fig. 3

Steven M. Hoefflin M. D., FACS, is more than just a well-known surgeon; as a lecturer and author, his fame has spread well beyond the borders of the U.S. © Private archive Steven M. Hoefflin M. D.

fig. 4

The surgeon's wife Pamela is his personal standard of beauty. © Private archive Steven M. Hoefflin M. D.

look 60. It makes a big difference in her life. The same with men: Why do men colour their hair now, why do they want to get rid of fat and grey hair? Because they want to feel good about themselves and be attractive to the opposite sex!

8. HAVE YOU HAD AESTHETIC SURGERY AND WHAT PROCEDURE?

For now I am comfortable with my appearance. But I would not hesitate to have something done if I needed it or wanted it.

9. DID YOU PERFORM SURGERY ON YOUR WIFE/PARTNER OR CHILD, AND WHICH?

I can't discuss what I've done to whom. But it is not uncommon for plastic surgeons to operate on their staff and on their family. Ethically speaking, it probably is not best to provide medical care to first-degree family members, but it's done.

10. CAN YOU AGREE TO EVERY DESIRE OF YOUR PATIENTS FOR CHANGE?

No. We as plastic surgeons are doctors first, surgeons second, and plastic surgeons third. My priorities are a safe, painless and pleasant experience, and an exceedingly good result.

11. WHAT IS THE MOST UNUSUAL REQUEST THAT YOU'VE EVER UNDERTAKEN?

Each of the last three decades has provided one distinctly unusual request. In the 1970s, to reattach eight amputated fingers and a hand, which was successful. In the 1980s, to rebuild the entire face of a young girl who had a seizure of her face because of a campfire. In the 1990s, to repair the nose and cheeks of another plastic surgeon who did his own surgery.

12. WHAT ARE THE REACTIONS OF THE PATIENTS AFTER THEIR OPERATIONS?

Most of them are tremendously happy, thrilled. And that has been the case since I entered this field, even though people were not that open about it 30 years ago. Phyllis Diller brought it to people's attention, when most people were still hiding cosmetic operations. It is very important for patients to realise that plastic surgery is serious medicine and not a visit to a beauty parlor. There are potential risks and a recovery period. Choosing a properly trained surgeon and anesthesiologist, ensuring the use of a certified operating theatre and staff and being properly prepared are extremely important.

13. COULD YOU NAME YOUR FAMOUS CLIENTS?

No. I can't really, because, as a physician, I have taken the Hippocratic oath, and I have to keep the names of my patients confidential.

14. ARE YOU AFRAID OF BECOMING OLDER?

No. I think the fear most people have in growing old is the maladies that accompany it. I have four very close acquaintances now that have cancer. Once you turn 50, you start to see women who have breast cancer, men have prostate cancer, people have heart attacks, and you are aware of all kinds of medical problems. It is wonderful that most people do age with good health, and I think that's the way it should be. I'm not sure people want to live to 120. Some people do, but I think almost everybody would like to be in good health in the middle and late years of their life. One should take care of the inside as well as of the outside.

15. DO YOU BELIEVE THAT BEAUTY COMES MAINLY FROM YOUR INSIDE?

Yes, *feeling* beautiful comes from the inside, *looking* beautiful comes from the outside. A woman's quest for beauty is stronger than a man's quest for power, money or success. It is genetic. Just recently, a "grooming gene" was discovered in mice. In laboratories, they are generally clean animals: They live in clean cages, keep themselves clean and groom themselves like a cat. If you extract this gene, they become slobs: They tear their hair out, and so on. We have an innate attraction to beauty, and this applies to all living things. Let me give you an example: Why are flowers beautiful? Because the most beautiful flower attracts the insects, and they will help pollinate it, and then beautiful flowers create beautiful flowers over and over again. The most beautiful part of a person is inside.

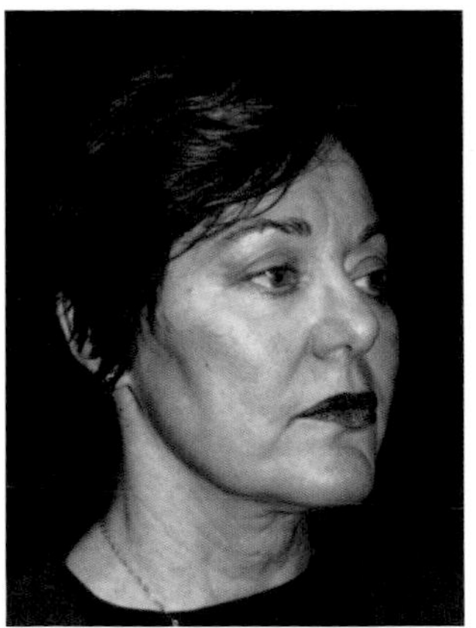

fig. 5 a

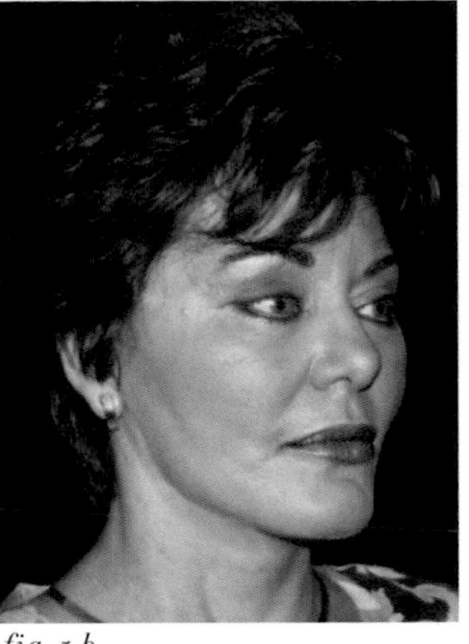

fig. 5 b

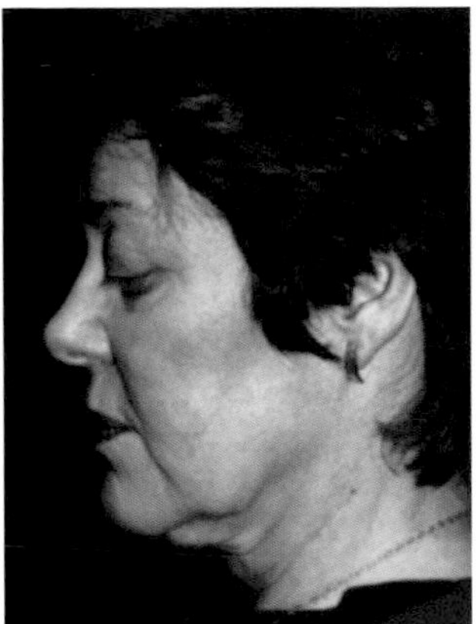

fig. 5 c

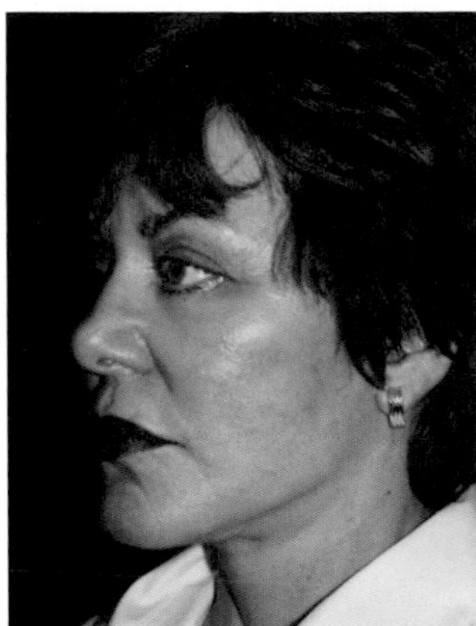

fig. 5 d

fig. 5 a–f

Originally specializing in nasal, breast and body sculpting corrections, Dr. Steven M. Hoefflin has focused on developing new successful techniques and publishing his work on facelifts over the past 15 years. © Private archive Steven M. Hoefflin M. D.

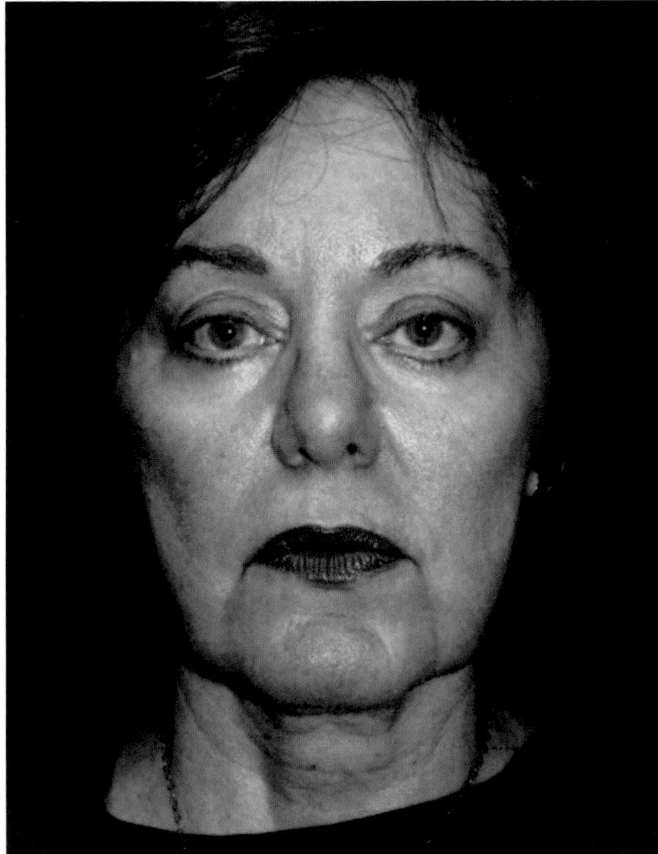

fig. 5 e

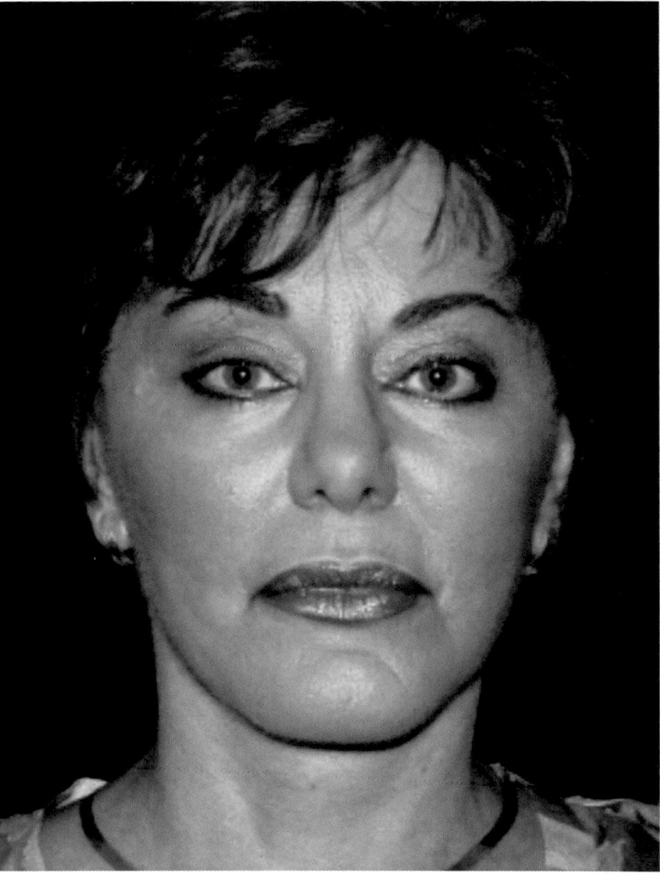

fig. 5 f

16. DO YOU BELIEVE A MORE BEAUTIFUL PERSON IS HAPPIER AND HAS A BETTER LIFE?

It depends on the individual, how they feel about themselves. Certainly somebody who is handsome or beautiful is much happier than somebody who is *un*attractive. We live in a world where 40% of the population has no electricity – so, is somebody with electricity happier than somebody without electricity? We'd say yes, but there may be circumstances where that's not the case.

17. DO YOU THINK A BEAUTIFUL PERSON HAS A BETTER SEX LIFE?

I would imagine so, yes. I believe the most beautiful part of a person is the heart, soul and mind. External beauty complements inner beauty. There have been surveys that people who are more attractive get better jobs, they tend to be more popular, they tend to have more active social lives and naturally have a more active sex life.

18. WHAT IS THE FUTURE OF AESTHETIC SURGERY?

First of all, the volume is going to increase. About eight million cosmetic procedures were performed last year in the United States, and that includes Botox injections and collagens and things like this. Baby boomers are more concerned about getting older, appearing older, acting older and getting diseases, so plastic surgery is more common. I think it has also become much safer.

Interview: Richard Rushfield, Los Angeles

"Plastic Surgery is the most creative speciality in medicine"

GARY J. ALTER, Los Angeles

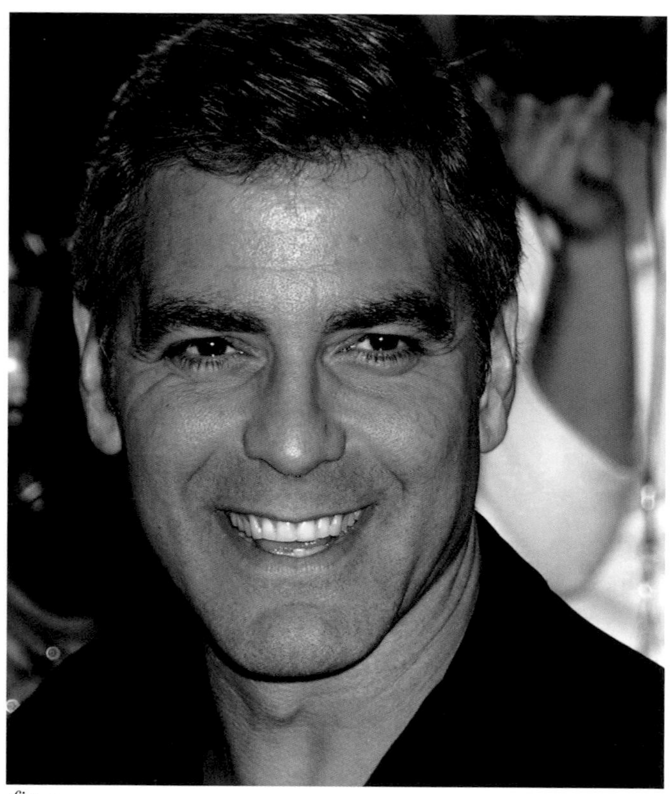

fig. 1

1. WHAT FASCINATES YOU MOST ABOUT BEING AN AESTHETIC SURGEON?

Plastic surgery is, at least in my opinion, the most creative specialty. In many of the surgical specialties of medicine, specific techniques are taught. Plastic surgeons learn principles, because there are many different solutions to a problem. Thus, each surgeon decides the best approach to a problem depending on his prejudices, imagination, training and experience. Each surgeon can — within reason — explore his creativity.

2. WHAT IS YOUR SPECIALISATION?

I have a very unique, diverse practice. Probably about a third of my practice is aesthetic surgery: liposuction, breasts, face, etc. I also perform these procedures on transgender patients who desire facial and body feminisation. About 50 percent of my practice is plastic surgery of the genitalia. Genital plastic surgery includes many different areas from reconstruction of congenital or acquired deformities to sex changes. I also do a large amount of aesthetic genital surgery on both men and women. I perform penis reconstruction to make the penis look or function better. I devised a revolutionary new technique for female labia minora (vaginal inner lip) reduction, and — believe it or not — there's really a major demand for it. I perform male to female sexual reassignment and some female to male sexual reassignment techniques.

3. DO YOU CONSIDER YOURSELF AN ARTIST?

Yes and no. I think a good plastic surgeon has to have an artistic eye, but that is not enough. The excellent surgeon must also be compulsive to insure that the operation is performed meticulously. Otherwise, problems can occur. In addition, the surgeon can't allow his imagination or desire to go beyond what is technically possible or aesthetically pleasing.

4. WHAT IS YOUR IDEAL OF BEAUTY? HOW WOULD YOU SEE THIS IN ART?

There's a classical ideal of beauty, which is obviously based more on the Caucasian culture, but each ethnic group has its own concept of beauty. For example, somebody with a large nose may not be considered beautiful in our culture but may be attractive in another culture. Opinions of beauty also change with time. For example, a thin woman may now be considered more attractive than a full-figured Rubenesque woman of the past.

5. WHAT LIVING MAN OR WOMAN FOR YOU IS THE MOST BEAUTIFUL?

I always thought Michelle Pfeiffer has a beautiful face. I think a man such as George Clooney is good-looking, because he's masculine in addition to being handsome. However, I find some actors that other people consider good-looking aren't as masculine.

6. DO YOU BELIEVE YOURSELF TO BE ATTRACTIVE AND WHY?

I think I am ... better than average-looking — because

fig. 1

George Clooney has featured on "sexiest men alive" lists for years. To Gary J. Alter, the Hollywood hunk's pervasive masculinity helps make him so attractive. © picture-alliance

fig. 2

Gary Alter had his nose surgically reduced partially to increase his creativity towards patients wanting rhinoplasty. © Private archive Gary J. Alter M.D.

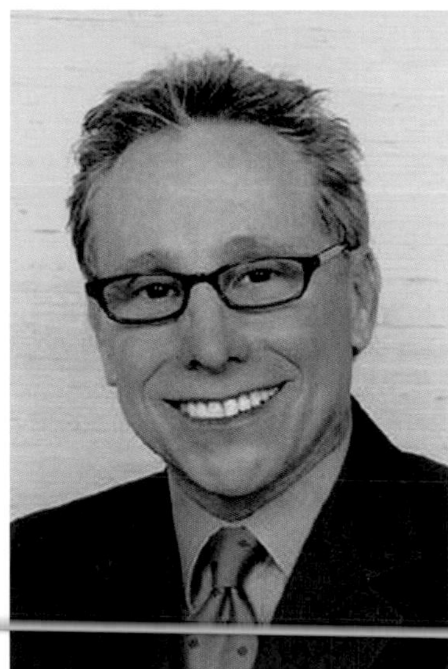

fig. 2

people tell me so. You talk to models, and they don't think *they* are good-looking. Everybody is telling them they are beautiful, but they look in the mirror and see multiple flaws. They might be spectacularly beautiful, but they don't see it. Their insecurity illustrates the insecurities present in most of us.

7. WHAT DOES AGING MEAN TO YOU?

Well, some people — including women — look better as they age. Aging is classified as the deterioration of tissues. I think that if you are obsessed with counteracting aging, as are some plastic surgery addicts, you will always fight a losing battle. Plastic surgery enables someone to look refreshed or better. Aging does not have to be an enemy, because an older person can still look good.

8. HAVE YOU HAD AESTHETIC SURGERY AND WHAT PROCEDURE?

I had a rhinoplasty at age 40 just prior to starting my plastic surgical training. I always wanted to have it done, anyhow. I reasoned that a plastic surgeon with a large nose would not be credible if he recommended a rhinoplasty to a patient.

9. DID YOU PERFORM SURGERY ON YOUR WIFE/PARTNER OR CHILD, AND WHICH?

I don't have a wife or a child, but I have performed plastic surgery on girlfriends. It is much more difficult to deal with the emotional aspects and to be unaffected. If a complication occurs, it's more stressful. That's why, generally speaking, you don't like to operate on family members, loved ones or friends.

10. CAN YOU AGREE TO EVERY DESIRE OF YOUR PATIENTS FOR CHANGE?

If it's beyond the realm of what I consider good taste or if the request is unreasonable, I won't do it.

11. WHAT IS THE MOST EXCEPTIONAL DESIRE THAT YOU'VE EVER UNDERTAKEN?

In terms of genital cosmetic surgery, I would say I have done some unusual procedures, but they were not unreasonable. I have performed some genital plastic surgical operations that other surgeons wouldn't do, because I knew hat it was possible and that I could achieve the patient's expectations.

12. WHAT ARE THE REACTIONS OF THE PATIENTS AFTER THEIR OPERATIONS?

They're very happy, generally, extremely happy. I'm straightforward and honest with my patients, so I tell them the pros and the cons. I explain what they can expect, so I have few problems with patients having unrealistic expectations. I have a very happy practice.

13. COULD YOU NAME YOUR FAMOUS CLIENTS?

No.

14. ARE YOU AFRAID OF BECOMING OLDER?

In some respects I am, mainly because I want to maintain my health and energy. In terms of my physical looks, I think I'm better-looking than I was 20 years ago. And I'm in good shape. The key is that you have to take care of yourself. I'd be terrified if I was eating unhealthy foods, was overweight and was ill. Thank God I'm not. A youthful attitude also helps keep you young.

15. DO YOU BELIEVE THAT BEAUTY COMES MAINLY FROM YOUR INSIDE?

Physical beauty is important, but you wouldn't want to be around or married to someone who's physically beautiful and unpleasant. Internal beauty makes someone more attractive physically.

16. DO YOU BELIEVE A MORE BEAUTIFUL PERSON IS HAPPIER AND HAS A BETTER LIFE?

I think a more beautiful person has more opportunities in many respects. Many studies have shown that attractive people are treated more favourably than unattractive persons. However, that does not imply that a beautiful person is happier or has a better life. Happiness is internal, and life is what you make of it.

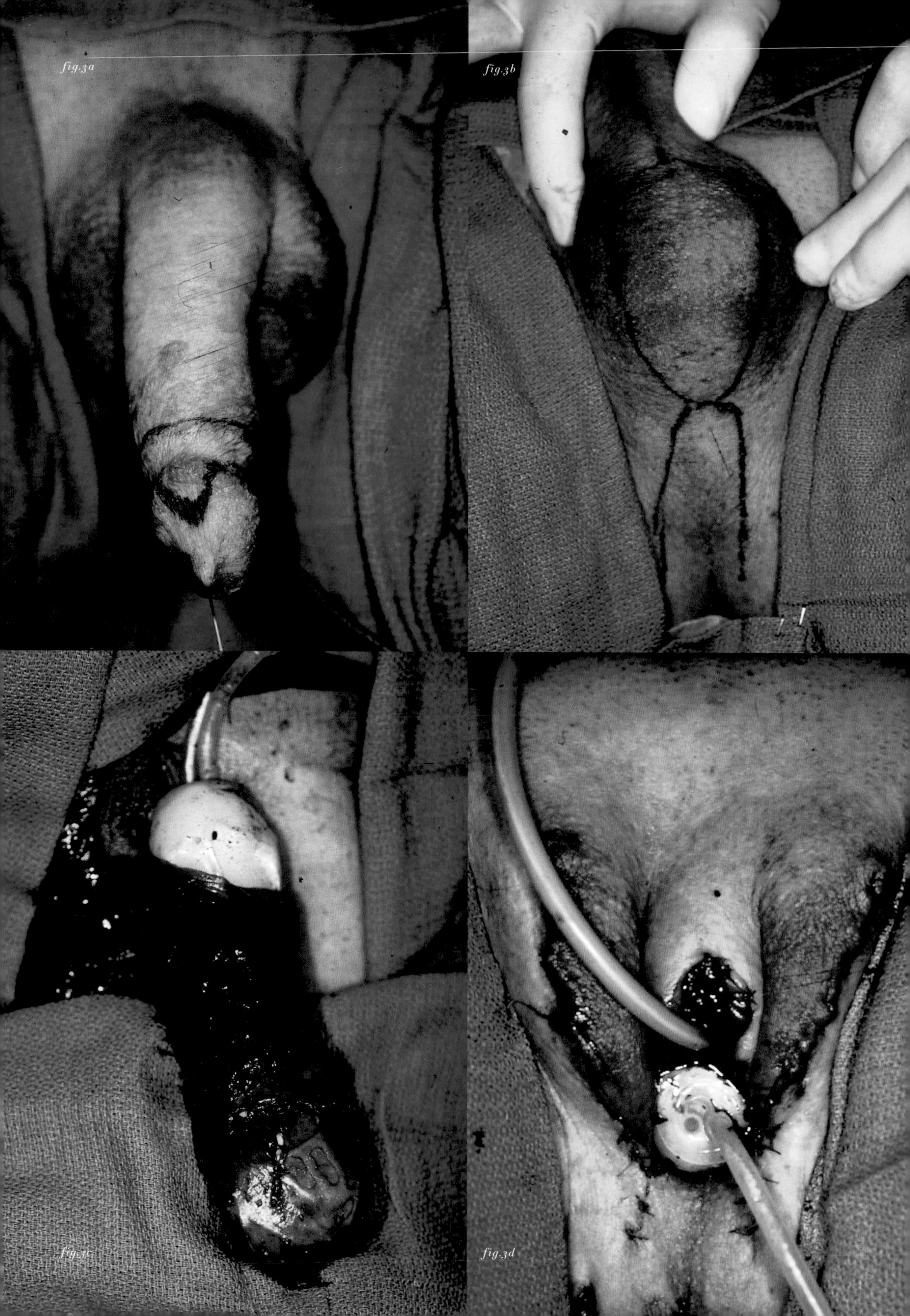
fig.3a
fig.3b
fig.3c
fig.3d

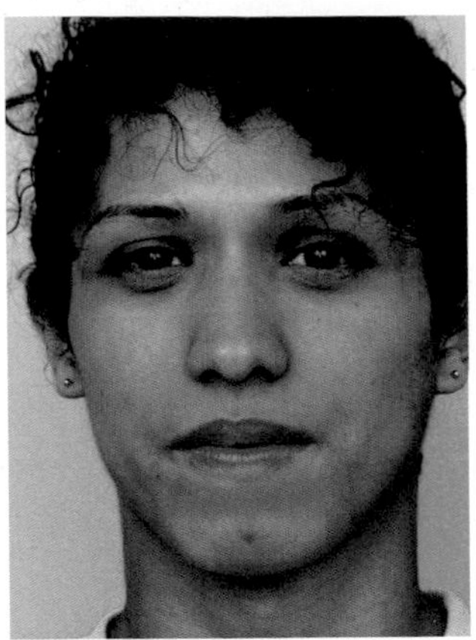

fig. 4 a

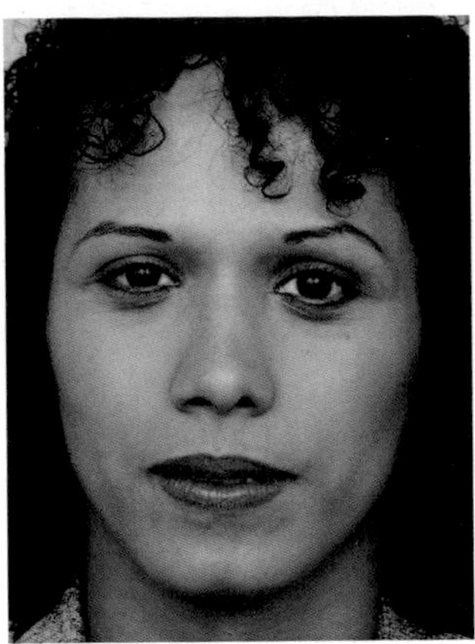

fig. 4 b

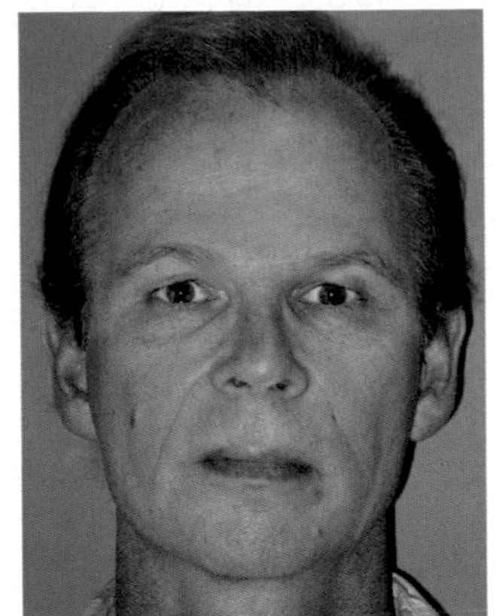

fig. 5 a

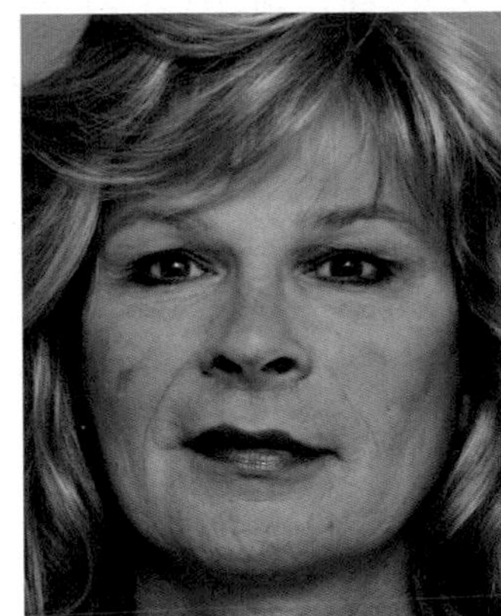

fig. 5 b

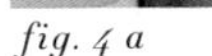

50 percent of the procedures performed by Gary J. Alter are genital surgeries. He specialises in transforming male genitals into female genitals — as shown by these photos (3 a–d). Below, the same patient three months after the operation. The top photos (3 e+f) show the patient's vagina when she is standing up (left) and lying down (right). The two bottom photos with a dilator in the vagina show a vaginal depth of at least six inches. © Private archive Gary J. Alter M.D.

fig. 4 a+b & 5 a+b

Two before-and-after photos of patients that Gary J. Alter has performed a sex change on. The surgeon mostly turns men into women, not vice versa. © Private archive Gary J. Alter M.D.

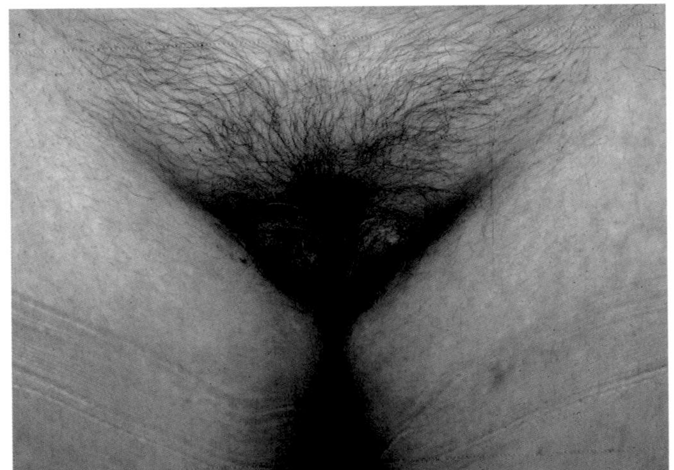

fig. 3 e

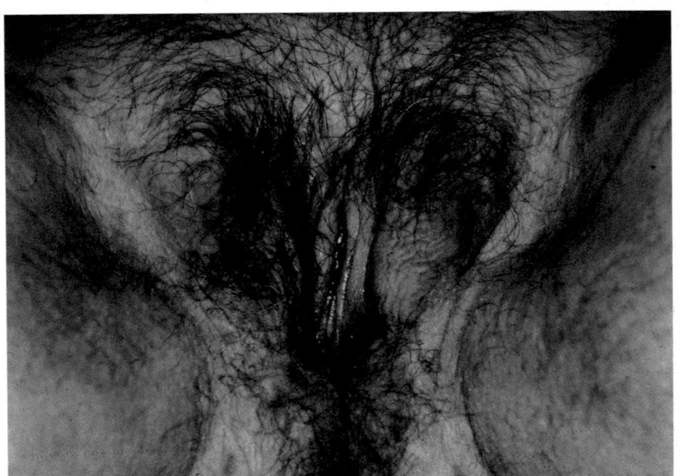

fig. 3 f

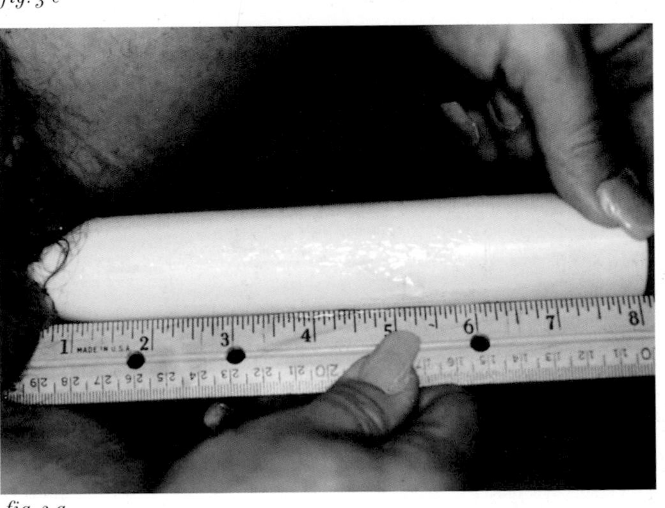

fig. 3 g

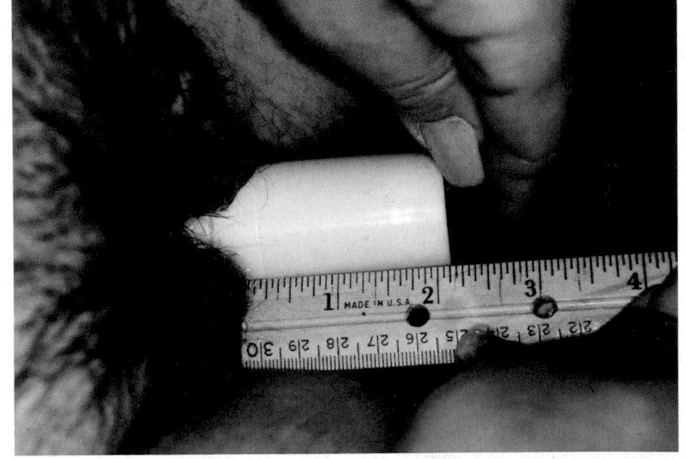

fig. 3 h

fig. 6 a+b

Preoperation – revealing normal female external genitalia with a large clitoris. Postoperation – after a metaidoioplasty and insertion of testicle implants into the labia majora. The urethra was not extended. Extra surgical techniques were used to straighten the new penis. © Private archive Gary J. Alter M.D.

fig. 7 a+b

An example of reducing the labia minora (inner vaginal lips): The photos show a patient's vagina with asymmetrical and large labia, before the procedure and six months after. © Private archive Gary J. Alter M.D.

17. DO YOU THINK A BEAUTIFUL PERSON HAS A BETTER SEX LIFE?

No, I wouldn't make that presumption. I think a good sex life is chemistry between two people, both physically and emotionally. I don't think it matters how a person looks except if it makes that person feel more confident and uninhibited. It would be very shallow to think beautiful people are having better sex than unattractive people. Everybody has his or her own needs and desires and who he or she considers sexually desirable.

18. WHAT IS THE FUTURE OF AESTHETIC SURGERY?

Well, everything gets better. Medicine, generally, in the last ten years has had changes in almost every speciality. In plastic surgery, the techniques have improved. There are more non-invasive procedures that allow people to look better with smaller incisions. In my opinion, plastic surgeons are among the most creative, innovative specialists in medicine. There are always surgeons trying new things, attacking new problems and improving operations.

Interview: Richard Rushfield, Los Angeles

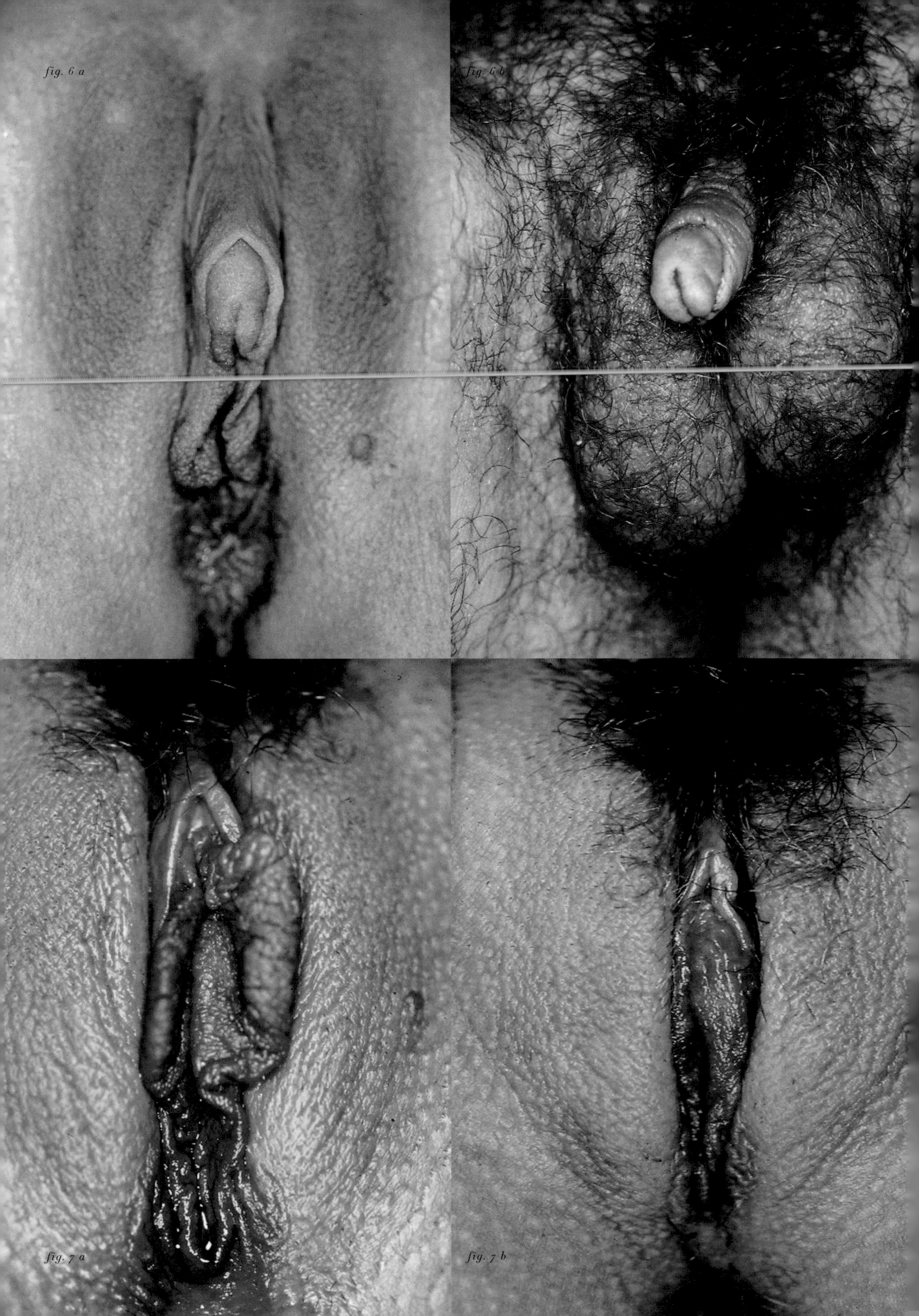

fig. 6 a

fig. 6 b

fig. 7 a

fig. 7 b

"I view it as a privilege to do what I do"

ALAN M. ENGLER, New York

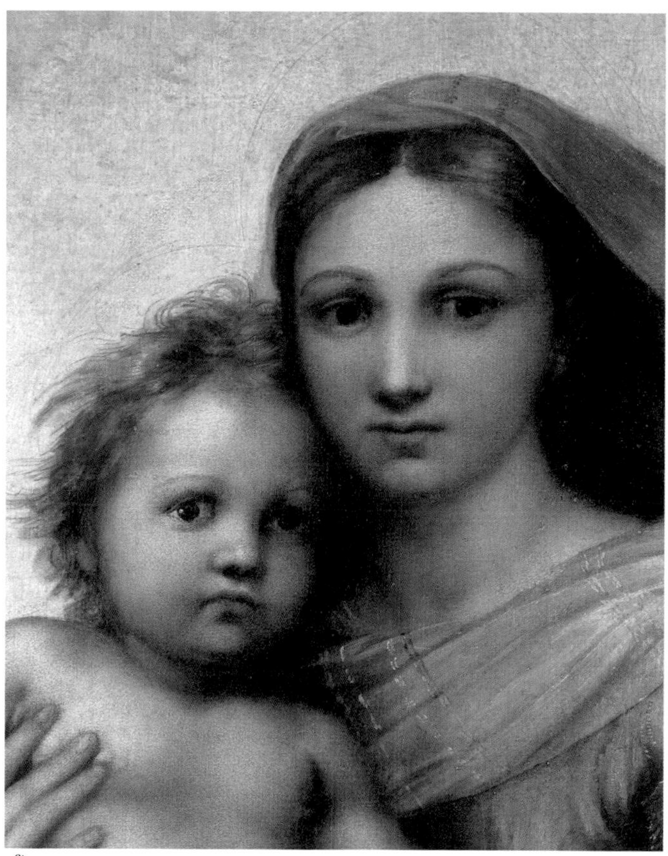

fig. 1

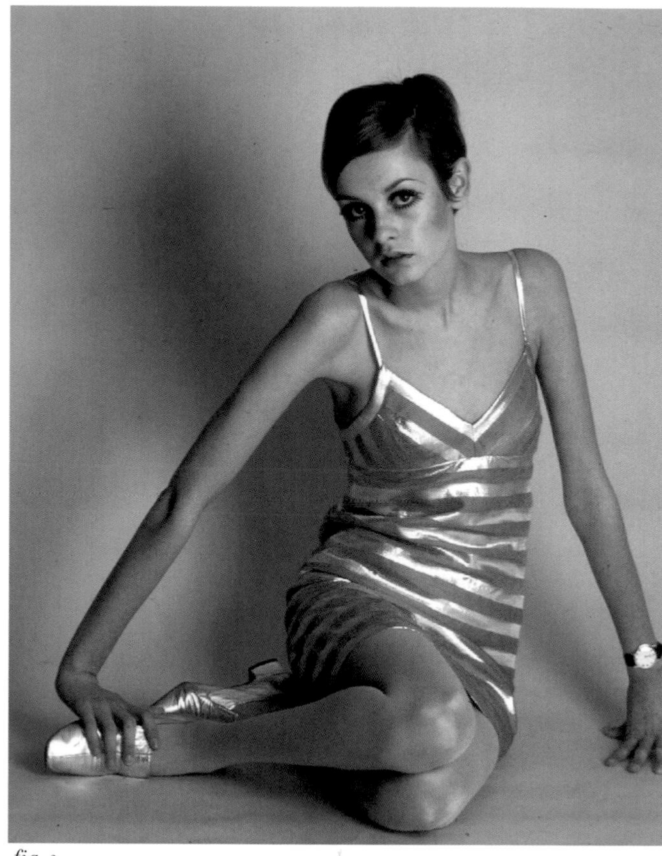

fig. 2

1. WHAT FASCINATES YOU MOST ABOUT BEING AN AESTHETIC SURGEON?

I like to be able to take the human tissues, from a purely technical standpoint, and to change them and mold them in a way that both the patient and I find aesthetic, attractive, proportional. It's really a joy to be able to do that. We saw a patient yesterday who had had a tummy tuck five days ago. She came in, we opened up the dressing, she looked down at her stomach and she burst into tears, in front of the nurse and me. She went out, and an hour later she had a big bouquet of flowers sent over to the office. That's very rewarding, to be able to do that technically — and something I enjoy — that affects the quality of life for these people. I view it as a privilege to be able to do what I do.

2. WHAT IS YOUR SPECIALISATION?

I actually do a wide range of aesthetic procedures of the face and the body. But since my book, "BodySculpture", came out in 1998 and generated a lot of interest, I focus on surgery of the body, including breast surgery, liposuction and tummy tucks.

3. DO YOU CONSIDER YOURSELF AN ARTIST?

I think I do consider myself that, and I think any patient having this surgery would care very much that their surgeon, their plastic surgeon is artistic. There are many plastic surgeons who do actual artwork and display it in their offices — sculptures and paintings or things like that — and I think that's completely consistent with what we do all day long.

fig. 1 & 2

A close-up of Raphael's "Sistine Madonna" from c. 1513 (1). British super model Twiggy, who was "the world's most expensive beanstalk" in the 1960s (2). © akg-images (1), picture-alliance (2)

fig. 3, 4 & 5

Alan M. Engler's line-up of the world's most beautiful people include Hollywood icons Brad Pitt and Charlize Theron, and the fashion model Paulina Porizkova, whose extraordinary face he especially admires. © Getty Images (3), picture alliance (4), Steve Azzara / CORBIS SYGMA (5)

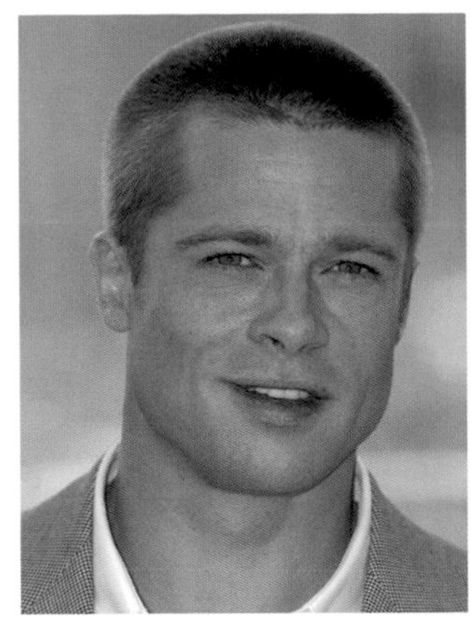

fig. 3

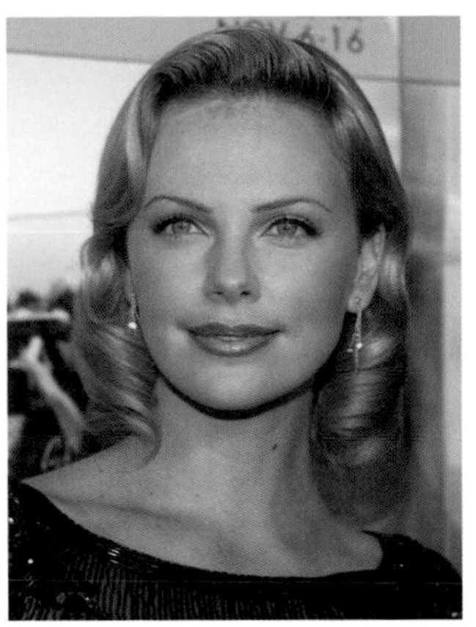

fig. 4

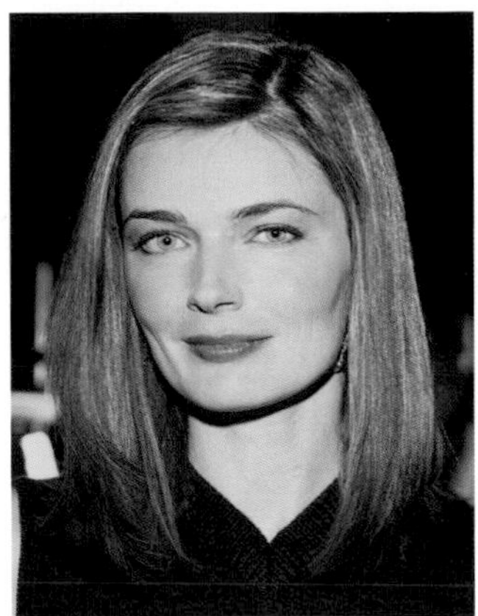

fig. 5

4. WHAT IS YOUR IDEAL OF BEAUTY? HOW WOULD YOU SEE THIS IN ART?

If you go through societal forms of beauty, you can see that it depends on where you are and what time period it is. In our own society, Raphaelian beauties were voluptuous — and then a few hundred years later, Twiggy was considered beautiful. Beauty is actually a relative term, and it comes in many different shapes and sizes, and even hues.

5. WHAT LIVING MAN OR WOMAN FOR YOU IS THE MOST BEAUTIFUL?

I would probably list the following three women as the most beautiful right now: Halle Berry, Charlize Theron, and the model Paulina Porizkova, who I think has just an exquisite face. Of course, these are all a little bit younger — you could also go with Catherine Deneuve for a slightly older group. And among men, I would probably put Sean Connery in all his stages; George Clooney and Brad Pitt — most people probably have them on their list.

6. DO YOU BELIEVE YOURSELF TO BE ATTRACTIVE AND WHY?

I wouldn't really say it's my best asset, perhaps unfortunately. That's just the way it is, not at least according to standards of beauty that I imagine most of my patients adhere to.

7. WHAT DOES AGING MEAN TO YOU?

Aging is a difficult process for all involved. There are societies throughout history that have made it easier to age than ours does. Our society really puts a premium on youth and vigor, enthusiasm and energy, and all of that makes it harder to get older. In Chinese society, for example, where aging might have been revered, worshipped, respected to a greater extent, the signs of aging are easier to tolerate. For us it's a little bit harder. You don't want to see things starting to sag, and excess folds, because our society puts a premium on youth.

8. HAVE YOU HAD AESTHETIC SURGERY AND WHAT PROCEDURE?

I have not, but I would not hesitate to do so, and I suspect that the first thing I will do — when and if it's appropriate — is eyelid surgery.

9. DID YOU PERFORM SURGERY ON YOUR WIFE/PARTNER OR CHILD, AND WHICH?

I won't answer this question because I would consider this issue confidential, but: yes, I would perform cosmetic procedures on those people and would perform them on various members of my family.

10. CAN YOU AGREE TO EVERY DESIRE OF YOUR PATIENTS FOR CHANGE?

Definitely not. Not all things are possible for all people. You have to really look at what the patient has, what the patient wants, and try to be very honest about it. And I think — aside from the fact that you can't always do things — it's potentially quite dangerous for all involved to suggest something that's unrealistic to patients. You may do a very good surgical procedure with a good result, but if it's not what they thought they were getting, they'll be unhappy. Aside from any of the aesthetic and ethical issues, this is a litigious age that we live in, and a plastic surgeon who promises something that's not feasible, is likely to cause grief for many people.

11. WHAT IS THE MOST UNUSUAL REQUEST THAT YOU'VE EVER UNDERTAKEN?

I don't think I've ever done anything unusual and probably wouldn't. I think that the vast majority of the requests patients have come in with have been reasonable, and it's been relatively easy to try to accommodate them.

12. WHAT ARE THE REACTIONS OF THE PATIENTS AFTER THEIR OPERATIONS?

Excluding those times and conditions in which they're physically uncomfortable with it, within the first day or so, there is typically this wonderful euphoria that patients have when they get a look and can see the results. Now, that's more with some procedures than others. For example, liposuction: you may not see that dramatic a result right away, because it takes a while for the skin to shrink back down, but the other extreme is breast implants. On

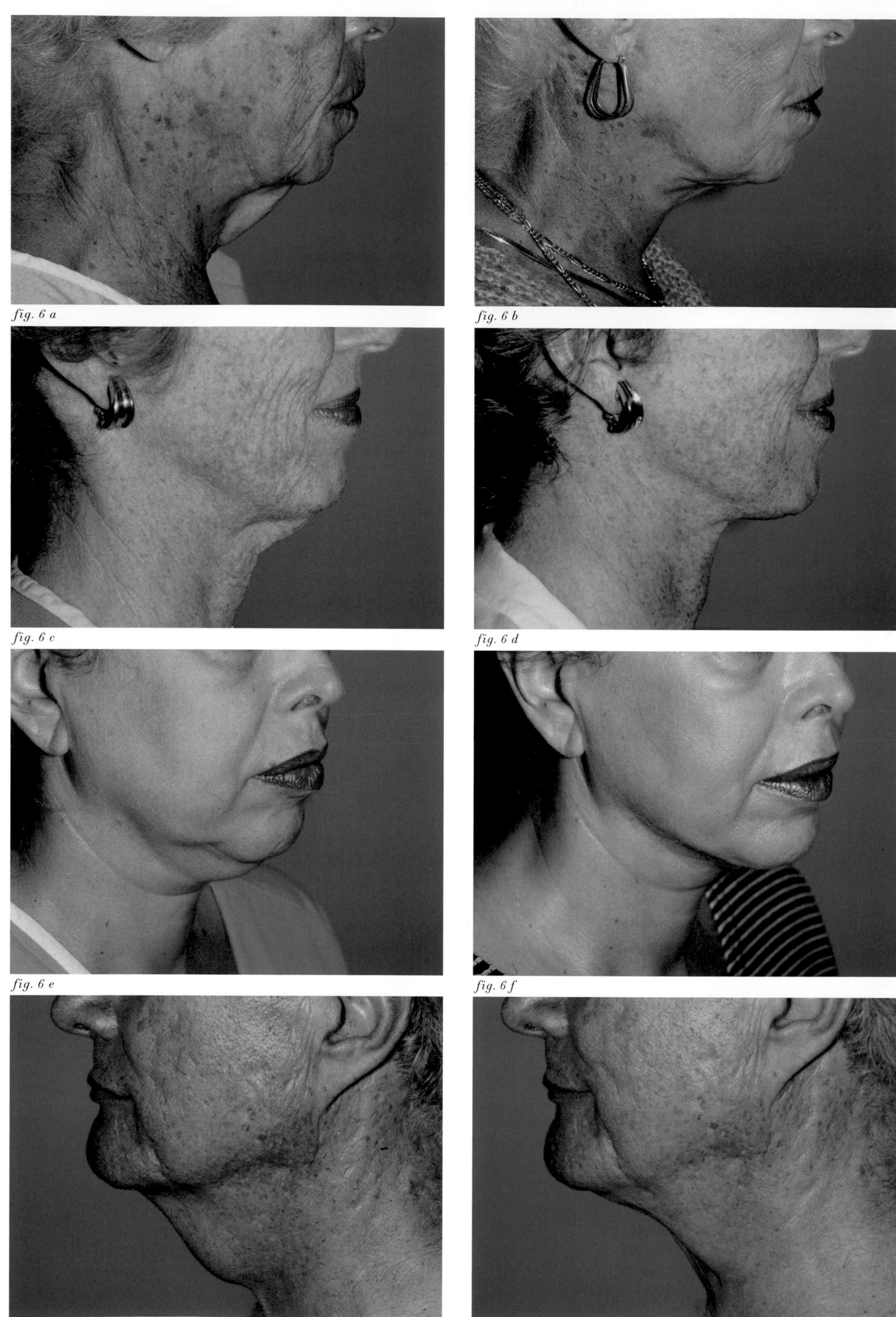

fig. 6 a

fig. 6 b

fig. 6 c

fig. 6 d

fig. 6 e

fig. 6 f

fig. 6 g

fig. 6 h

fig. 6 a–h

Alan M. Engler specialises in aesthetic operations on the face and the neck. A selection of before-and-after images (6 a–d) show patients who have had lower face lifting as well as neck liposuction and chin contouring (6 e–h). According to Engler, the physical improvements of this combination procedure last for approximately seven to ten years. © www.bodysculpture.com

fig. 7 a–f

The eyes are usually the first to show signs of aging – frequently when people reach their mid to late thirties. Alan M. Engler smoothes patients' wrinkles and lachrymal sacs in one or two hours, returning their "youthful looks" to them in a single operation. © www.bodysculpture.com

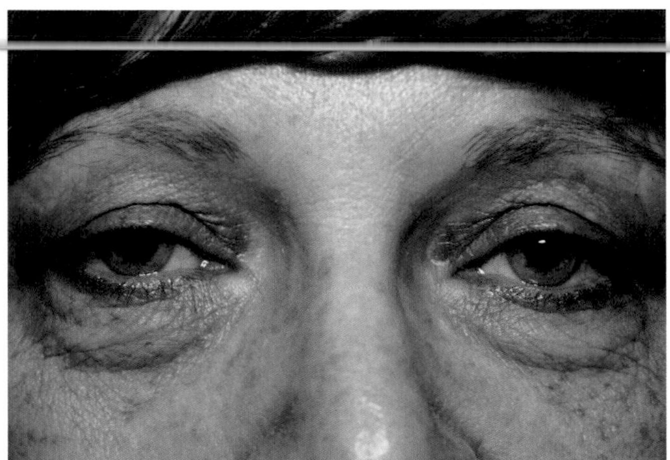

fig. 7 a

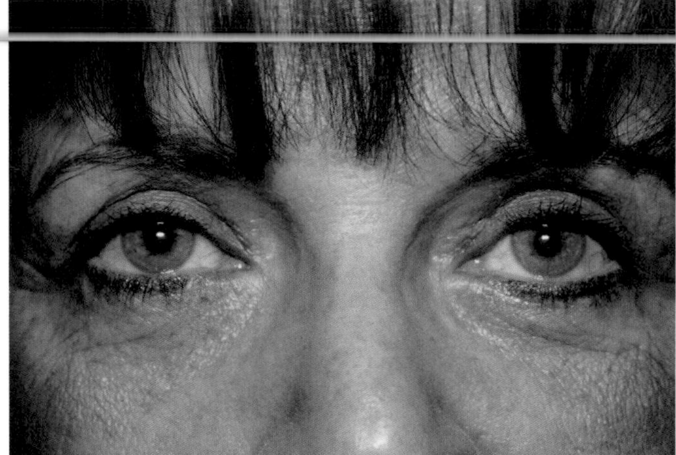

fig. 7 b

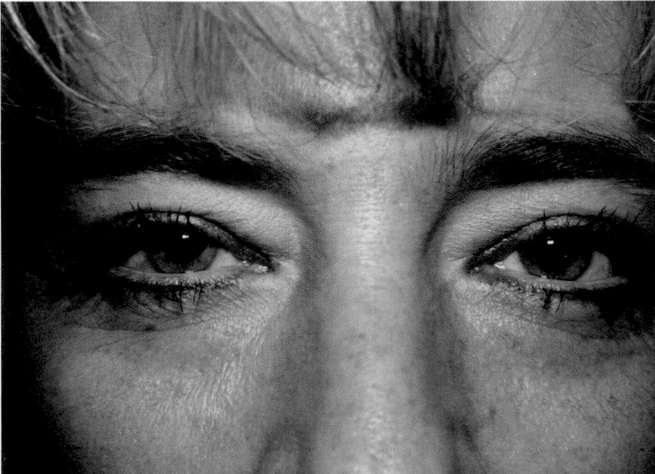

fig. 7 c

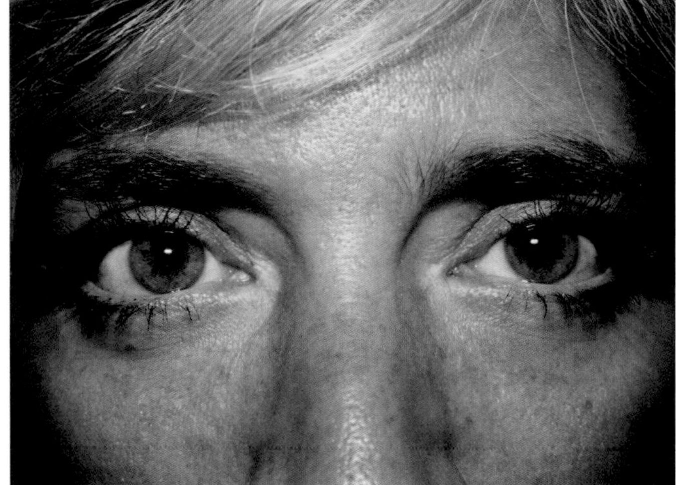

fig. 7 d

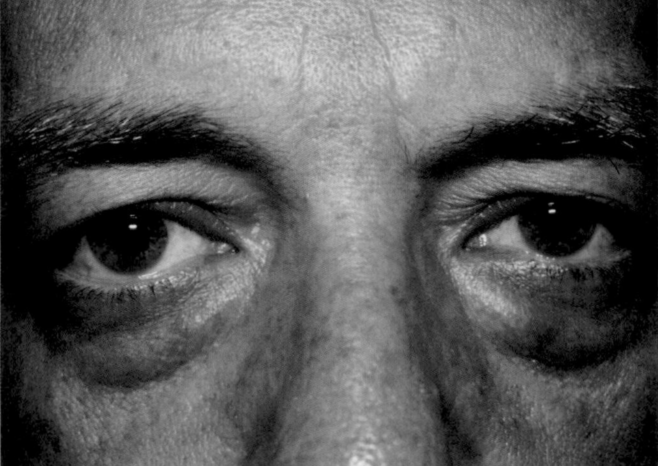

fig. 7 e

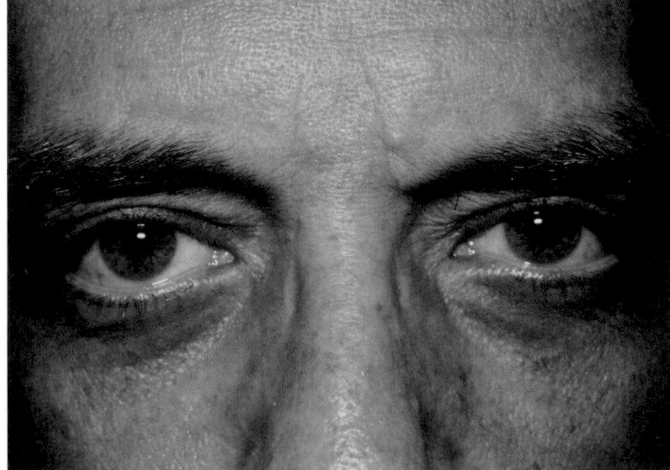

fig. 7 f

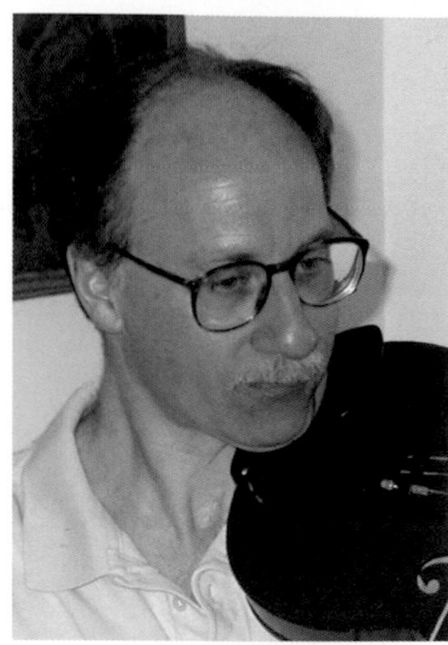

fig. 8

fig. 8

Alan M. Engler is not only a medical practitioner and amateur musician but also an author: In 1998, he published "BodySculpture", which has become a Health & Beauty bestseller. © Private archive Alan M. Engler M.D.

fig. 9 a+b

An upper arm liposuction, carried out by Alan M. Engler. © www.bodysculpture.com

fig. 10 a+b

Liposuction is one of the most widespread surgical techniques in the US. As the incisions in the skin are very small, there are no visible scars after the operation. © www.bodysculpture.com

fig. 11 a+b

Many female patients combine the so-called "tummy tuck" with liposuction to remove excess abdominal flab. © www.bodysculpture.com

some occasions, it's literally a euphoria, a very joyous occasion, as they have been able to realise the change that they desperately wanted.

13. COULD YOU NAME YOUR FAVORITE CLIENTS?
No, next question. I have some, I know, and if I named them they would not be happy.

14 ARE YOU AFRAID OF BECOMING OLDER?
Again, I would say I don't think there's a lot that's wonderful to look forward to. I'm not necessarily terrified of it. What's the alternative, anyway? So from that standpoint, I'll take getting older. I'll sort of roll with the punches as they come.

15. DO YOU BELIEVE THAT BEAUTY COMES MAINLY FROM YOUR INSIDE?
I think it's both. There are certainly some people that can literally take your breath away. Paulina Porizkova is the perfect example, because she's not famous as an actress — although I don't know if she would like it if I say that —, but I know of her as a model of perfume fragrances. I don't know anything else about her, but you just look and go: Oh, that's so beautiful! And other people's beauty is enhanced as you find out a little bit more about them, so for them it certainly comes at least partly from the inside. It's really a combination, I think.

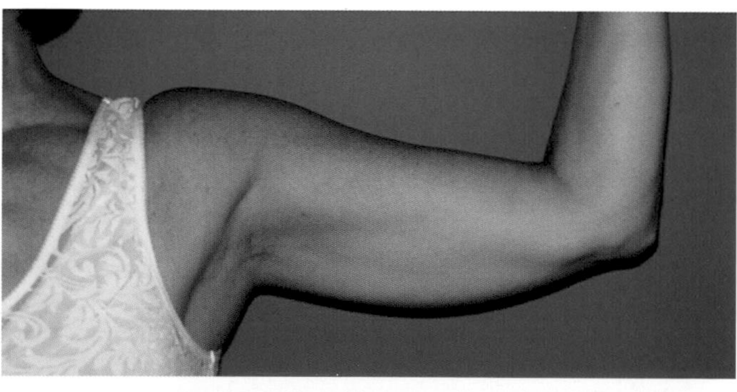

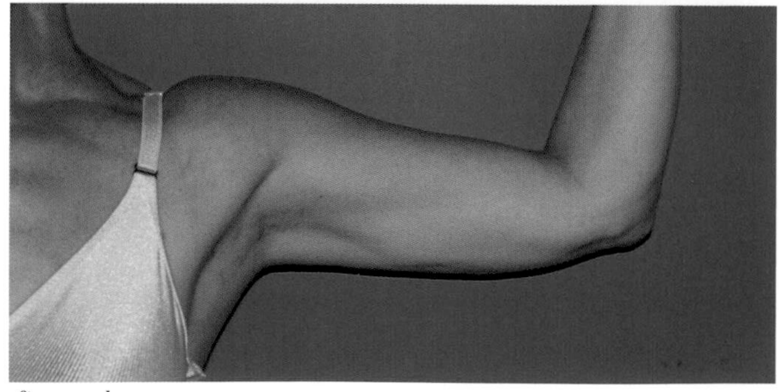

fig. 9 a+b

16. DO YOU BELIEVE A MORE BEAUTIFUL PERSON IS HAPPIER AND HAS A BETTER LIFE?
Happiness is a difficult thing to define. It's largely a state of mind. It's not necessarily related to other people's views of you, and just because somebody thinks you're beautiful doesn't mean you're happy. Hollywood is full of examples of people who can have everything going for them — beauty, success and fame, riches — and yet they're miserable, sometimes to the point of ending their lives.

17. DO YOU THINK A BEAUTIFUL PERSON HAS A BETTER SEX LIFE?
I don't think there necessarily is any correlation. I could be wrong, I'm not a sex therapist. I think that, although it doesn't necessarily make your sex life better, it's feeling better about yourself that makes everything more pleasurable, including intimate relationships, probably.

18. WHAT IS THE FUTURE OF AESTHETIC SURGERY?
I think plastic surgery is going to have more surgery through smaller incisions, and we've seen some of these trends already. With endoscopic procedures, with liposuction, with small instruments, more and more can be done. The other trend is more computer guidance of procedures — and again we've started to see this: lasers, for example, always — or almost always — use computers to deliver precise amounts of energy to certain areas. Now, it's not very far to think that by extension you can have them direct beams of light to just be absorbed by certain tissues. When you combine the two — small incisions, more computer-guided procedures —, I think that's the future.

Interview: Richard Rushfield, Los Angeles

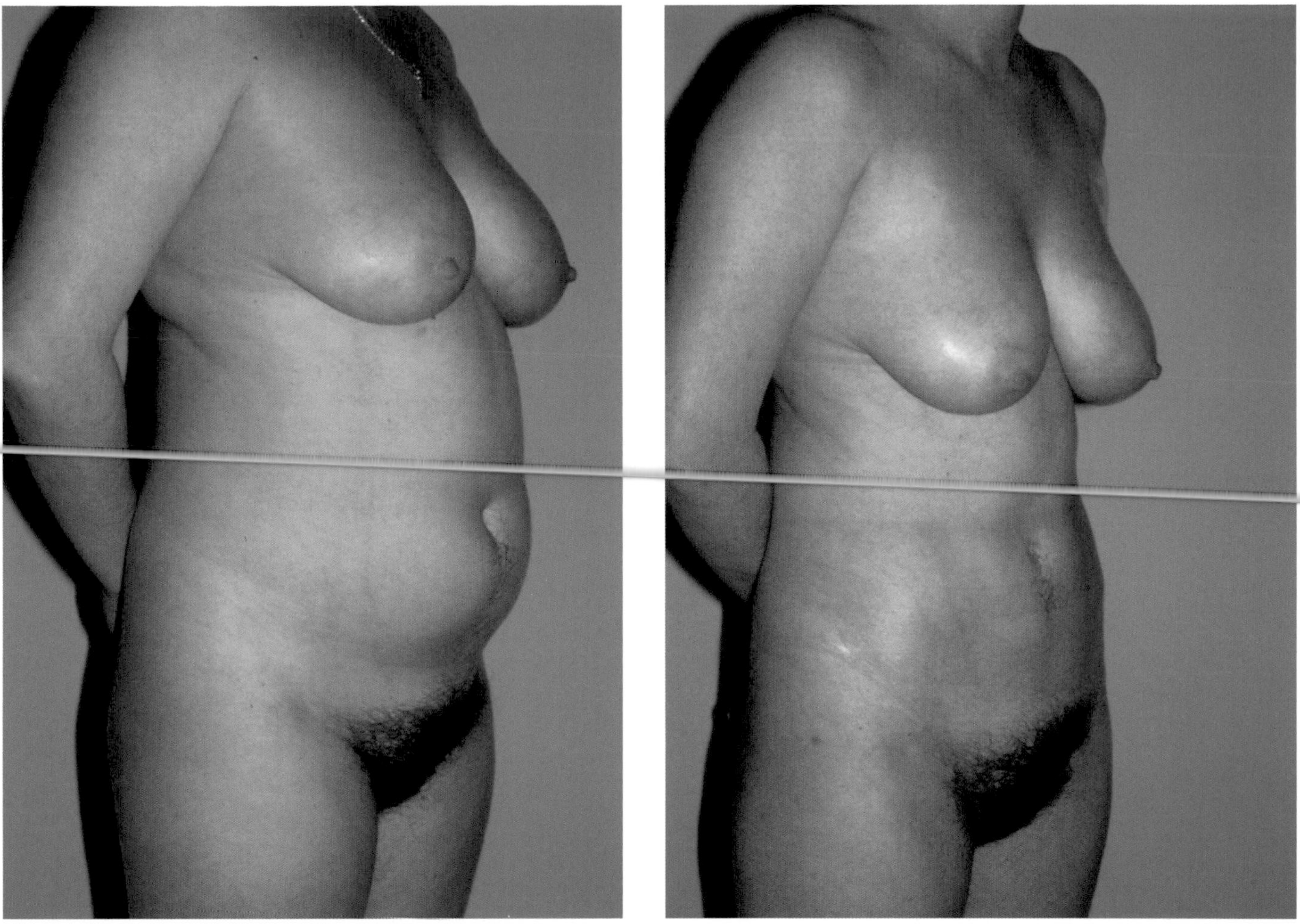

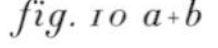

fig. 10 a+b

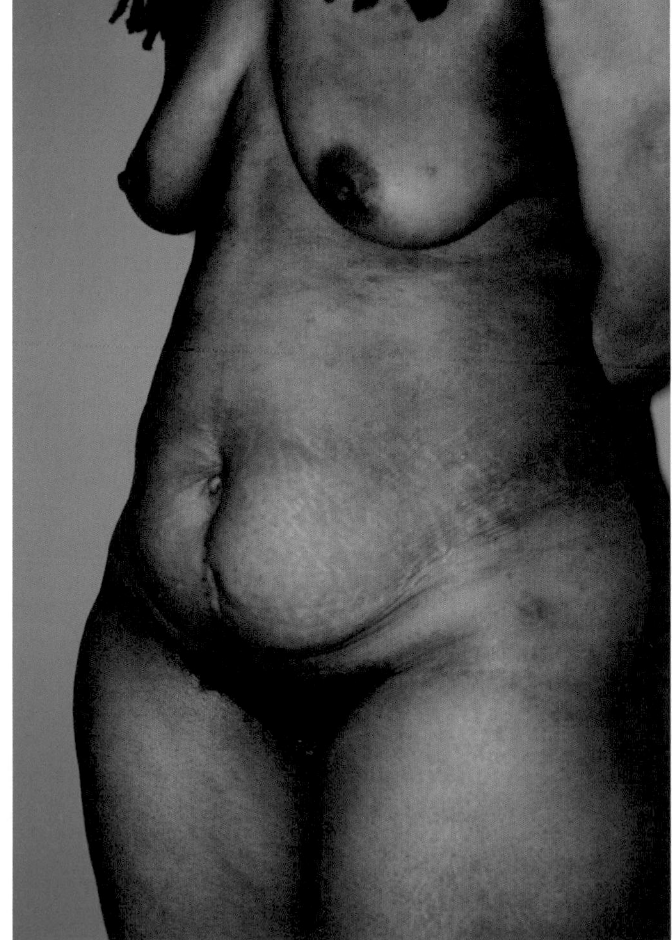

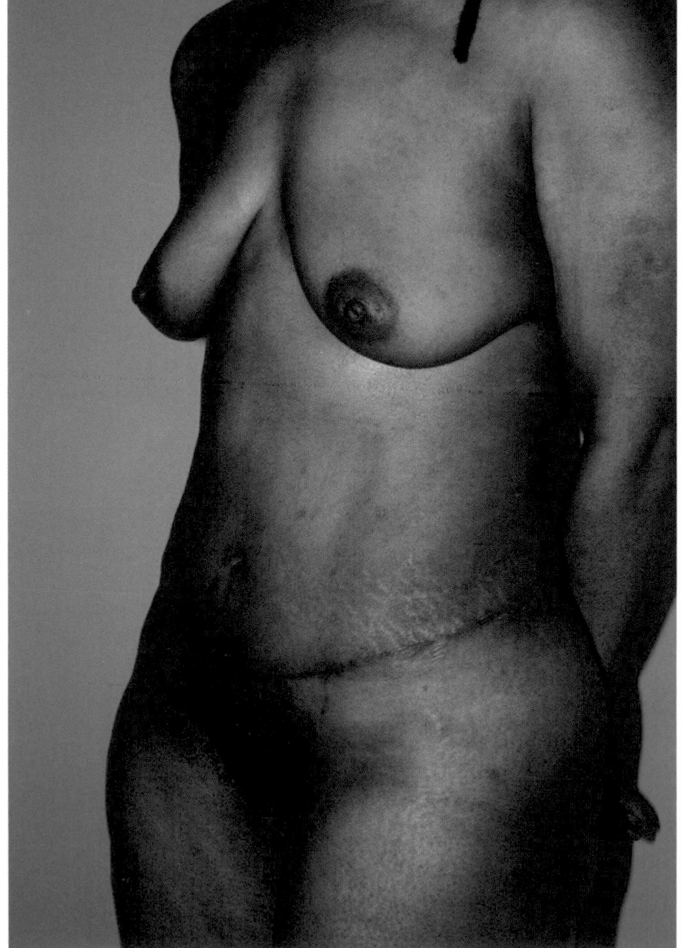

fig. 11 a+b

"There is always room for your imagination"

GERALD H. PITMAN, New York

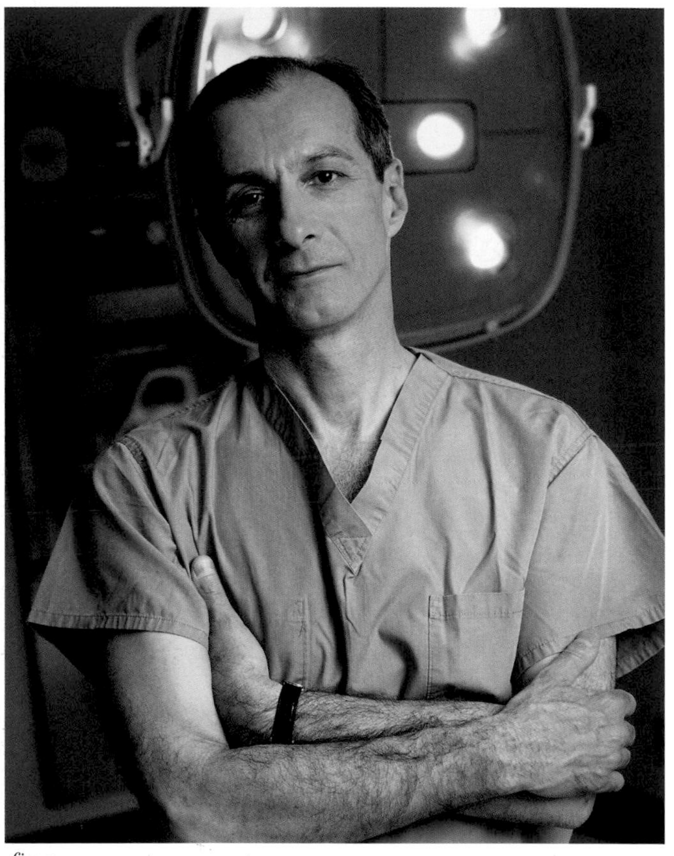

fig. 1

1. WHAT FASCINATES YOU MOST ABOUT BEING AN AESTHETIC SURGEON?

To me, aesthetic surgery is more intellectual and creative than other medical specialities, including some specialities that are traditionally considered intellectual, such as internal medicine. Psychiatry is the only speciality which has equal intellectual stimulation. In fact, I often describe what I do as "psycho-surgery," because I am operating to improve the patients' emotional state. I want to help them feel better about themselves. I love that what I do combines science, anatomy, medicine and artistry. Patients come to me with featural imperfections, and I translate in my mind's eye how the patients' underlying anatomy is expressed as a surface imperfection; and, then, design and execute an operation to correct the deformity. Aesthetic surgery is continually stimulating and still excites me every day.

2. WHAT IS YOUR SPECIALISATION?

I have two areas of speciality — facial rejuvenation and liposuction. I first became known for liposuction when I wrote a textbook on the subject. My goal in writing the textbook was to establish and promulgate a scientific basis for liposuction. In many ways, the textbook defined the field of liposuction and is still useful today, although I wrote it more than ten years ago.

Many of my liposuction patients retained me as their surgeon when they aged and wanted facial rejuvenative surgery. I was forced to consider this area of aesthetic surgery with the same rigorous scrutiny I gave to liposuction. My goal was to produce natural, long-lasting results. I believe I was successful, and now, my practice is evenly divided between facial and body. I have just published a chapter on face-lifts for the principal textbook of aesthetic plastic surgery in the United States.

3. DO YOU CONSIDER YOURSELF AN ARTIST?

Of course. As a plastic surgery resident-in-training, I took courses at the New York Art Students League. I particularly liked drawing, and still carry a sketch pad with me. Drawing the human form makes you look very carefully and precisely at human features. I have to absorb in my mind and eye all of the contours of the human face and body before I can commit them to paper. Drawing is a wonderful discipline and has certainly made me a better surgeon.

4. WHAT IS YOUR IDEAL BEAUTY? HOW WOULD YOU SEE THIS IN ART?

Beauty is certainly in the eyes of the beholder, and the beauty of the human face and figure, while timeless in many ways, is also subject to the dictates of fashion. In the 19th century, full-bodied, voluptuous women, such as those depicted in Renoir's "The Bathers" (Les Baigners), epitomised sexual desirability. In the early 21st century, a thinner, yet more muscular, athletic woman is the feminine ideal of beauty. The actress Uma Thurman is a good example.

For me personally, a very wide range of physical features can be beautiful. Much of beauty lies in the carriage and attitude of the object of desire.

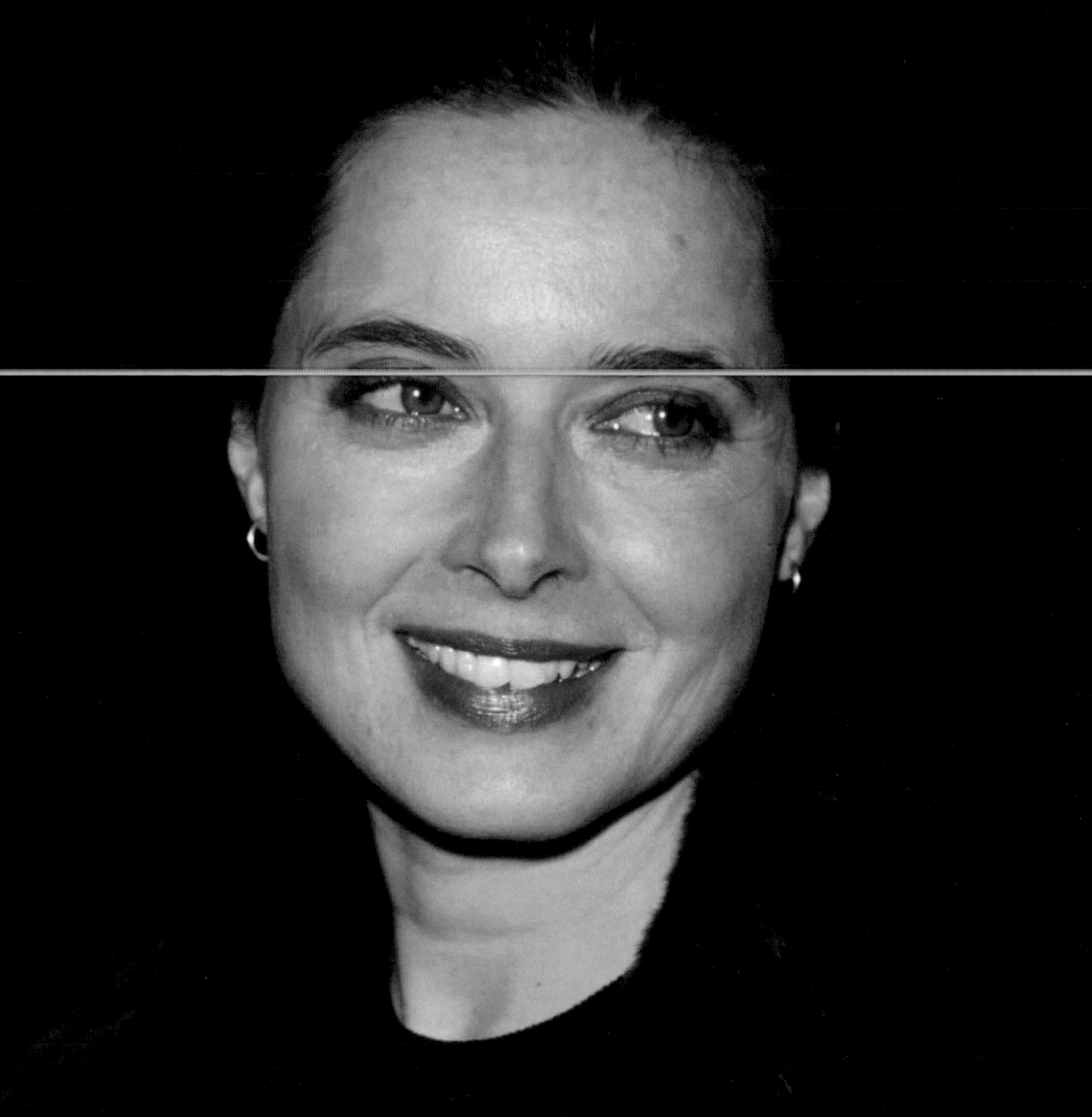

fig.2

fig. 1

Gerald H. Pitman in his private clinic operating theatre © Private archive Gerald H. Pitman M.D.

fig. 2

To Gerald H. Pitman, Isabella Rossellini is a striking beauty who combines both intelligence and sexuality. © Getty Images

fig. 3

Gerald H. Pitman and his wife, Nancy. © Private archive Gerald H. Pitman M.D.

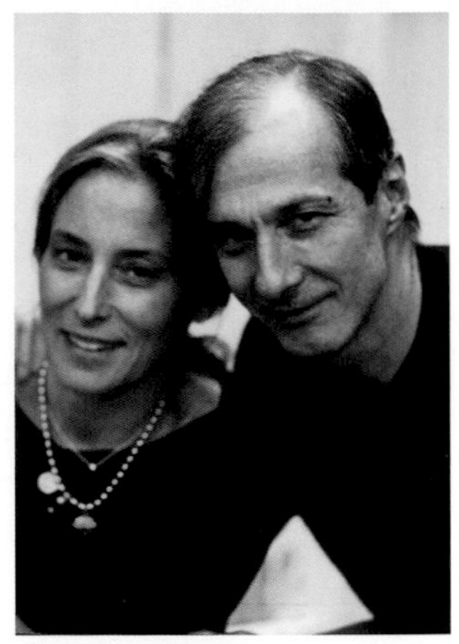

fig. 3

5. WHICH LIVING WOMAN AND/OR MAN ARE, FOR YOU, THE MOST BEAUTIFUL?

Isabella Rossellini is devastatingly beautiful. She combines intelligence and sexuality in a unique way. Penelope Cruz is elegant, yet has an underlying insouciance, which makes her irresistible.
Among men, Tom Cruise and Leonardo DiCaprio are quite opposite in appearance, but both exemplify rugged male sexuality and romanticism.

6. DO YOU BELIEVE YOURSELF TO BE ATTRACTIVE AND WHY?

Of course I consider myself attractive. I've never thought of myself as exceptionally handsome, but I'm happy with the way I look, and being happy with the way you look is essential to overall happiness. Notice I don't say "being beautiful is essential to happiness." I am saying something different. "Being happy with your appearance is essential to overall happiness." Why else would people go to plastic surgeons?

7. WHAT DOES AGING MEAN TO YOU?

Aging is the inevitable loss of youthful vigour and vitality. We all eventually have to face it. But now, at the beginning of the 21st century, the concept of aging is totally different than it was even 50 years ago. In the mid-20th century, 50 was old. Today, even 60 is not old for some people.
Men in their sixties and older compete in triathlons. Aging occurs later and later in life. People are not just living longer lives, but they're more active and healthier lives. One of the biggest segments of my patient population is middle-aged people who feel young and want to look as young as they feel. They want to bring their physical appearance into harmony with their youthful physiologic and emotional state.

8. HAVE YOU HAD AESTHETIC SURGERY AND WHAT PROCEDURE?

No, I haven't. I'm still happy with the way I look. But if ever I'm not happy, I'll do it in a heartbeat.

9. DID YOU PERFORM SURGERY ON YOUR WIFE/PARTNER OR CHILD, AND WHICH?

I would not perform elective surgery on an immediate family member. One of the essential requirements to being a good surgeon is to have complete objectivity and be dispassionate as you subject the patient to a surgical procedure. You can't be dispassionate if you're operating on a loved one.

10. CAN YOU AGREE TO EVERY DESIRE OF YOUR PATIENTS FOR CHANGE?

No. Some changes will not emotionally benefit the patient and some may be harmful. I refuse to operate on approximately ten percent of patients seeking consultation.

11. WHAT IS THE MOST EXCEPTIONAL DESIRE THAT YOU'VE EVER BEEN ASKED TO PERFORM?

I can't answer that question because it might identify the patient.

12. WHAT ARE THE REACTIONS OF YOUR PATIENTS AFTER THE OPERATIONS?

There are several reactions. I'll tell you the good ones. "Gee, it was nothing. You know, I thought it would be much worse. I thought I would have a lot of pain." Thankfully, most of the plastic surgery I do is only minimally painful.
As far as the physical changes resulting from the surgery, most patients love them. Plastic surgery has a magical quality to it.
Of course, not all operations turn out as planned, and occasional patients have complications. Before offering surgery, I always take time to explain the limitations and possible complications of the surgery as well as the expected improvements.
It would be impossible, however, for me to perform surgery on a regular basis unless most of my patients were happy and satisfied with the results. Typical comments from patients are, "Big change." "Changed my life. I feel much, much better." "Gee, I look great, I'm happy with it." "Thank you."

fig. 4 a+b

Patient of Gerald H. Pitman's before and after face lift, brow lift, eyelid operation and dermabrasion of lips. © Private archive Gerald H. Pitman M.D.

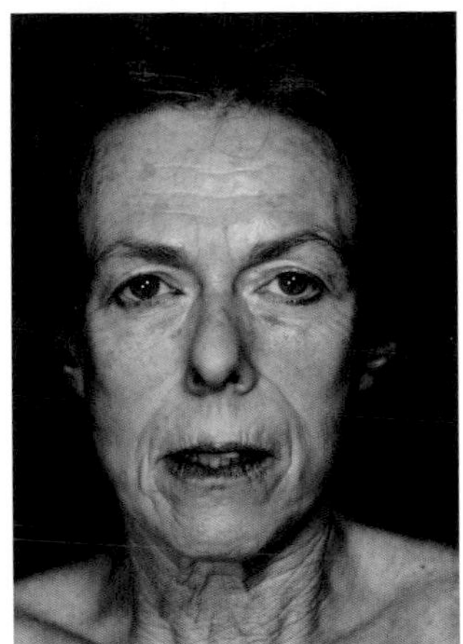

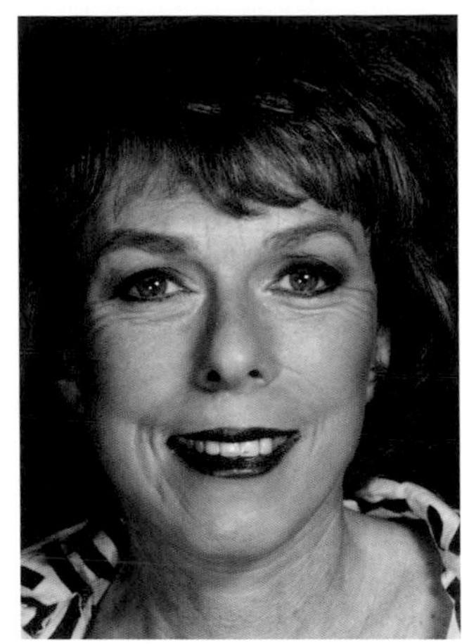

fig. 4 a+b

13. COULD YOU NAME YOUR FAMOUS CLIENTS?

No.

14. ARE YOU AFRAID OF BECOMING OLDER?

I'm not afraid of it. I'm very accepting of it. But I keep myself in terrific shape. And I believe being in good shape not only makes me feel better, but makes me a better person for my family and my patients.

15. DO YOU BELIEVE THAT BEAUTY COMES MAINLY FROM INSIDE?

Absolutely, yes. You are beautiful if you see yourself as beautiful.

16. DO YOU BELIEVE A MORE BEAUTIFUL PERSON IS HAPPIER AND HAS A BETTER LIFE?

No. Some very beautiful people have very unhappy lives. But it's a huge advantage to your self-esteem to consider yourself beautiful – not to *be* beautiful, but to *consider* yourself beautiful. Many people who have plastic surgery don't look much different after the surgery, but they feel different inside. They feel better about themselves. That's a huge advantage in life.

17. DO YOU THINK A BEAUTIFUL PERSON HAS A BETTER SEX LIFE?

Absolutely not. Beauty does not give you a better sex life. In fact, some very unremarkable looking people have active and gratifying sex lives. I once had a patient whom most people would consider homely. He was out of shape and overweight. His wife was similar, very plain. The first thing the husband said to me as I was putting his dressing on was: "How long until I can have sex with my wife?" I loved that! Sex was obviously an important and satisfying aspect of his life. You don't have to be beautiful to enjoy sex.

18. WHAT IS THE FUTURE OF AESTHETIC SURGERY?

The future of aesthetic surgery is in wellness centers – a more global and holistic approach to keeping people young and healthy. It's impossible to be beautiful if you're not healthy. Eat in moderation; exercise regularly; reduce stress in your life. Staying healthy permits you to be vigorous and active. A healthier population won't put plastic surgeons out of business. In fact, a healthier population will result in more people wanting aesthetic surgery to look as young as they feel.

Interview: Richard Rushfield, Los Angeles

"Our substance, the body, is divine"

JUAREZ AVELAR, São Paolo

1. WHAT FASCINATES YOU MOST ABOUT BEING AN AESTHETIC SURGEON?

Rebuilding the patient both physically and mentally. Every patient is a new challenge to me.

2. WHICH AREAS DO YOU SPECIALISE IN?

Ever since my residency and training in plastic surgery I was fascinated by several fields, however to create a new auricle was a challenge that intrigued me particularly. I was very concerned about all problems involving patients with severe physical abnormalities and the consequent suffering of their families. All these circumstances motivated me to devote a lot of time to research, in order to find a solution for each specific organic imperfection. In the last 30 years, I performed more than 800 ear reconstructions, published articles, took part in several international congresses and courses and I also published a book, "Creation of the Auricle". In aesthetic surgery, I predominantly do facelifts, rhinoplasty, breast surgery, abdominoplasty, eyelid corrections and liposuction.

3. DO YOU REGARD YOURSELF AS AN ARTIST?

Yes. This is a central issue. As well as our technical skill and our anatomical knowledge, we also need imagination, creativity and a sense of aesthetics. Otherwise, we cannot successfully practice our profession. Artists, however, can select the substance they work on, and also reject or change it. The material we work with is arguably divine. As we don't have alternative materials, we have an enormous responsibility in what we do with it.

4. WHAT IS YOUR CONCEPT OF BEAUTY?

My concept of beauty is based on the harmony between the face and the body — and I mean every single part of it. The nose, for example, should be in harmony with the proportions of the entire face. Brazil has practically dedicated itself to the beauty cult. This is, of course, due to the tropical climate, where going to the beach is a way of life, and our population has a very high proportion of young people. In my opinion, far too much attention is paid to the ideal figure and attractiveness. Current fads include large breast implants and buttock lifts. Aesthetic surgery is an ongoing media favourite, but really they should be focusing more on reconstructive surgery.

5. IN ART HISTORY, WHAT IS YOUR FAVOURITE NOTION OF BEAUTY?

Every historical period has a different beauty ideal with its own specific characteristics. I find them all very exciting, and I don't want to choose one above the others.

6. TO YOU, WHO ARE THE MOST BEAUTIFUL WOMAN AND MOST BEAUTIFUL MAN ALIVE?

I think Elizabeth Taylor was very beautiful for quite a number of decades.

7. DO YOU REGARD YOURSELF AS ATTRACTIVE?

Physically, I'm normal. But I believe I become attractive to people when they talk to me and get to know me.

8. WHAT DOES AGING MEAN TO YOU?

It's a wonderful process. I may not be as fit as 20 years ago, but I know that I have lived as intensely as I could.

9. ARE YOU AFRAID OF GETTING OLDER?

Not at all. I enjoy it. I'm a happy person. I have always made the best possible decisions for myself, and because of this, aging is a joy to me.

10. HAVE YOU EVER UNDERGONE AESTHETIC SURGERY YOURSELF? IF SO, WHAT WAS IT FOR?

Not yet. But I'm planning to get my eyelids worked on.

11. HAVE YOU EVER OPERATED ON YOUR WIFE/PARTNER AND/OR CHILDREN? IF SO, WHY?

Yes. I did a facelift for my wife.

12. CAN YOU JUSTIFY EVERY OPERATION AND PATIENT REQUEST, OR IS THERE A POINT WHEN YOU REFUSE TO DO AN OPERATION?

I generally refuse to operate on patients that have exaggerated expectations of the outcome. Some of them seem to believe that a successful operation could help them secure a new job or a new partner. These expectations are

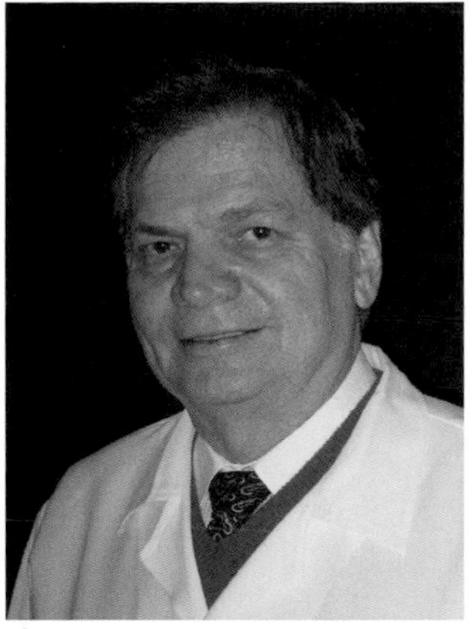
fig. 1

fig. 1

The body beautiful: Juarez Avelar works in Brazil, a country where physical beauty is cultivated with greater assiduity than almost anywhere else.

fig. 2

To Juarez Avelar, the youthful Elizabeth Taylor was one of the most beautiful women in the world. This photo dates from 1956 and shows Taylor as Leslie Lynnton in "Giant."

completely unrealistic. All we can do for our patients is to bolster their self-confidence.

13. WHAT IS THE MOST UNUSUAL REQUEST FOR SURGERY YOU HAVE ENCOUNTERED IN YOUR CAREER?

There are always patients that want to look exactly like another person — a celebrity or anyone else for that matter. But you can't increase your physical attractiveness by altering your facial features.

14. WHAT ARE YOUR PATIENTS' REACTIONS FOLLOWING SURGERY?

If the patients have understood the realistic possibilities of improving the physical harmony between their body and their face beforehand, they come out of the operation feeling satisfied. But if they have inflated expectations of aesthetic surgery, it can happen that the result of the operation does not match their preconceived ideas. It is crucial for us to assess the psychological state of a patient carefully in the consultation sessions preceding the operation.

15. COULD YOU NAME SOME OF YOUR MORE WELL-KNOWN PATIENTS?

No. My professional duty to maintain confidentiality prevents me from disclosing any names.

16. DO YOU BELIEVE THAT BEAUTY LARGELY EMANATES FROM WITHIN?

Yes. People have more self-confidence when they believe their appearance reflects their inner self.

17. DO YOU THINK THAT BEAUTIFUL PEOPLE ARE HAPPIER AND LEAD MORE FULFILLED LIVES?

Yes, I'm sure. A person who believes in his or her attractivity feels more self-confident, and also happier. This improves their life greatly.

18. DO BEAUTIFUL PEOPLE HAVE BETTER SEX?

The answer to this question is similar to the last answer. Again, when a person is more in balance with their inner self, their life as a whole improves. Among other things, this means they can enjoy their sexuality more fully.

19. WHAT DOES THE FUTURE HOLD FOR AESTHETIC SURGERY?

It's an open playing field. There are four kinds of patients that require our help: those with birth defects (which will sadly never be completely prevented), those with traumatic amputations, those whose skin, extremities or organs have been destroyed by cancer, and finally those who are aging. For all of them, we have to continue to search for the best possible solutions.

Interview: Eva Karcher, Munich

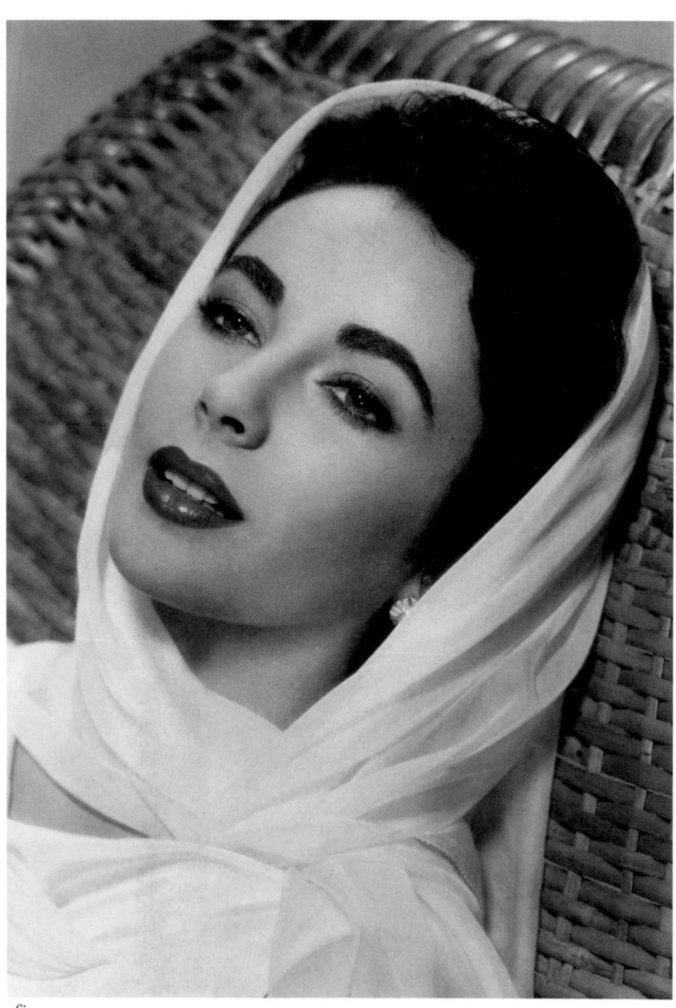
fig. 2

fig. 3 a–f

Anatomical disseccion on a female cadaver to demonstrate the level of subcutaneous tunnelization on face and neck. The vessels, nervs and connective tissues are preserved during the no traumatic procedure which is very useful to perform during rhytidoplasy (3 a-e). Photo during rhytidoplasty on a female patient showing the right side of the neck. The right ear is pulled forward and the cutaneous flap is pulled backward in order to expose the lateral side of the neck with preservation of all anatomical structures (3f).

fig. 4 a–f

Photo during rhytidoplasty on a female patient showing the lateral of the face on right side. The skin is already dissected showing all vessels preseeved (4 a). Photo during surgery showing the cutaneous flap is dissected all around the left ear (4 b).
The cutaneous flap is pulled forward in order to demonstrate that the vessels and nervs are preserved in order to provide good blood supply and natural sensitivity to the skin of the face after surgery (4 c).
Photo during rhytidoplasty on the right side of the face. The cutaneous flap is pulled forward to show the anatomical level of the operation (4 d).
One can see all vessels and nervs are preserved during surgery. Rhytidoplasty procedure is performed all around of the ear (4 e).
Suture of the muscles after cutaneous tunnelization which is very useful procedure during rhytidoplasty (4 f).

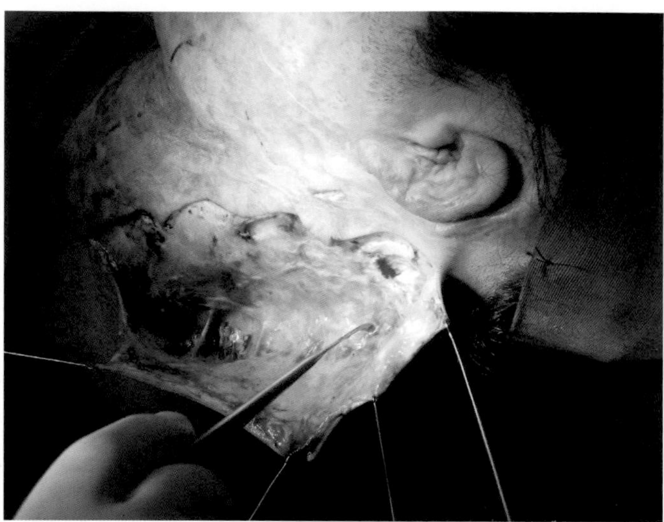

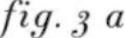

fig. 3 a

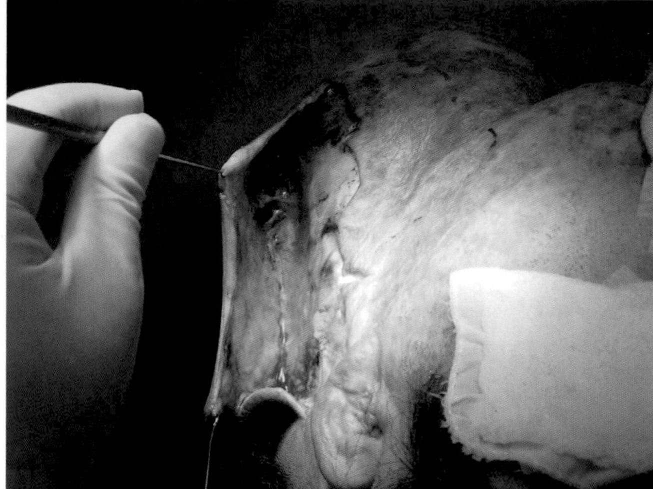

fig. 3 b

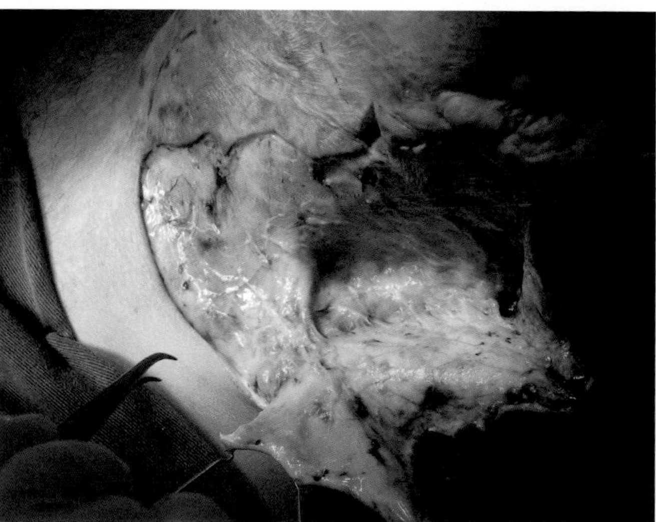

fig. 3 c

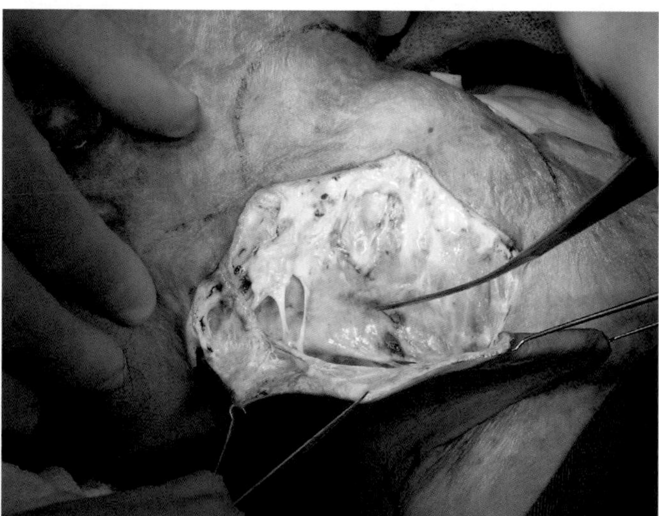

fig. 3 d

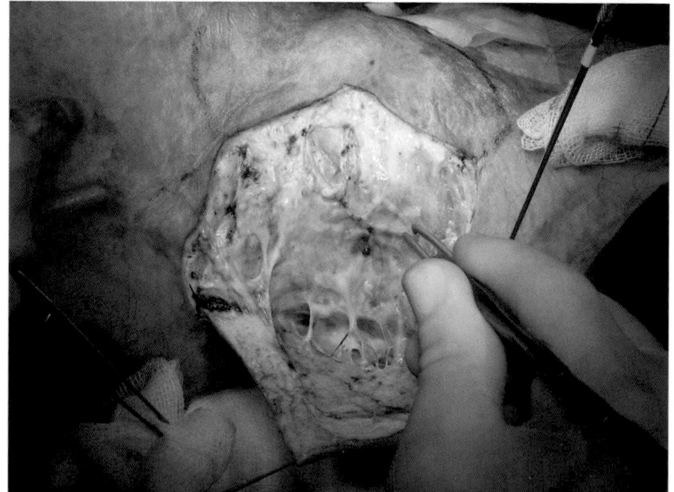

fig. 3 e

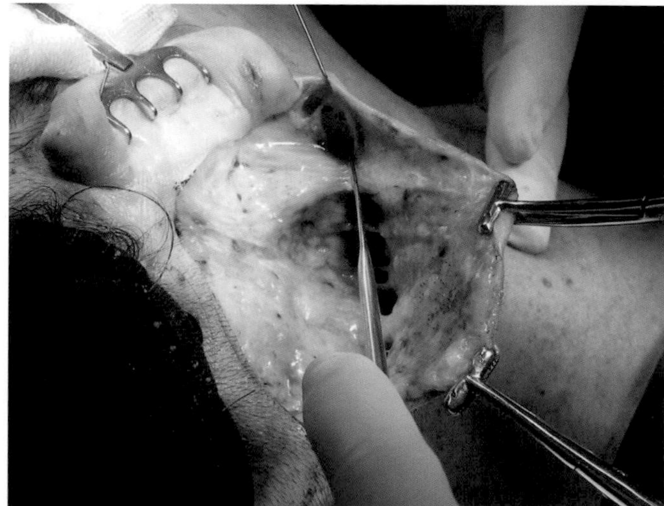

fig. 3 f

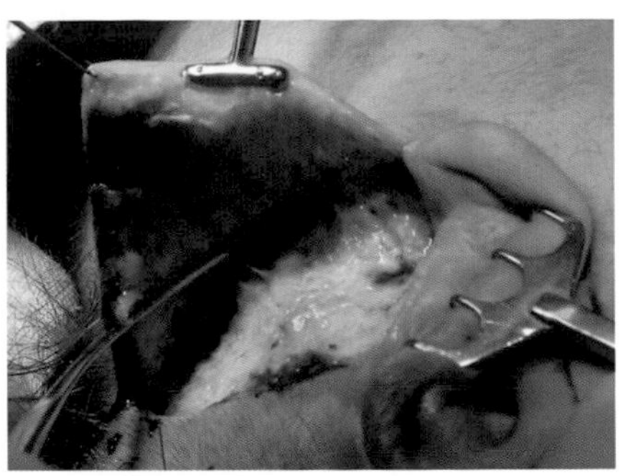
fig. 4 a

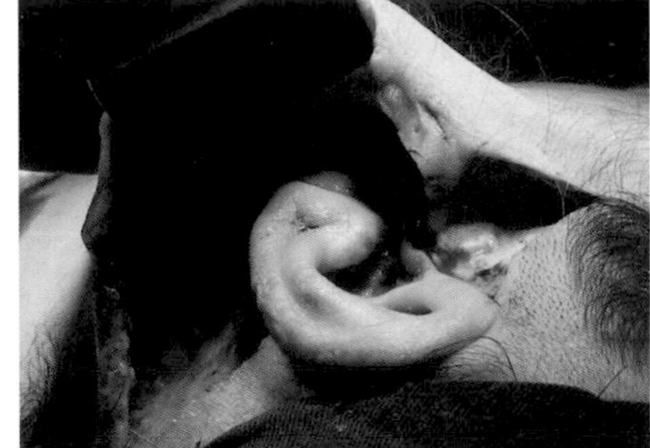
fig. 4 b

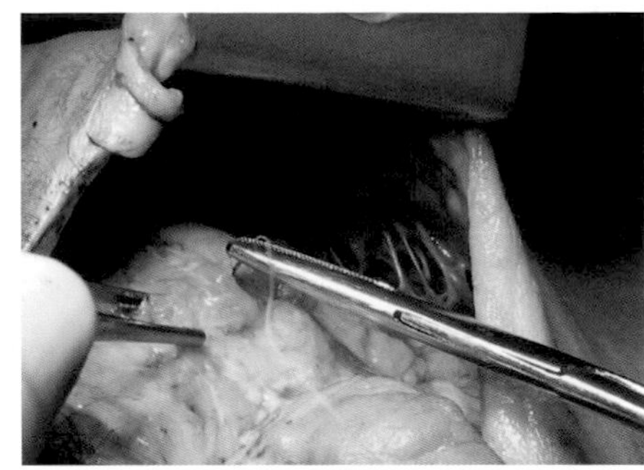
fig. 4 c

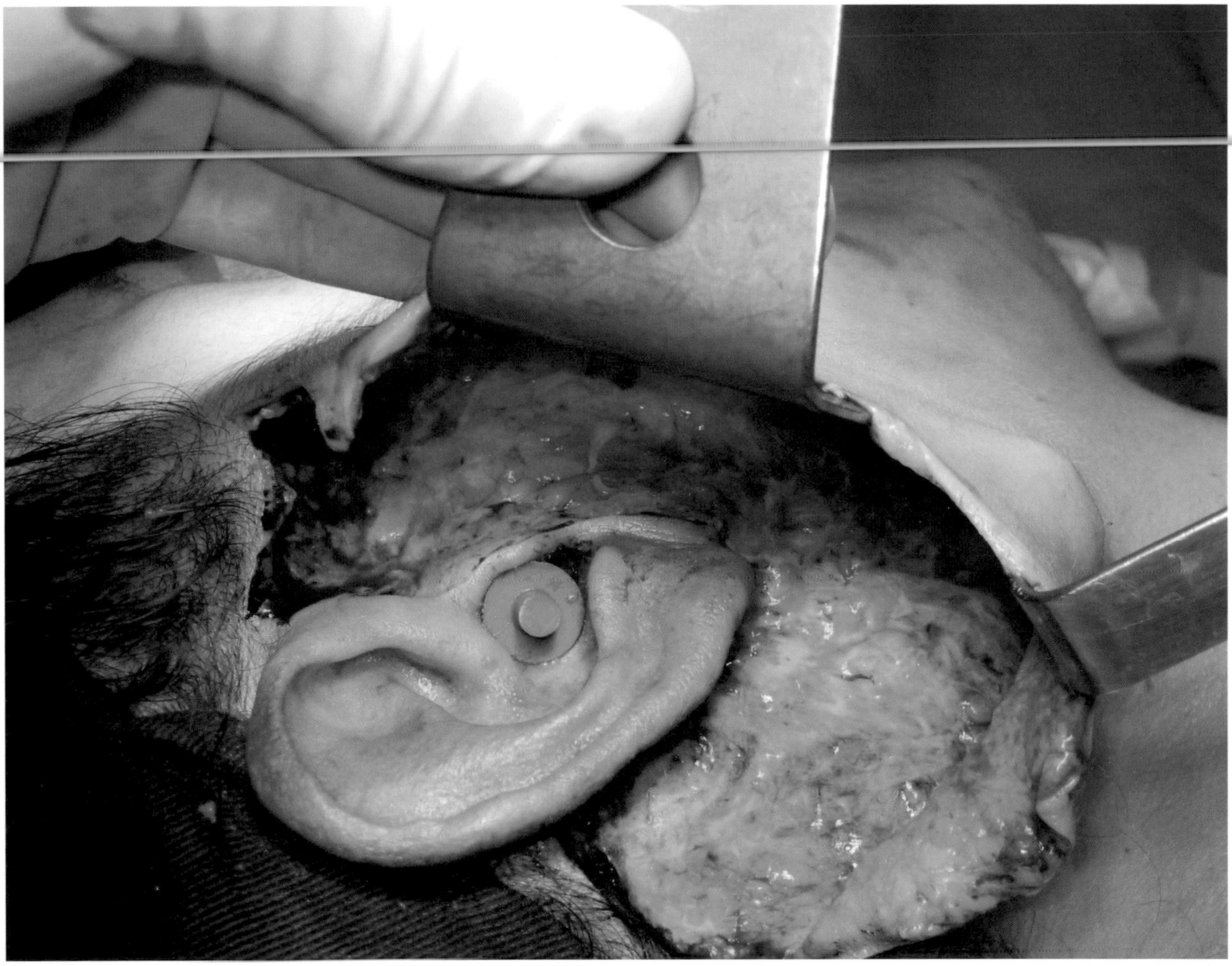

fig. 4 d

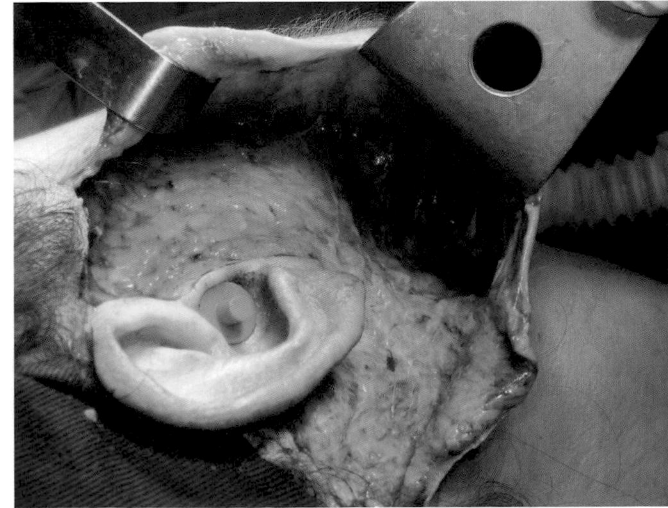
fig. 4 e

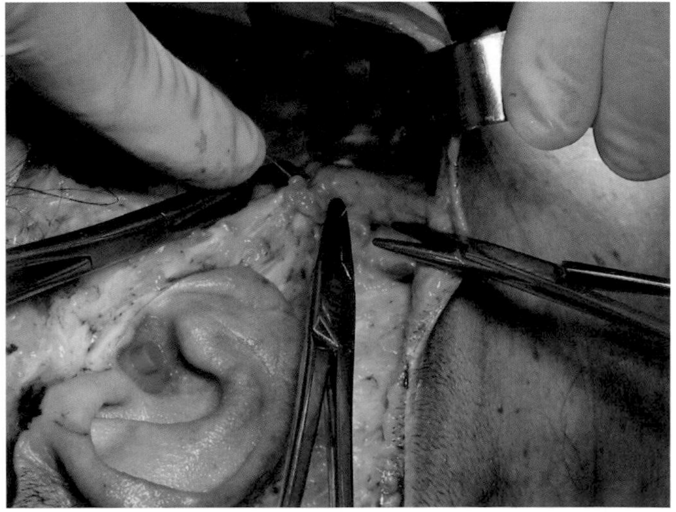
fig. 4 f

"Choose only one master – nature!"

JORGE HERRERA, Buenos Aires

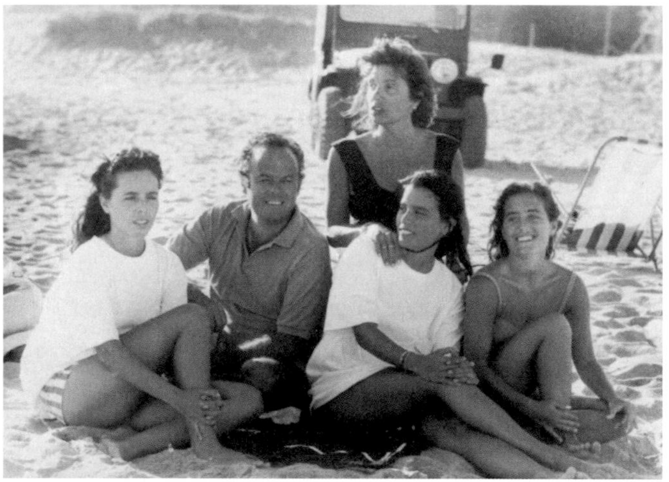
fig. 1

1. WHAT FASCINATES YOU MOST ABOUT BEING AN AESTHETIC SURGEON?

The same that fascinates me about being a reconstructive surgeon – the ability to help people and improve their quality of life. After more than 30 years of practising, I have also realised that my work has always made me happy because I've never stopped researching and learning. I am still able to refine my methods and techniques and achieve better results every year.

2. WHICH AREAS DO YOU SPECIALISE IN?

Breast enlargements and reductions, eyelid corrections, eyebrow lifts and facelifts, i. e. facial rejuvenation procedures. For breast reductions, I have developed a technique with minimal scar formation; furthermore, I have developed special peelings to smoothen wrinkles and creases, as well as a method to rejuvenate aged upper lips.

3. DO YOU REGARD YOURSELF AS AN ARTIST?

No. I am a medical professional. Unfortunately, our profession is being romanticised considerably by the media and to some degree also by our surgeons. Certainly some aesthetic surgeons are artists, just like some architects or lawyers make an art of their profession. But you don't need to be a good artist to be a good aesthetic surgeon or vice versa!

4. WHAT IS YOUR CONCEPT OF BEAUTY?

Proportion, balance and harmony. However, I'm not an art collector, despite being a great admirer of art and owning a number of works, especially of Spanish painters such as Garcia Uriburu, Galofre and Pergolla.

5. IN ART HISTORY, WHAT IS YOUR FAVOURITE NOTION OF BEAUTY?

I love the Renaissance. Take Leonardo da Vinci's world-famous drawing of the "Vitruvian Man," for example. To me, it brings together ideas from art, architecture, human anatomy and symmetry in one clear and complete image. This illustration is a symbol of the idea of perfect balance, which I see as the ultimate aesthetic principle.

6. TO YOU, WHO ARE THE MOST BEAUTIFUL WOMAN AND MOST BEAUTIFUL MAN ALIVE?

To me, beauty is not limited to external appearance. It only comes to life when coupled with intelligence, warmth, integrity, activity and charisma. This applies to women as well as men. Without these additional characteristics, beauty can be very blank and boring.

7. DO YOU REGARD YOURSELF AS ATTRACTIVE?

I've never thought much about this question – I haven't had the time!

8. WHAT DOES AGING MEAN TO YOU?

Like every other aspect of life, aging has its advantages and disadvantages. The inevitable processes of deterioration the body experiences and its drop in vitality are definitely disadvantages. The main benefit I can see is the opportunity to celebrate life in a new way: to be more relaxed, more balanced, and even a little wiser. It is often said that grandchildren can bring you more joy than your own children. Age is a question of attitude. I hope that my spirit will remain young and that I can continue to realise my projects and ideas.

9. ARE YOU AFRAID OF GETTING OLDER?

No. The only thing I could imagine being afraid of is losing my passion for life.

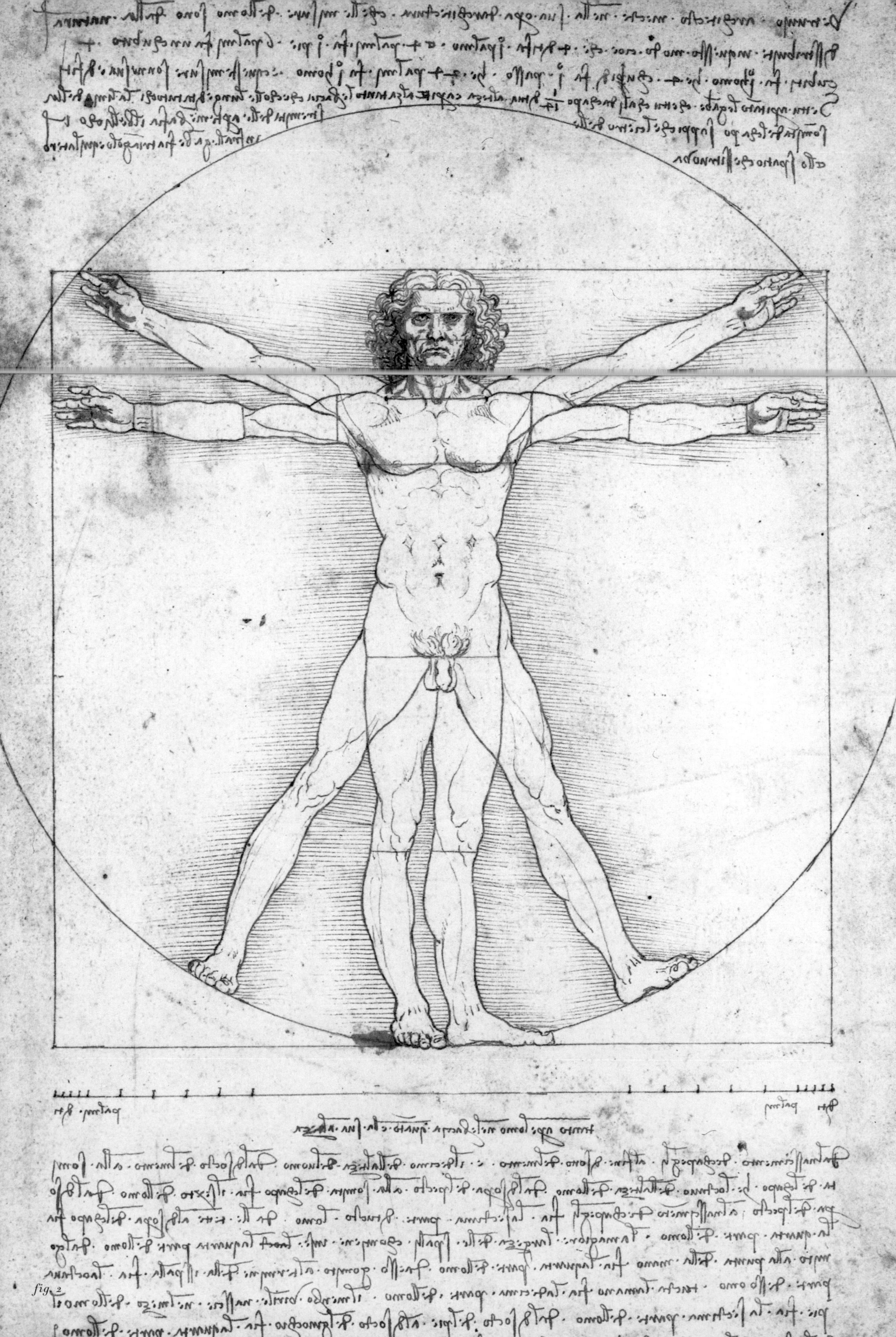

fig. 2

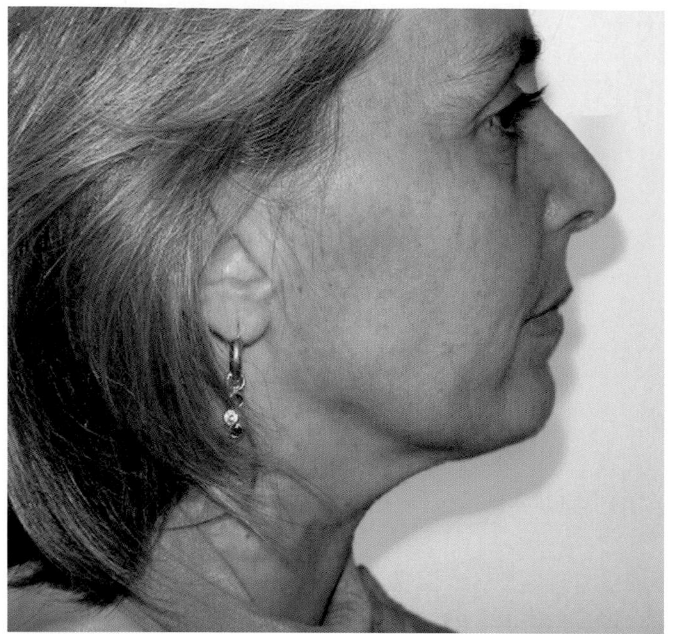

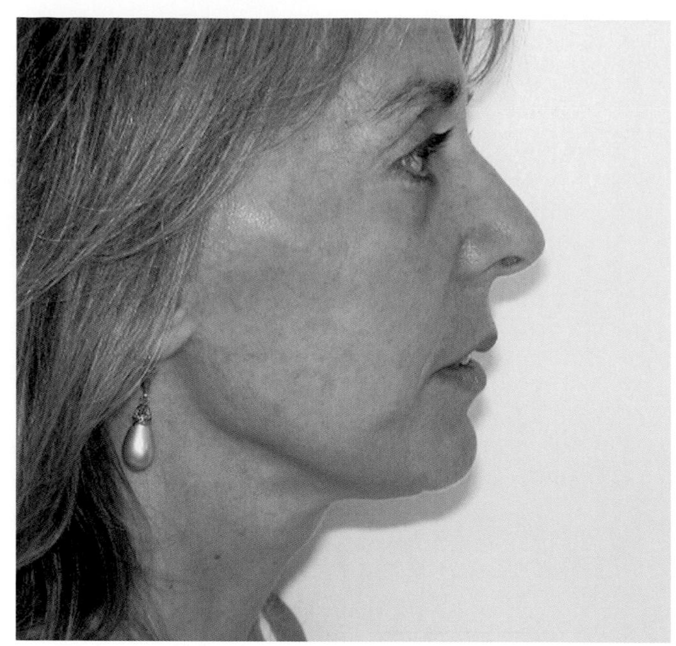

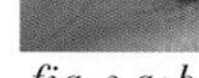

fig. 3 a+b

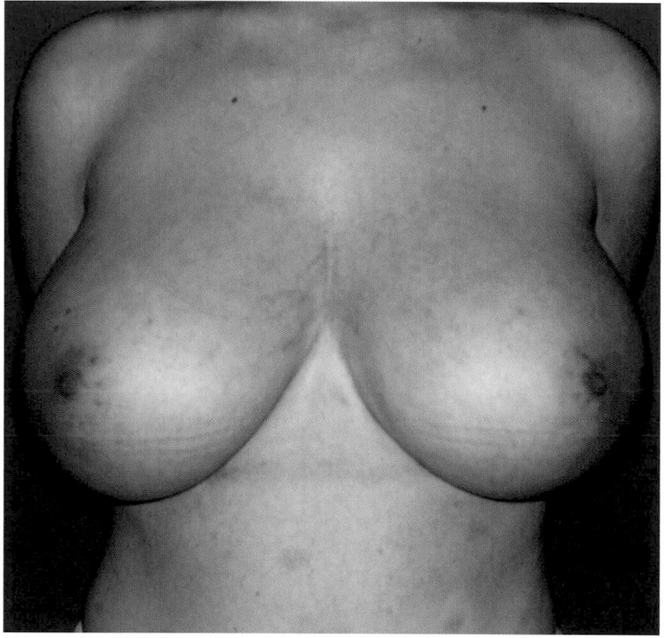

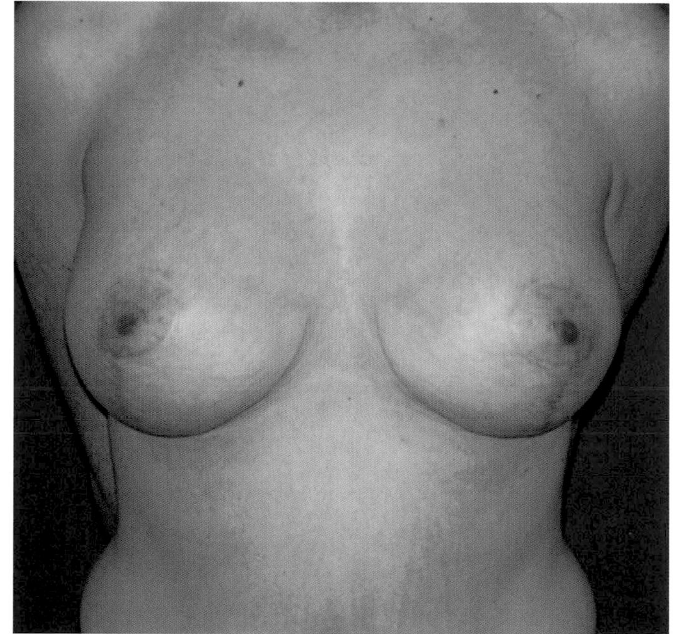

fig. 3 c+d

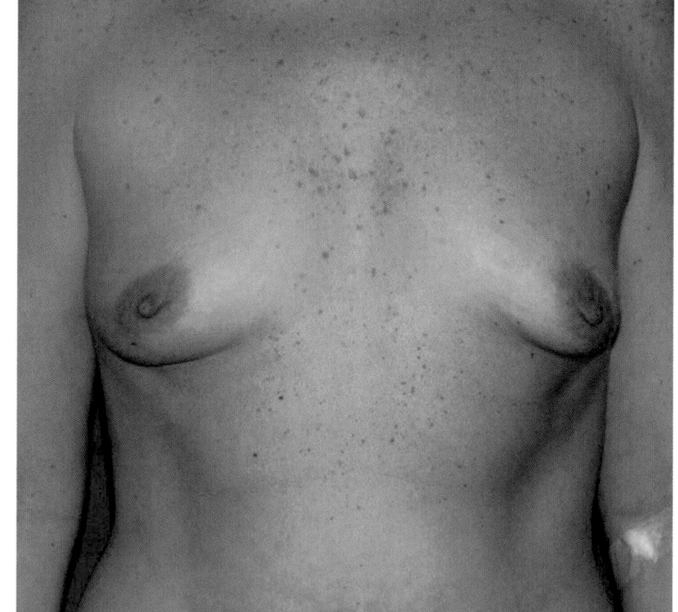

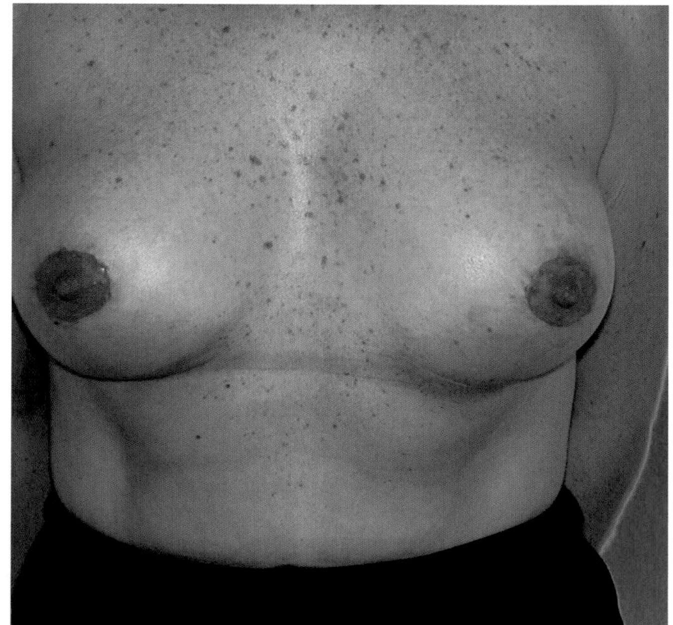

fig. 3 e+f

fig. 1

Jorge Herrera with his family. He is convinced that nature is the best source of beauty and inspiration. © Private archive Dr. Herrera

fig. 2

The sketch of the "Vitruvian Man" by Leonardo da Vinci (1452–1519) is the essence of "perfect balance" – the ultimate aesthetic quality in the mind of Renaissance enthusiast Jorge Herrera. © Venice, Galleria dell'Accademia

fig. 3 a–f

Jorge Herrera is a specialist for facelifts and breast reductions/enlargements. He has developed his own breast reduction technique with reduced scarring. © Private archive Dr. Herrera

fig. 4

"I'm a surgeon, not an artist," Jorge Herrera emphasises. "Unfortunately, our profession has been considerably romanticised by the media – and to some degree also by ourselves." © Private archive Dr. Herrera

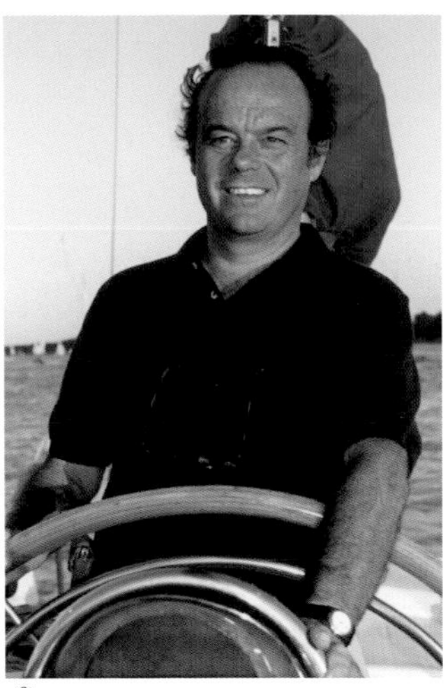

fig. 4

10. HAVE YOU EVER UNDERGONE AESTHETIC SURGERY YOURSELF? IF SO, WHAT WAS IT FOR?

No.

11. HAVE YOU EVER OPERATED ON YOUR WIFE/PARTNER AND/OR CHILDREN? IF SO, WHY?

My wife had a facelift and an eyebrow correction, and I did a breast enlargement for one of my daughters.

12. CAN YOU JUSTIFY EVERY OPERATION AND PATIENT REQUEST, OR IS THERE A POINT WHEN YOU REFUSE TO DO AN OPERATION?

Again and again, there are patients I try to convince that the procedure they are envisioning will fail. My talking is usually futile, but I never agree to operate on them.

13. WHAT IS THE MOST UNUSUAL REQUEST FOR SURGERY YOU HAVE ENCOUNTERED IN YOUR CAREER?

There haven't been any requests that were overly extreme. What I desire for every single one of my surgical patients is a result that is as natural-looking as possible. In this, I share Rembrandt's philosophy: "Choose only one master – nature." I am thoroughly convinced that nature is the best source of both beauty and inspiration. Aesthetic surgery should always follow nature's lead.

14. WHAT ARE YOUR PATIENTS' REACTIONS FOLLOWING SURGERY?

The most interesting final result and ultimate goal is to see patients strengthen their self-esteem considerably.

15. COULD YOU NAME SOME OF YOUR MORE WELL-KNOWN PATIENTS?

No.

16. DO YOU BELIEVE THAT BEAUTY LARGELY EMANATES FROM WITHIN?

I believe in a balance of interior and exterior beauty – beauty doesn't exist without the soul, regardless of the miracles performed by a plastic surgeon. Still, when I am presented with a charismatic person who has physical problems, I do my best to make him or her look more attractive.

17. DO YOU THINK THAT BEAUTIFUL PEOPLE ARE HAPPIER AND LEAD MORE FULFILLED LIVES?

What does that mean, "beautiful people"? Beautiful in comparison to whom? Beautiful for whom? Beauty only exists in the eye of the beholder, after all. I imagine that beauty can make a whole lot of things easier in life, but it certainly isn't the big jackpot for a happy, fulfilled life.

18. DO BEAUTIFUL PEOPLE HAVE BETTER SEX?

No. People who feel loved and accepted, and also accept themselves, have the best sex. Admittedly, however, attractiveness and being an object of desire can contribute quite significantly to a satisfying sex life.

19. WHAT DOES THE FUTURE HOLD FOR AESTHETIC SURGERY?

The possibilities of aesthetic surgery are boundless. As long as people continue to lose their physical suppleness and fitness with age despite an ever-improving array of preventive treatments, aesthetic surgery will remain indispensable. Techniques and technologies will become increasingly sophisticated, so problems can be addressed more quickly and reliably with more durable effects.

Interview: Eva Karcher, Munich

"Beauty has to touch us and take our breath away"

Woffles Wu, Singapore

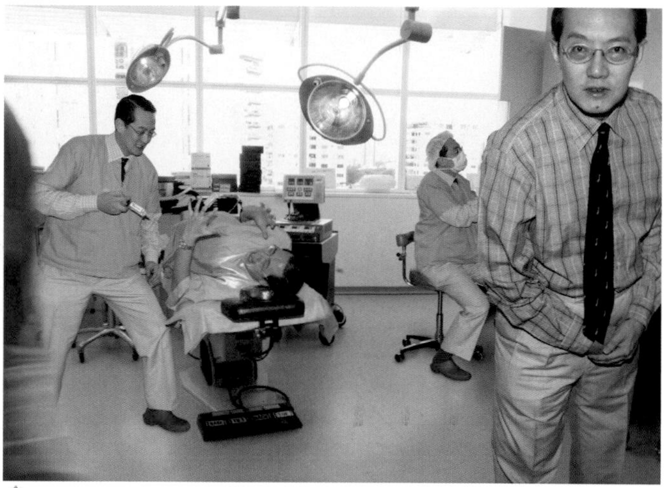
fig. 1

1. WHAT FASCINATES YOU MOST ABOUT BEING AN AESTHETIC OR COSMETIC SURGEON?

Aesthetic surgery incorporates art, architecture and medicine. It is fascinating to have the power to remodel a person's face, their body, and even their self-esteem. In a way, it's psychiatry with a knife. Being an aesthetic surgeon requires not only a high level of technical proficiency but also a great sense of responsibility, and ultimately also humility. What I love most about my work is to see the improvement in the patients' confidence, well being and relationship with others as they become more beautiful, younger looking and more whole. This is especially so when you see an introverted child with a hideous cleft lip deformity suddenly blossom into a vibrant, bubbly person after the lip and nose are corrected. It's like magic and sometimes I feel like a magician. (see fig.9 a+b)

2. WHICH AREAS DO YOU SPECIALISE IN?

I am originally a craniofacial surgeon specialising in facial contouring and rhinoplasty but over the years, I have developed a widely respected method of non-surgical facial rejuvenation using Botox, filler injections, IPL and laser treatments and a unique non-surgical facelift using specially designed barbed threads called "Woffles Threads". I call this the 4-R-Principle and it consists of four steps – "relax, restore, resurface, redrape." Firstly, I use Botox to relax the facial muscles that have become unattractive. Next, I restore the fullness of the face by injecting synthetic fillers into key areas. Then I resurface or retexturise the skin using innovative programs of Intense Pulsed Light and laser treatments, and finally I stretch and smoothen the facial and neck skin (redrape) using a special nonsurgical technique I developed called the "Woffles Lift": in this I insert unique, barbed "Woffles Threads" into the subcutaneous tissue of the face via a long needle and elevate and suspend these tissues to the dense tissue of the scalp.

I also specialise in breast enlargements, for which I have developed my own method called the Invisible WW Stealth Technique which places a zigzag incision on the areola margin, making the resultant scar imperceptible.

I also frequently do breast enlargements, for which I have developed my own method as well.

3. DO YOU REGARD YOURSELF AS AN ARTIST?

Totally! Without a deep passion for beauty, form and harmony, as well as the balance between them, I couldn't possibly do what I do! I love Modernist art and contemporary art, the sculptures of Henri Moore, Alexander Archipenko, Constantin Brancusi, Ju Ming and Zhan Wang, but also the paintings of Pablo Picasso, Fernand Léger, Le Corbusier, Andy Warhol, Roy Lichtenstein and James Rosenquist. Surrealism is less important to me, although I very much admire René Magritte and Giorgio de Chirico. I used to collect mostly paintings, but my focus has recently shifted to sculpture. I enjoy their three-dimensionality and physicality, and they are great in the garden. I'm also becoming increasingly fascinated with contemporary art from China which is challenging and politically charged. I have myself been working on a series of psycho-erotic works on Chinese paper for the last 20 years and will be having a major retrospective exhibition next year as well as a commemorative book chronicling my art.

4. WHAT IS YOUR CONCEPT OF BEAUTY?

I don't have one. In the face, beauty is all about symmetry, proportions, balance and harmony. Naomi Campbell, Kate Moss, Maggie Cheung and Iman are all beautiful, but in completely different ways. Iman's nose in Elizabeth Tay-

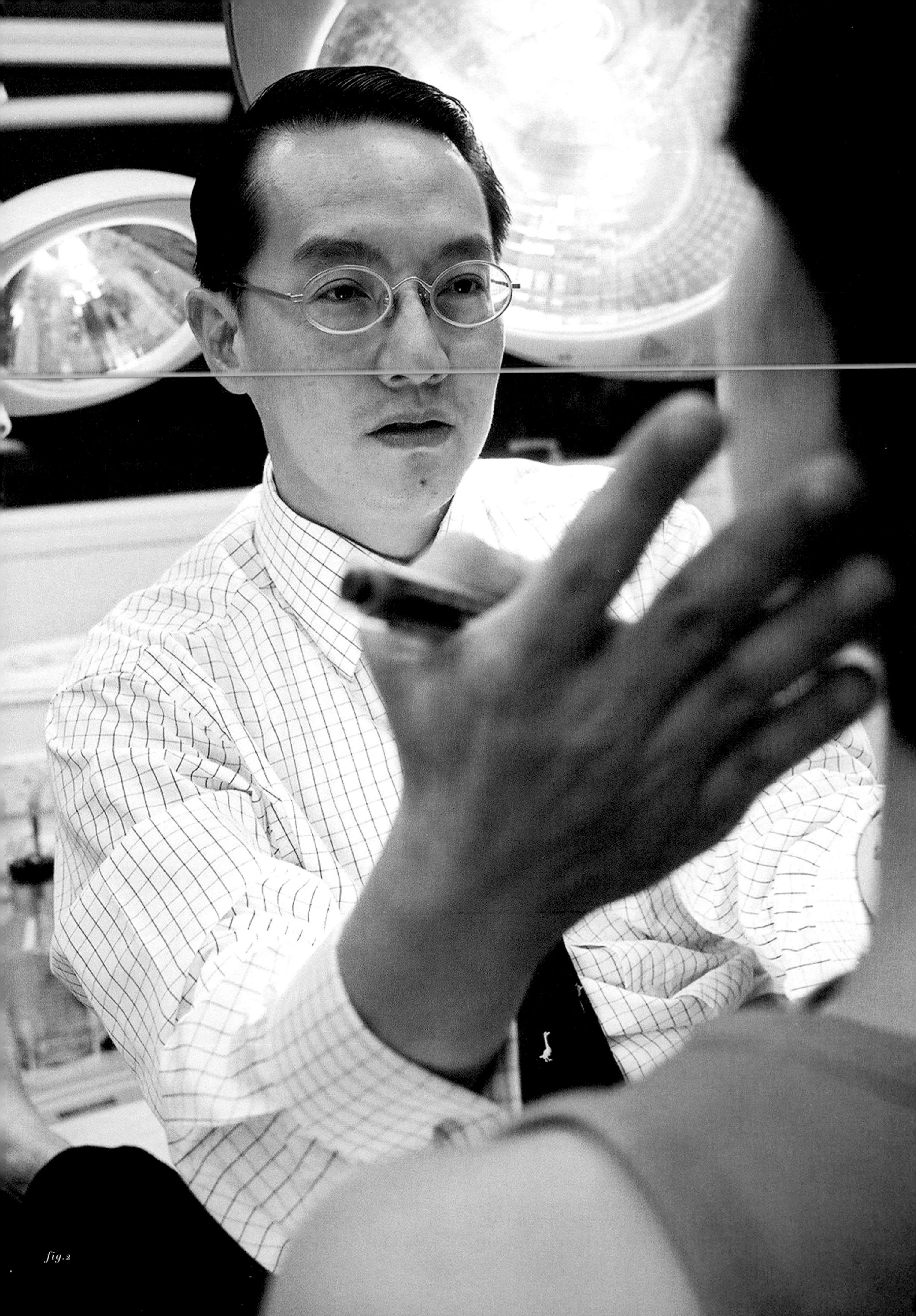

fig.2

fig. 1

Woffles Wu at his practice in Singapore, where he operates on numerous international clients. © Private archive Dr. Woffles Wu

fig. 2

Woffles Wu has developed his own technique for facial rejuvenation, popularly known as the "Woffles Lift." The technique consists of four completely non-invasive stages, employing Botox, laser treatment and injections. © Private archive Dr. Woffles Wu

fig. 3

Sandro Botticelli's "Birth of Venus" (c. 1482) in the Galleria degli Uffizi. © akg-images / Erich Lessing

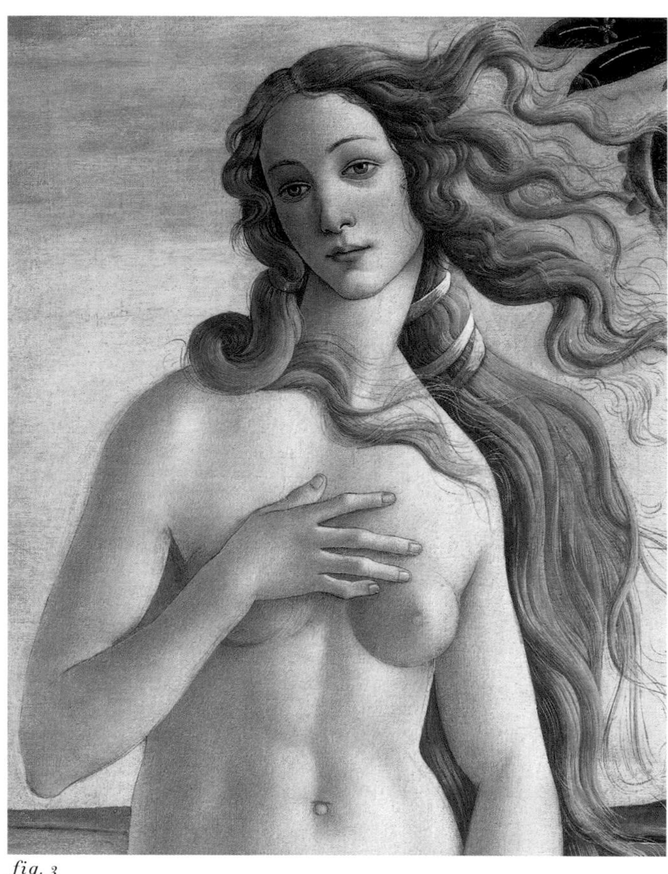

fig. 3

lor's face would look terrible and vice versa. I think that beauty has to touch us and take our breath away. True beauty is more than good looks, it has an ethereal, enchanting, spiritual and almost divine dimension. And it is very rare. Beauty is a phenomenon that is difficult to capture in words, but when we see it, we recognise it instinctively.

In architecture and interior design however, asymmetry may be more appealing than symmetry, take Frank O. Gehry's Guggenheim in Bilboa for example.

5. IN ART HISTORY, WHAT IS YOUR FAVOURITE NOTION OF BEAUTY?

I like feminine, sensual women with sex appeal- not skinny, skeletal women! My notion of beauty is best illustrated by Sandro Botticelli's "Birth of Venus." Michelangelo's "Pietà" possesses a similar symmetry and harmony. In contrast to these, I never thought the "Mona Lisa" to be very beautiful – she's too masculine and not at all erotic. I would be frightened to go to bed with her!

6. TO YOU, WHO ARE THE MOST BEAUTIFUL WOMAN AND MOST BEAUTIFUL MAN ALIVE?

Elizabeth Taylor and Ava Gardner when they were young. Of the current beauties, my picks are Penelope Cruz, Naomi Campbell, Kate Moss and Iman. In my eyes, the most beautiful man of all times was Elvis Presley. He had a seductive face, soft and masculine at the same time. Of today's men, I regard Tom Cruise, Johnny Depp and Jude Law as particularly attractive.

7. DO YOU REGARD YOURSELF AS ATTRACTIVE?

I've never thought of myself as attractive but I guess I must be because many people tell me so. They say I belong in a 1930's movie. I would say I am attractive but not in a startling, handsome way. I have a clear-cut face, expressive eyes and a well-trained body. But I don't think my looks are above average.

8. WHAT DOES AGING MEAN TO YOU?

The face and body becoming wrinkled, with dry, papery skin. It also means becoming clumsy, losing strength, concentration, memory, energy and, most scarily of all, virility.

9. ARE YOU AFRAID OF GETTING OLDER?

Yes. I'm especially scared of losing my vitality and not being able to do what I want. This thought is more frightening than the thought of my external attractiveness dwindling.

10. HAVE YOU EVER UNDERGONE COSMETIC SURGERY YOURSELF? IF SO, WHAT WAS IT FOR?

I've already started on non-invasive treatments. I inject Botox into my brow and fillers into my lips and cheeks. I use a combination of laser treatments, microdermabrasion, Radiofrequency therapy, chemical peelings and *fig. 4, 5, 6*

Woffles Wu considers Iman, Naomi Campbell and Kate Moss to be among the world's most beautiful women. To him, these women possess more than good looks; they also have plenty of spirit. © Getty Images (4,5), O'Neill Terry / CORBIS SYGMA (6)

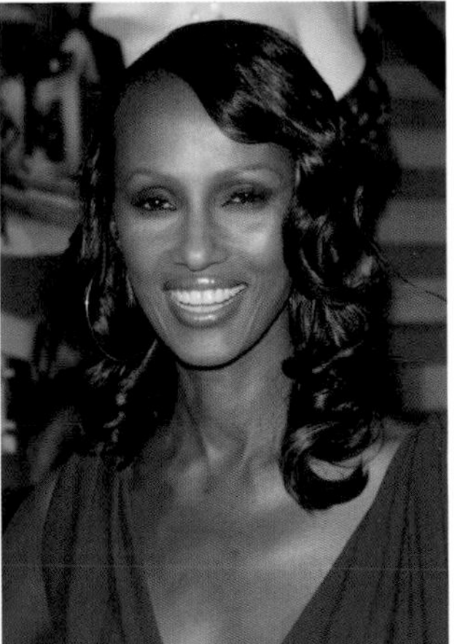

fig. 4

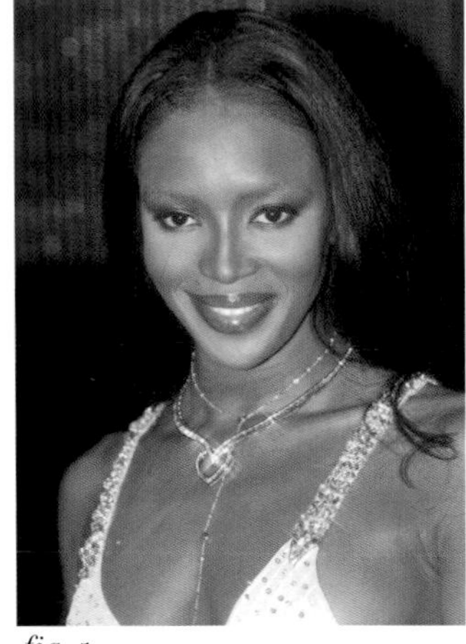

fig. 5

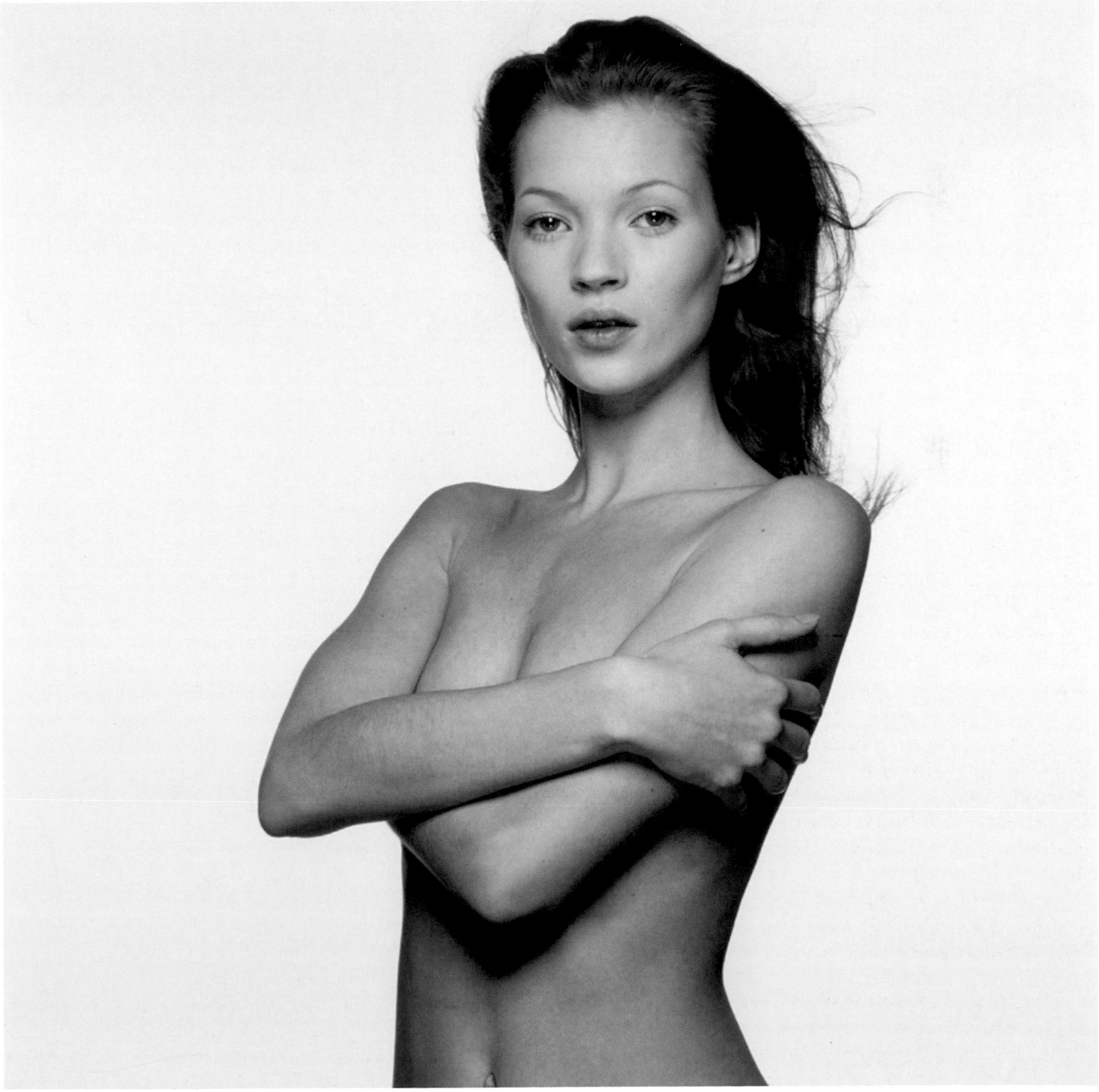

fig. 6

fig. 7 a+b, 8 a+b, 9 a+b

As well as purely aesthetic surgery, Woffles Wu also performs reconstructive operations. This is a selection of before/after photographs of patients with harelips. After the procedure, the upper lip and nose are fully separate and properly shaped – with almost no scars. © Private archive Dr. Woffles Wu

beauty creams to preserve the tension of my facial skin. I had my nasal septum straightened 25 years ago.

11. HAVE YOU EVER OPERATED ON YOUR WIFE/PARTNER AND/OR CHILDREN? IF SO, WHY?

My wife receives the same treatments as me. She also wants me to work on her breasts and tummy, should it become necessary, and do a "Woffles lift" on her face.

12. CAN YOU JUSTIFY EVERY OPERATION AND PATIENT REQUEST, OR IS THERE A POINT WHEN YOU REFUSE TO DO AN OPERATION?

I do some times turn away patients who have irrational requests or don't understand the limitations of plastic surgery. Some of these may suffer from Body Dysmorphic Disorder (BDD), which means they only imagine that they are ugly; no treatment could ever satisfy them. Others want to look exactly like somebody else, which often implies an infatuation or lack of maturity in which case their satisfaction with the eventual results may be shortlived. By and large, most patients today know from the information cycle what plastic surgery can and cannot do for them and are fairly realistic about their expectations.

13. WHAT IS THE MOST UNUSUAL REQUEST FOR SURGERY YOU HAVE ENCOUNTERED IN YOUR CAREER?

A 19-year-old girl desperately wanted me to make her look like an Alien – with square eyes, an enlarged head, fairy-like ears, a sloped brow, a pointed nose and narrower cheekbones. I sent her to a psychiatrist to find out what was bothering her.

Then there was a short, overweight, dark-skinned man with a Southern Indian face – he wanted to look like Brad Pitt, even the skin colour. I explained to him it was just imposible and sent him away. He returned the next day having lightened his skin tone with make-up and wearing a blond wig! Obviously, I refused to work on him.

14. WHAT ARE YOUR PATIENTS' REACTIONS FOLLOWING SURGERY?

They are generally surprised how well it went, they are very grateful and their self-esteem improves – which is evident in their body language, their make-up and in the way they dress. Breast enlargements in particular make shy, timid women very confident, almost overnight.

15. COULD YOU NAME SOME OF YOUR MORE WELL-KNOWN PATIENTS?

I can't, for ethical reasons. I can tell you however that some of my patients feel quite at home on the red carpet at the Oscars.

16. DO YOU BELIEVE THAT BEAUTY LARGELY EMANATES FROM WITHIN?

Certainly! The inner core of a person is where true beauty resides but unfortunately many people don't get beyond the exterior shell because this is what attracts or repels first. This is where our profession can help. Of course there are many beautiful people who appear cold, dull or superficial. Beauty is always a mixture of interior and exterior qualities – this is a well-known fact.

17. DO YOU THINK THAT BEAUTIFUL PEOPLE ARE HAPPIER AND LEAD MORE FULFILLED LIVES?

This is often the case, because they receive more compliments which is ego and confidence boosting. This makes them more self-confident, and as we all know, self-confidence is the key to success which in turn breeds a form of happiness. However, some people become obsessed with the pursuit of beauty because of what it represents and the promises it may fulfil: a better life, better spouse, better career. I don't think these people are realistic and I find they are often not happy.

18. DO BEAUTIFUL PEOPLE HAVE BETTER SEX?

Not necessarily. I'm sure they receive more offers, and often will end up having more sex than the average person but more often than not, this will make things more complicated and the sex may not necessarily be better. In many cases, they cannot actually fulfil the sexual promise suggested by their beautiful face. Beautiful people are also more easily exploited.

19. WHAT DOES THE FUTURE HOLD FOR COSMETIC

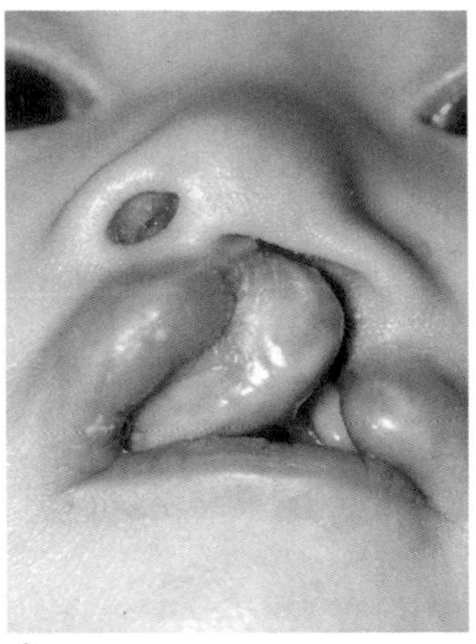

fig. 7 a

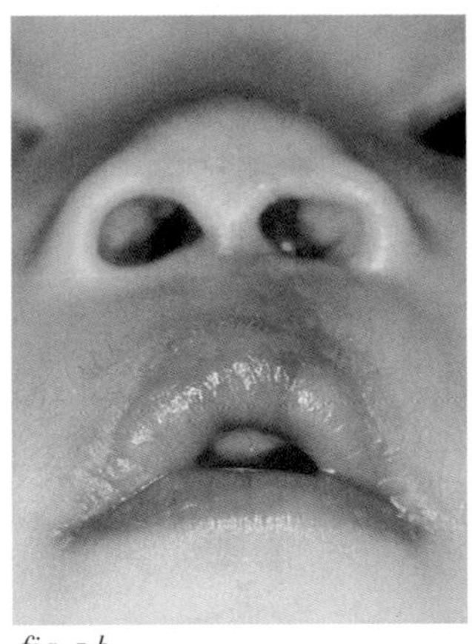

fig. 7 b

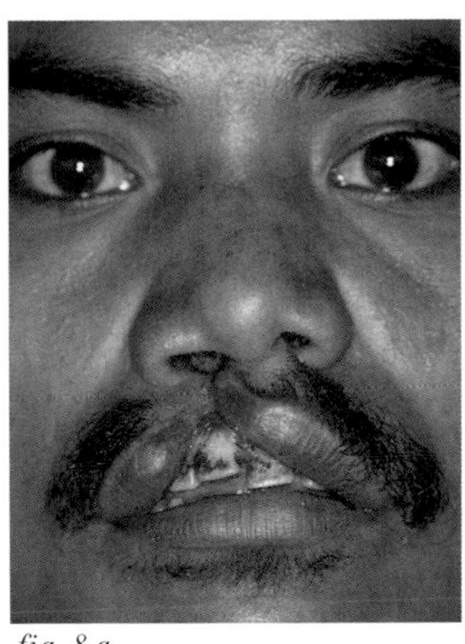

fig. 8 a

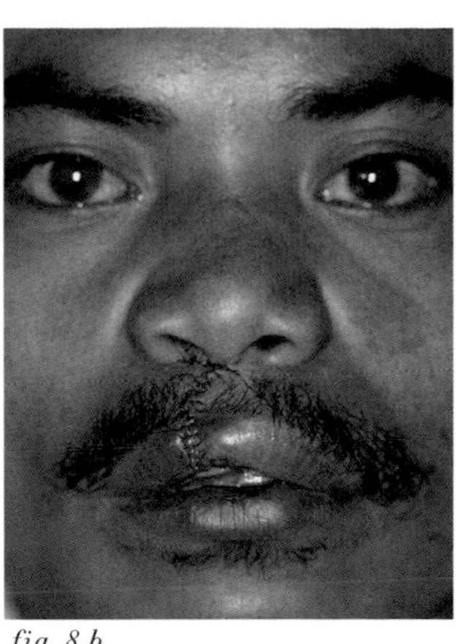

fig. 8 b

SURGERY?

It will be predominantly non-invasive and without scars. More and more people will demand cosmetic procedures but will want to spend less time on them. I believe my "Woffles lift" will revolutionise facial rejuvenation! In terms of aesthetics, I think the so-called "global" look will be prevalent, a look I also describe as "pan-ethnic." It fuses the European and Asian concepts of beauty, featuring a straight nose, large, almond-shaped eyes, high cheekbones and full lips.

Interview: Eva Karcher, Munich

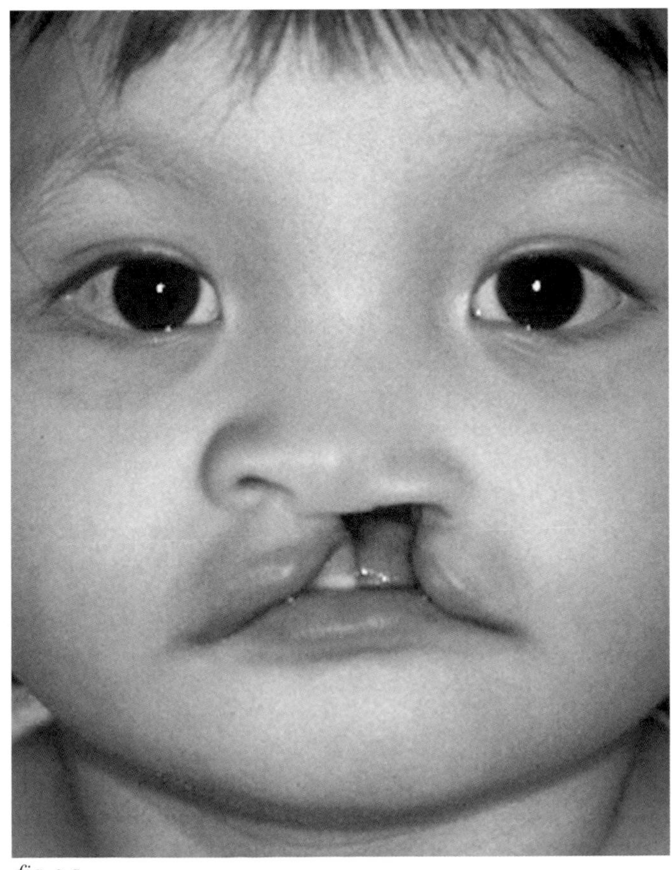

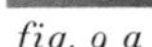

fig. 9 a

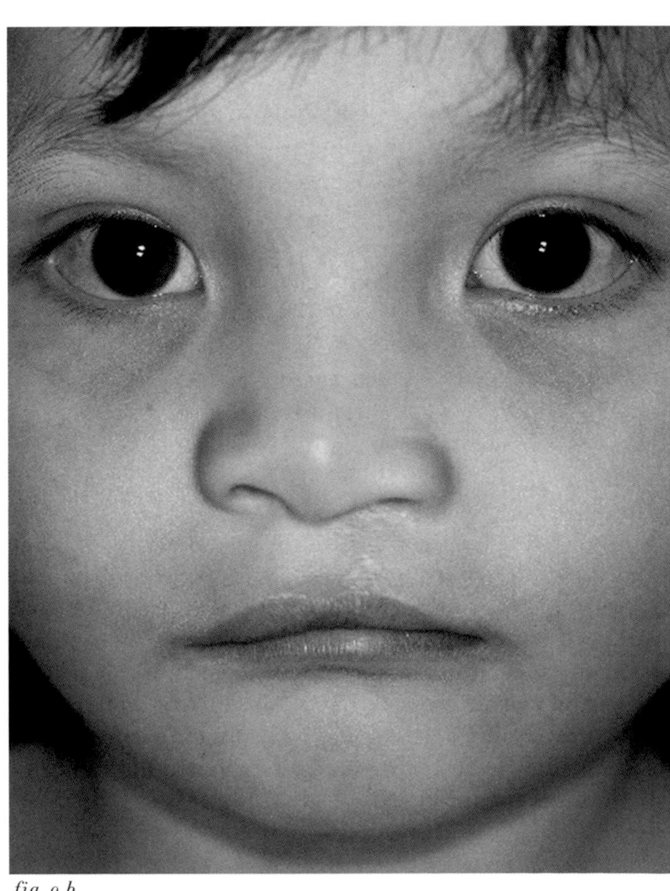

fig. 9 b

"A beautyful face is more than the sum of its attractive parts"

KEIZO FUKUTA, Tokyo

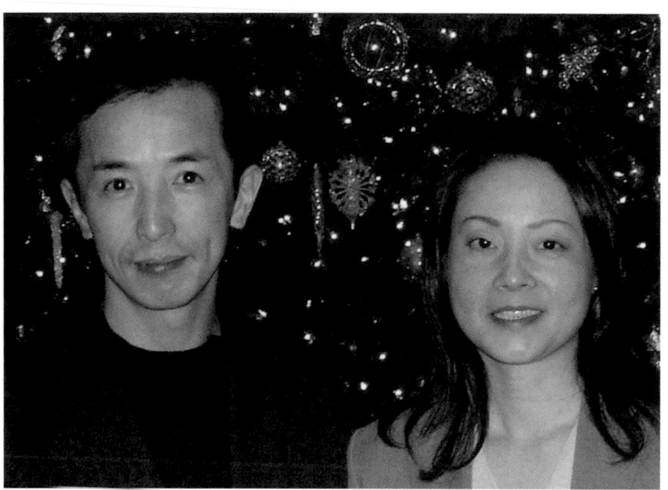

fig. 1

1. WHAT FASCINATES YOU MOST ABOUT BEING AN AESTHETIC SURGEON?

This occupation requires the utmost discipline and concentration, as well as ongoing training in analysis, diagnosis and technique. Every time I stand at the operating table, I imagine that I'm in a sword fight. My work presupposes talent and a trained sensibility for beauty. To me, it remains a constant challenge, and that's what makes it fascinating.

2. WHICH AREAS DO YOU SPECIALISE IN?

Facial surgery – predominantly correcting Asian noses and eyelids, but also performing facelifts.

3. DO YOU REGARD YOURSELF AS AN ARTIST?

If you think of an interior designer as an artist, then I am one too. Painters and sculptors create their works from scratch; an interior designer, on the other hand, needs to work with the architecture, the budget and the client's taste. My work process is akin to this – I similarly take the ideas and possibilities offered by my clients and optimise them aesthetically. It is important to me to convey to my clients that what I aim for is harmony, not a perfect anatomical construct.

4. WHAT IS YOUR CONCEPT OF BEAUTY?

Harmony, harmony and harmony. During my training, I kept asking myself what makes a face look beautiful. At first, I thought it was the nose. Then, the eyes seemed more important; I thought big, round eyes were particularly attractive. Later, I focused on the mouth and the lips. But after many years of experience, I have learnt that they all need to work together. The perfect shape of one facial feature alone does not make the entirety of a face beautiful.

5. IN ART HISTORY, WHAT IS YOUR FAVOURITE NOTION OF BEAUTY?

I am fascinated by Bushido, the ethical culture of the Samurai warrior cast that developed in the 17th century. It is one of the spiritual foundations of the Japanese tea ceremony, which I love very much. In fact, I collect objects associated with this ritual, especially from the Edo period of the 18th century. In contrast to this, the house my wife and I have decorated and live in is kept in a Western, American style. We do have Japanese antiques, but also Modernist paintings and sculptures from around the world.

6. TO YOU, WHO ARE THE MOST BEAUTIFUL WOMAN AND MOST BEAUTIFUL MAN ALIVE?

My wife. Tom Cruise in "The Last Samurai."

7. DO YOU REGARD YOURSELF AS ATTRACTIVE?

Yes. I think it is very important to see yourself as attractive, because otherwise you won't be! I impress this upon my patients as much as I can, before the operation and especially after.

8. WHAT DOES AGING MEAN TO YOU?

It means to gain maturity as a human being. We may lose our physical strength, but we keep growing mentally and spiritually. If we look too old or tired, we can correct our appearance using the cosmetic methods we have developed.

9. ARE YOU AFRAID OF GETTING OLDER?

No. If anything, it scares me that one day I might not be able to do my work anymore, that I won't be able to live up to my own standards.

fig. 1

Keizo Fukuta and his wife. The Japanese surgeon specialises in correcting Asian noses and eyelids. © Private archive Dr. Fukuta

fig. 2 & 4

Fukuta is fascinated by the ethical culture of the samurai – maybe one of the reasons he regards Tom Cruise in the role of "The Last Samurai" as one of the world's most beautiful men. © Warner Bros./defd (2), "Samurai brandishing sword" by Felice Beato © Historical Picture Archive/CORBIS (4)

fig. 3

A portrait of Keizo Fukuta. In his practice and his home, he likes to combine the aesthetics of Eastern and Western design. © Private archive Dr. Fukuta

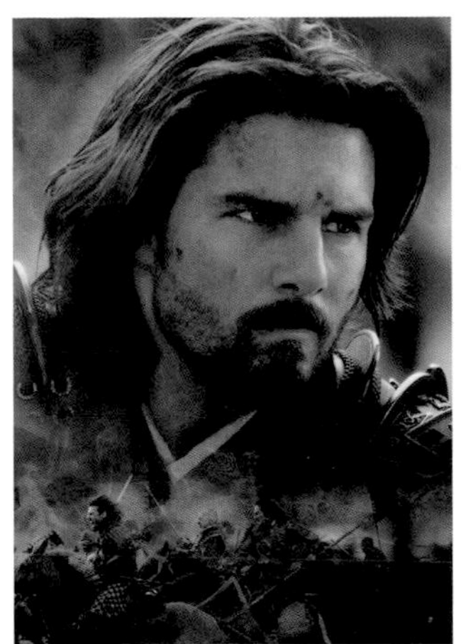

fig. 2

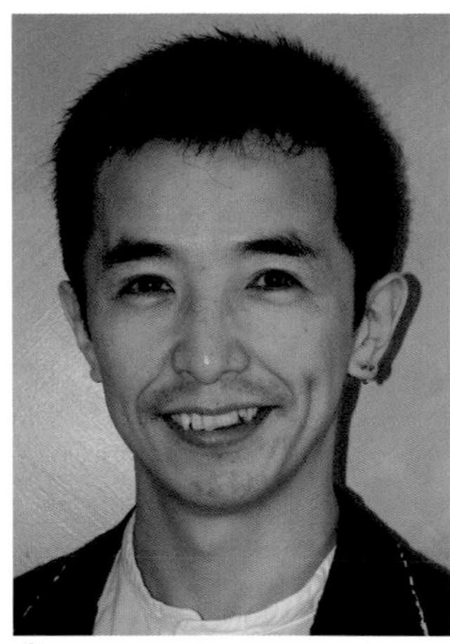

fig. 3

10. HAVE YOU EVER UNDERGONE AESTHETIC SURGERY YOURSELF? IF SO, WHAT WAS IT FOR?

Yes, I had my eyelids corrected.

11. HAVE YOU EVER OPERATED ON YOUR WIFE/PARTNER AND/OR CHILDREN? IF SO, WHY?

No.

12. CAN YOU JUSTIFY EVERY OPERATION AND PATIENT REQUEST, OR IS THERE A POINT WHERE YOU REFUSE TO DO AN OPERATION?

Obviously, I refuse to perform an operation if it is unrealistic, or if the person wanting it has a distorted self-perception. I generally try to comply with a patient's requests as much as possible, assuming he or she is open to my professional advice and reservations. An attractive outcome always results from a successful team effort between the patient and myself.

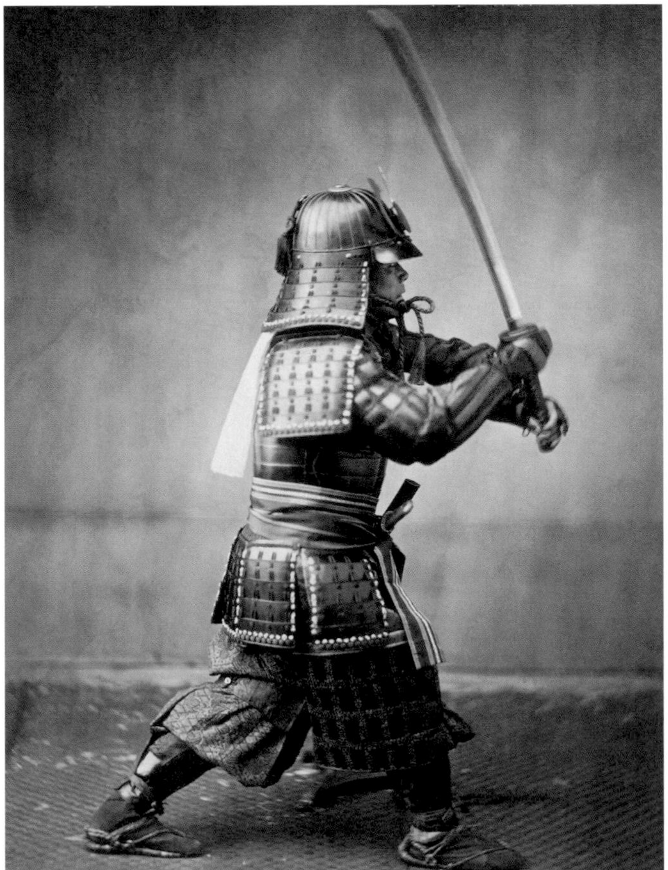

fig. 4

13. WHAT IS THE MOST UNUSUAL REQUEST FOR SURGERY YOU HAVE ENCOUNTERED IN YOUR CAREER?

A Japanese couple approached me about an operation. The man had a face not unlike a gorilla, the poor chap! His wife showed me a photo of Brad Pitt and begged me to make her husband look like him. The unfortunate man didn't even know who the actor was! The sad thing about this story is that bizarre requests like this are not isolated incidents. Usually, however, they come from American clients, sometimes also from Europeans. The Japanese generally prefer procedures that can go unnoticed and have very natural results.

14. WHAT ARE YOUR PATIENTS' REACTIONS FOLLOWING SURGERY?

Straight after the procedure, some are surprised or angry, even shocked. This is due to the swellings, reddened skin or bruises that typically appear after an operation. Of course I point out these skin reactions to my patients well before operating on them, but many simply choose to suppress this information. In such instances, I like to tell them that they are going through a cocooning stage, a necessary station on their way to becoming a butterfly. Indeed most of them are completely happy once the healing stage is completed. It is very rare that a patient is dissatisfied in spite of the procedure being a surgical success. In these cases, I try to find out what the patient still finds disturbing and then address the problem in a follow-up operation.

15. COULD YOU NAME SOME OF YOUR MORE WELL-KNOWN PATIENTS?

As a matter of principle, no.

16. DO YOU BELIEVE THAT BEAUTY LARGELY EMANATES FROM WITHIN?

First impressions always focus on external appearance.

fig. 5 a+b

A 30-year-old female underwent breast augmentation with silicone gel implants and body sculpture of the flank and thigh with liposuction. She also had augmentation rhinoplasty with a silicone implant to the dorsum and ear cartilage graft to the tip. Her chin was highlighted with a small silicone implant. © Private archive Dr. Fukuta

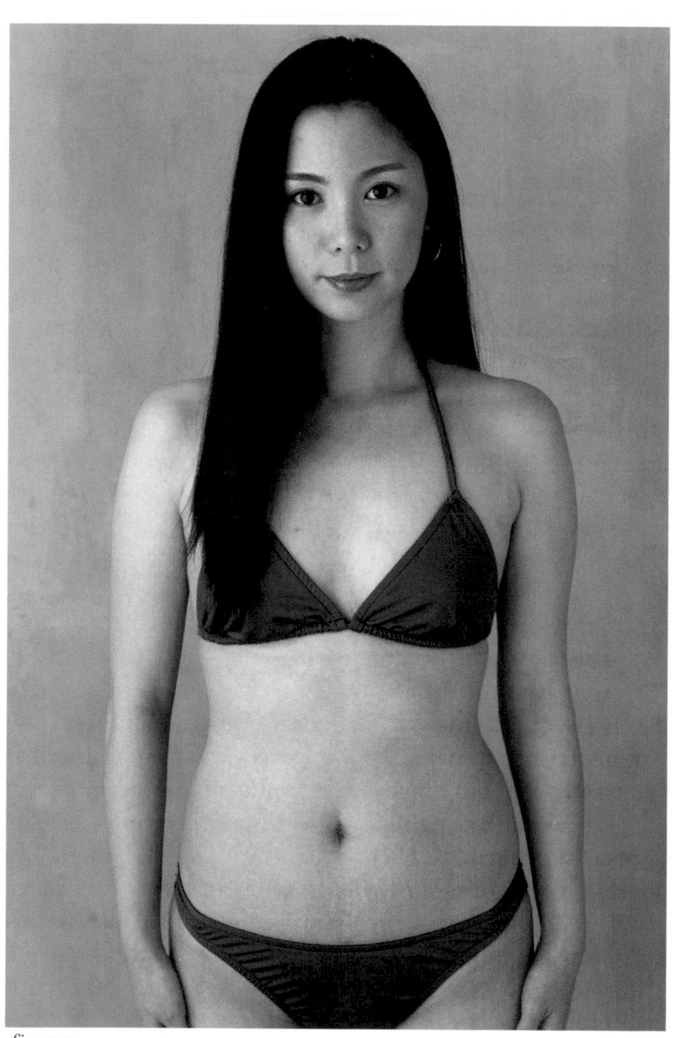

fig. 5 a

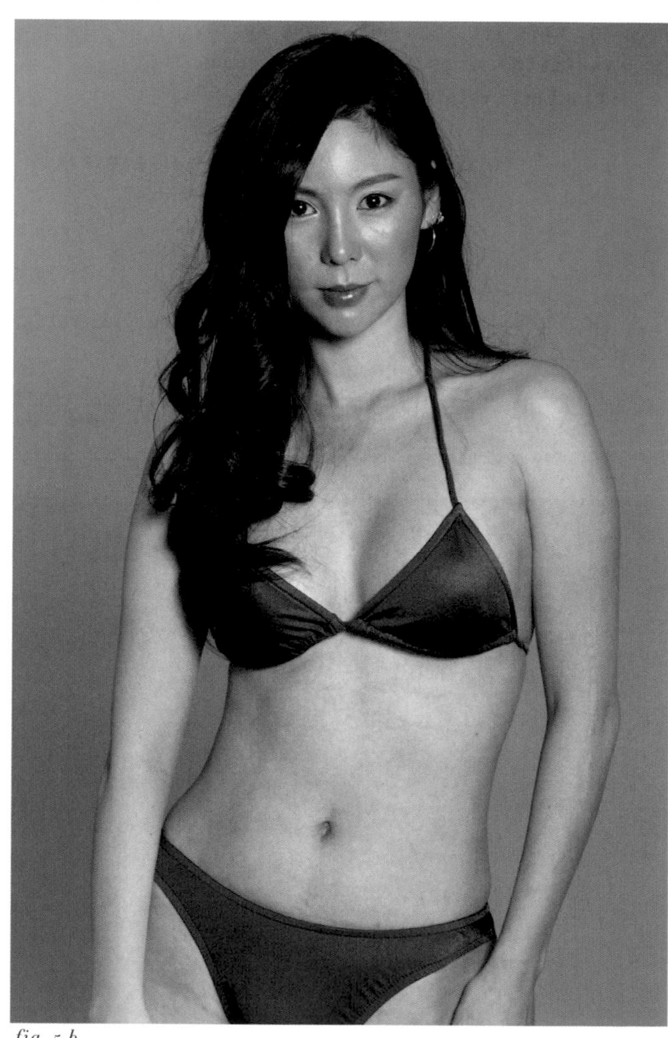

fig. 5 b

We see the proportions of a face, the colour and texture of the skin. It is only natural that delicate and symmetrical faces attract us more than roughly drawn ones. But in the long run, other qualities are more significant – the charisma and character of a person. In a relationship, these become much more important than external appearance. An arrogant person with a perfect face is not at all attractive. Yes, I believe that inner beauty will ultimately prevail over external beauty.

17. DO YOU THINK THAT BEAUTIFUL PEOPLE ARE HAPPIER AND LEAD MORE FULFILLED LIVES?

The real question is: Who or what determines a person's happiness? I think it's always the person. Without fail, people with positive attitudes lead happier lives. Most of my patients approach me for surgery hoping to become happier as a result of their enhanced attractiveness. And rightly so – when they feel better and more self-confident after a successful operation, this also makes them happier. Good looks can indeed heal minor complexes.

fig. 6 a+b

A 19-year-old female presented with a short nose deformity and depression at the alar base. She underwent augmentation of the nasal dorsum and alar base with silicone implants. Her short nose was corrected with a septal elongation procedure with a rib cartilage graft.

fig. 7 a+b

A 20-year-old Japanese male sought for a Caucasian look. The patient underwent the epicanthoplasty and upper blepharoplasty. The rib cartilage graft was used for the augmentation of the glabella and nasal dorsum and the septal elongation of the nose. It was important to create the deep set of the eye in relation with the nose and forehead to achieve the Caucasian look.

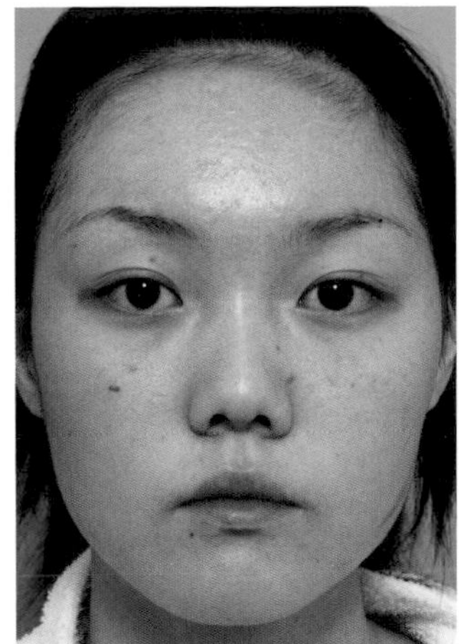
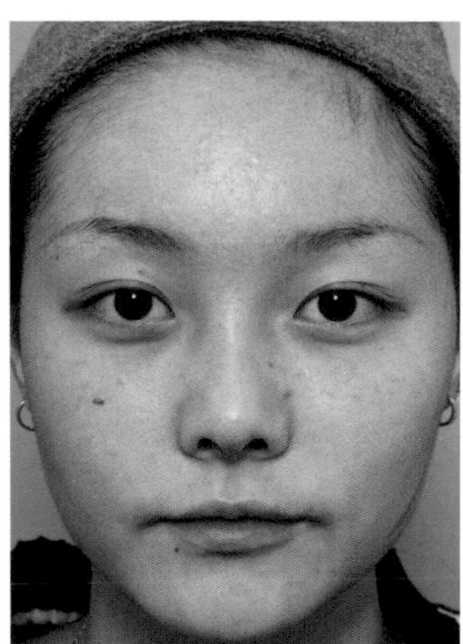

fig. 6 a+b

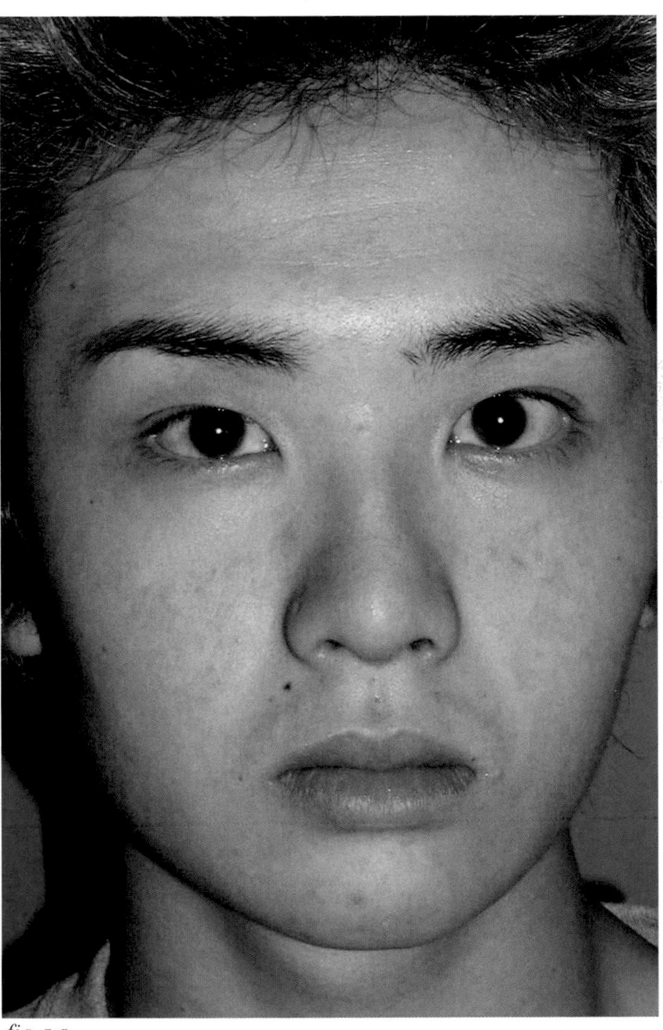

fig. 7 a

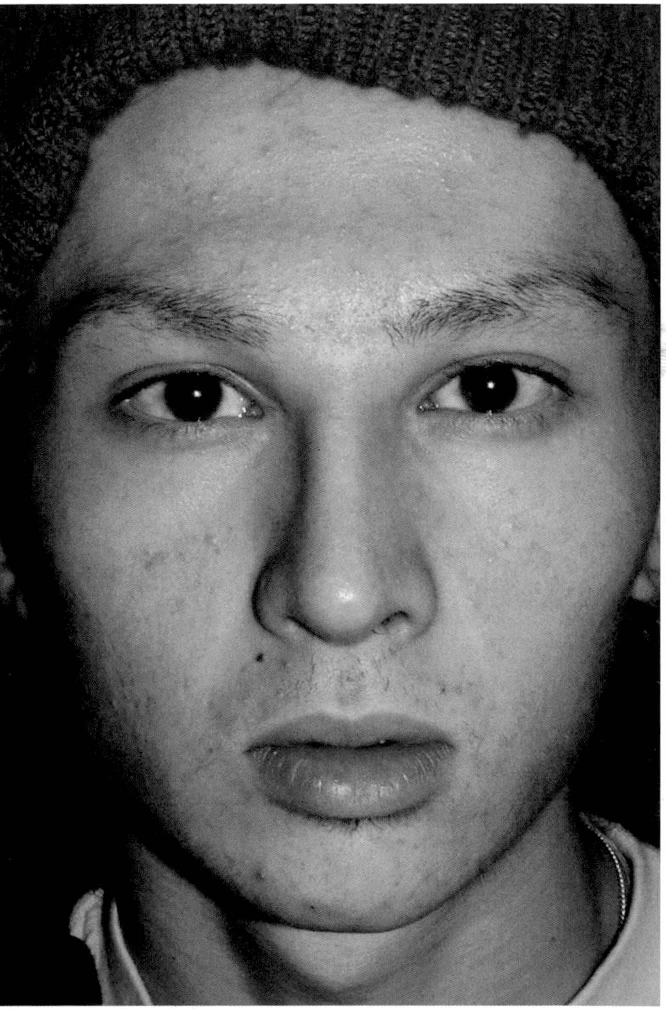

fig. 7 b

18. DO BEAUTIFUL PEOPLE HAVE BETTER SEX?

What is good sex? If this question asks whether a beautiful person has a better chance at getting a large number of sexual partners, then the answer would have to be yes. But I don't believe that a good sex life depends on good looks.

19. WHAT DOES THE FUTURE HOLD FOR AESTHETIC SURGERY?

Technical advances and innovations will result in aesthetic surgery becoming less invasive, i. e. scalpels being used less, and in operations being performed faster and with a shorter recuperation period. General surgical standards will reach a higher, uniform level all over the world. The Japanese already prefer minimal surgical procedures, a tendency that may well spread to Europe and even the US in the long term.

Interview: Eva Karcher, Munich

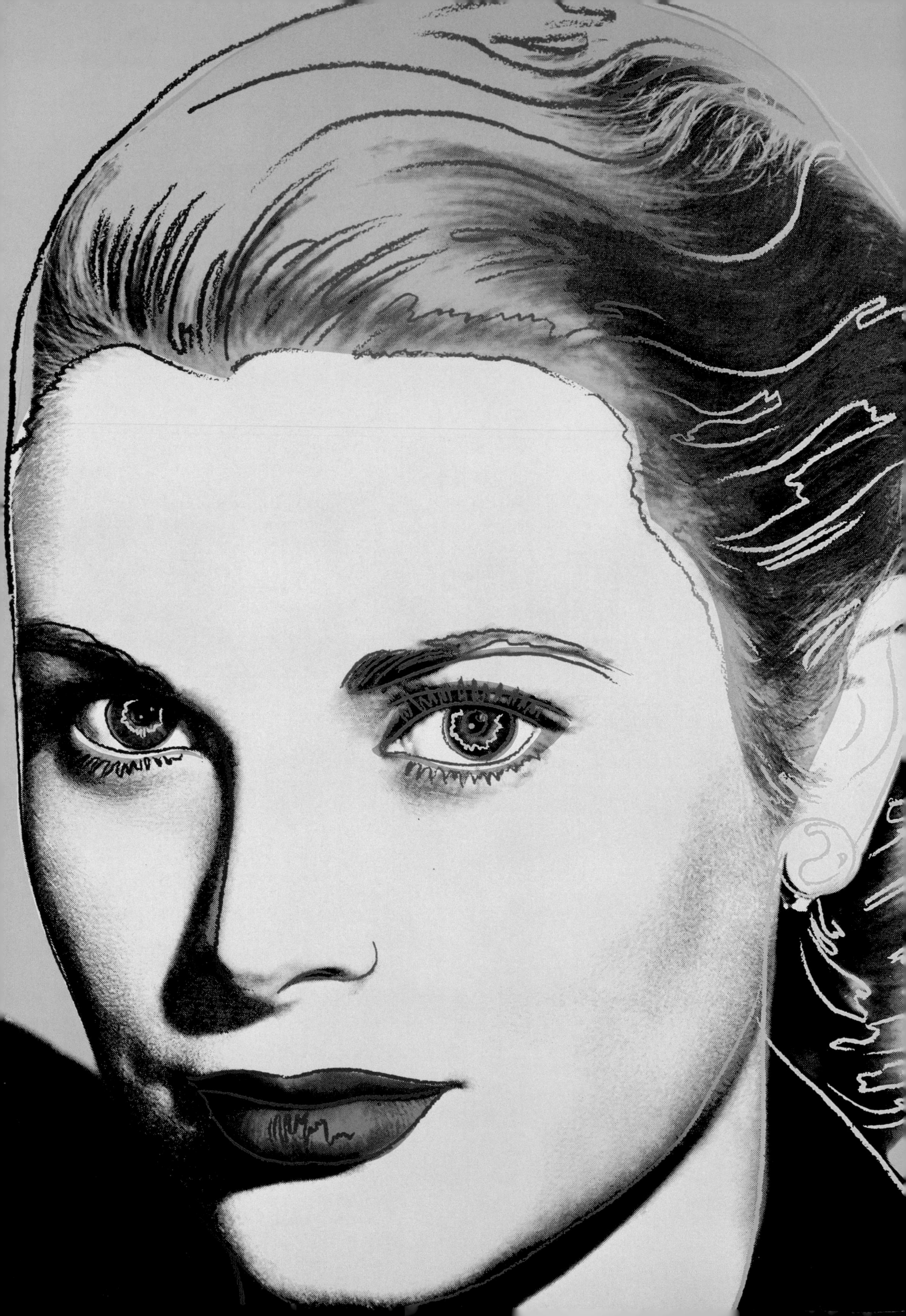

VIII.1

ABOUT BEAUTY

STATEMENTS BY THE WORLD'S MOST FAMOUS AESTHETIC SURGEONS

Ali Al-Numairy, Dubai; Sherrell J. Aston, New York; Bernhard Brinkmann, Hamburg; Johannes C. Bruck, Berlin; John F. Celin, London; Sydney R. Coleman, New York; Axel-Mario Feller, Munich; Carlo Gasperoni, Rome; Barry M. Jones, London; Ulrich K. Kesseling, Lausanne; Morten Kveim, Oslo; Dagmar Millesi, Wien; Egle Muti, Turin; Axel Neuroth, Düsseldorf; Rolf Rüdiger Olbrisch, Düsseldorf; Norman Orentreich, New York; Jean-Louis Sebagh, Paris; Antonio Tapia, Barcelone; Kiyotaka Watanabe, Tokyo; Christoph Wolfensberger, Zurich

About Beauty

When you look at popular magazines,
you quickly realise that today's aesthetics are
totally focused on appearance and superficiality.
The laws of capitalism are in full force here,
all that counts is a flawless façade.
This is highly regrettable.

Jean-Louis Sebagh, Paris

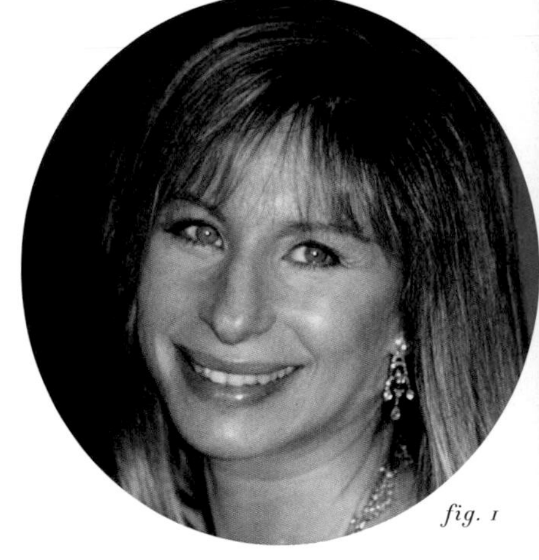

fig. 1

Barbra Streisand is beautiful even though she doesn't fit the standards at all!

Morten Kveim, Oslo

fig. previous pages
Andy Warhol, "Grace Kelly", 1967. © The Andy Warhol Estate
fig. 1 Barbra Streisand, 1982. Photo © Corbis
fig. 2 Michelangelo: The Dying Slave, 1513/15. Musée du Louvre, Paris.
fig. 3 Benvenuto Cellini: Narcissus, 1548. © Arte & Immagini srl / CORBIS
fig. 4 André de Dienes: Marilyn Monroe, 1949. © André de Dienes

To me, Michelangelo Buonarotti was the genius of harmonious proportions.

Egle Muti, Turin

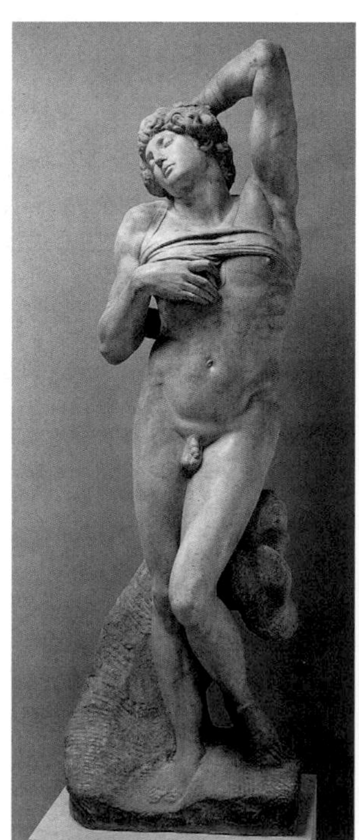

fig. 2

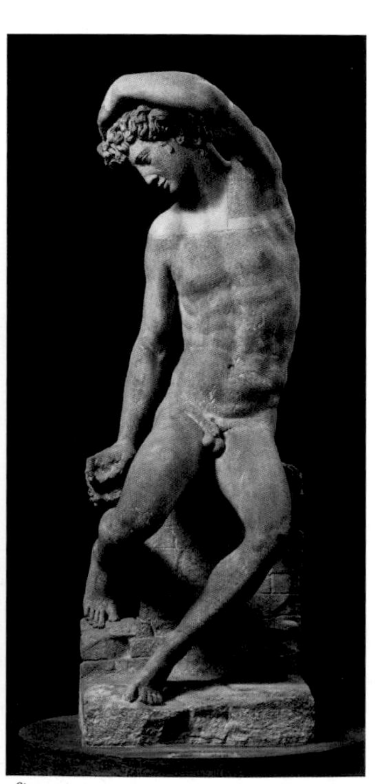

fig. 3

I love sculptors such as Auguste Rodin, Michelangelo Buonarroti or Benvenuto Cellini. They mean more to me than painters or architects — unsurprisingly, considering my profession.

John F. Celin, London

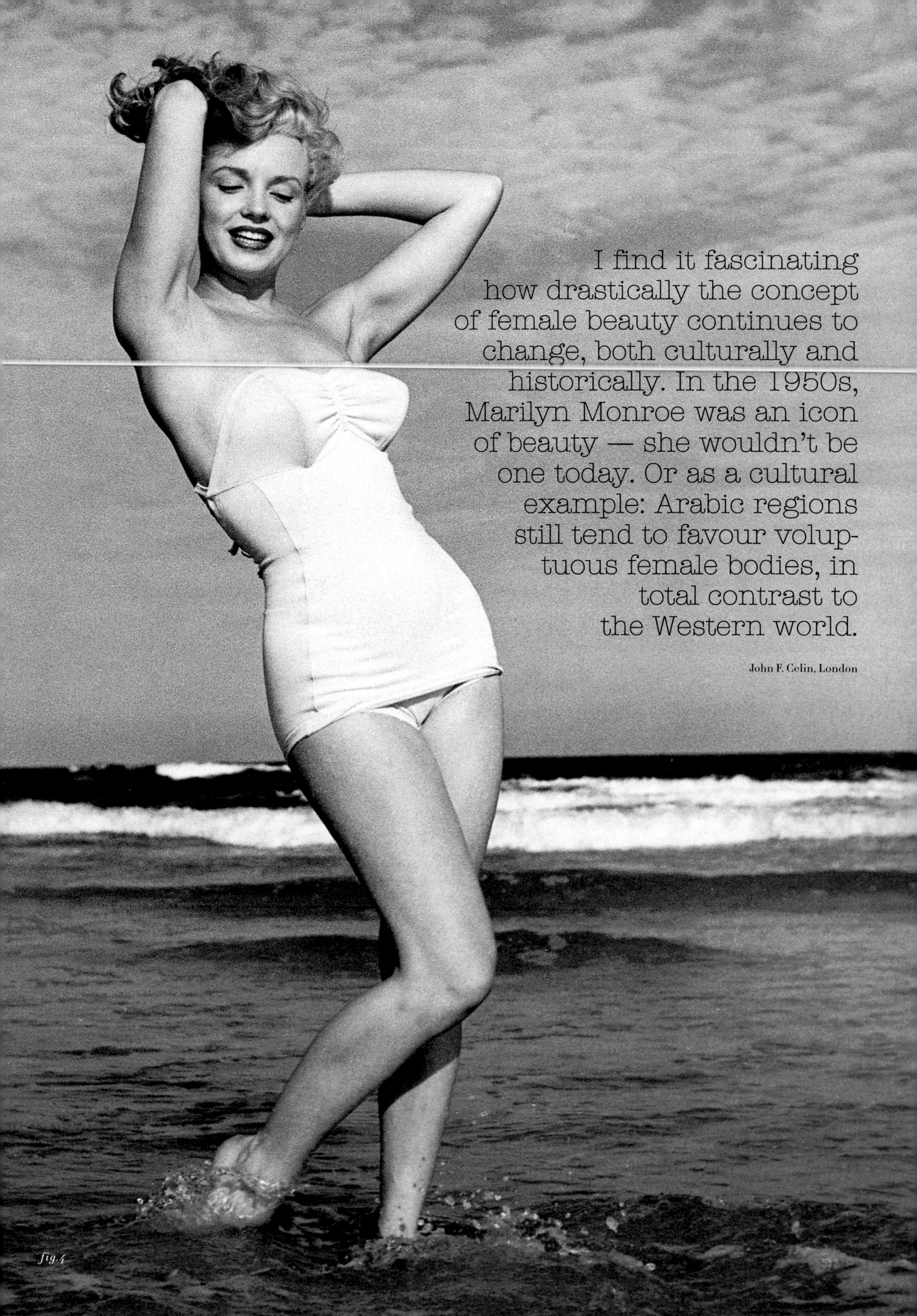

I find it fascinating how drastically the concept of female beauty continues to change, both culturally and historically. In the 1950s, Marilyn Monroe was an icon of beauty — she wouldn't be one today. Or as a cultural example: Arabic regions still tend to favour voluptuous female bodies, in total contrast to the Western world.

John F. Celin, London

fig.4

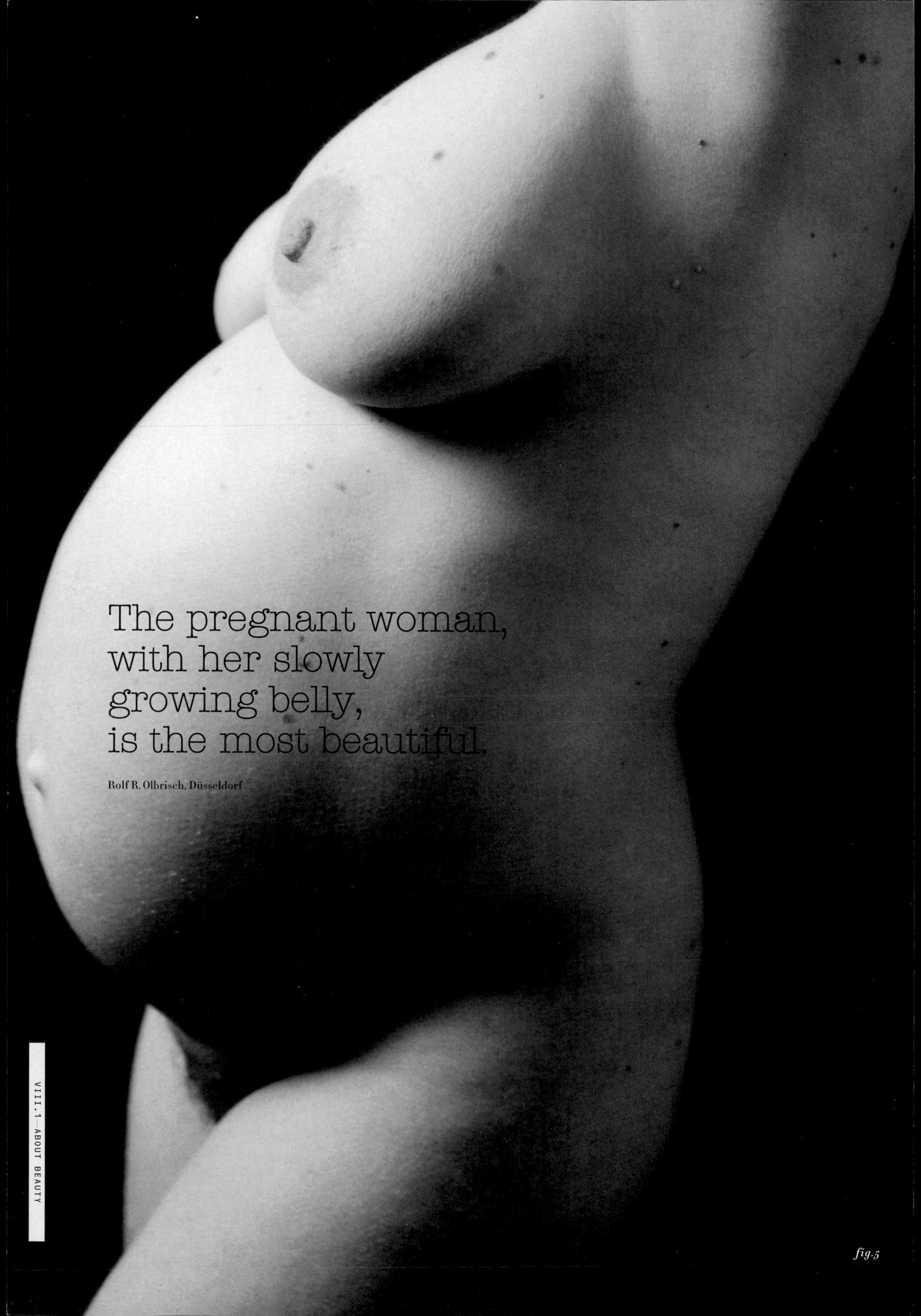

The pregnant woman,
with her slowly
growing belly,
is the most beautiful.

Rolf R. Olbrisch, Düsseldorf

fig.5

fig. 5 *Johnny Buzzerio: Pregnant Woman, c. 2001.*
© Johnny Buzzerio / CORBIS
fig. 6 *Michelle Pfeiffer, 1998.*
© picture-alliance / Picture Press / CAMERA PRESS / Gary Lewis
fig. 7 *Kevin Costner, 2003. © Getty Images*
fig. 8 *Sandro Botticelli: The Birth of Venus (detail), 1485.*
Botticelli © 1990, Photo Scala, Florence,
courtesy of the Ministero Beni e Att. Culturali

To me, Michelle Pfeiffer is the most beautiful woman alive, Kevin Costner the most beautiful man.

Dagmar Millesi, Vienna

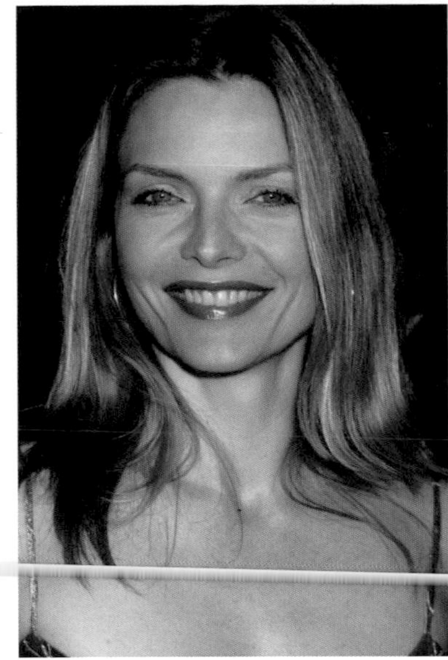

fig. 6

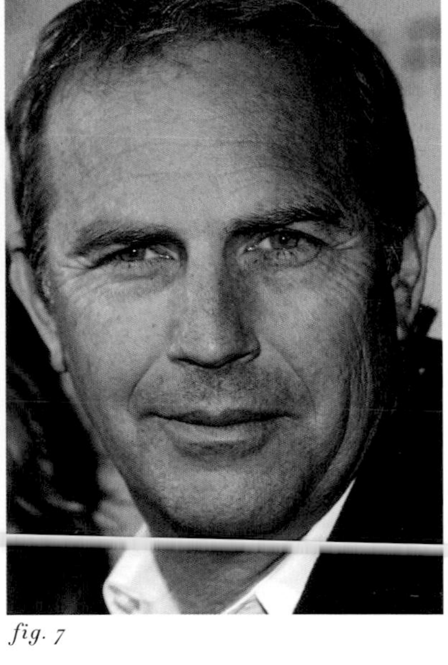

fig. 7

Beauty is the right balance of spirit, emotion and appearance. These three factors exist only in relation to each other and ceaselessly influence each other.

Antonio Tapia, Barcelona

I am suspicious of surgeons and doctors who claim there are universally valid measurements and proportions. It would be so boring to clone people according to a look that is currently in fashion. Beauty should never be allowed to reign supreme.

Jean-Louis Sebagh, Paris

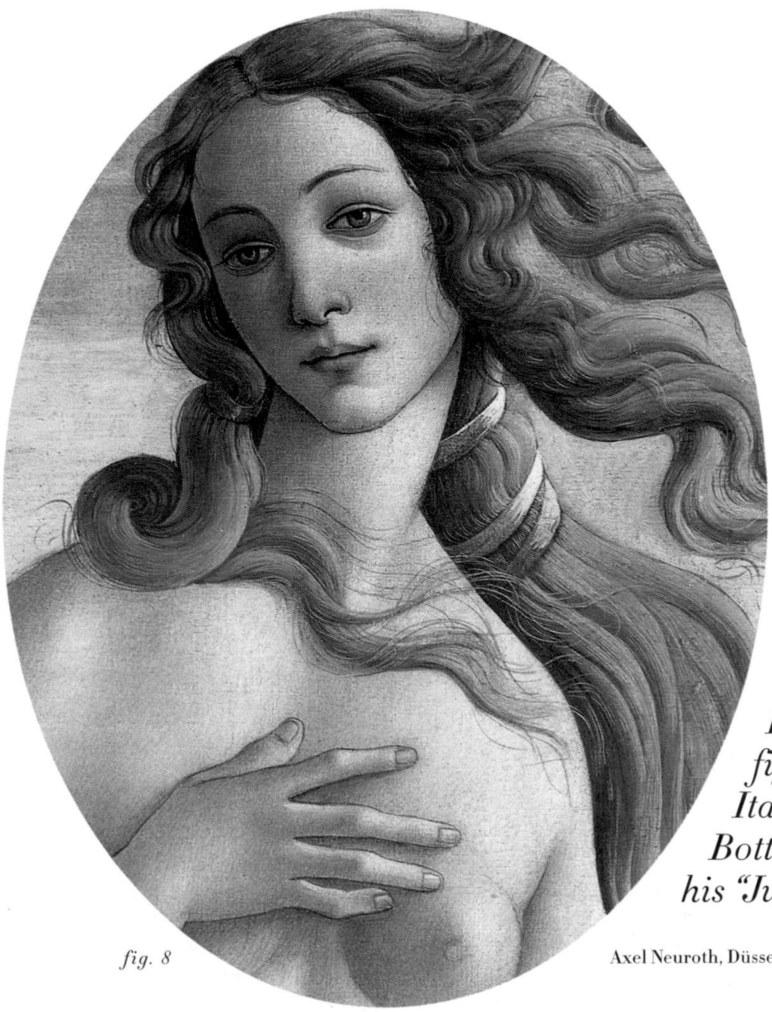

I have a weakness for the female figures depicted in the paintings of Italian Renaissance artist Sandro Botticelli, particularly his "Primavera", his "Judith" and his "Venus".

fig. 8

Axel Neuroth, Düsseldorf

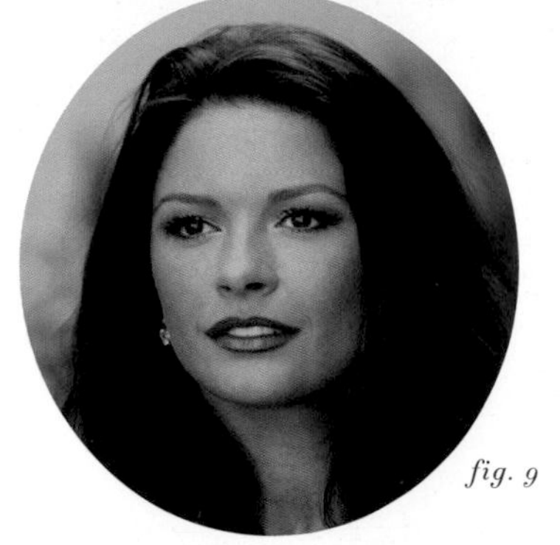

fig. 9

Quite possibly, it may be easier to be beautiful and unhappy than to be ugly and unhappy.

Jean-Louis Sebagh, Paris

fig. 10

To me, Grace Kelly is the goddess of beauty. Catherine Zeta-Jones is also very attractive, as is the Brazilian model Gisèle Bündchen. It's not so simple with men, on the other hand. Personally, I regard Gary Cooper as a particularly attractive man.

Carlo Gasperoni, Rome

fig. 11

If a person lives in harmony with his or her outward appearance, he or she is beautiful.

Johannes C. Bruck, Berlin

fig. 9 Catherine Zeta-Jones, 2003. © Getty Images
fig. 10 Gisele Bündchen, 2003. © Getty Images
fig. 11 Gary Cooper, 1940. © Getty Images / Hulton Archive
fig. 12 Grace Kelly, 1974. © Sunset Boulevard / CORBIS SYGMA
fig. 13 Audrey Hepburn, 1954. © Getty Images / Hulton Archive

I think you can have the most beautiful outside appearance and be the bitchiest, meanest person on the inside.

Norman Orentreich, New York

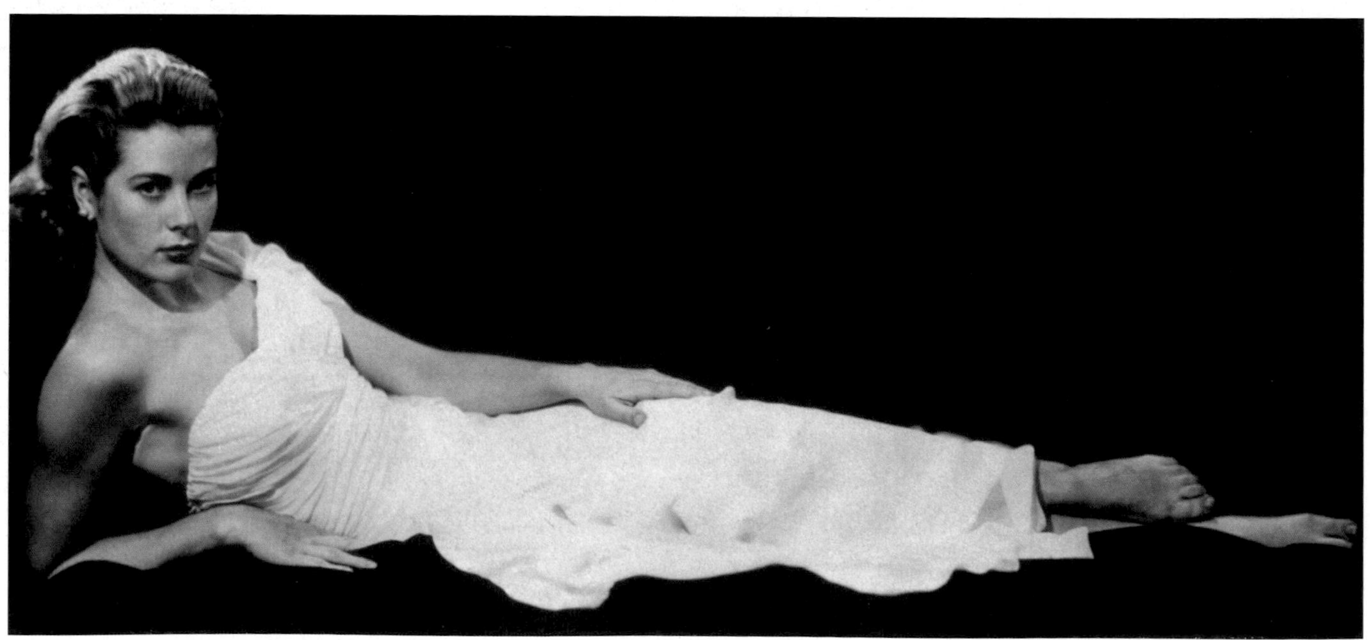

fig. 12

fig. 13

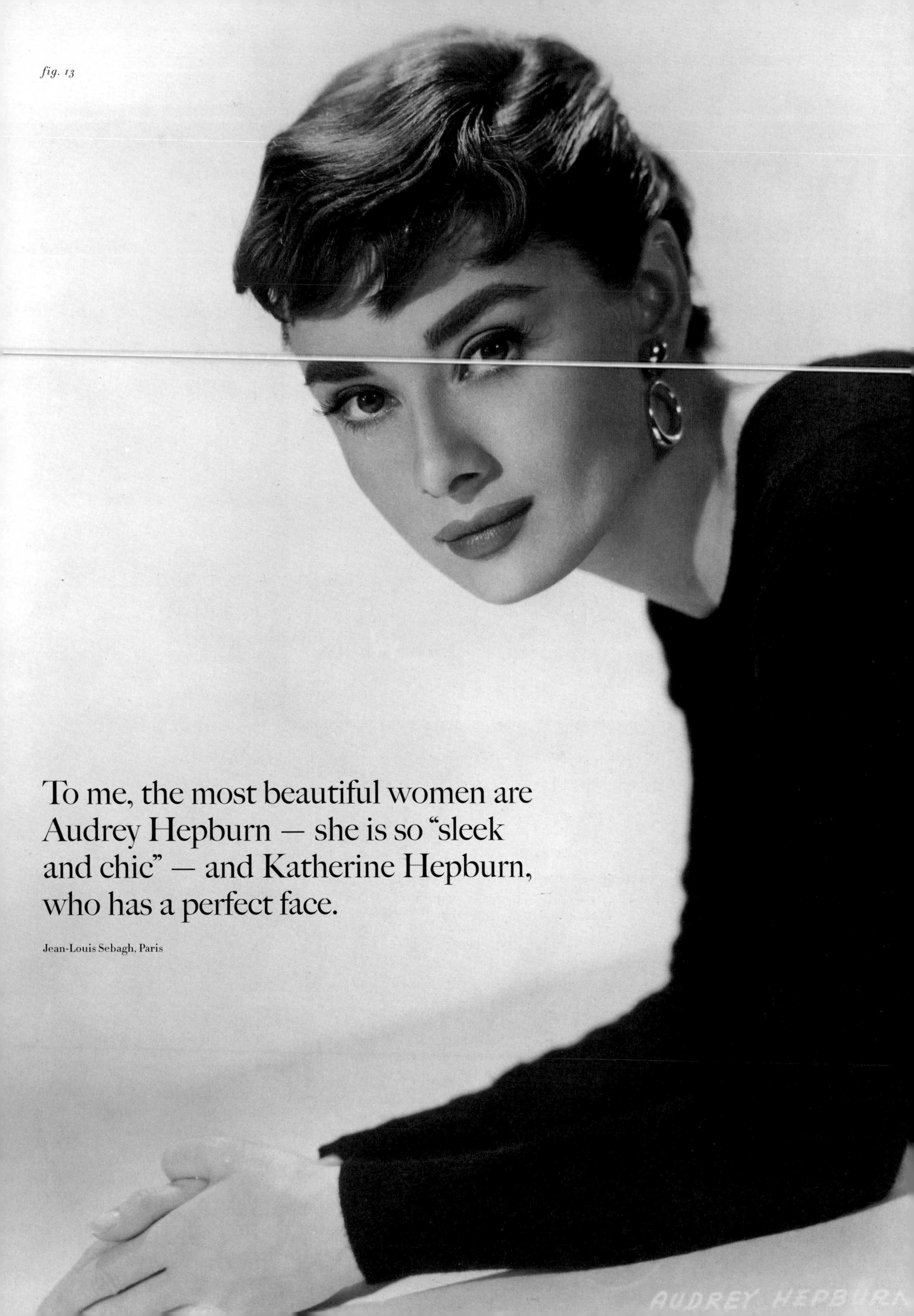

To me, the most beautiful women are Audrey Hepburn — she is so "sleek and chic" — and Katherine Hepburn, who has a perfect face.

Jean-Louis Sebagh, Paris

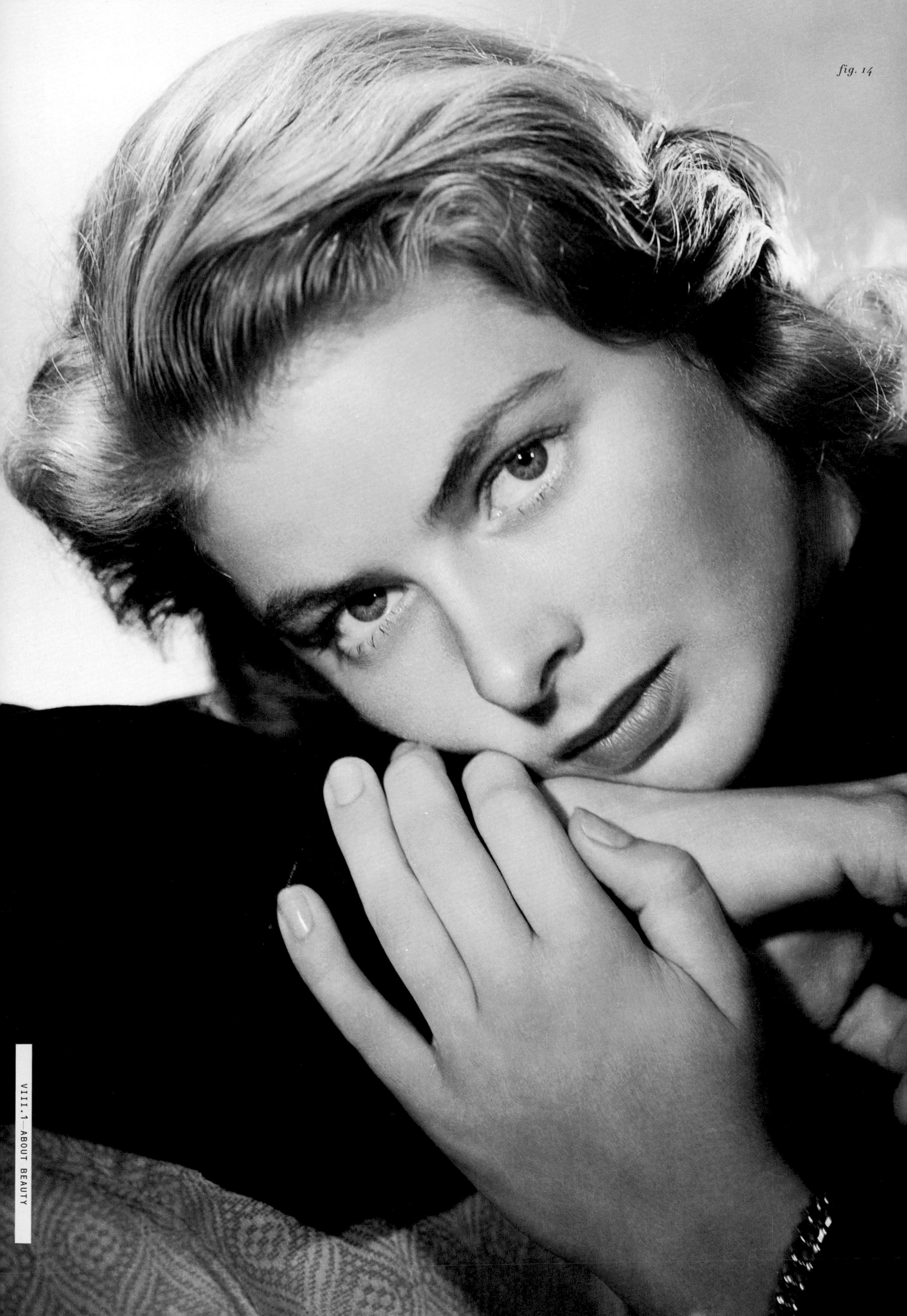

fig. 14

As a matter of principle, I reject those American-style, media-propagated blueprints for uniform faces and bodies.

Dagmar Millesi, Vienna

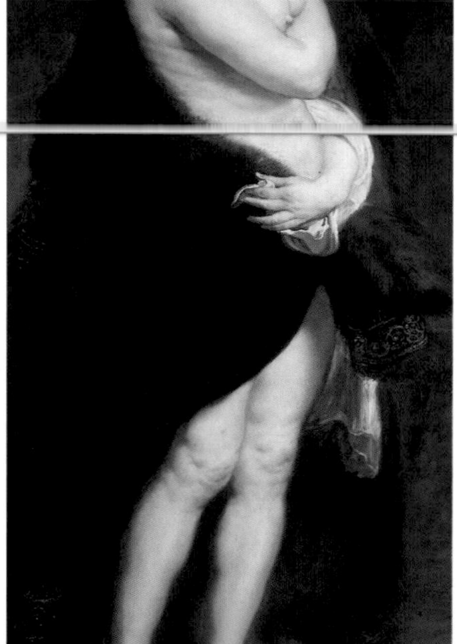

fig. 15

Then again there are attractive people who, sometimes with our own help, maintain the illusion that their outward beauty also reflects their personal qualities. However, once they start to voice their opinions, it soon becomes apparent that there isn't much substance behind their dazzling façade.

Axel Neuroth, Düsseldorf

Some people find obesity beautiful, and they consider a very fat woman something very sexually attractive.

Norman Orentreich, New York

I always regarded Ingrid Bergmann as particularly beautiful. Her physical appearance and her aura are beyond compare.

John F. Celin, London

It is well recognised that attractive people are generally treated more amicably and generously than people not considered good-looking.

Barry M. Jones, London

fig. 14 Ingrid Bergmann, 1956. © Getty Images / Hulton Archive
fig. 15 Peter Paul Rubens: The Little Fur (Helene Fourment), c. 1638. Kunsthistorisches Museum, Vienna.

When you have a beautiful inside and a beautiful outside, that's a remarkable person.

Norman Orentreich, New York

The woman of Ur, Nefertiti or a François Boucher nude for example, will always stimulate our aesthetic sensibilities.

Ali Al-Numairy, Dubai

fig. 16

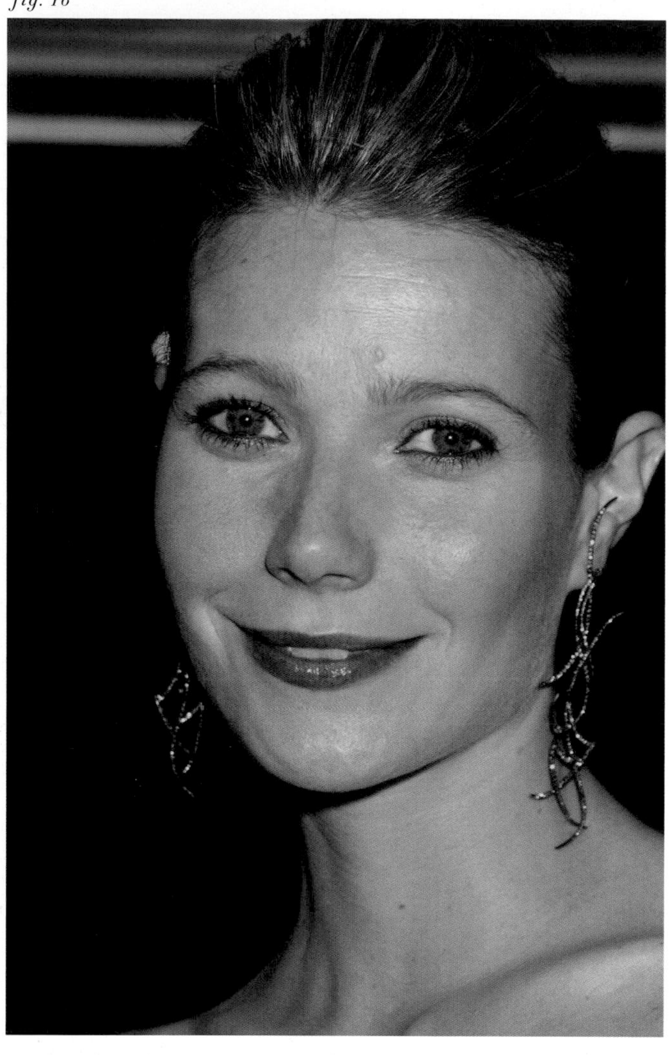

I've looked at my wife's face for 56 years of marriage. I've known her for 60 years, and she's still beautiful to me.

Norman Orentreich, New York

To me, the American film star Gwyneth Paltrow is one of the most beautiful women alive.

Johannes C. Bruck, Berlin

fig. 16 Gwyneth Paltrow, 2003. © Getty Images
fig. 17 Nefertiti, c. 1340 B.C. © Ruggero Vanni / CORBIS

We know people in various cultures who are beautiful, but the culture in which that person is living probably has a different sense of beauty than you and I. For instance, if you take the wife of a Masai warrior in Kenya, his appreciation for beauty is a lot different than yours and mine, probably. And he is likely not going to see a Hollywood starlet as being as beautiful as he sees his bride. Or in his case, one of his brides.

Sherrell J. Aston, New York

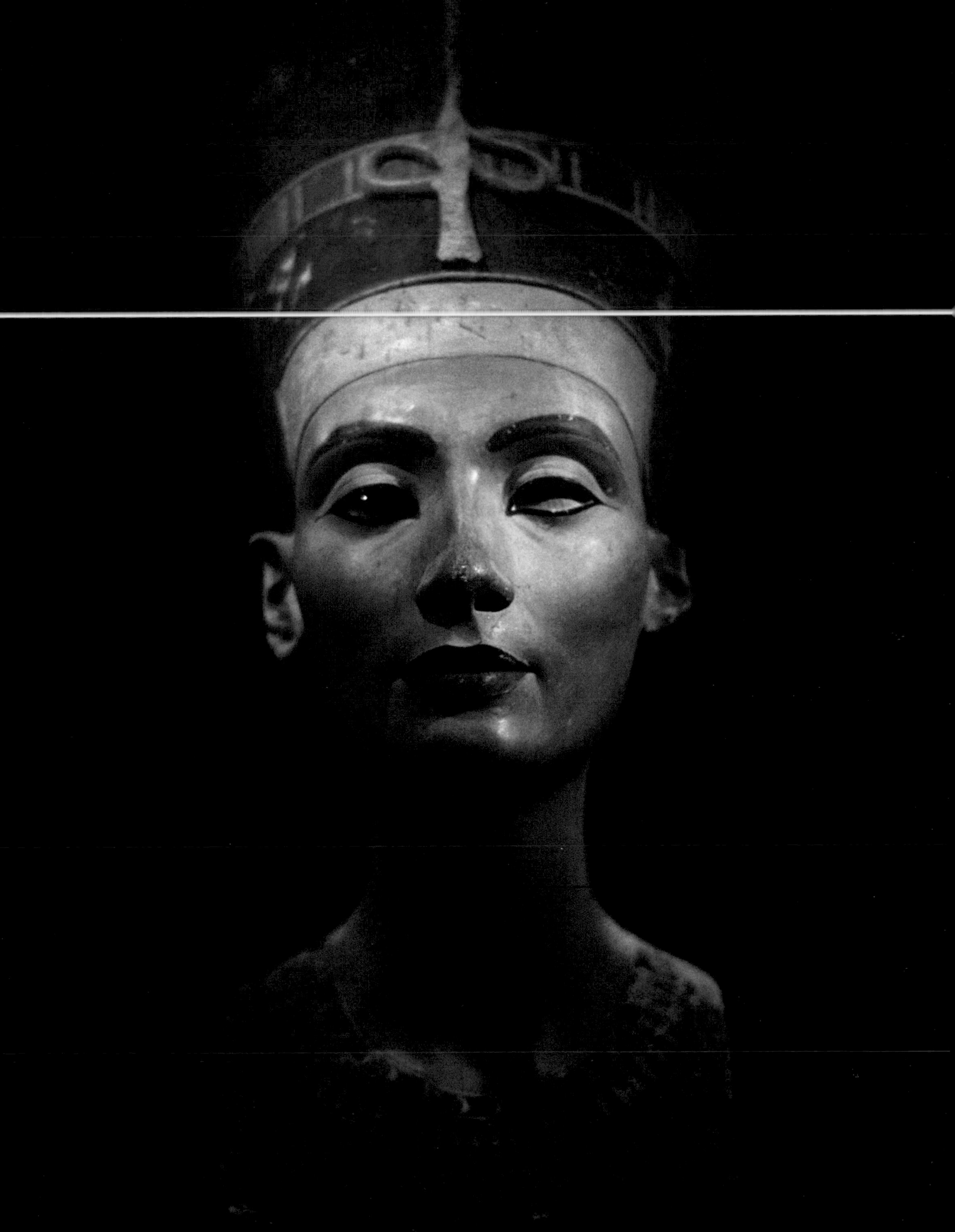

fig.17

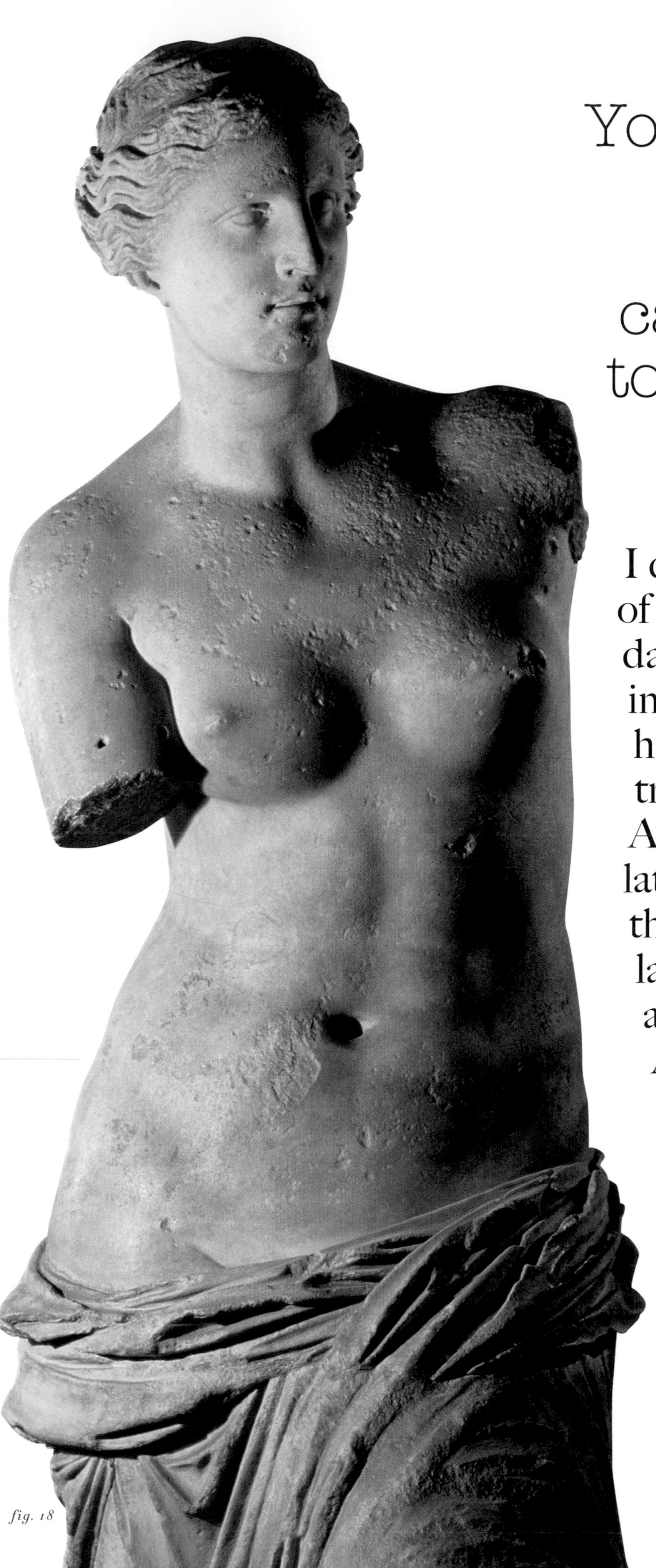

fig. 18

You can learn techniques, but you cannot learn to have a feel for beauty.

John F. Celin, London

I deal with harmonies of proportion every day. Essentially, all our insights into these harmonies can be traced back to the Ancient Egyptians, later the Greeks and the Romans, and even later the Renaissance and its timeless art. As the cradle of Western culture, the Mediterranean region and its art are a paramount influence even in my profession.

Christoph Wolfensberger, Zurich

fig. 18 Venus de Milo (detail), c. 150–100 B.C. Musée du Louvre, Paris. © 1990 Photo Scala, Florence
fig. 19 Halle Berry, 2002. © picture-alliance / Picture Press / Everett Collection / MGM

There are undeniable correlations between a person's spirit and their physiognomy. The soul is always reflected in the face.

Carlo Gasperoni, Rome

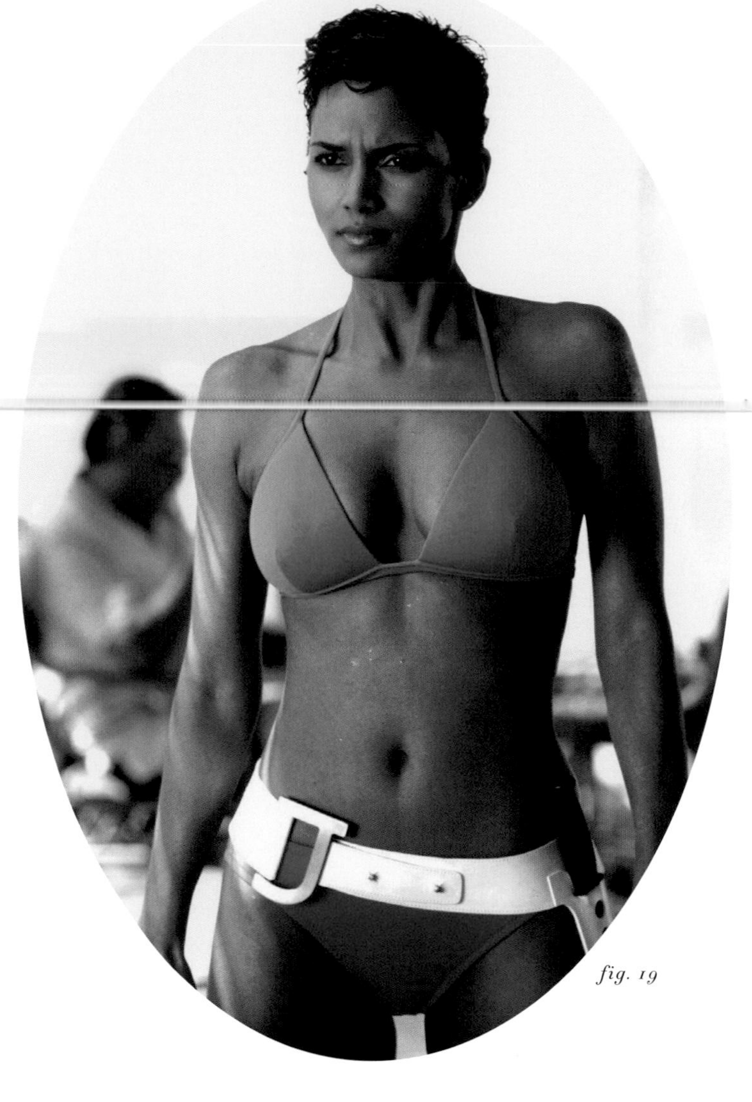

fig. 19

If all they've got is their, what I call book cover people, book cover, and there's no content, they're in trouble. And you're in trouble as a physician, too. Because no matter how good you make that book cover, you're not gonna have a happy book. You've got to have a good cover and a good content, as a patient.

Norman Orentreich, New York

Beauty and bliss are closely related, but neither one can guarantee the other.

Axel Neuroth, Düsseldorf

Experiments have shown that the perception of beauty is innate. When faced with a line-up of people, a three-year-old instinctively can point to the most beautiful one.

Ulrich K. Kesselring, Lausanne

Beauty makes some women happy and others unhappy.

Kiyotaka Watanabe, Tokyo

I think that Catherine Deneuve, in terms of her overall anatomy, is one of the most beautiful women.

Sherrell J. Aston, New York

The face is the window to the soul.

Sydney R. Coleman, New York

fig. 20 *Njemps tribeswoman, Kenya.* *© Brian A. Vikander / CORBIS*
fig. 21 *Catherine Deneuve, 1967.* *© picture-alliance / Picture Press / CAMERA PRESS / Alex Youssoupoff*

I don't subscribe to any particular notion of beauty. To me, the vital criteria for beauty are harmony and charisma. A Masai warrior, for example, can look very beautiful.

Axel-Mario Feller, Munich

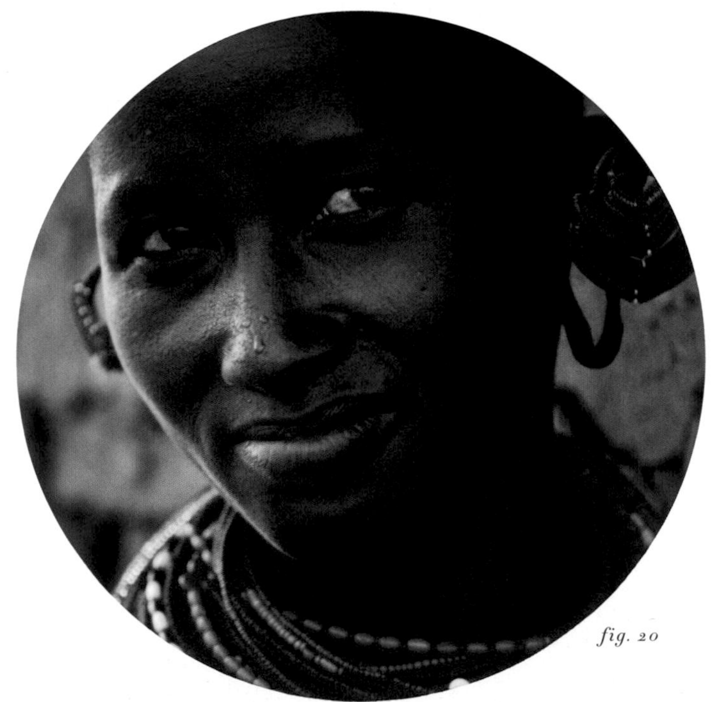

fig. 20

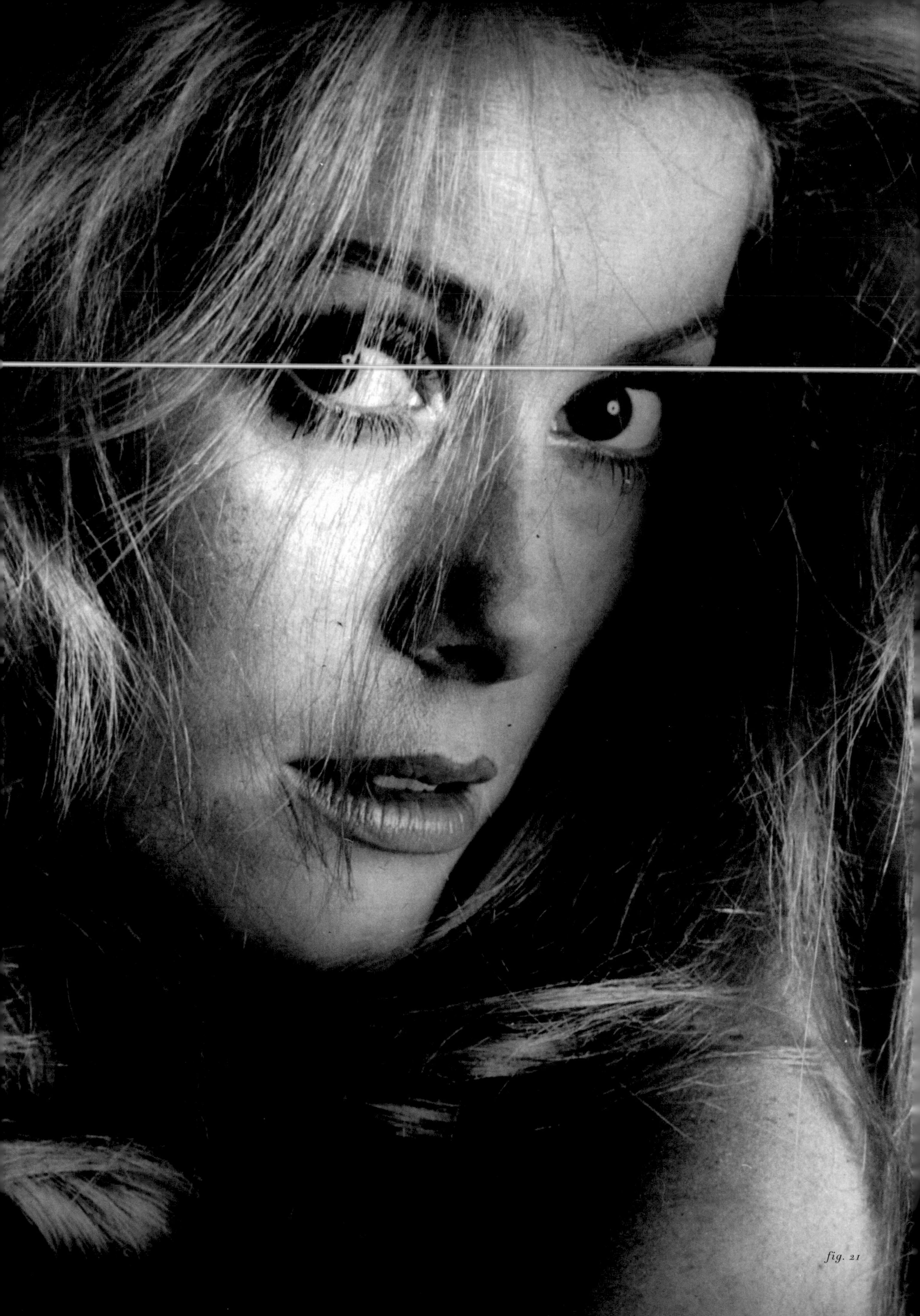

fig. 21

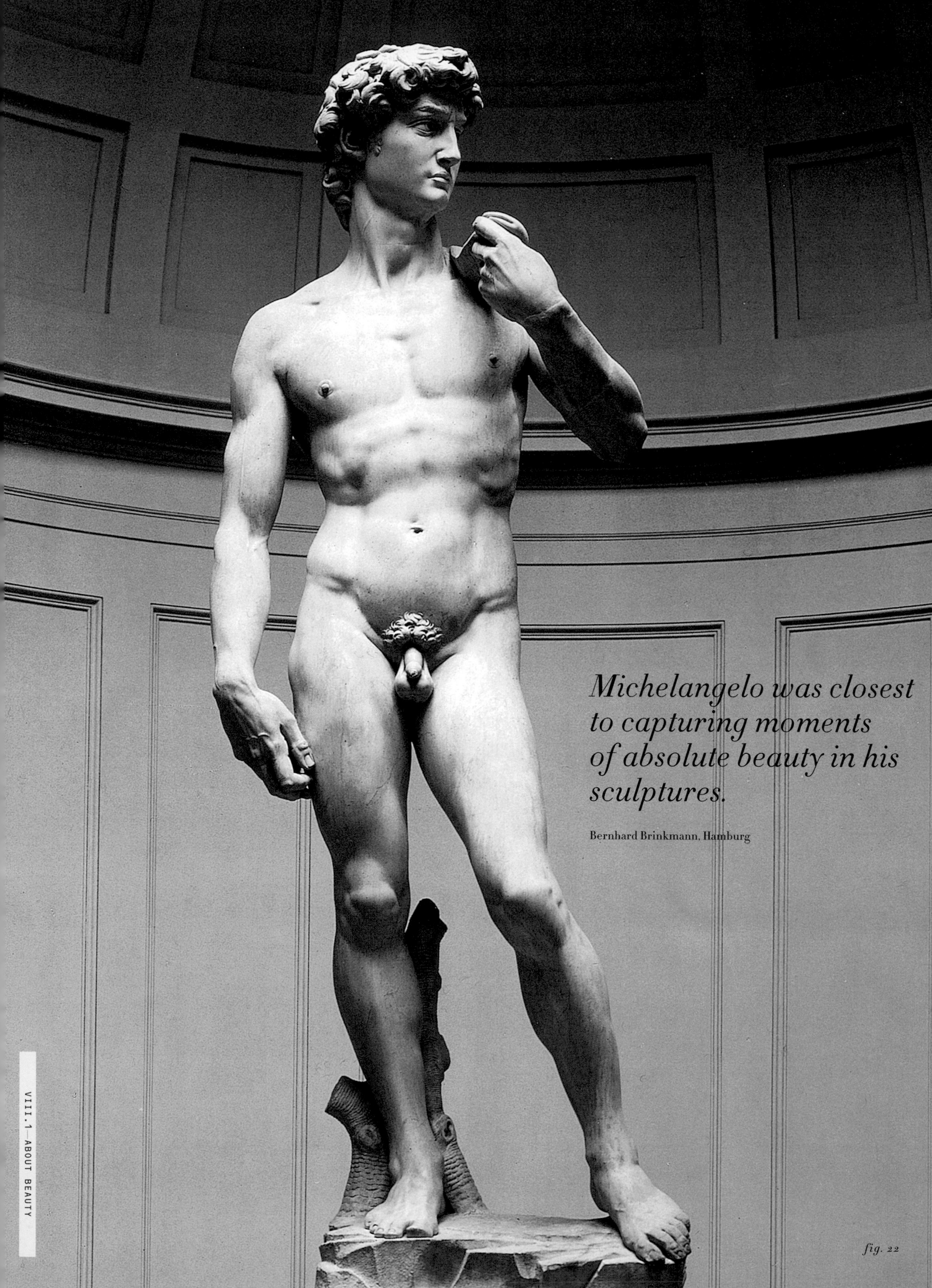

Michelangelo was closest to capturing moments of absolute beauty in his sculptures.

Bernhard Brinkmann, Hamburg

fig. 22

Be careful — there are some people, especially women, who will suddenly become arrogant or overconfident after a successful operation; they may even try to seduce their best friend's husband!

Egle Muti, Turin

Beauty can also mislead people in the way they regard and treat themselves and others.

Kiyotaka Watanabe, Tokyo

fig. 23

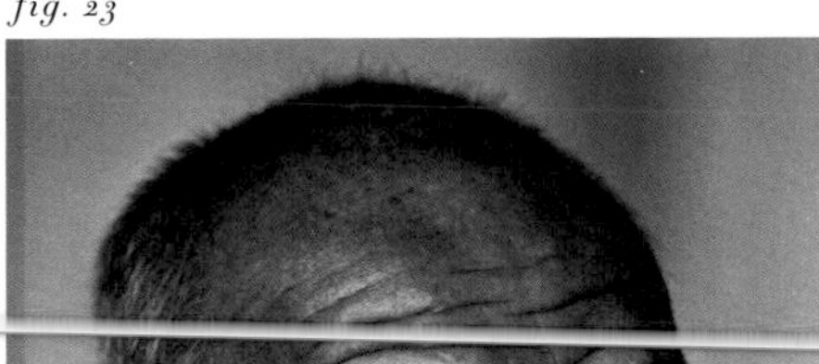

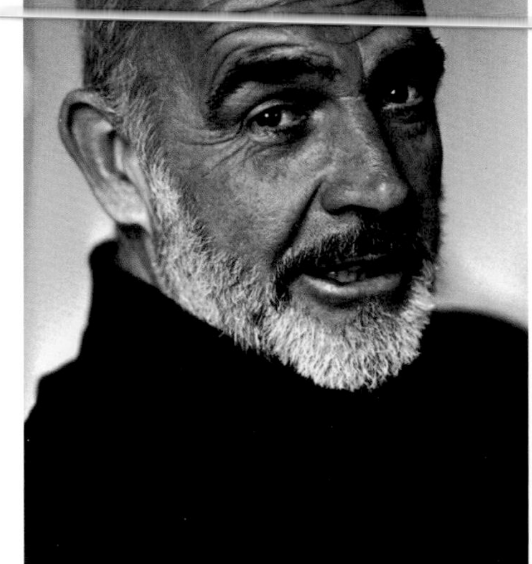

fig. 24

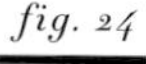

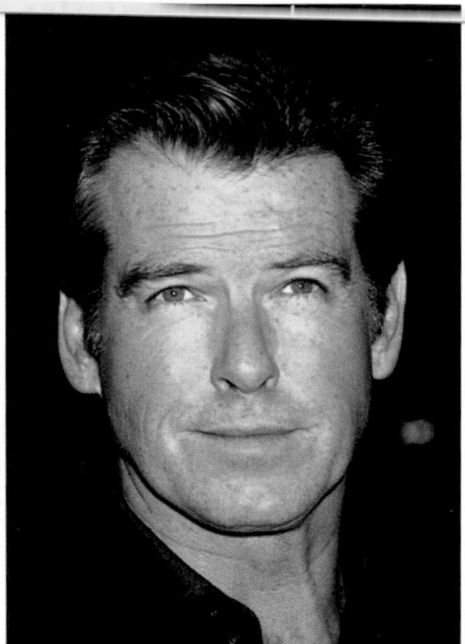

Usually, this is a rather superficial type of beauty, which I personally don't find very attractive. If I had to pick good-looking men, these would be Omar Sharif, Sean Connery and Pierce Brosnan (although it is widely claimed that Brosnan has already had a facelift).

Axel Neuroth, Düsseldorf

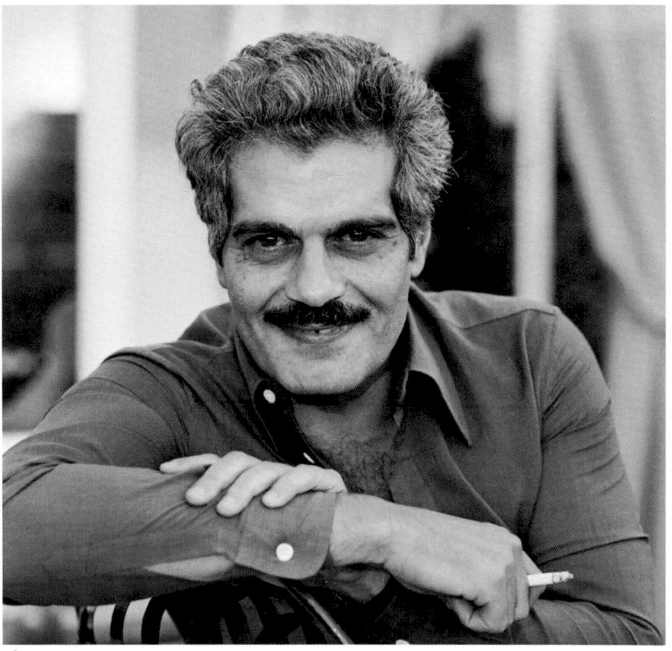

fig. 25

fig. 22 Michelangelo: David, 1501–04. Galleria dell'Accademia, Florence
fig. 23 Sean Connery, 1998. © picture-alliance / Picture Press / Camera Press / Frank Herrman
fig. 24 Pierce Brosnan, 2003. © Getty Images
fig. 25 Omar Sharif, 1974. © Getty Images / Hulton Archive

I think that symmetry and proportion, as far as ideal symmetry and ideal proportion go, are way overrated. The New York Times in particular has gotten carried away with it, and a lot of our media. But I think that the exotic proportions can often be the most attractive. (...) Often the really attractive person, especially in our modern culture, is the person with the little, quirky nose. I mean, the big, quirky nose. Or the jawline that's just a little bit too big.

Sydney R. Coleman, New York

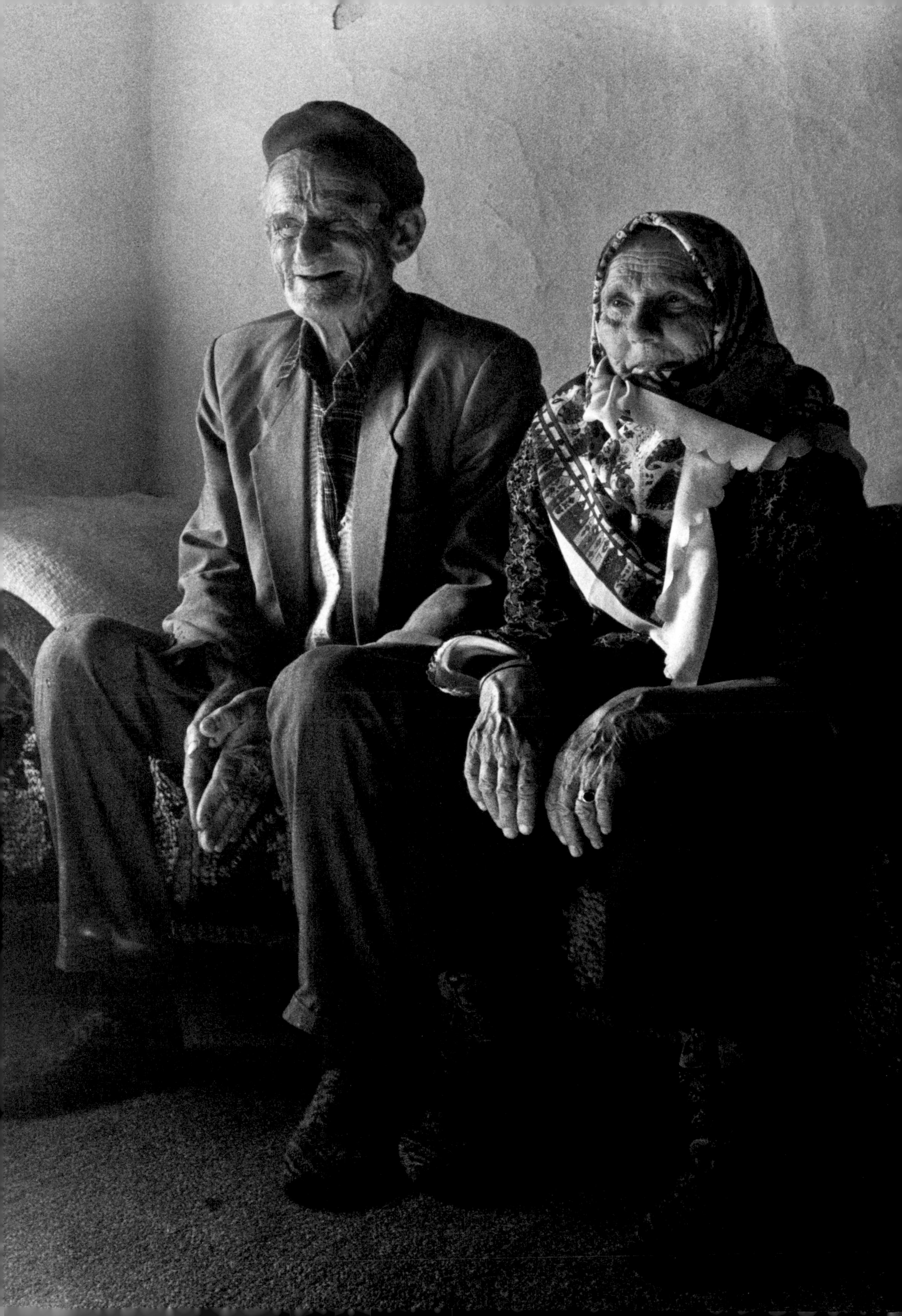

VIII.2

ABOUT AGING

STATEMENTS BY THE WORLD'S MOST FAMOUS AESTHETIC SURGEONS

Ali Al-Numairy, Dubai; Sherrell J. Aston, New York; Javier de Benito, Barcelone; Bernhard Brinkmann, Hamburg; Johannes C. Bruck, Berlin; John F. Celin, London; Bernard Cornette de Saint Cyr, Paris; Axel-Mario Feller, Munich; Carlo Gasperoni, Rome; Barry M. Jones, London; Ulrich K. Kesseling, Lausanne; Dagmar Millesi, Wien; Axel Neuroth, Düsseldorf; Antonio Tapia, Barcelone; Gerald H. Pitman, New York; Kiyotaka Watanabe, Tokyo

About Aging

fig. previous pages Couple in Bosnia, 2002
© 2004, Konrad R. Müller / Agentur Focus
fig. 1 Hercules and Old Age, greek vase. © akg-images / Nimatallah
fig. 2 Leonardo da Vinci: Old and Young Man in Profile, c.1495.
© akg-images / Rabatti - Domingie
fig. 3 Hans Baldung Grien: The Seven Ages of Woman, 1544.
© Christoph Sandig - ARTOTHEK

Aging equals living. Aging is a continual challenge that we cannot run away from and that we should meet with the utmost self-confidence and grace.

Bernhard Brinkmann, Hamburg

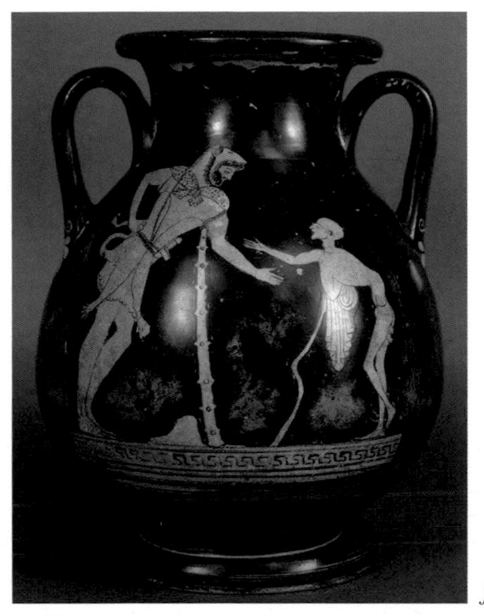

fig. 1

As we grow older, our personality shines through our appearance more strongly — the positive as well as the negative traits.

Axel Neuroth, Düsseldorf

As we cannot halt the aging process, we should attempt to lead our lives in accordance with our age.

Ali Al-Numairy, Dubai

I am convinced that
life and death are
deeply connected.
If I do not die,
my children will not live.

Johannes C. Bruck, Berlin

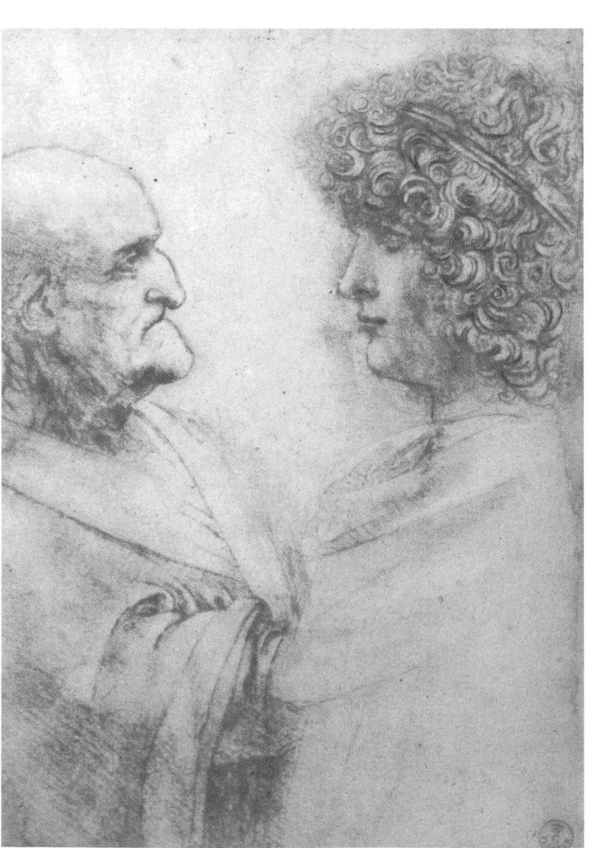

fig. 2

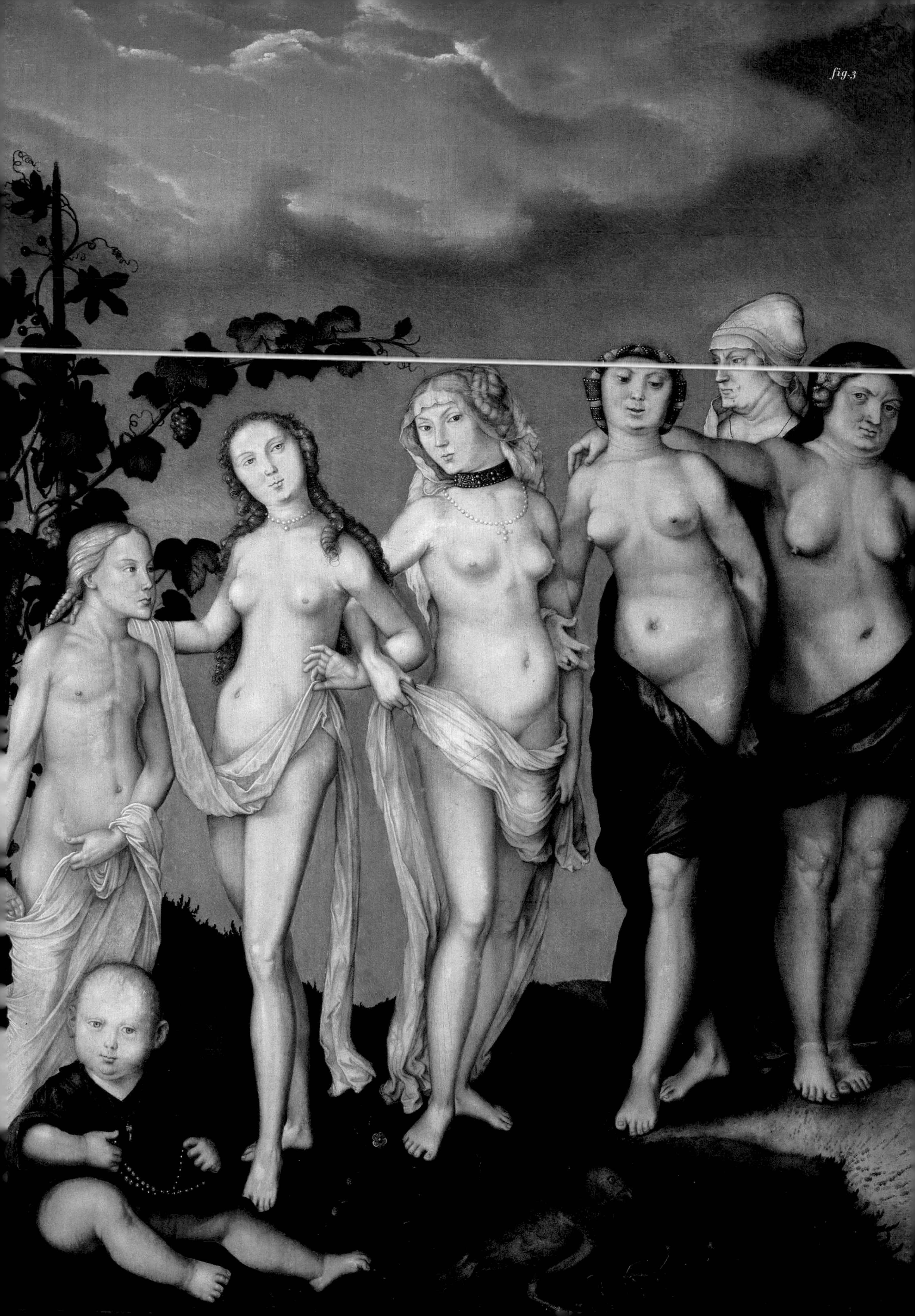
fig.3

I don't really have a fear of getting old, because it's certainly the better alternative.

Sherrell J. Aston, New York

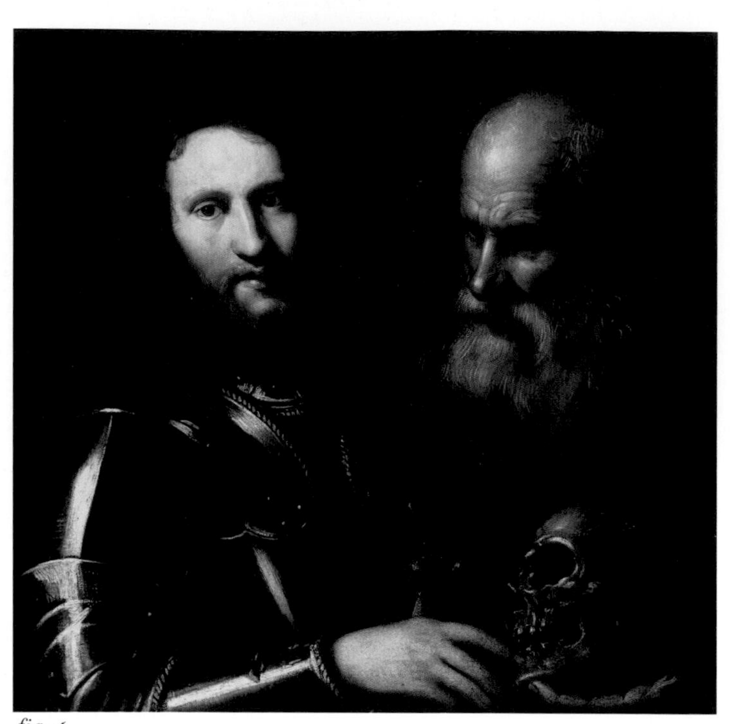

fig. 4

Unfortunately, aging is a process that deteriorates both mind and body. This scares me. (...) Luckily, my work keeps me fit and young.

Carlo Gasperoni, Rome

Aging means getting older! Looking on the bright side, it means that I will be wiser and more experienced — but also that I have to work harder on staying healthy, physically as well as mentally.

Barry M. Jones, London

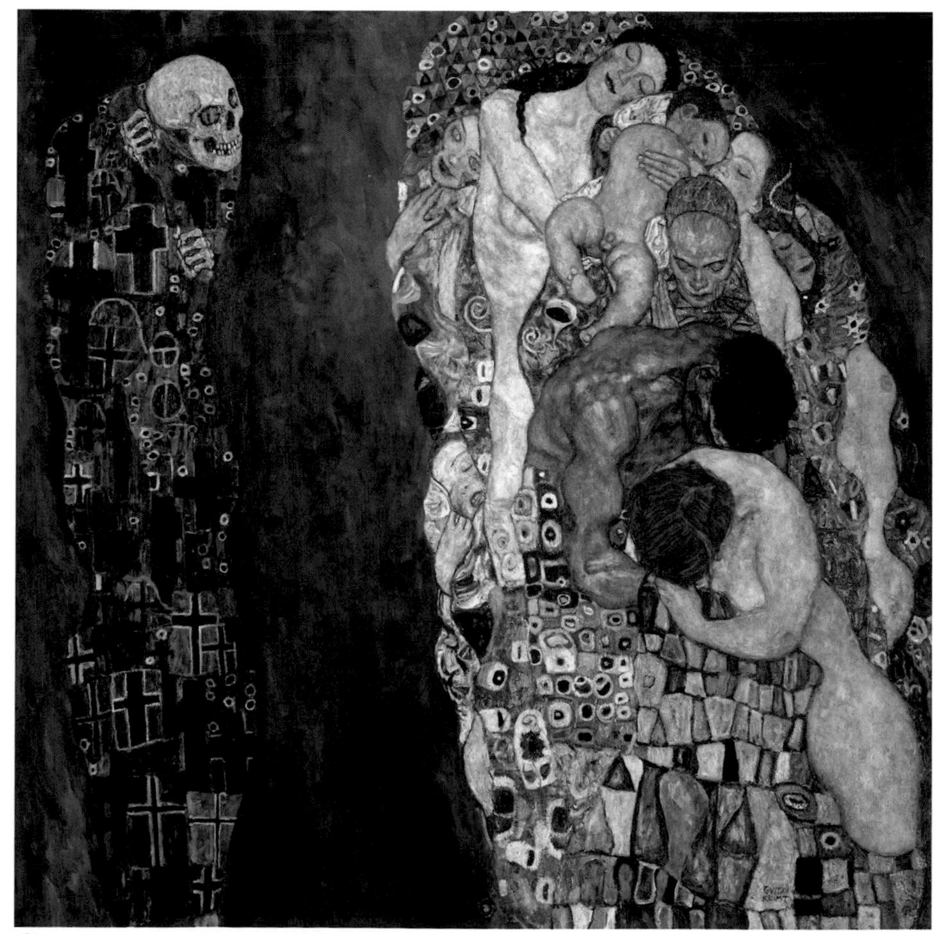

fig. 5

Aging is a biological process, one where a person ideally becomes more mature, more experienced and more understanding.

Javier de Benito, Barcelona

fig. 4 Tiziano: Allegorie Youth and Old Age, 1600. © akg-images / Cameraphoto
fig. 5 Gustav Klimt: Death and Life, [illegible] Leopold Collection Vienna. © akg-images / Erich Lessing
fig. 6 Hans Baldung Grien: The Ages of Life and Death, 1540. Museo del Prado, Madrid. © 1994, Photo Scala, Florence

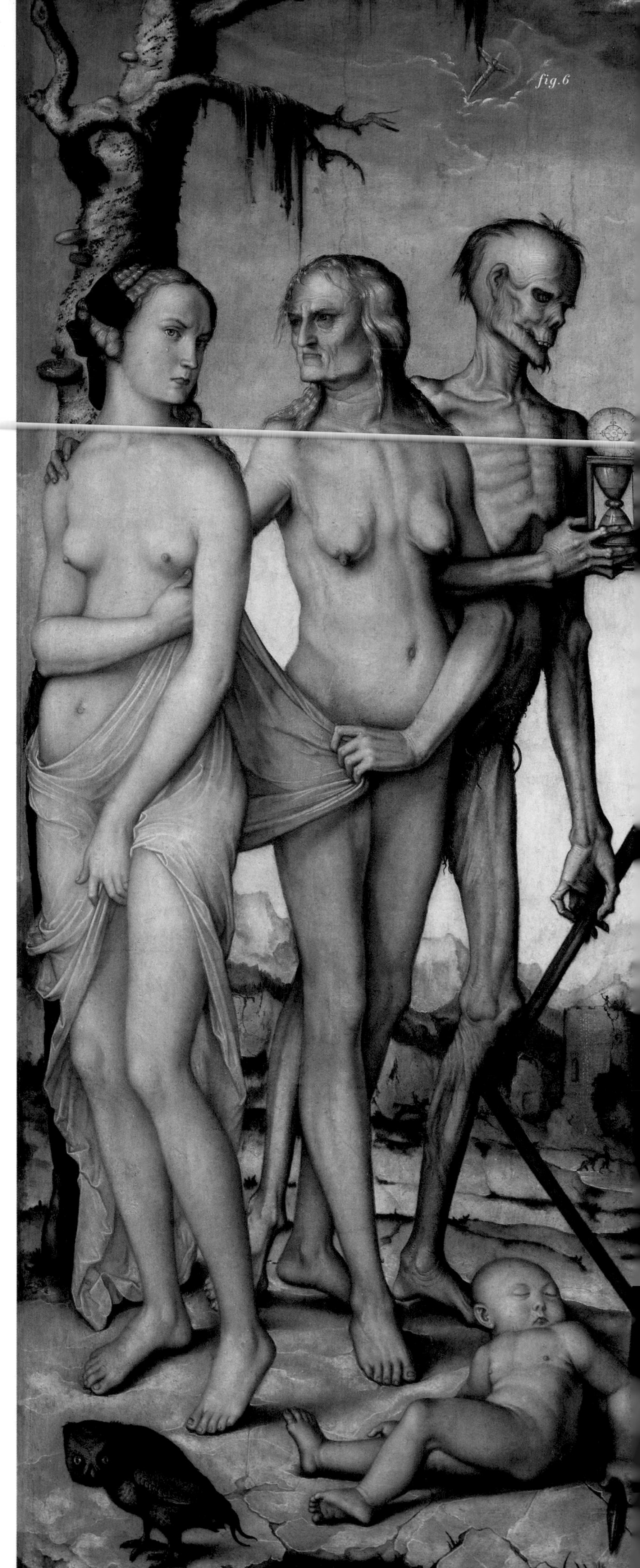

Unfortunately, aging is inexorably linked to a decline in physical ability. Our memory weakens and we cannot focus on things and people as well as we could when we were younger. At some point, we have to accept that we cannot realise all our ambitions and visions, none of us. Still, we should never stop pursuing our dreams.

Kiyotaka Watanabe, Tokyo

Looking at aging as a transitive process, it means that we need to confront our weaknesses and our mortality and come to terms with these aspects. Looking at it as an intransitive process means giving in to physical decay. This is one side of aging that can be countered with plastic surgery.

Johannes C. Bruck, Berlin

fig. 7

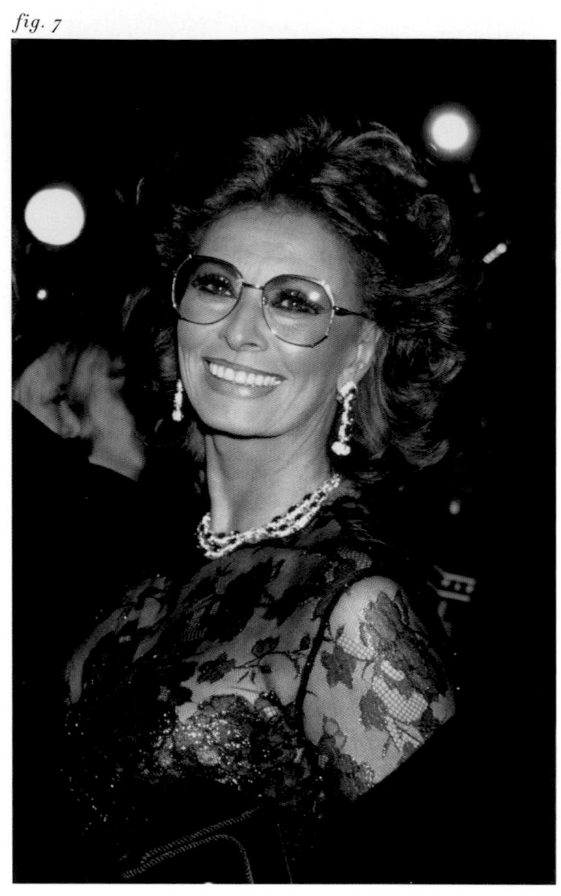

You cannot change your destiny. All you can do is live every day with as much awareness and optimism as possible.

Axel-Mario Feller, Munich

A few years ago, a very elegant lady and distinguished French aristocrat said to me, "Vous savez, Docteur, vieillir, c'est enmerdant." You know, Doctor, aging is bloody annoying.

Ulrich K. Kesselring, Lausanne

fig. 7 Sophia Loren, 1994. © Mitchell Gerber / CORBIS
fig. 8 Katherine Hepburn, c. 1948 © Underwood & Underwood / CORBIS
fig. 9 Katherine Hepburn, c. 2001 © Bryson John / CORBIS SYGMA
fig. 10 Sophia Loren, 1950s. © John Springer Collection / CORBIS

To me, like to everybody else, aging signifies a decline in bodily functions and a rise of physical ailments. For this reason alone, we should strive to retard and avoid the consequences of aging for as long as possible. Quite possibly the best way to do this is to combine a healthy lifestyle with anti-aging measures and cosmetic surgery.

Dagmar Millesi, Vienna

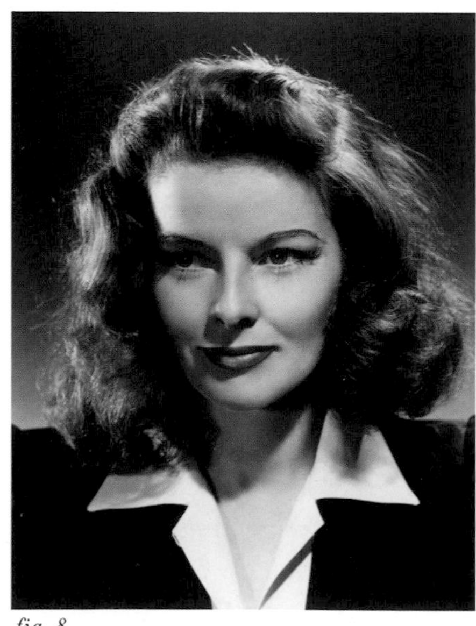

fig. 8

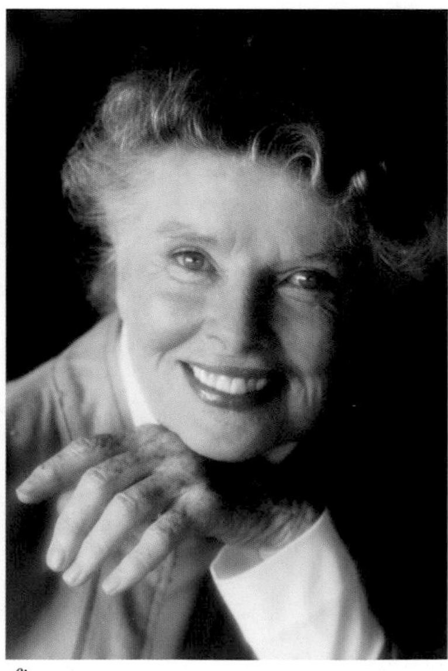

fig. 9

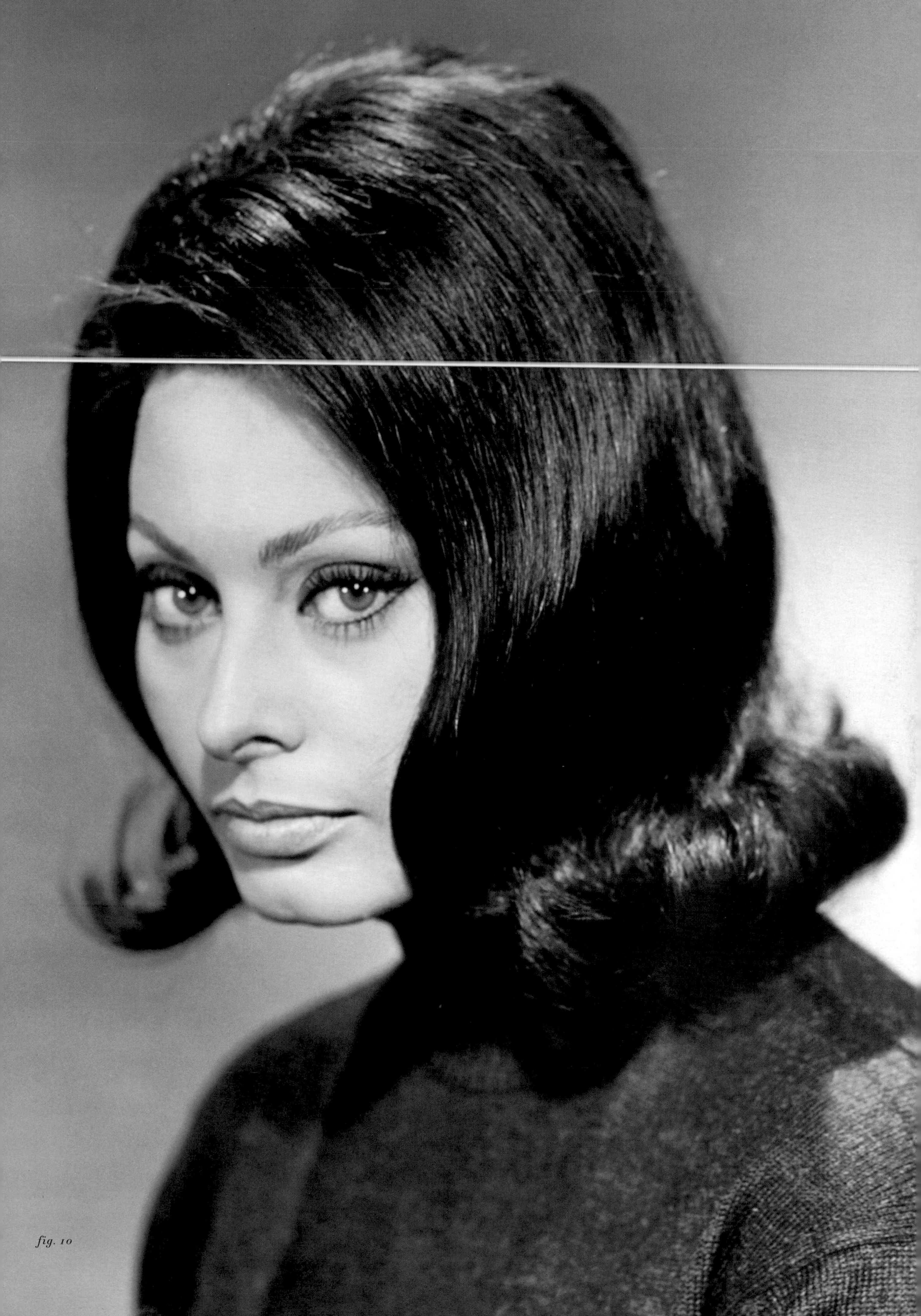

fig. 10

fig. 11

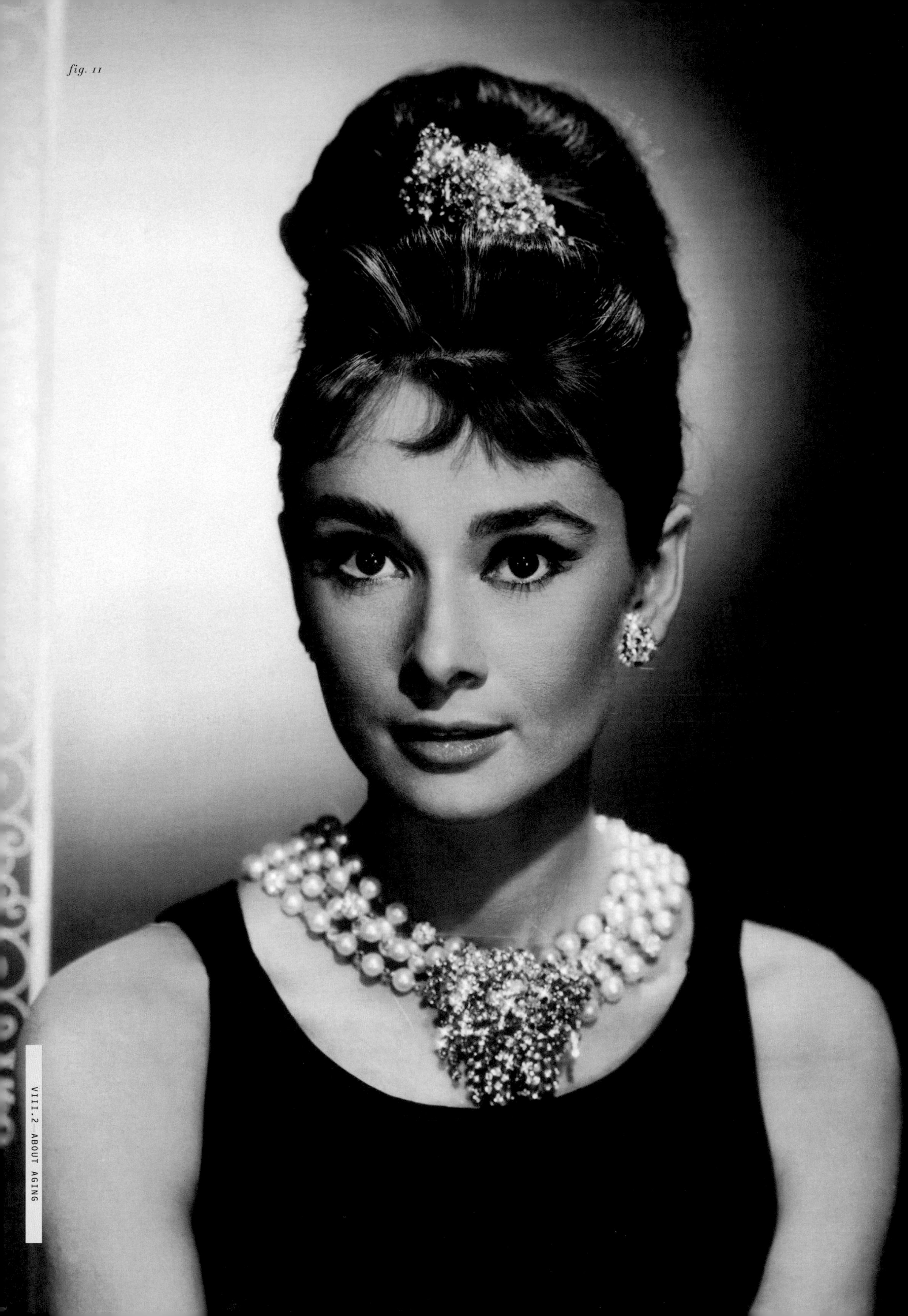

There are 25-year-olds who look frighteningly old and 55-year-old who are bursting with energy and vitality. Some men and women become more beautiful with age, others become less attractive. I think people have a lot of control over how they age.

Bernard Cornette de Saint Cyr, Paris

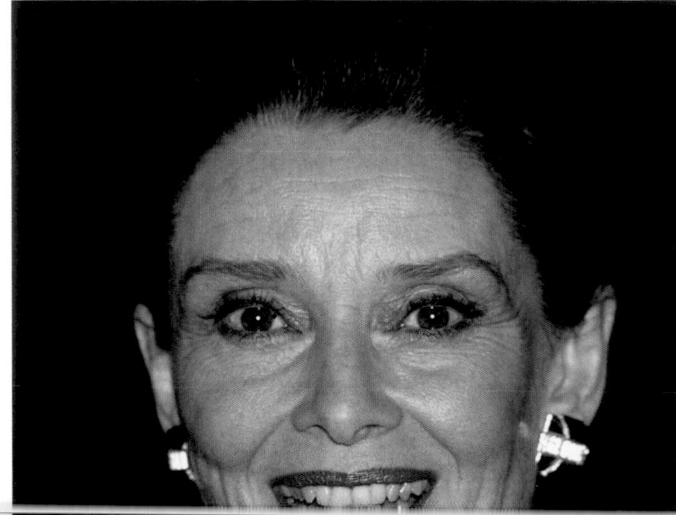

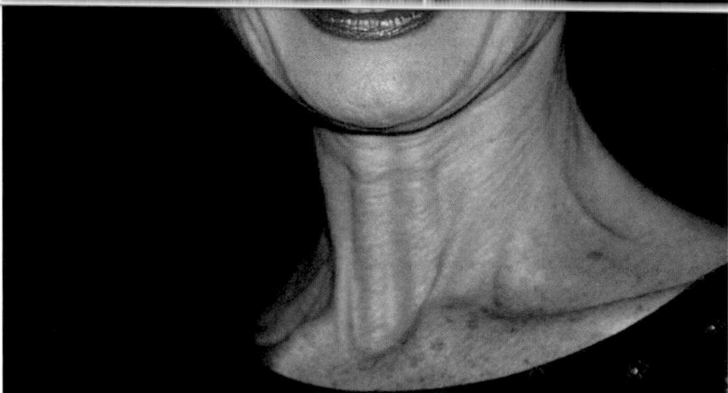

fig. 12

fig. 11 *Audrey Hepburn, 1961. © Underwood & Underwood / CORBIS*
fig. 12 *Audrey Hepburn, 1989. © Time Life Pictures / Getty Images*
fig. 13 *Omar Sharif, 1965. © Getty Images / Hulton Archive*
fig. 14 *Omar Sharif, 1995. © Matthew Mendelsohn / CORBIS*

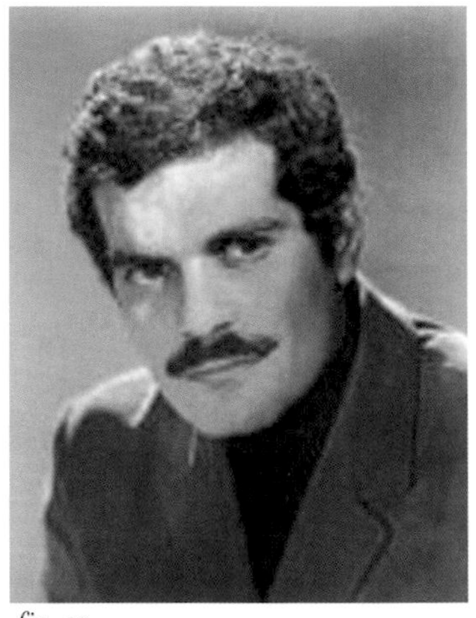

fig. 13

I think at the beginning of the 20th century, 50 was old. At the beginning of the 21st century, 60 is not old, for some people.

Gerald H. Pitman, New York

I live and work so intensely that I don't even have the time to be afraid of aging.

John F. Celin, London

The aging process is an accumulation of life experiences, and really a maturation of our personality and our emotional responses to life in general.

Sherrell J. Aston, New York

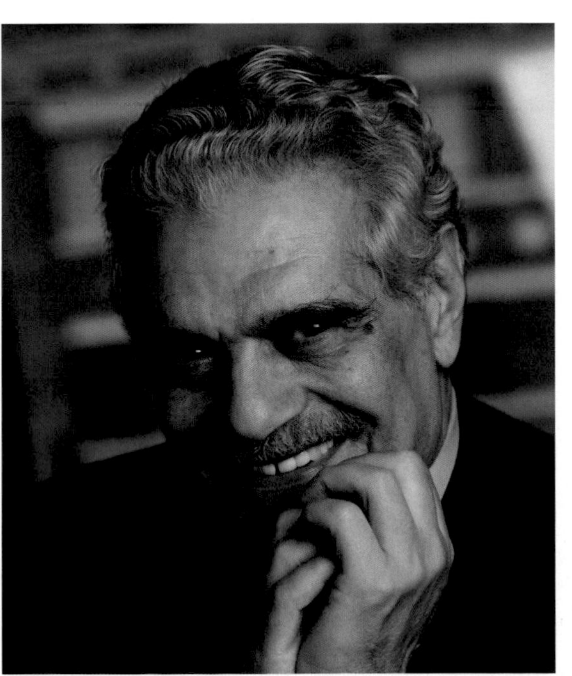

fig. 14

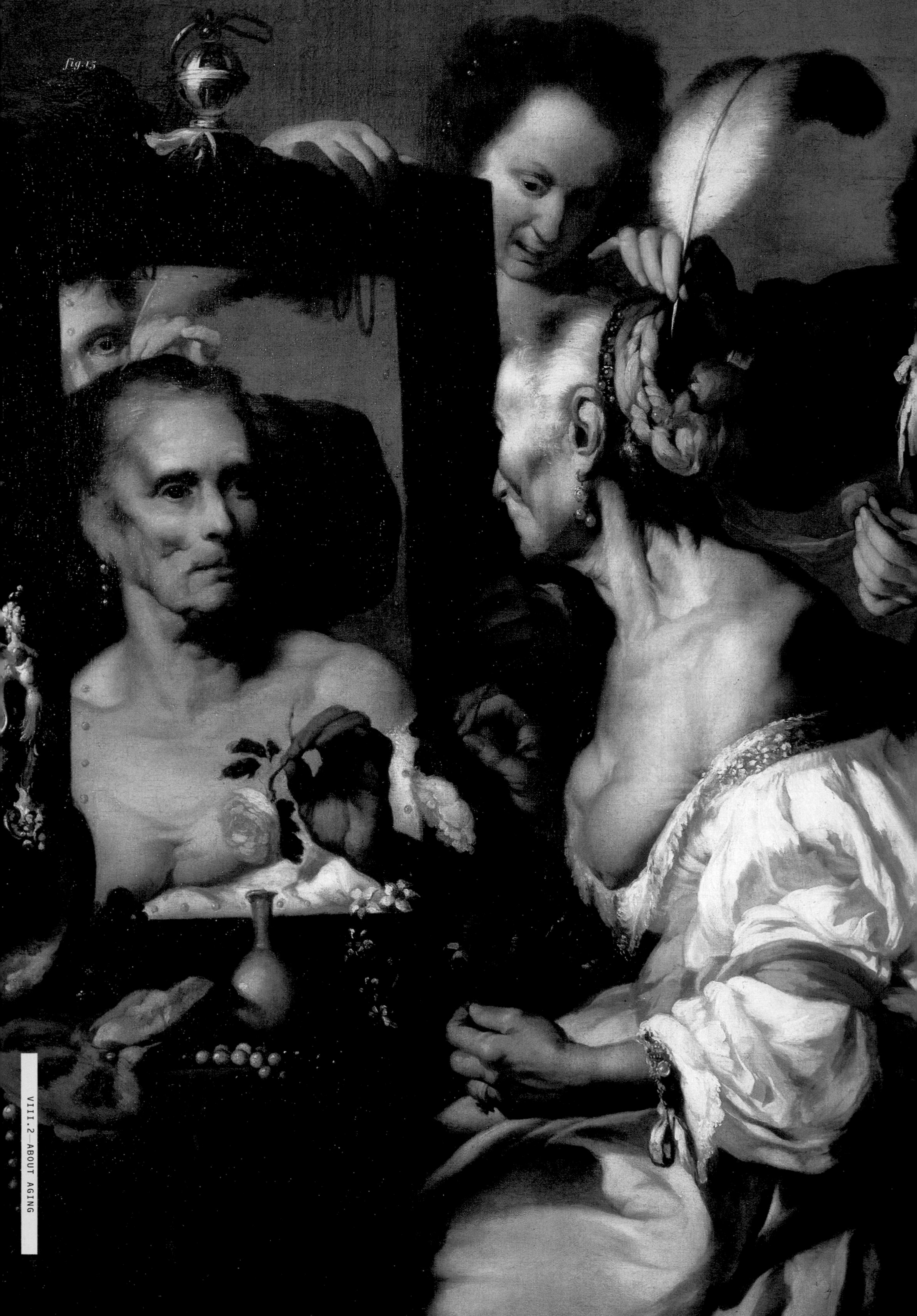

fig.15

Age is just another part of life. With the help of aesthetic surgery, it may run its course more smoothly — or not!

Antonio Tapia, Barcelona

fig. 16

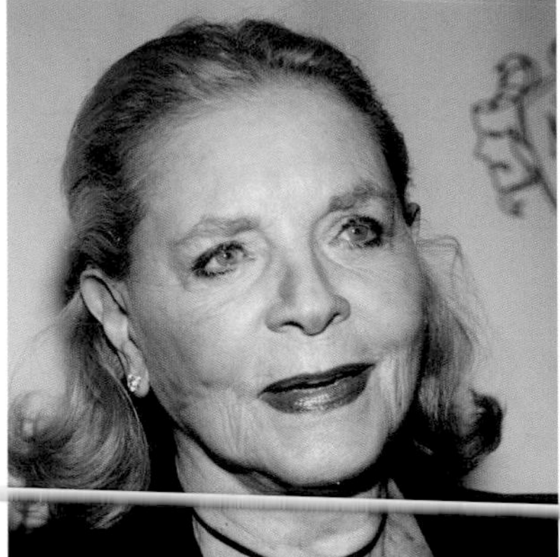

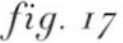

fig. 17

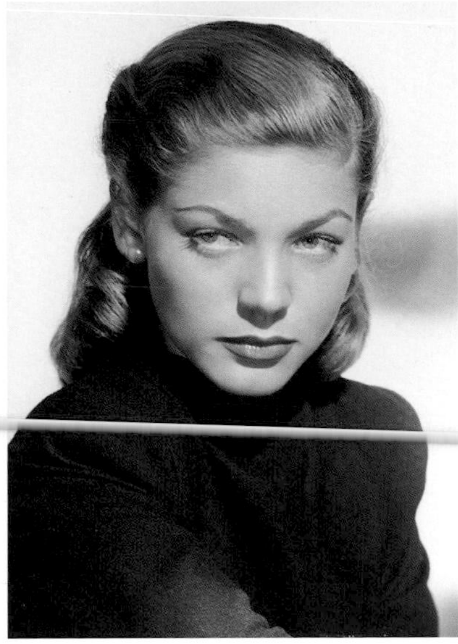

fig. [illegible] Strozzi: Vanitas, 1630. Pushkin Museum, Moscow. © ARTOTHEK
fig. 16 Lauren Bacall, 2004. © Getty Images
fig. 17 Lauren Bacall, 1945. © Getty Images / Hulton Archive
fig. 18 Martha Graham photographed by Andy Warhol, 1979. © Andy Warhol Foundation / CORBIS
fig. 19 Lucas Cranach the Elder: The Fountain of Youth, 1546. SPMK Gemäldegalerie, Berlin. © Joachim Blauel - ARTOTHEK

To me, beauty is not bound by age. Lauren Bacall, for example, is still exceptionally beautiful.

Barry M. Jones, London

Many of our qualities wane with age: beauty, charisma, power, sexual attractiveness. This leads to a loss in self-esteem, and because of this, a lot of old people are bad-tempered. If they didn't make other people notice them, they might soon become invisible.

Ulrich K. Kesselring, Lausanne

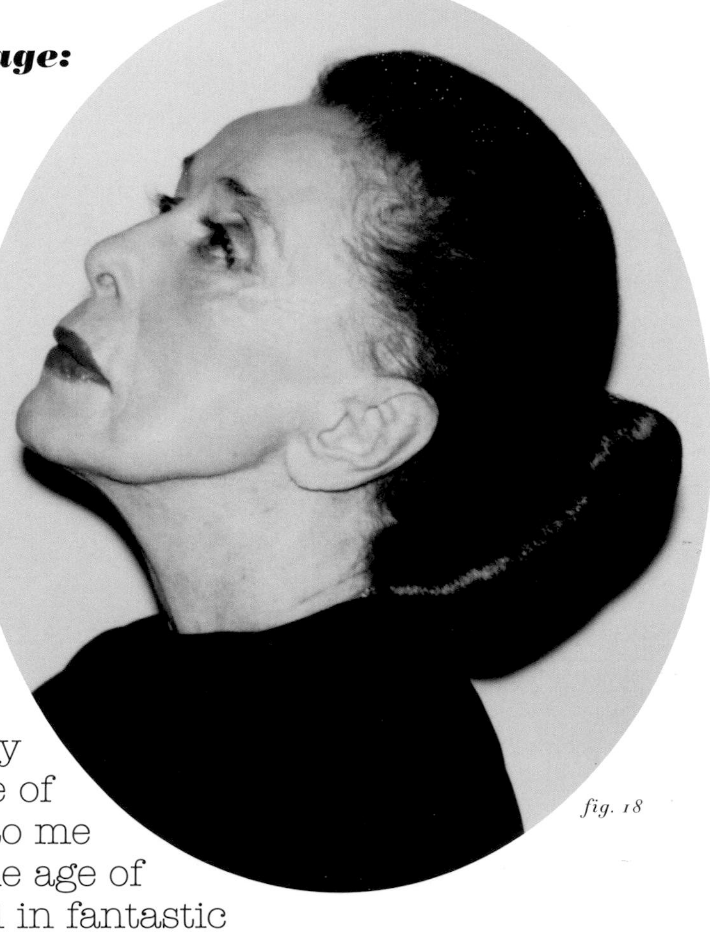

fig. 18

When Martha Graham, the most famous US choreographer and dancer of the 20th century and a founding force of American ballet, came to me for cosmetic surgery at the age of 84, her body was still in fantastic shape. She wanted her face to match her body's relentless energy. She died at the age of 97 in 1991.

John F. Celin, London.

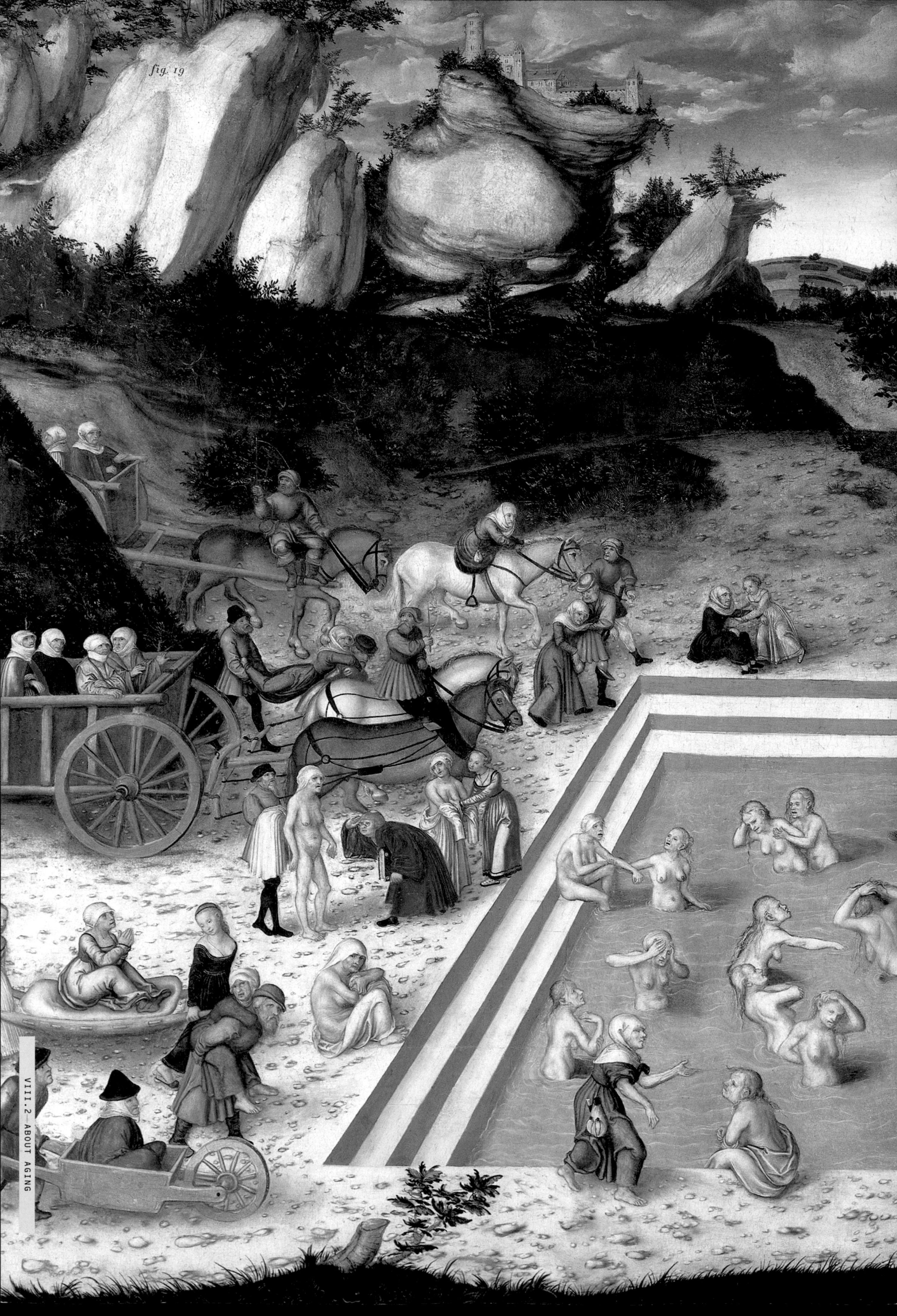

fig. 19

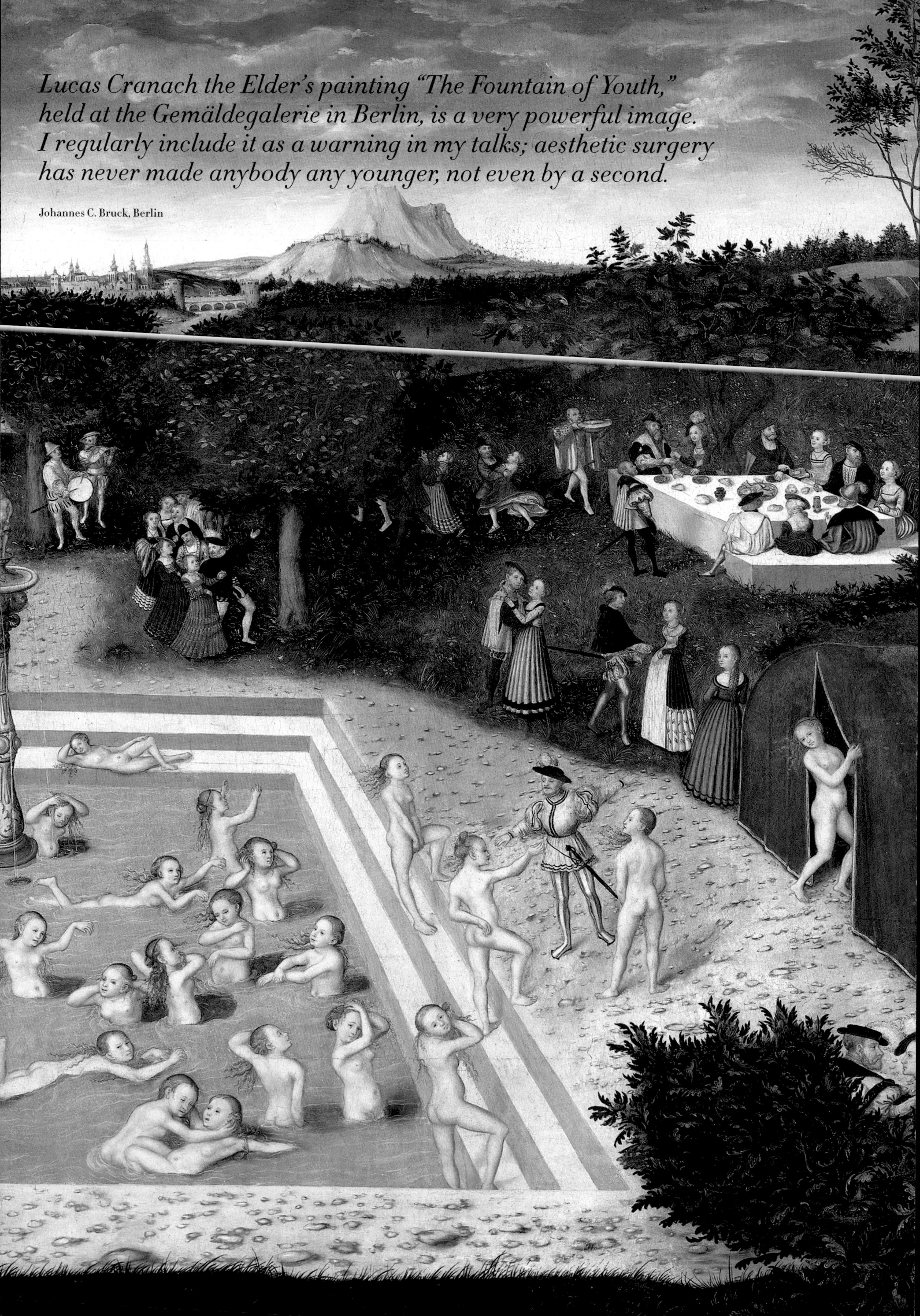

Lucas Cranach the Elder's painting "The Fountain of Youth," held at the Gemäldegalerie in Berlin, is a very powerful image. I regularly include it as a warning in my talks; aesthetic surgery has never made anybody any younger, not even by a second.

Johannes C. Bruck, Berlin

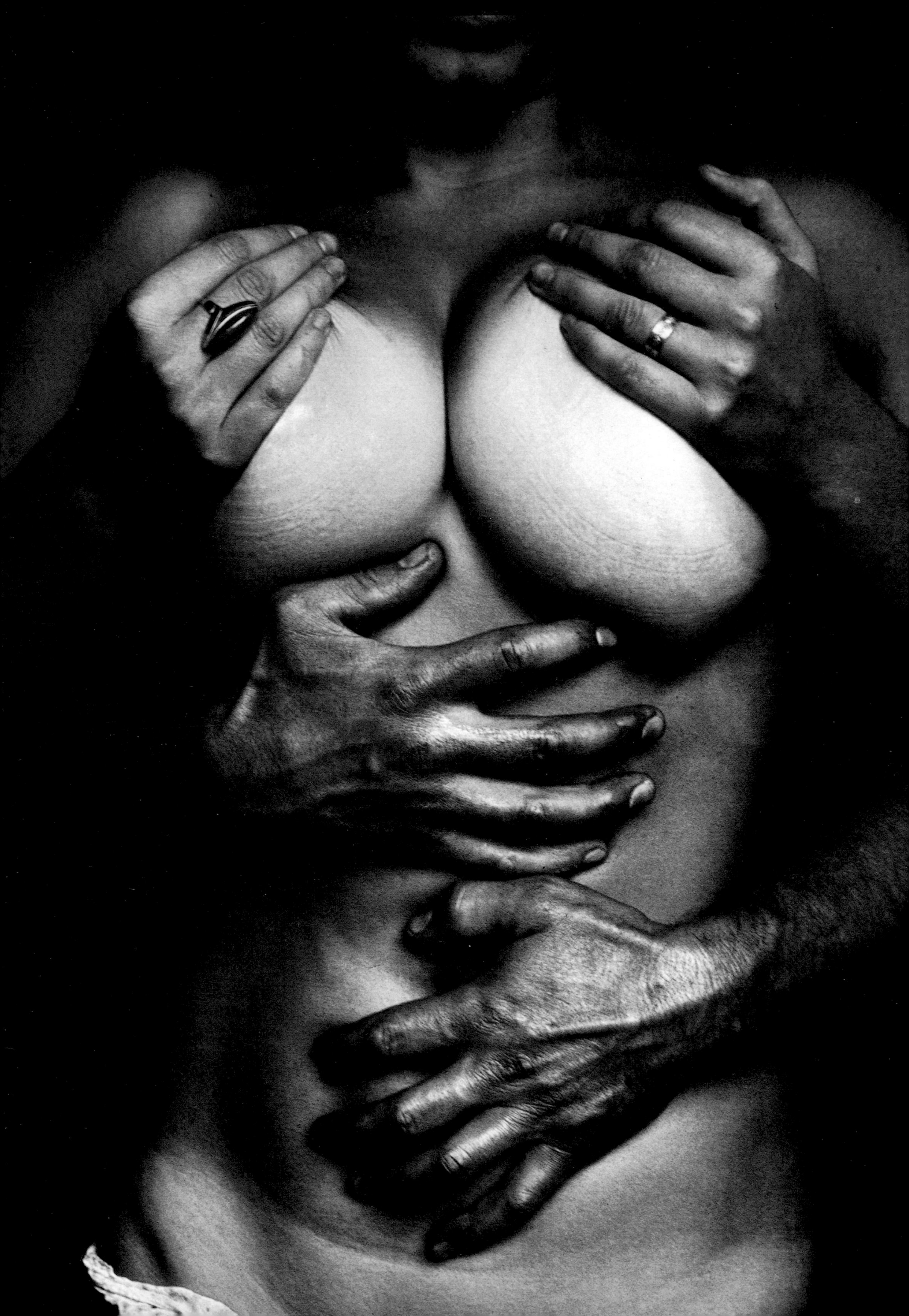

VIII$_3$

ABOUT SEX

STATEMENTS BY THE WORLD'S MOST FAMOUS AESTHETIC SURGEONS

Johannes C. Bruck, Berlin; John F. Celin, London; Axel-Mario Feller, Munich; Carlo Gasperoni, Rome; Jorge Herrera, Buenos Aires; Ulrich K. Kesseling, Lausanne; Daymar Millesi, Wien; Egle Muti, Turin; Axel Neuroth, Düsseldorf; Rolf Rüdiger Olbrisch, Düsseldorf; Jean-Louis Sebagh, Paris; Kiyotaka Watanabe, Tokyo

About Sex

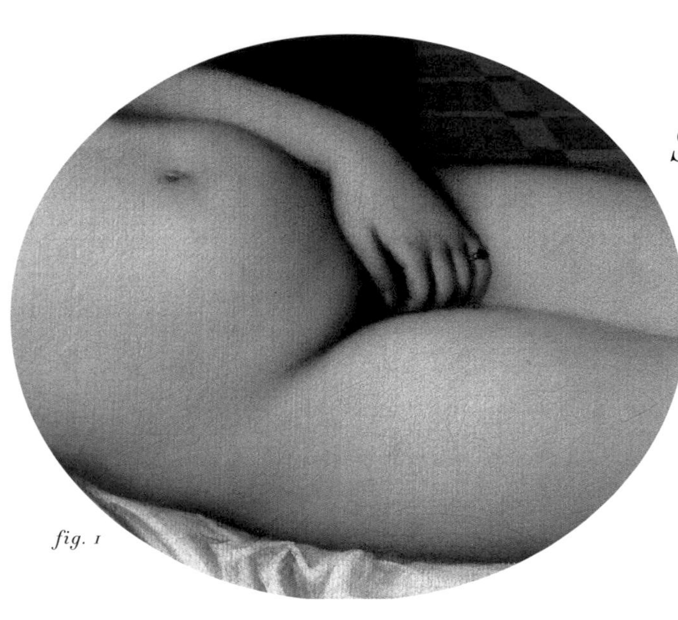

fig. 1

Sexuality is not linked to physical beauty. This is especially true for women.

Egle Muti, Turin

fig. previous pages
Jan Saudek: Those days of the Sixties, 1965
© Jan Saudek, Prague
fig. 1 Tiziano: Resting Venus (The Venus of Urbino), Detail, c.1538. Oil on canvas, 119 x 165 cm. Galleria degli Uffizi, Florence.
© Photo Scala, Florence
fig. 2 Roman Mosaik: Erotic Scene (Satyr and Nymph, House of the Fauno), from Pompeii, 100 A. D. Museo Nazionale Acheologico, Naples.
© 2003, Photo Scala, Florence / Fotografica Foglia
fig. 3 Man Ray: Restored Venus (Vénus restaurée), 1936. Plaster, rope. Height: 71 cm. Private Collection, Milan. Man Ray
© akg-images / Piero Baguzzi

A beautiful woman certainly receives more sexual offers. However, this does not necessarily mean she has a better sex life.

Ulrich K. Kesselring, Lausanne

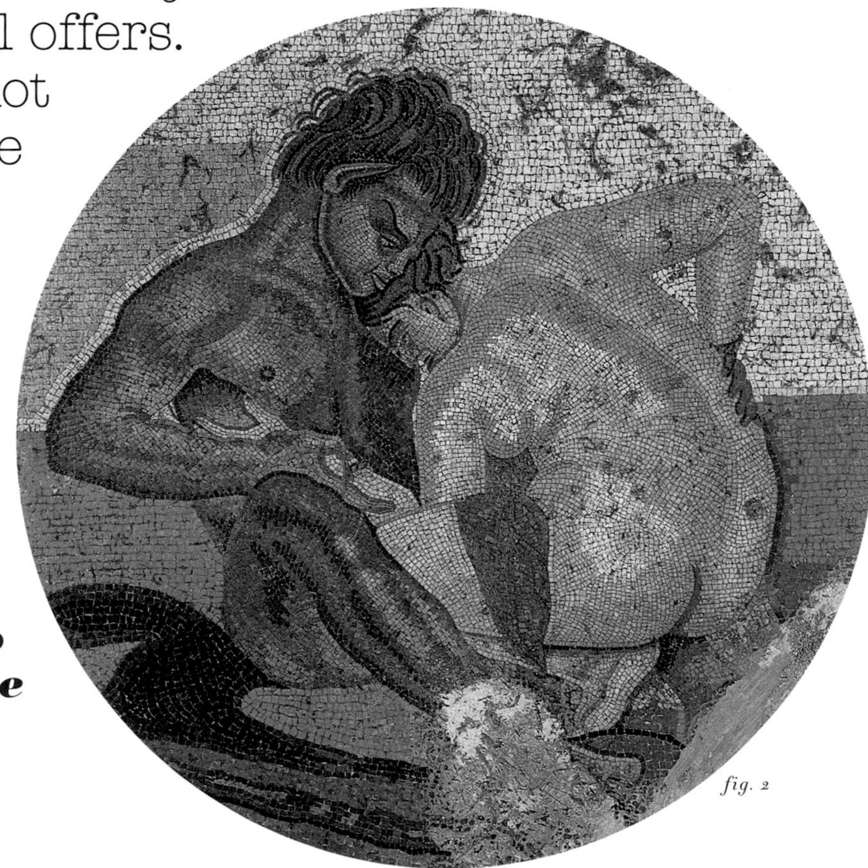

fig. 2

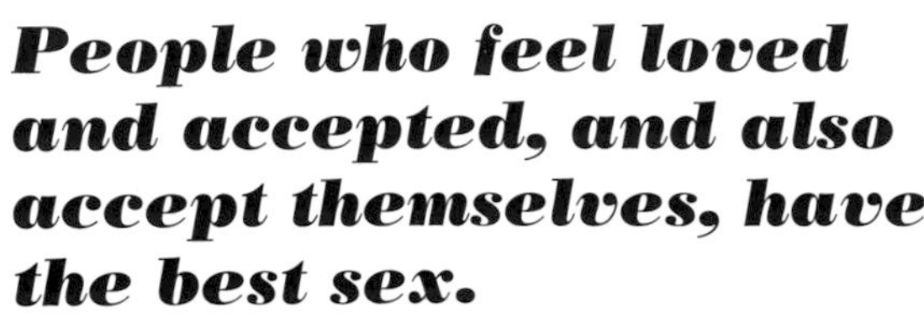

People who feel loved and accepted, and also accept themselves, have the best sex.

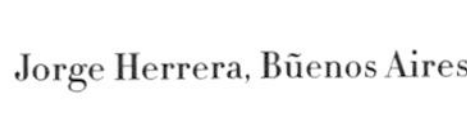

Jorge Herrera, Būenos Aires

You can have great sex at any age. The prerequisite is not beauty but self-esteem. Sex symbols don't necessarily have good sex; often they feel very objectified and have surprisingly little self-confidence.

Jean-Louis Sebagh, Paris

Sex takes place in your head. For a beautiful person, it is probably easier to have sex — but not to have better sex. To the contrary, sex may well be more difficult for beautiful people because their partners expect more from them.

Axel-Mario Feller, Munich

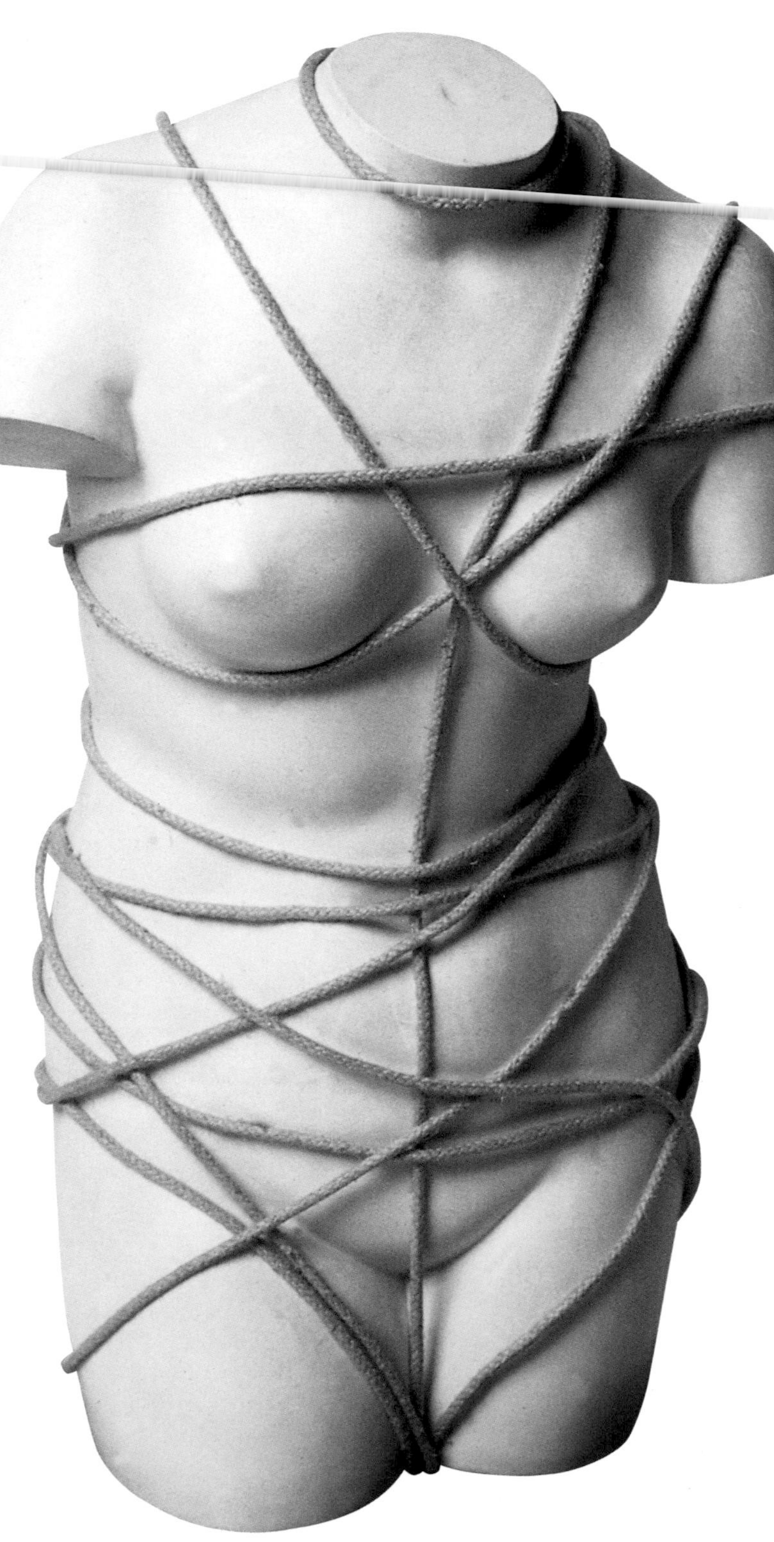

Beauty can also get in the way of good sex if it invites fears of failure.

Axel Neuroth, Düsseldorf

fig. 3

Beauty and a fulfilling sex life have nothing to do with each other. I even believe that beauty and sexual appetite are diametrically opposed! Beautiful people may often be the object of lust or desire, but this is probably not what they want.

Carlo Gasperoni, Rome

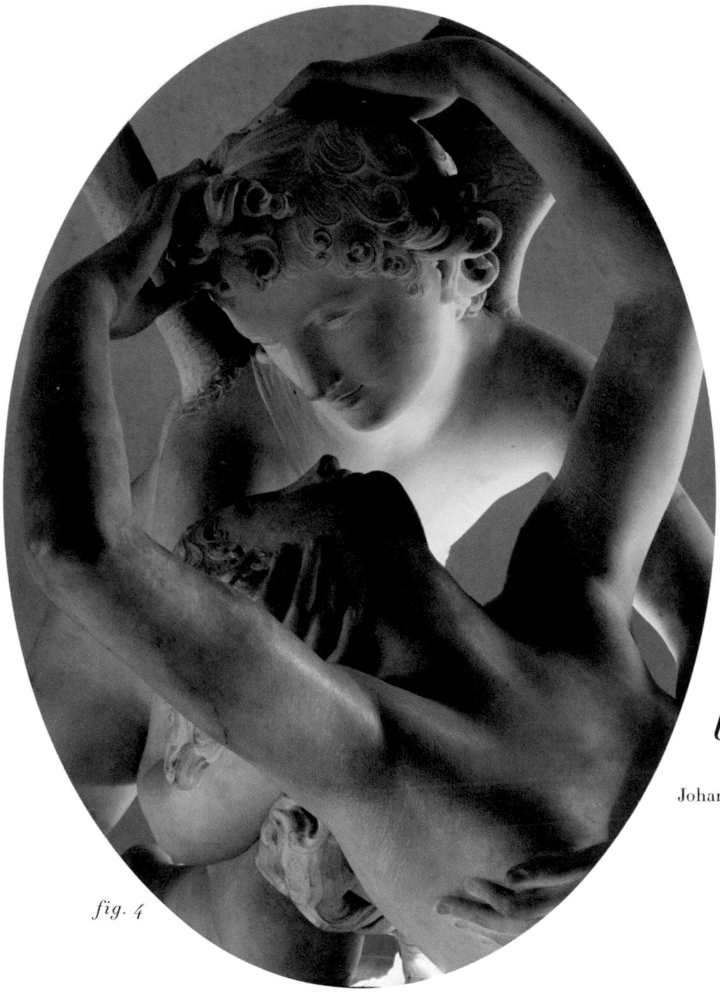

Every sexual act is a glimpse of immortality. If you are happy with your body, you will be more relaxed during sex.

Johannes C. Bruck, Berlin

fig. 4

fig. 4 Antonio Canova: Cupid and Psyche, Detail, 1787–93. Marble, height: 155 cm. Musée du Louvre, Paris. © akg-images / Erich Lessing
fig. 5 Terry Richardson: Untitled. © Terry Richardson, New York
fig. 6 Kim Basinger in Nine 1/2 Weeks, 1986. © M. G. M. / United Artist / Album / Akg

People who feel attractive find it easier to attract others. This doesn't, however, make the sex any better.

John F. Celin, London

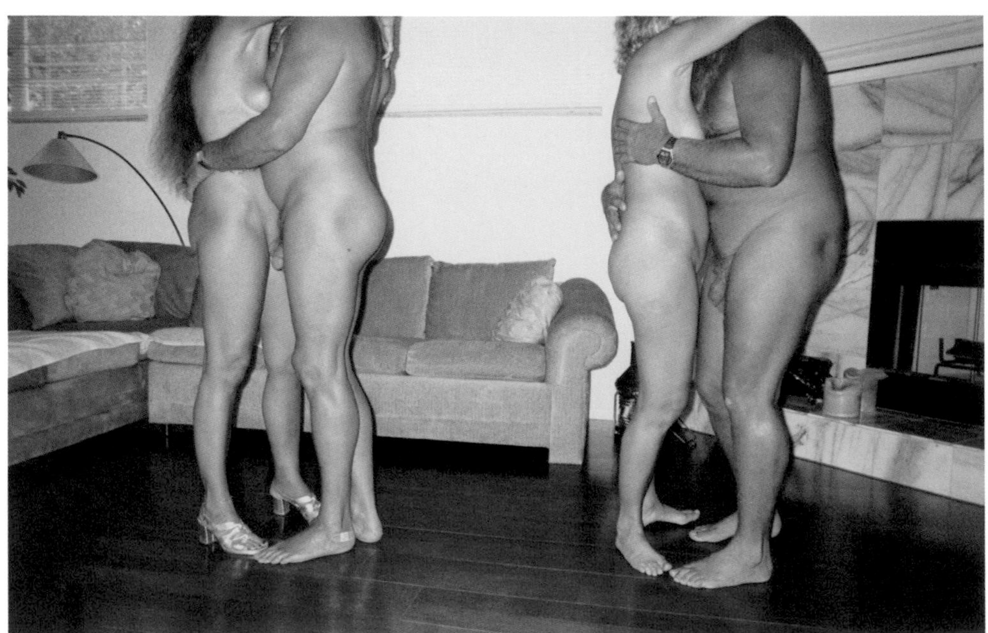

fig. 5

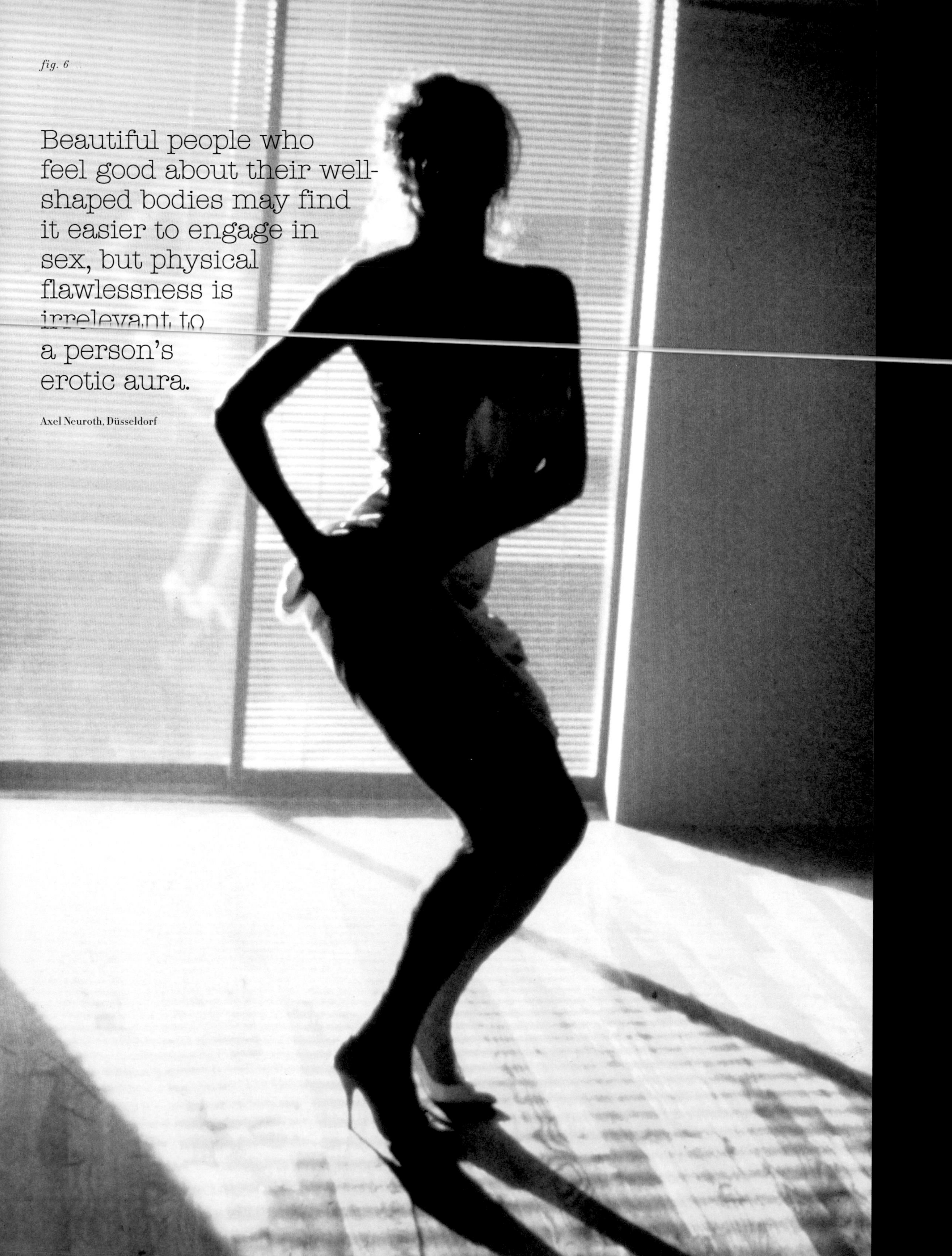

fig. 6

Beautiful people who feel good about their well-shaped bodies may find it easier to engage in sex, but physical flawlessness is irrelevant to a person's erotic aura.

Axel Neuroth, Düsseldorf

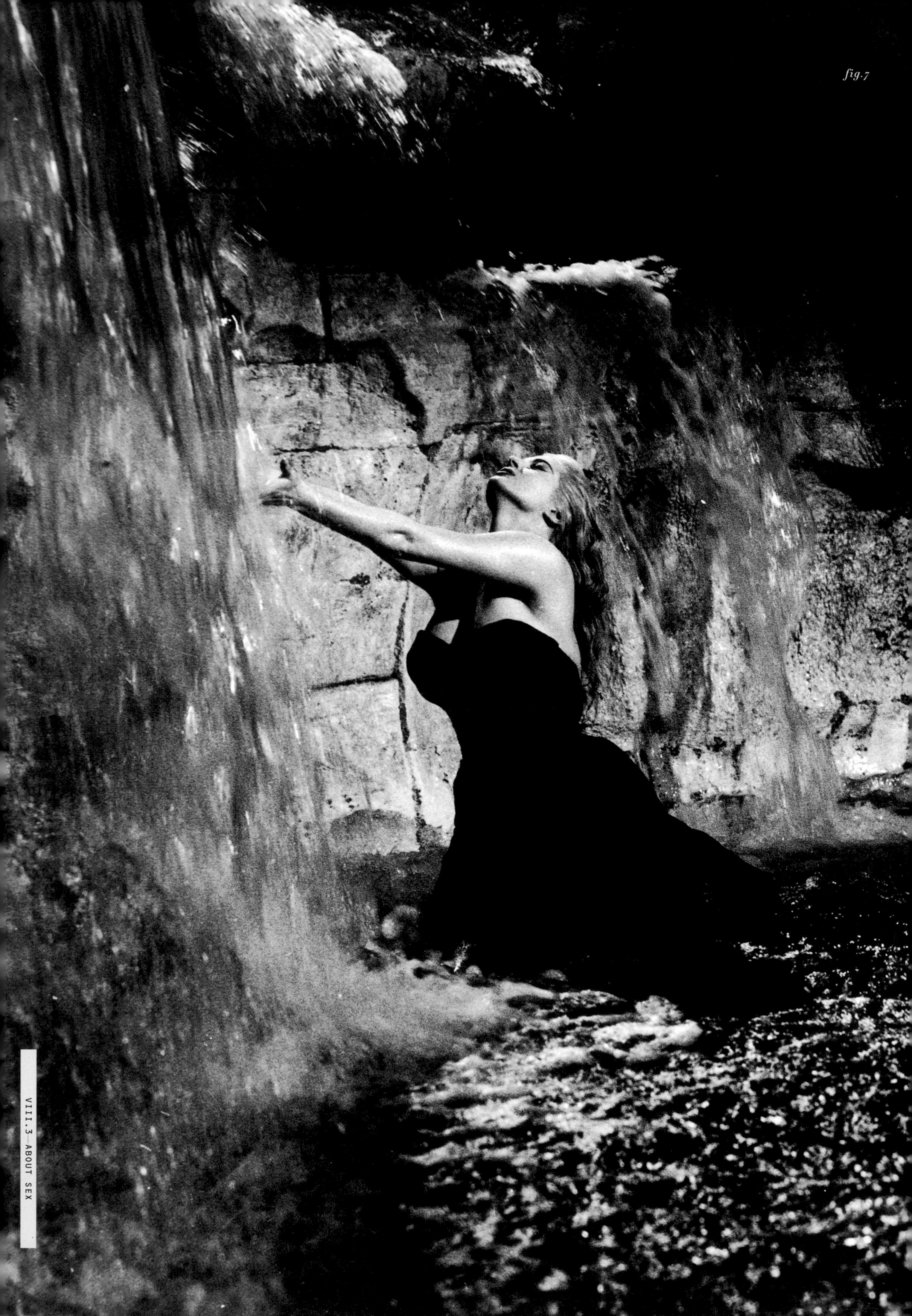

fig.7

One fact is certain: Beauty and sex are independent of each other.

Axel Neuroth, Düsseldorf

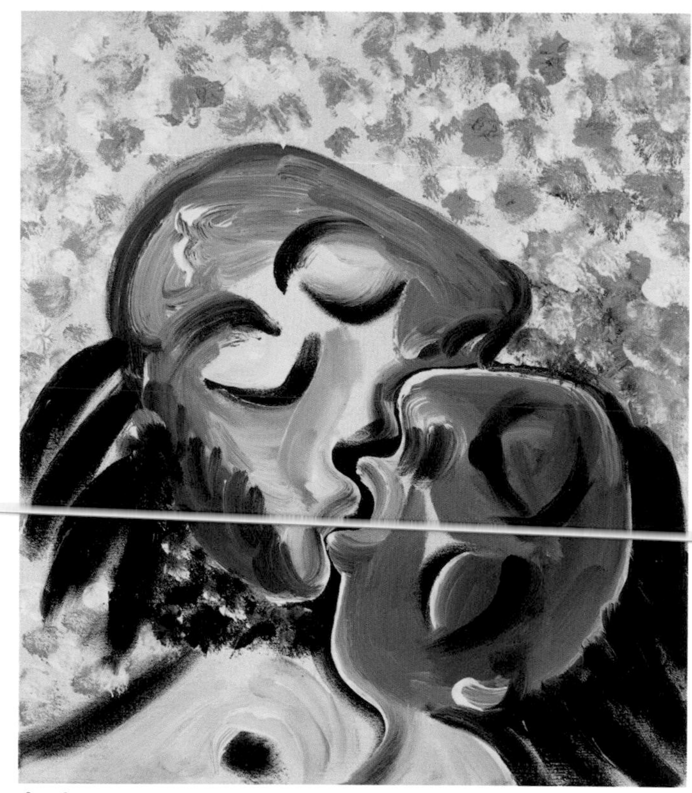

fig. 8

I don't see any connection between beauty and sex.

Kiyotaka Watanabe, Tokyo

As a person's self-esteem grows together with his or her beauty, I could imagine that some patients who had previously been shy in bed — possibly due to a subjective flaw — suddenly develop much greater self-confidence after their operation and are then able to enjoy a more fulfilled love life.

Dagmar Millesi, Vienna

fig. 7 Anita Ekberg in Federico Fellini's La Dolce Vita. © defd
fig. 8 Pablo Picasso: The Kiss, 1969. Oil on canvas, 46 x 38 cm. Private Collection. Picasso© Pablo Picasso / DACS
fig. 9 Jack Nicholson and Jessica Lange in "The Postman Always Rings Twice", 1981. © Paramount Pictures / Album / akg

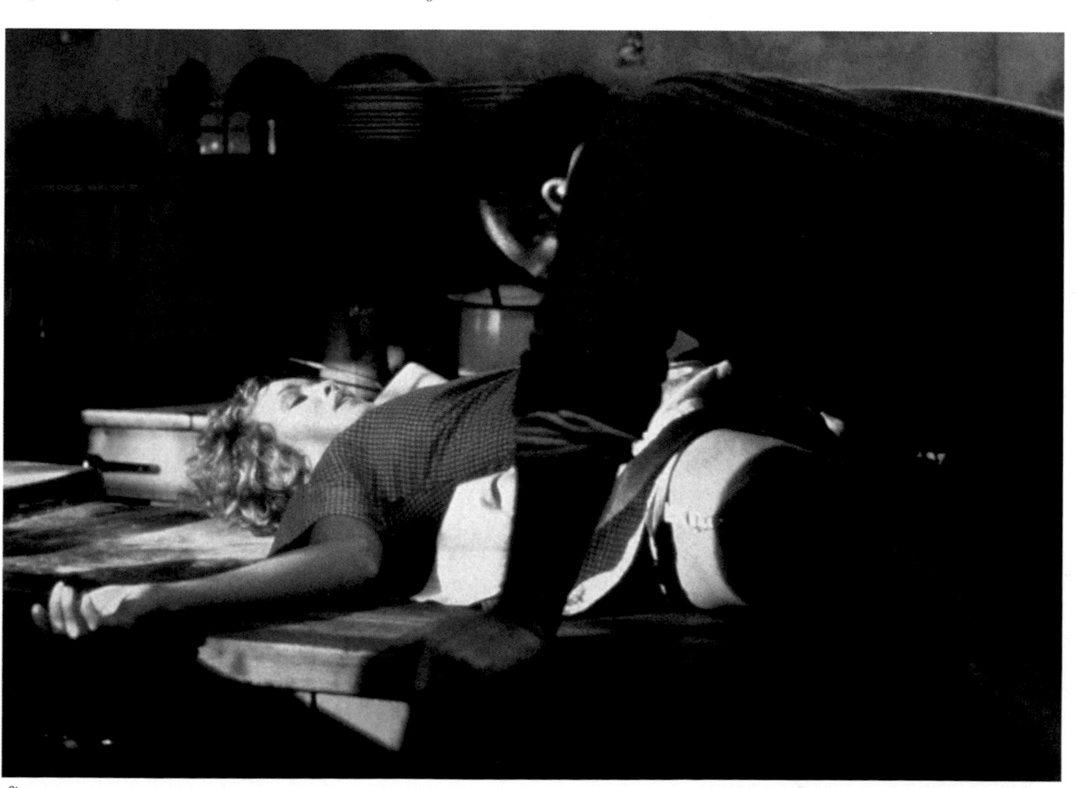

fig. 9

Our animal instinct is our strongest urge, regardless of beauty.

Rolf R. Olbrisch, Düsseldorf

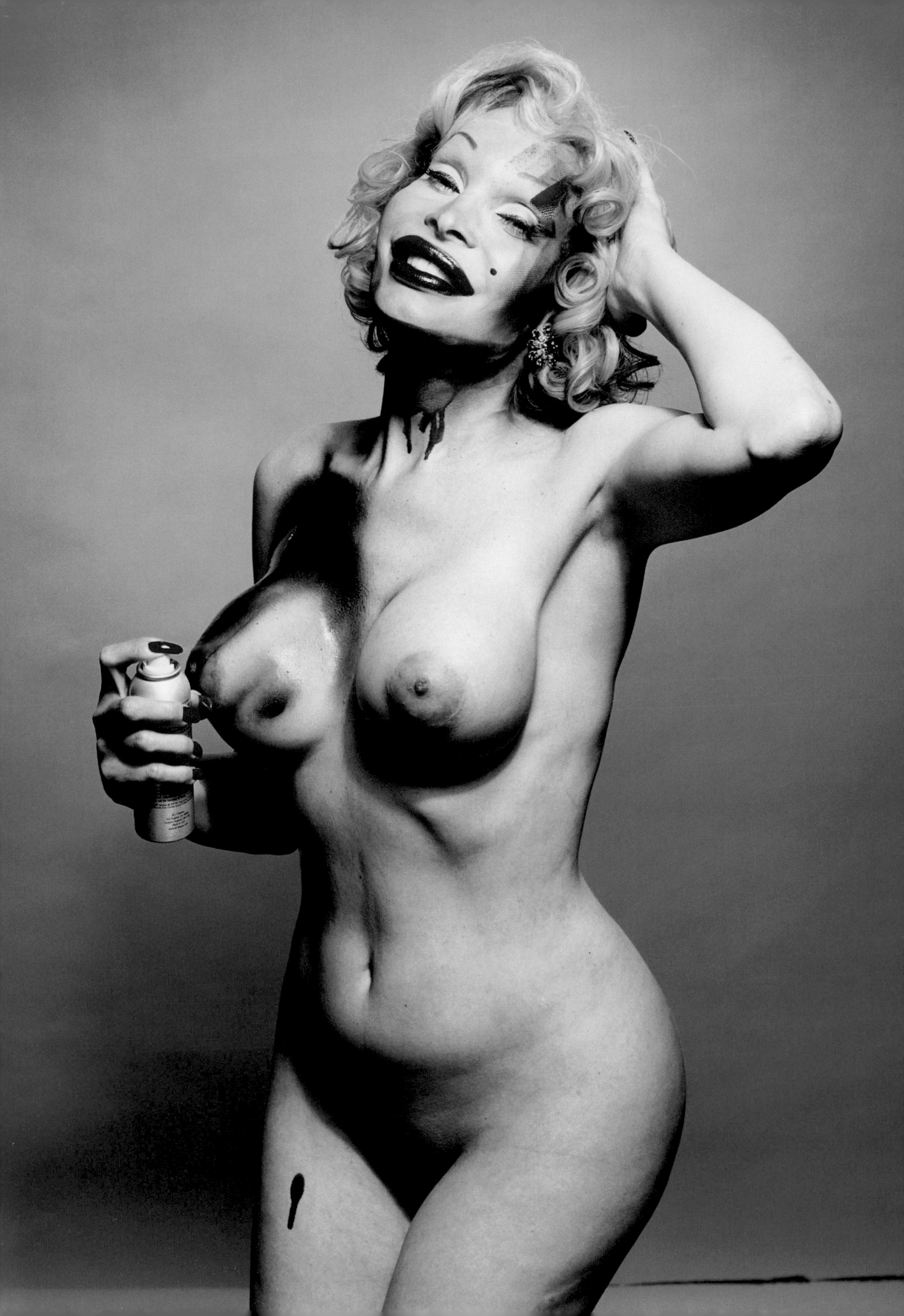

VIII.4

ABOUT EXTREMES

STATEMENTS BY THE WORLD'S MOST FAMOUS AESTHETIC SURGEONS

Johannes C. Bruck, Berlin; Sydney R. Coleman, New York; Axel-Mario Feller, Munich; Carlo Gasperoni, Rome; Ulrich K. Kesseling, Lausanne; Dagmar Millesi, Wien; Egle Muti, Turin; Axel Neuroth, Düsseldorf; Rolf Rüdiger Olbrisch, Düsseldorf; Gerald H. Pitman, New York; Jean-Louis Sebagh, Paris

About Extremes

Because of my particular niche in plastic surgery, I'm probably asked for a lot of the more unusual things. Recently, I would say, nipple augmentation in really normal, attractive boys has become very sort of bizarrely trendy.

Sydney R. Coleman, New York

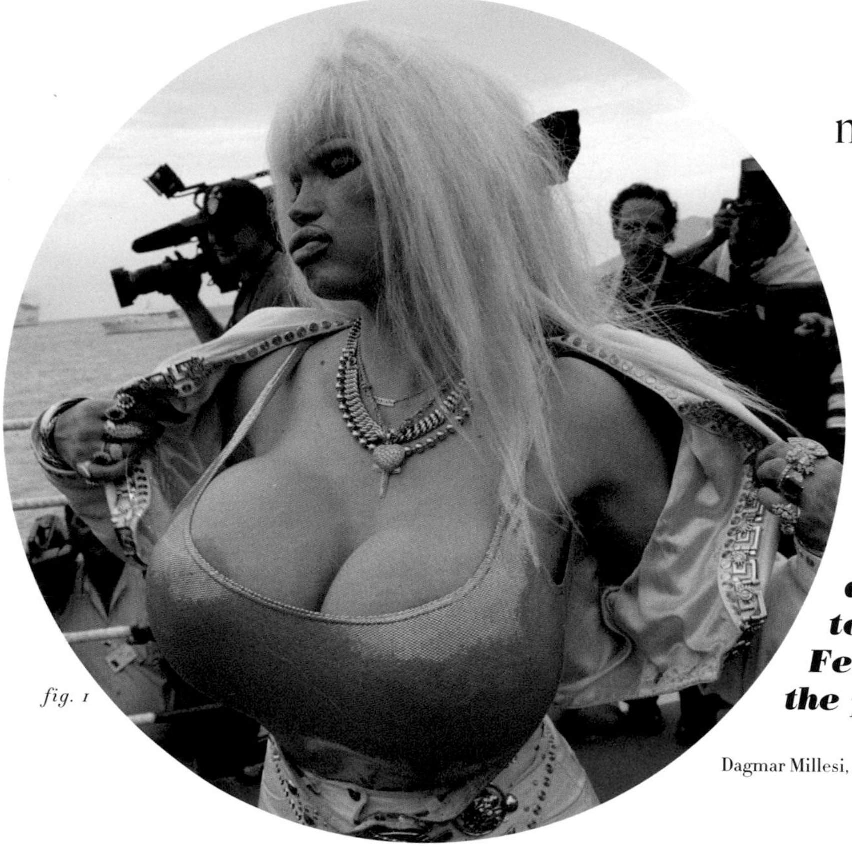

fig. 1

If I realise that the desired operation is not the patient's own idea, for example if a husband wants his wife to have huge tits à la Lolo Ferrari, I refuse to work on the patient.

Dagmar Millesi, Vienna

It is usually the female patients who have unrealistic requests — the men are generally more rational and have precise, feasible ideas.

Axel-Mario Feller, Munich

My husband Aldo once told me the following true story: One day, a woman with a monstrous nose approached him for surgery. "Doctor, I've got a problem," she said to him, to which he replied, "I can tell, it's your nose." Indignantly, she answered: "Whatever gave you that idea? I want to have a breast enlargement!"

Egle Muti, Turin

fig. previous pages Warhol's Amanda with spray paint, 2002. © David LaChapelle, New York
fig. 1 Lolo Ferari (Eve Valois) 1996 in Cannes. © AFP / Getty images
fig. 2 Amanda Milkshake, 2003. © David LaChapelle, New York

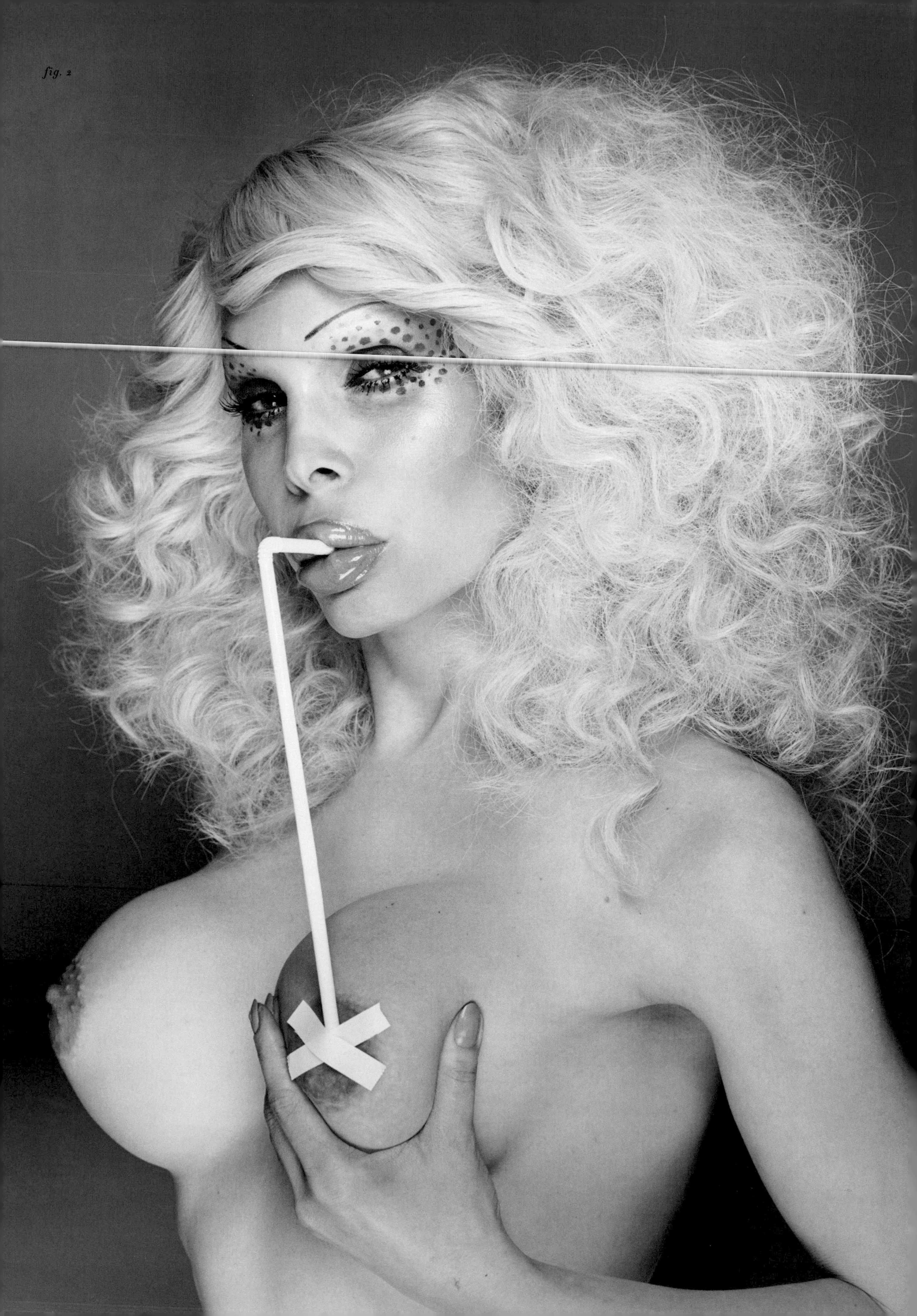

fig. 2

fig. 3 Alessandra, 1995. © 2004 Andres Serrano. Photograph courtesy of the Paula Cooper Gallery
fig. 4 Parlor Tatto, 2003. © David LaChapelle, New York

A young man came to me wanting a new face. Apparently, he looked just like his father, whom he hated. I didn't do it, as he would have become a different person.

Rolf R. Olbrisch, Düsseldorf

A transvestite who wanted to have bigger breasts brought along some plaster-cast models to the consultation. They were absolutely monstrous, totally beyond the normal range of anatomical proportions. I refused.

Johannes C. Bruck, Berlin

One time, a man approached me wanting to have a scar cut into his face! He worked as a diamond prospector in Brazil and wanted to look harder and more masculine. I did not do it.

Jean-Louis Sebagh, Paris

A transvestite approached me once, a very nice person. He wanted to have a smaller, more feminine chin. I operated on him. When I checked on him two hours after the operation, he was sitting on his bed knitting. Beaming with joy, he said: "Look doctor, I've knitted this already!" On the other hand, I never operate on transsexuals. We normally refer sex change patients to specialist surgeons in Bern or Casablanca.

Axel Neuroth, Düsseldorf

fig. 3

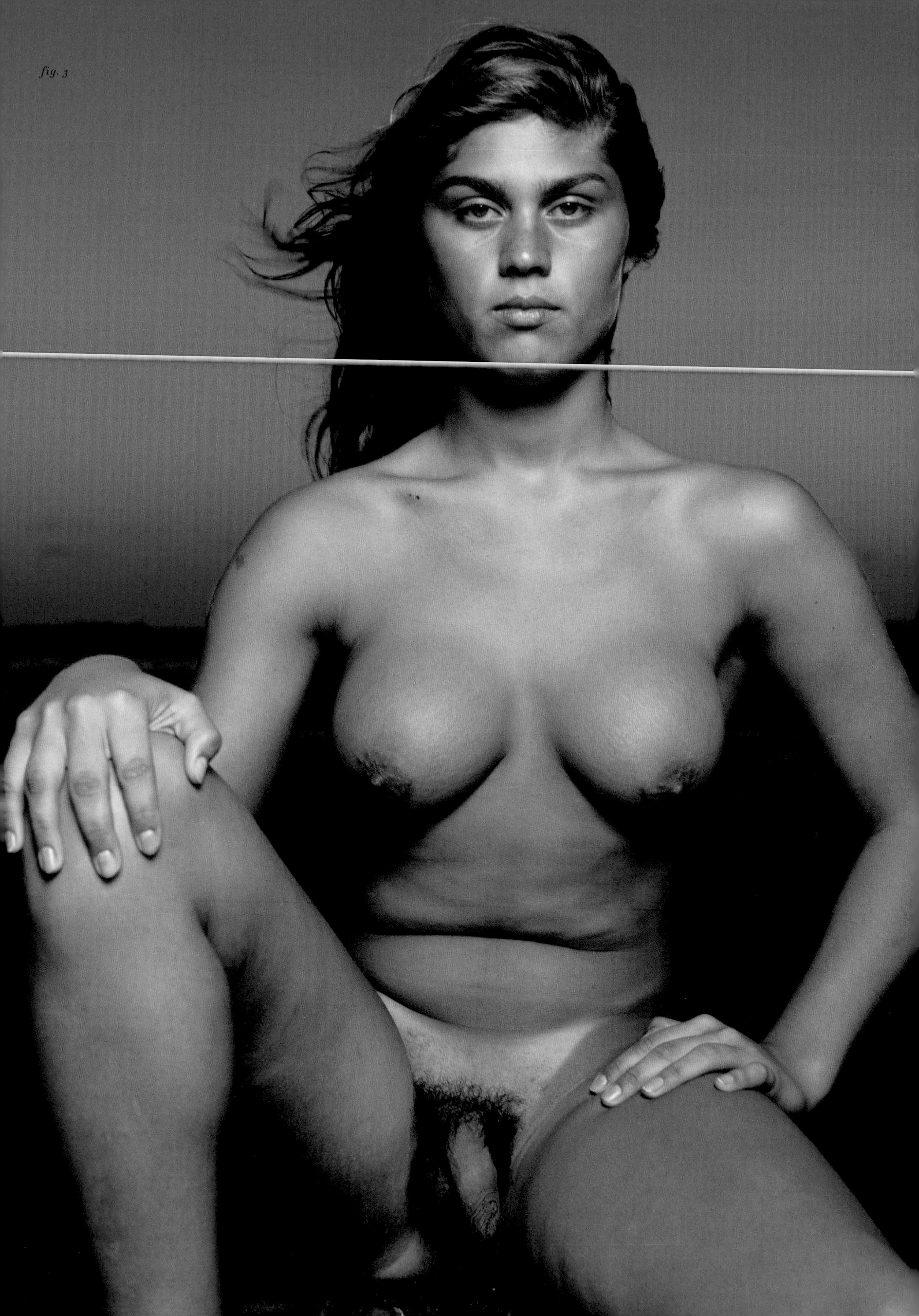

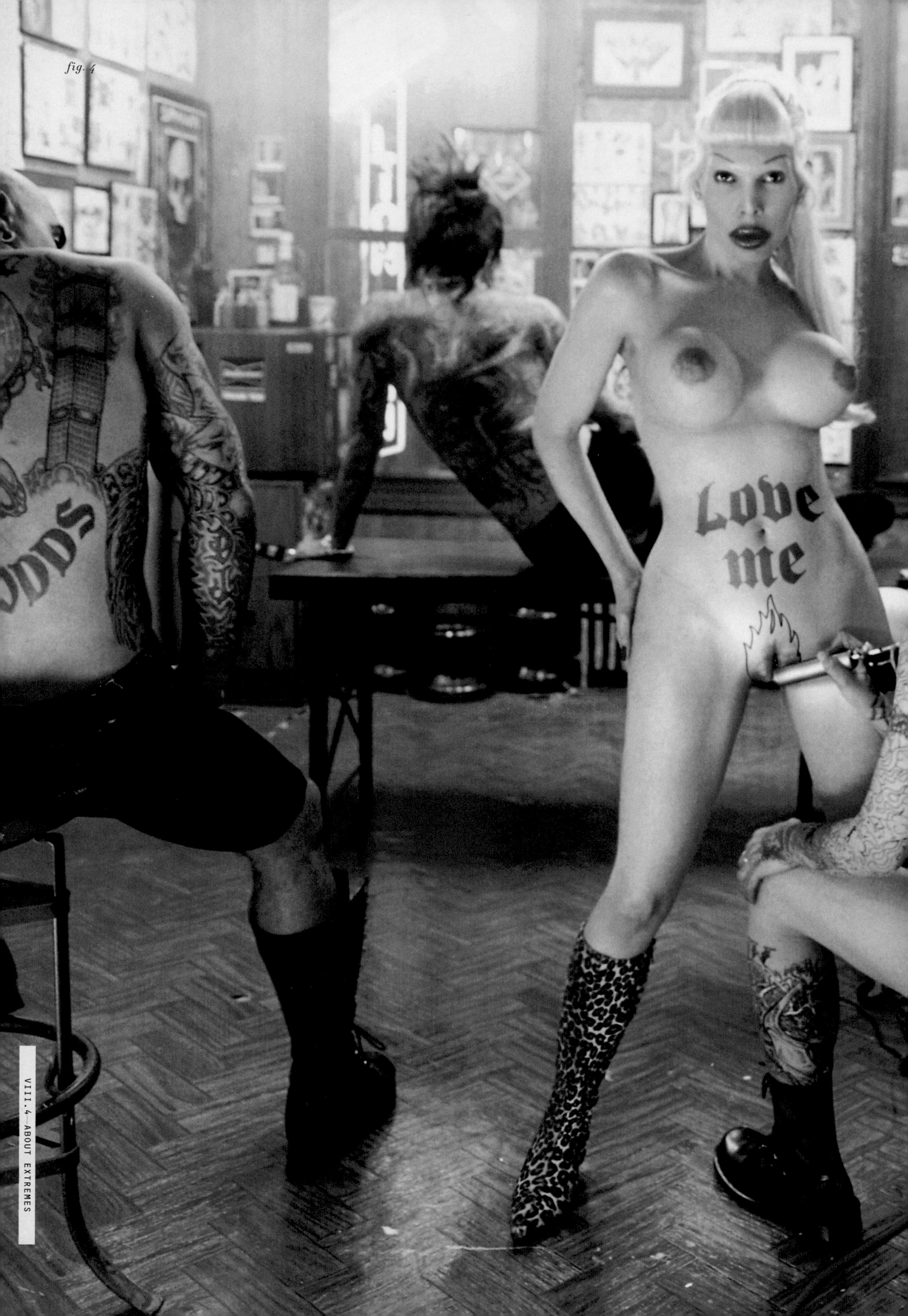

fig. 4

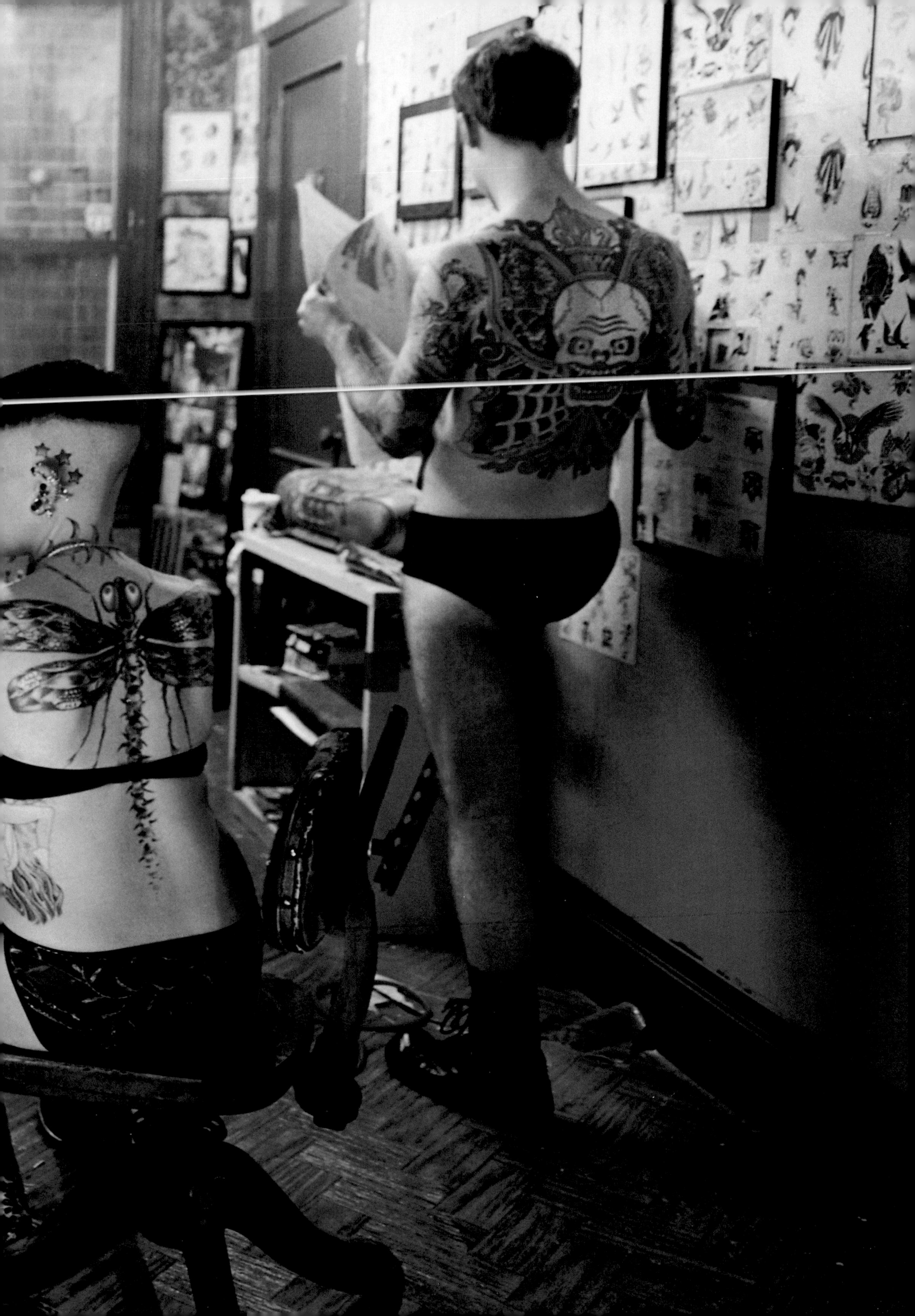

An extreme request I sadly receive at an increasing frequency is patients who ask me to cure their obesity with liposuction. Some of these people hardly fit through the door! Then there are people who approach me with photos of film stars, wanting me to turn them into their replicas. Increasingly, I also get very young patients who want facelifts or breast enlargements.

Axel-Mario Feller, Munich

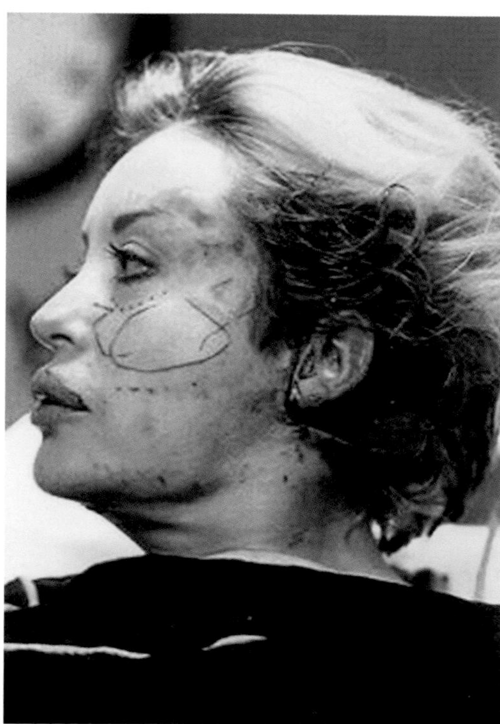

fig. 6

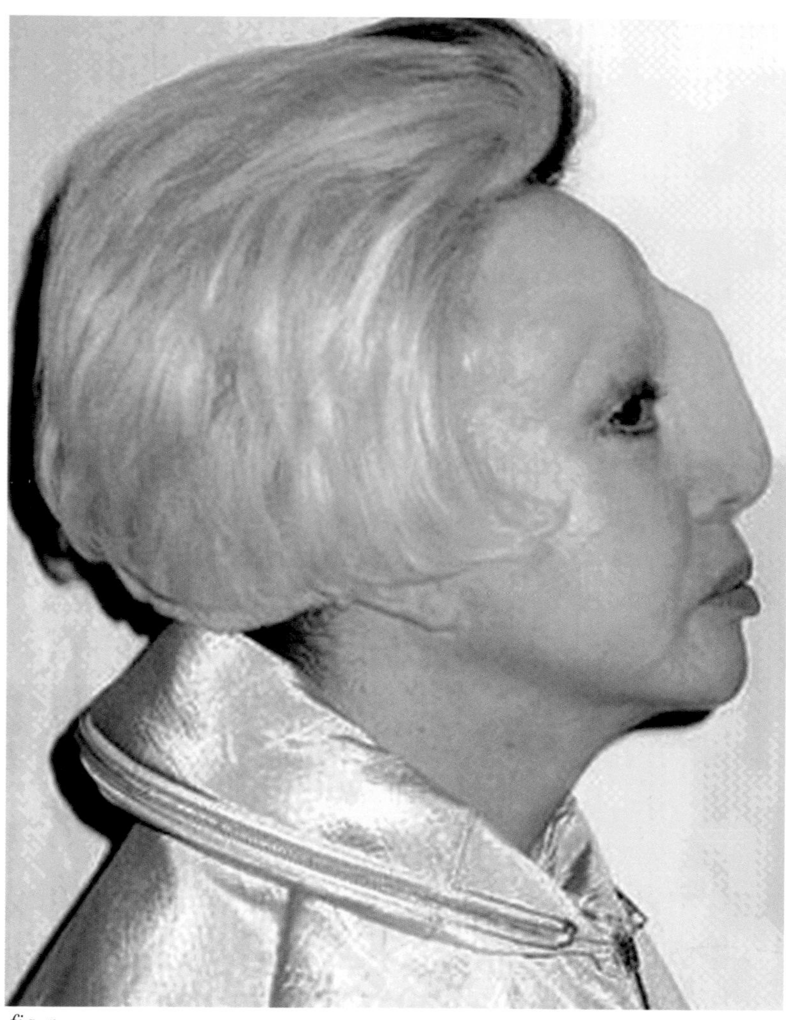

fig. 5

It's awful when 14-year-old girls — accompanied by their parents! — ask me to enlarge their breasts.

Carlo Gasperoni, Rome

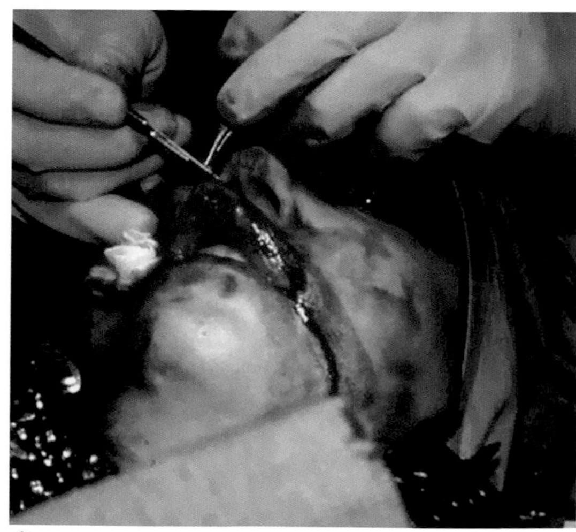

fig. 7

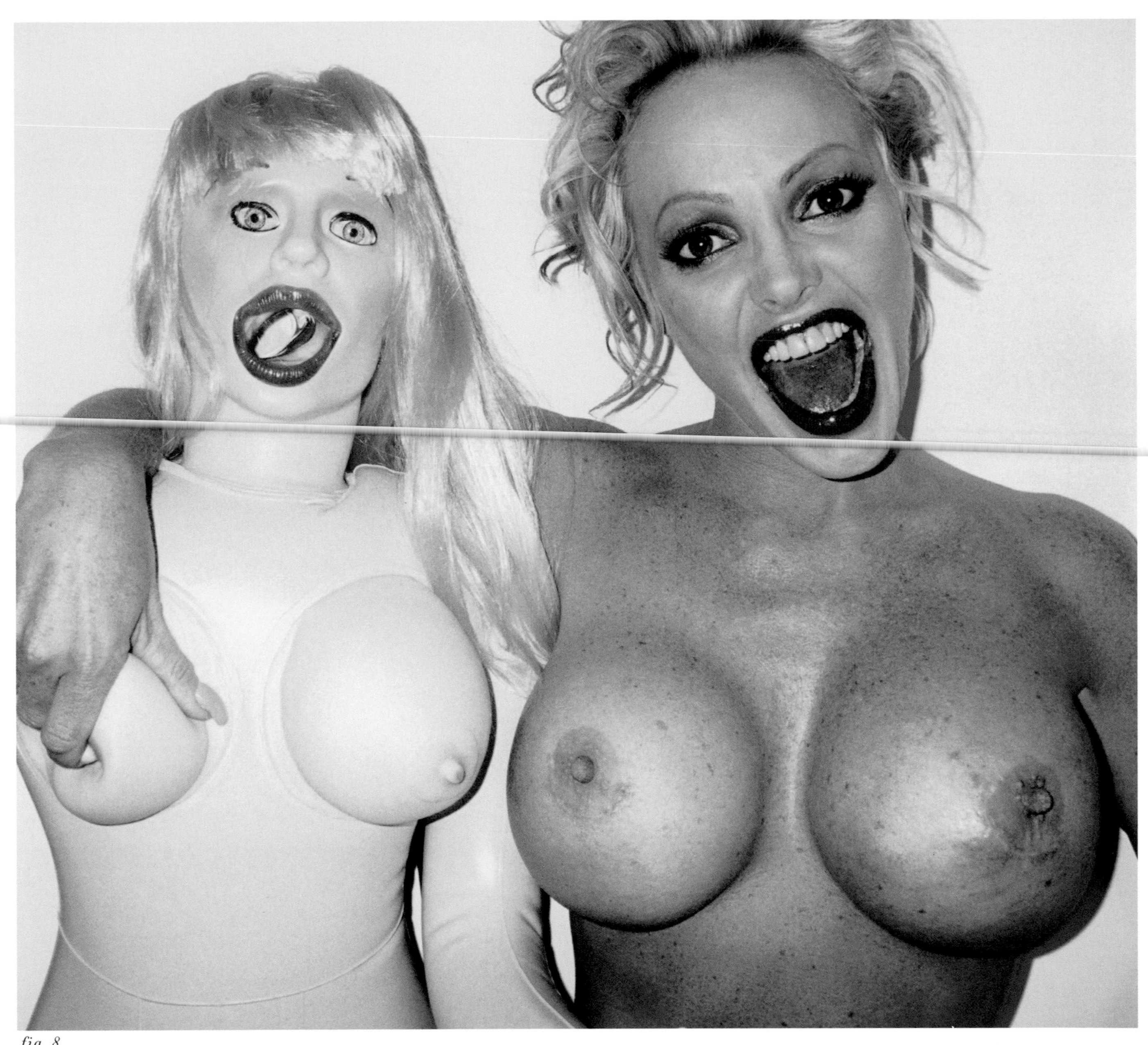

fig. 8

Unfortunately, about ten percent of the patients that approach me are addicted to plastic surgery. They always want something else — bigger cheekbones, breasts, mouths, you name it. If I complied with all their bizarre requests, I could no longer respect myself.

Jean-Louis Sebagh, Paris

... asked to do liposuction on people who are either too fat or too thin. Actually, more frequently too thin.

Gerald H. Pitman, New York

fig. 5 © *Orlan, Paris*
fig. 6 © *Orlan, Paris*
fig. 7 © *Orlan, Paris*
fig. 8 *No title.* © *Terry Richardson, New York*

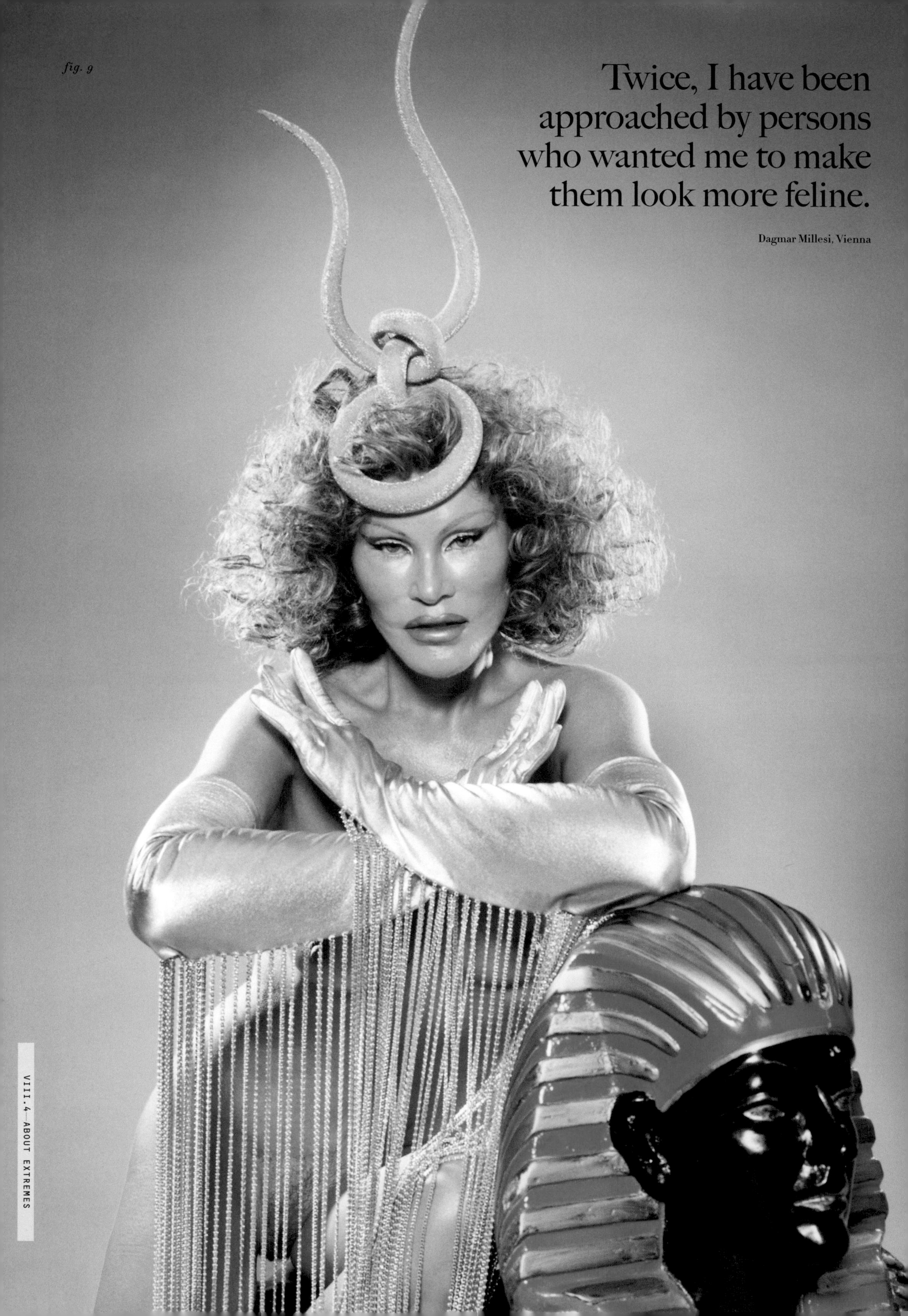

fig. 9

Twice, I have been approached by persons who wanted me to make them look more feline.

Dagmar Millesi, Vienna

One day, I was approached by a dark-skinned man of African descent. He showed me a photo of a pale-skinned Japanese man with a tiny nose and told me he wanted to look just like him. Obviously, I sent him straight to a psychologist.

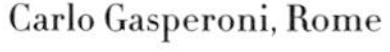

Carlo Gasperoni, Rome

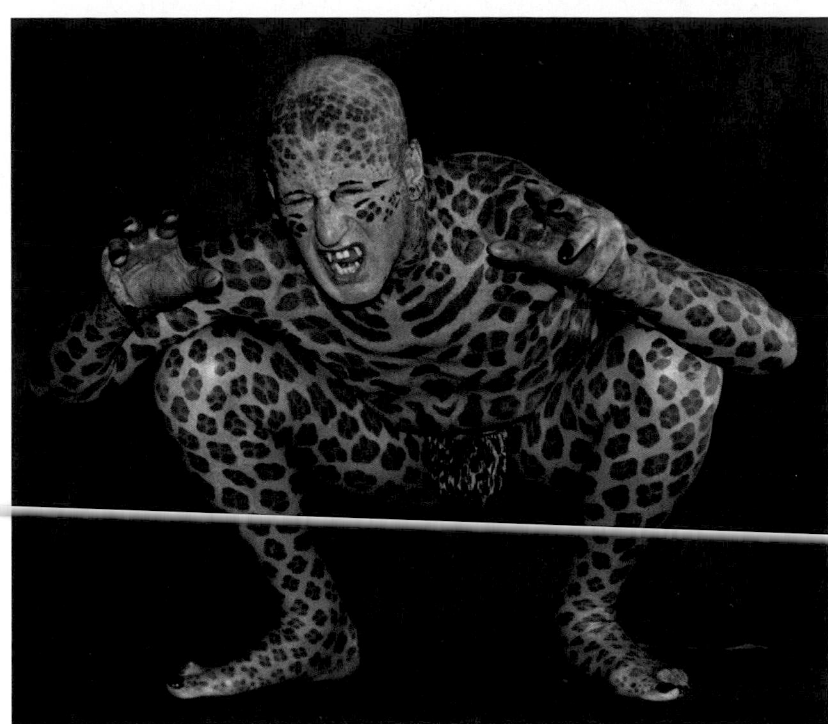

fig. 10

A beautiful young woman, about 30 years of age, desperately wanted to have a bigger nose. There was nothing wrong with her nose as it was, so I gave her a lump of putty and asked her to sculpt me the nose she was after. She produced something that looked like the nose of a rhinoceros. I told her: "You realise this isn't normal. Please, go see a psychiatrist." She did, but the psychiatrist sent her straight back to me — claiming the woman would kill herself if she didn't get a new nose! So I implanted a gigantic amount of silicone rubber into her nose, making it as monstrous as she had wished. I also told her that she should come back if she didn't like her new nose anymore. She returned to my practice several times over the next ten years. Each time, I removed some of the silicone, and after ten years, it was all taken out. Fortunately, her nose also shrank back to its normal size.

Ulrich K. Kesselring, Lausanne

fig. 9 *Jocelyn Wildenstein and Sphynx – New York, 1999.* © *David LaChapelle*
fig. 10 *"Leopard man" Tom Leppard, 1996.* © *picture-alliance / dpa*

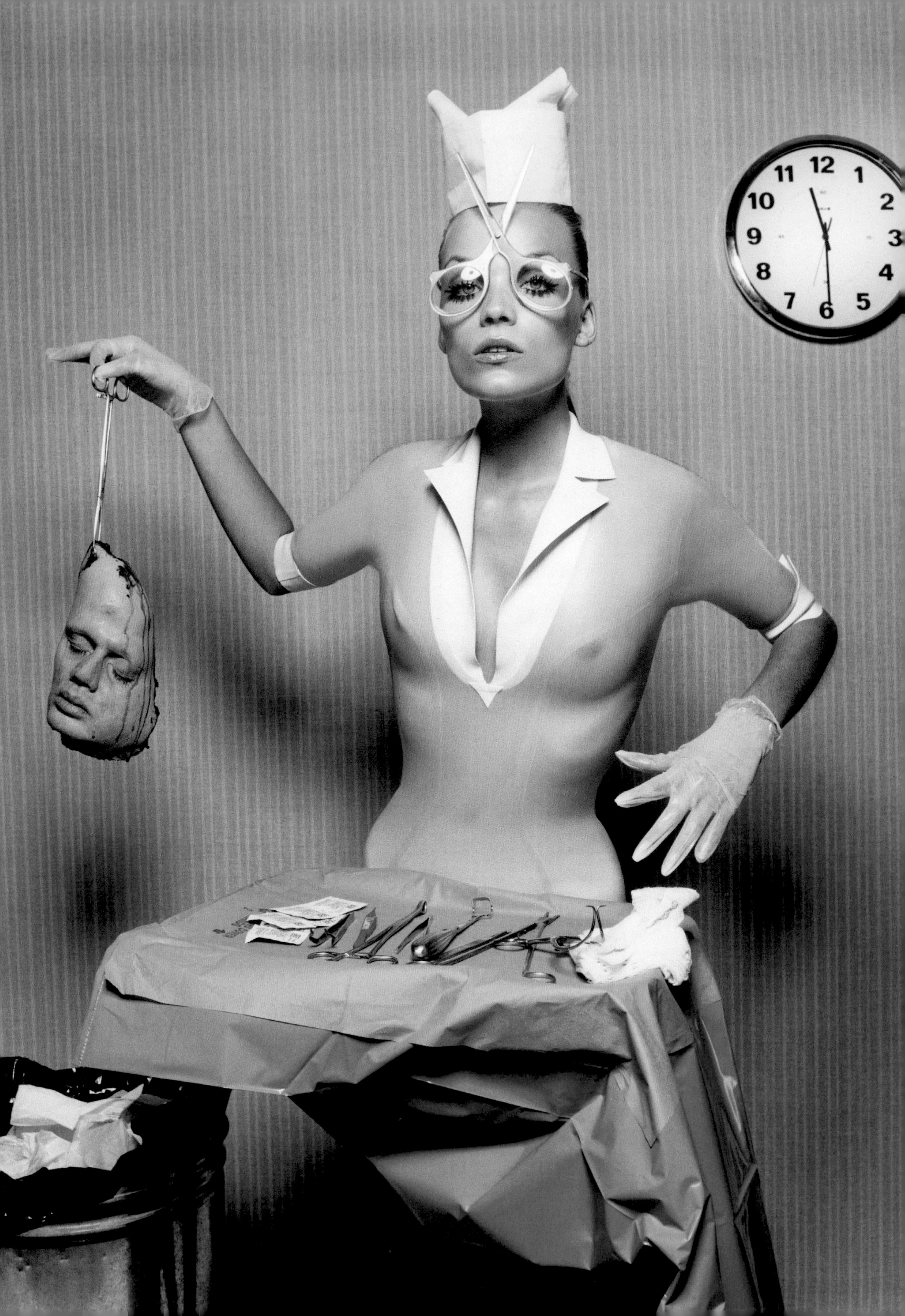

IX.

METHODS AND TECHNIQUES A—Z

Text by

EVA KARCHER

Photos by

BODENSEEKLINIK PROF. MANG

Illustrations by

BLUE BRAIN BELGIUM

THE BIG RULE

!

Beauty only manifests itself in the unique flaws, the microscopic irregularities of a face and a body. Symmetrical features and sculptural smoothness don't exist in nature. You keep your body fit and healthy through regular exercise. The same applies to your face — it needs training. After a facelift, you should ensure that you don't lose your facial expressions and characteristics! Laugh, smile and enjoy life!

IX.

The golden rules for a successful aesthetic procedure

EVA KARCHER, Munich

1.

Find out if your aesthetic surgeon or cosmetic practitioner respects the human body, regardless of it being male or female, and if his offer to help you is sincere. If he refuses to do an operation and offers you sound medical reasons for his decision, this is usually a sign of professional integrity. To find an aesthetic surgeon in your region visit www.isaps.org or www.ipras.org.

2.

The aesthetic-plastic, minimally invasive or cosmetic remodelling of your beauty should not be aimed at making you look photogenic but at making you more attractive. Your face and body need to be in harmony with each other, according to your own unique proportions and contours. It should never be your objective to look like another person, especially not a celebrity!

3.

Beware of doctors who make you sign an agreement that your photos can be published in print or broadcast on TV. Be equally wary of surgeons who frequently appear on commercial TV channels or in tabloid celebrity magazines. This apparent popularity is usually due to the efforts of a PR agency, a sign that many of these practitioners are more concerned with the fortunes of their business than with their patients' welfare. Although there are always exceptions to the rule, discreet promotion is a much better indicator of professional quality. Beware of aesthetic surrgons who show photos or image simulation, they demonstrate the possible changes but not the result on you.

4.

Be suspicious of promises such as "eternal youth" or permanent results. Age is not some kind of demon, nor is it a taboo – it is a stage of human life that can be as exciting as youth! Surgeons and practitioners are primarily there to help you feel healthy and good for as long as possible. Your getting older should be as much fun as your growing up, a process you may still be in now or that you have already completed – and hopefully enjoyed.

5.

Distrust medical professionals who treat every procedure, be it surgical, minimally invasive or cosmetic, as a minor routine. The more detail a surgeon provides about an operation, its risks and possible complications, the more professional he is. Ideally, you should be consulting a number of different surgeons by way of comparison. Remember you also have the option of employing a respectable, discreet professional consulting agency to support you, or seeking advice from an association like IPRAS, ISAPS, etc.

6.

Be sceptical of magazine advertisements, and never trust promotional websites on the internet! Almost invariably, these sites use manipulated photos to win over their unsuspecting victims. Never randomly pick a surgeon from the telephone directory!

7.

Surgeons who claim that women should have their first facelift in their late 30s or even their late 20s are highly questionable. It is a medical fact that every facelift needs to be renewed in a cycle of 10–15 years. What will you do when you reach 60 and your skin tissue has already been subjected to so much tightening in previous operations that it would be too risky to have another procedure?

8.

Try to double-check all surgeons recommended by friends. When going to consultations, take a person you really trust.

9.

Don't restrict your search for the most suitable surgeon or practitioner to your area; you should also look abroad. If you have a specific problem or request, there may well be an established specialist somewhere who is experienced in minimising any potential risks. Only follow recommendations if they can ensure the utmost discretion and professionalism.

10.

Prepare for every cosmetic or surgical procedure as carefully as possible. Four, ideally six weeks before an operation, you should stop drinking alcohol and smoking. A comprehensive preoperative health check is mandatory! Especially your lungs need to be in excellent condition! Surgical risks may arise if you have diabetes, blood clotting problems, or a drug addiction – this also includes heavy drinking and smoking. If at all possible, you should refrain from consuming any alcohol or nicotine the week before a facial injection, a laser treatment or a peeling, and you should absolutely not have any alcohol or nicotine the days before and after the operation.

11.

Be patient: After cosmetic as well as surgical procedures, you will have bruises, swellings and recurring spells of pain. For at least three, ideally six weeks, you should avoid all strenuous physical activities, including sports and sun-tanning. Also try to abstain from alcohol and cigarettes. After any operation, there are a number of risks: allergies, secondary haemorrhages, raised scarring (keloids), infections, localised paralysis or alteration of sensation, breathing problems after rhinoplasties, visible physical asymmetries, temporary deafness, and wound healing problems (caused by bad circulation of the skin, a common smokers' problem). The most severe reaction is necrosis (tissue death).

12.

Ascertain that your anaesthetist, the person who takes care of your sedation during the operation, is reliable and trustworthy. If you have any uncertainties, request a personal talk with your anaesthetist before the operation.

13.

Regardless of what the procedure is, make sure to receive a detailed contract in advance and in writing. This should specify all costs – for the operation, preoperative consultations, clinic care and accommodation, and postoperative support. Follow-up operations for corrections or to resolve subsequent complications should always be included in the price of the operation. Surgeons wishing to receive their entire fee in advance are unprofessional! An advance payment of no more than 50 percent is acceptable, provided that it will be refunded if the operation has to be cancelled due to unforeseeable circumstances. If unsure, seek advice from your lawyer or a qualified consultant well in advance.

14.

Be sure to discuss the details of the procedure with your surgeon before signing the informed consent of the procedure and with the anaesthetist if the procedure needs general anaesthesia or sedation.

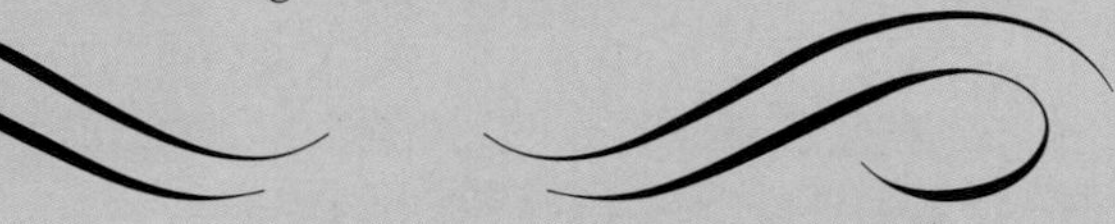

Anti-Aging
Age Prevention

EVA KARCHER, Munich
in collaboration with DR. THOMAS KLOSTERHALFEN, Munich

Aging is not a disease. It is the natural course run by a long life. There are, however, different ways of aging: your objective should be to maintain your physical and mental agility for as long as possible.

"**Anti-aging**" is a term that suggests age is a disease, to be avoided at all costs. "**Active aging,**" a synonym for anti-aging, describes the aims of anti-aging medicine without any negative connotations: to slow down the weakening and aging processes displayed by the body once it has reached a certain age (approx. 40 years) with preventive individual diagnoses and therapies.

"**Age prevention**" is the step that should precede any anti-aging procedure, be it cosmetic, minimally invasive or surgical. Ideally, age prevention complements the services provided by your general practitioner or specialist. It also makes sense to undertake age prevention in parallel to cosmetic, minimally invasive or surgical procedures. Surgeons and practitioners working in the field of aesthetic medicine are increasingly adopting this approach.

The four pillars of anti-aging medicine are:
— *Lifestyle* (how you choose to live your life)
— *Nutrition* (different diets, nutritional supplements, micronutrients, antioxidants etc.)
— *Fitness* (physical and mental activity, training your physical strength and stamina, meditation, gymnastics, dance)
— *Hormone replacement therapy* (addressing hormonal imbalances; aesthetic endocrinology).

European and American practitioners who specialise in age prevention are usually also gynaecologists and / or endocrinologists, i. e. hormone experts. Hormone therapy is based on a wide range of diagnostics:

— *Anamnesis of symptoms* that have been identified as "aging" indicators: osteoporosis, arthritis, heat flushes, age-related cardiac problems, breast formation (men), breast growth and sagging breasts (women), decreases in libido, hair loss, weight gain, cellulite, loss of vitality, skin laxity and dryness, wrinkles and lines, bouts of depression, sporadic insomnia and memory impairment.
— *Diagnostic body check* to determine the patient's biological age and compile an individual quality-of-life and risk profile.
— The patient's biological, that is functional age denotes possible deviations from his or her chronological age. The deviations are assessed using an
 · *age scan test*, which is based on computerised analysis and an extensive reference database. Test subjects include
 · Memory power
 · Response to auditory and visual signals
 · Muscle response
 · Physical coordination
 · Lung function (PFT – Pulmonary Function Test)
 · Accommodation of the eyes (focusing capabilities)

NOTE: The validity of the age scan test is disputed by some specialists.

— To compile the patient's individual quality-of-life and risk profile, visual and chemical analyses (e. g. examining the blood composition) may additionally be performed:
 · Endoscopy, colonoscopy
 · Bone density test
 · Fat/muscle ratio analysis
 · Analysis of the calcification and flow velocity in the coronary arteries; determination of aortic elasticity
 · Assessment of heart attack, arteriosclerosis and thrombosis risks.

— Further diagnostics may include:
 · Osteoporosis test
 · Tumour marker tests: these provide information about which organs are susceptible to a tumour or other form of attack within the next ten years – colon, prostate gland, breasts, testicles, ovaries, lungs, thyroid gland, skin, pancreas, liver
 · Fat/moisture content of the skin

fig. on page 312

From the series "Make-over (Surgery Story)" by David LaChapelle. © David LaChapelle, New York

· Body mass index (BMI)
· Polymorphism diagnostics (the "gene chip")
· Vitamin levels
· Hormone status testing: the hormonal levels of estrogens, androgens, DHEA-S (dehydroepiandrosterone, identified as an anti-stress hormone that also bolsters the immune system), pregnenolone (the most potent transmitter of neuronal brain activity), thyroid hormones, somatotropin (HGH or Human Growth Hormone that controls cell regeneration), serotonin (affects sleep, mood and the fat metabolism), melatonin, leptin (regulates body weight), glutathione (employed by many detoxification processes), peroxides and malondialdehyde

— *Therapies* usually combine
· Medication (hormones, vitamins, minerals)
· Special treatments for hair loss or cellulite
· Nutritional advice
· Lifestyle advice (meditation, autogenic training, Psychotherapy)
· program of physical exercises, fitness and sport advice
· Minimally invasive (facial injections – see Section B) and/or surgical procedures (see Section C) as needed.

NOTE:

— Again and again, hormone therapy has been proclaimed as the most crucial component of anti-aging medicine. This industry-driven focus on hormone replacement should be viewed critically. Some specialists claim that dosages, e. g. of the rejuvenating growth hormone, can be set according to individual requirements. After a person has reached 25 years of age, the growth hormone level supposedly

— decreases by 50 percent every seven years. Similarly, the levels of the sexual hormones estrogen and testosterone are claimed to decrease dramatically with age, both in women and men; a cream-based therapy is now widely endorsed.

— Experts also recommend to keep hormone dosages as low as possible and warn of the increased risks of long-term therapy, including heart attacks, strokes and tumours in the breasts, ovaries or uterus. The effectiveness of hormone therapy to treat osteoporosis has also become debatable.

— **The most sensible approach is to only take hormones your body is undeniably low on**. To facilitate more accurate hormone level assessments, diagnostic systems have been developed to measure the
· long-term estrogen stress on women, i. e. the increased breast cancer risk, and the
· genetically higher risk to men of developing prostate cancer.

— **Long-term experience is still lacking**. One of the difficulties of gathering objective criteria is that a person's hormone levels fluctuate several times a day on an individual basis.

Nonsurgical (minimally invasive) procedures

EVA KARCHER, Munich
in collaboration with DR. STEFAN DUVE, Munich

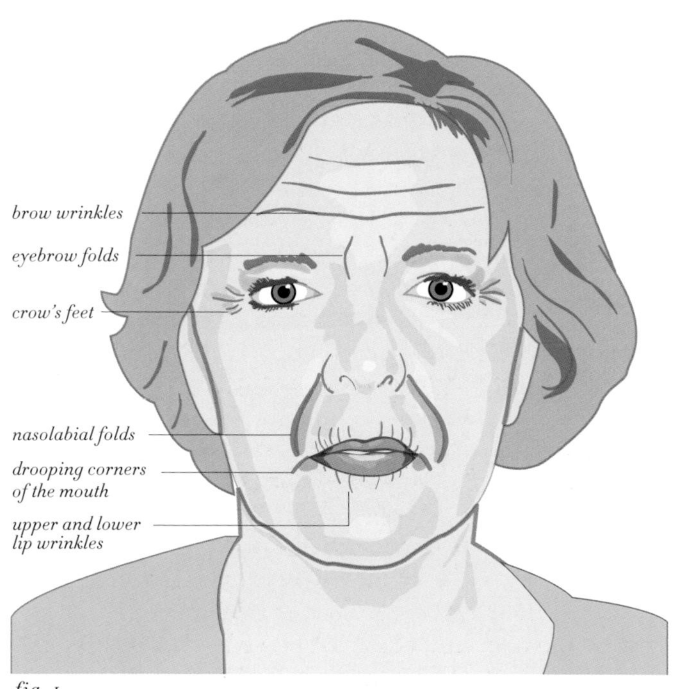

fig. 1

Wrinkle treatments

The treatments described in this chapter are increasingly being used in conjunction with surgical procedures.

Always remember: *Dosis sola facit venenum* – Dosage alone makes the poison! The substances and methods described below are only to be administered or applied by experienced specialists. As a rule, dosages should always be low and injected only with the greatest accuracy. Only this way can risks and side-effects be minimised. A treatment in stages, stretched over several sessions, is much more advisable than a single session with a dosage that is potentially too high with irreparable consequences.

Injections

Substances used and their properties:

A) *Biological substances: Botox, hyaluronic acid, autologous fat*
These substances break down within 3–12 months.

1. Botox (Botulinum Toxin A): A bacterial neurotoxin. Neurologists first discovered Botox as a way to relax muscle cramps; since the 60s, doctors have been using it to treat dystonic children with spasmodic torticollis. Today, Botox is increasingly being used to eliminate dynamic wrinkles in the face. These wrinkles are created by long years of muscular activity in the face, particularly in the brow, next to the eyes (crow's feet), above the mouth and around the neck. Botox is also an effective treatment against excessive sweat gland activity of the hands, feet and armpits. It blocks the neurotransmitter that triggers sweating for 6–18 months. Botox can even be used to relieve symptoms of migraine and post-stroke paralysis.

NOTE: Botox may never be injected into muscles used for motoric functions – these include the eyelids and the lips! For other types of wrinkles and creases, such as the nasolabial folds on either side of the nose, Botox is not effective. These need to be treated with gel-based fillers (see Section B).

Application

- Using a very fine needle, Botox is injected directly into the muscle or muscle area in short intervals over a period of approx. 20 seconds. The contractions of the muscles treated are reduced to a degree where the surrounding wrinkles flatten out or disappear altogether. The puncture pain is negligible, although a stinging or burning sensation may be perceived briefly. For the brow area, an experienced practitioner uses five injections; for the eye areas only two or three. Depending on the composition of the skin, dosages range from 0.05 ml to 0.1 ml per injection.
- On the day of the procedure, the skin areas treated should not be touched, as the Botox may otherwise

fig. 1

Botox is used to treat folds and wrinkles on the brow, above the root of the nose, around the eyes and in the mouth/neck area. The nasolabial folds remain unaffected by the toxin, which is why they need to be treated with other injection fillers. © Blue Brain Belgium

fig. 2

Botox is injected directly into the muscle underneath the problem area. The toxin's smoothing effect is noticeable after two to five days and lasts for three to six months – time for the next injection. © laif

fig. 3 a+b

In the face of this 38-year-old patient, the skin is beginning to show signs of aging around the nasolabial and lip areas. The photo on the right shows the face six months after an injection therapy involving lactic and hyaluronic acids. The lactic acid is injected deeply into the skin; the hyaluronic acid is injected intradermally into specific skin areas. Together, they produce a natural-looking revitalisation.
As both substances are organic, they break down naturally. The revitalising effect lasts for approx. six to eight months, then it needs to be refreshed with further injection sessions.
Despite this, it is always more sensible to use organic substances than alloplastic, i. e. artificial substances, such as silicone or acrylic microbeads. Although these substances are more durable, they can also have undesirable side effects, such as lumps, tissue hardening and infections. © Bodenseeklinik Prof. Mang

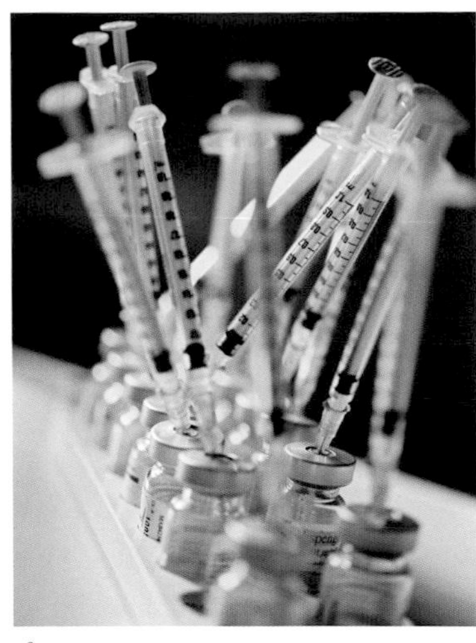

fig. 2

be spread. Facial massages, beauty creams and cleansing lotions are to be avoided altogether. You should not go to bed for at least four hours following the treatment.

— Botox works by blocking (i. e. paralysing) specific nerve impulses of the muscles treated. Other nerve functions, e. g. for sensory perception, are not affected by the procedure. The smoothing effect is usually discernible after two days, but sometimes only after five. After three to six months, the injection's effects gradually lessen. If the treatment is repeated, the skin smoothness will last six to nine months before a new injection is needed. Permanent smoothness is usually granted by two treatments a year.

— *Chemical brow lift:* An alternative to the conventional Botox treatment, as developed by Professor Dr. Martina Kerscher (Hamburg University): Depending on the type of wrinkles to be treated, the substance is injected immediately above the eyebrow or immediately below the hairline. The aim is to preserve the patient's natural facial expressions.

2. *Collagen:* A large part of our connective tissue consists of collagen, an animal protein. It is won from bovine skin and tendons, which is done in the US using strictly-controlled, CJD-free cow herds. To prevent allergic reactions, which occur in approx. Three percent of the patients and cause reddened skin or swellings, a test injection should be administered in the lower arm a month before the treatment. With multiple treatments, the allergy risk increases slightly.

— Suitable for augmenting thin lips, superficial and normal wrinkles around the eyes, nasolabial folds.

3. *Hyaluronic acid:* This organic substance is won from cockscombs. It also occurs naturally in the human body. Its ability to bind water gives the skin added volume; the compound consists of cross-linked molecules. The most popular brands are *Hylaform*, *Restylane*, *Hyal-System* and *Perlane*. There are different mixtures for different types of treatment, e. g. with larger gel particles for adding volume to thin lips, or with smaller particles to smooth fine wrinkles. Any reddened skin or haematomas disappear within two days.

— Suitable for nasolabial folds and fine upper lip wrinkles, as well as for augmenting lip contours.

— Some experts inject the compound, which breaks down naturally, from the inside of the lips. A local anaesthetic is used for this procedure. Practitioners claim that the natural red of the lips is accentuated and that the lips don't look artificially inflated.

— In combination with Botox, the liquid hyaluronic product *Hyal-System* can be used to treat wrinkles and lines on the décolleté. Four treatment sessions are required, one per month. The treatment has to be renewed every three months.

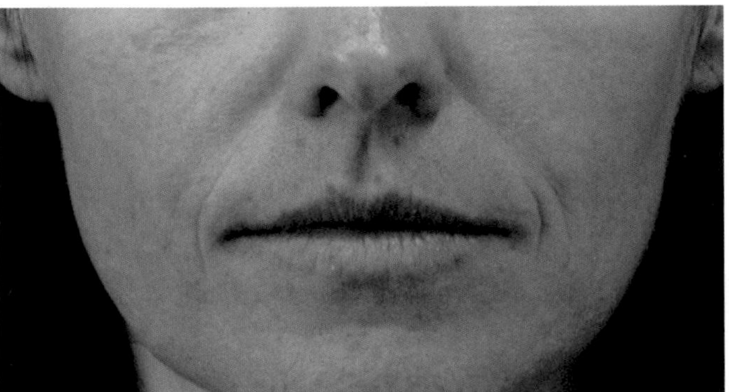

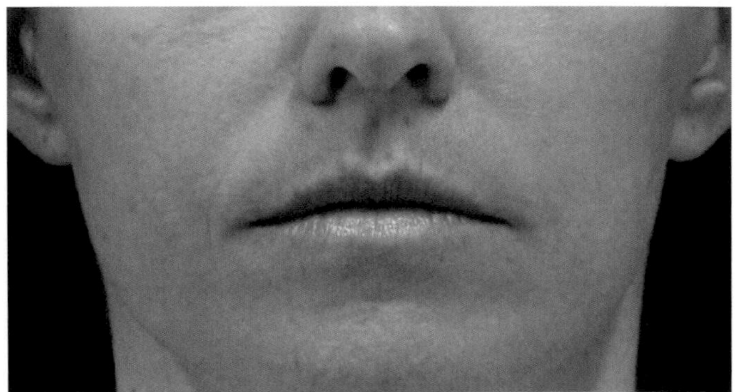

fig. 3 a+b

fig. 4

Autologous fat can also be used for facial injections. The surgeon harvests the fatty tissue from the patient's buttocks, abdomen, hip or upper thigh, cleanses it, filters out the unbroken cells and transplants these using microscopically fine cannulas. © *Blue Brain Belgium*

4. *Autologous fat* (a treatment also known as *lipostructure*): Autologous fat is taken from the patient's own body, e.g. the buttocks, abdomen, hip or upper thigh. Because of this, the patient will not display any adverse physical reactions to the substance. Thanks to improved harvesting and grafting techniques, the treatment is effective for up to a year. However, the substance can only be harvested in a surgical procedure. While the patient is sedated, the fat is extracted using a suction technique and subsequently cleansed of oils and tissue liquids using a specialised rinsing process. The intact fat cells are filtered out, and using microscopically fine cannulas, they are grafted under the folds. Usually, several portions of autologous fat are harvested and deep-frozen for later use (in a so-called "fat bank"). The treatment can lead to temporary swellings in the face.

— Suitable for pronounced nasolabial folds, augmentation of the lips, rounding the cheeks, rejuvenating the hands.

NOTE: In most cases, the fat isn't reabsorbed completely – irregular contours or small chalk deposits may form after a period of time.

5. *Lactic acid* (also known as *New Fill*): Synthetically produced polylactic acids that break down into autologous substances. New Fill can be applied very evenly and over large areas. Thanks to the cross-link injection method used, it acts like a support grid under the skin. To achieve the desired smoothing effect, several treatments are required, spaced two to six weeks apart.

— Suitable for padding hollow cheeks, reinforcing chin contours, padding large scar areas and smoothing deep nasolabial folds. The treatment should be effective for several years.

B) Artificial compounds, e.g. *hyaluronic acid* or *collagen* combined with *sugar-based* or *lactic acid-based acrylic microspheres*.

— One of the best products available is *Artecoll*, a mixture of collagen and tiny acrylic beads (PPMA). The result is permanent. However, this advantage can turn out to be a disadvantage if the practitioner injects the substance wrongly! The little beads may then be discernible by touch or visibly thicken the skin.

— Another popular and widely compatible substance is *Reviderm Intra*, a mixture of hyaluronic acid and flexible carbohydrate-based particles. This compound stimulates the body to form new connective tissue,

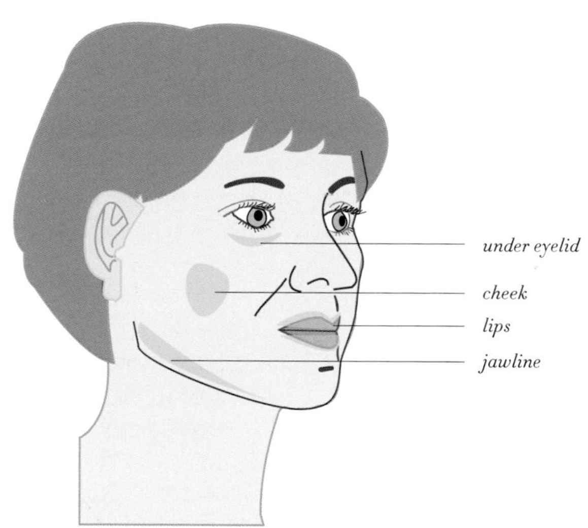

fig. 4

which smoothes the wrinkles from underneath. *Reviderm Intra* is a semi-permanent substance, which means that it is effective for two to four years.

— *Aquamid* is a gel made of water and polyacrylamide, a compound also used to manufacture soft contact lenses. It has very natural-looking results.

— *Goretex* and *SoftForm (fibrillated polytetrafluorethylene)* are plastic fibres that are woven into the skin as extremely thin threads using a needle. A local anaesthetic is administered, and the surgeon creates a tunnel in the tissue under the fold using a cannula. The thread is then inserted with a blunt needle. The tiny puncture wounds are sealed with a tissue adhesive. After the treatment, the areas operated on will display heavy swelling and reddened skin for two to three days.

NOTE: *Goretex* or *SoftForm threads* under the skin can be discernible by touch or even visible. If they are not positioned completely accurately, this may result in asymmetries, inflammation or even paralysis. In this case, the plastic fibres need to be surgically removed.

— *Aptos threads* are regarded as one of the most promising future alternatives to scalpel-based facelifts. The procedure was developed by the Moscow dermatologist Dr. Marlen Sulamanidze, which is why the threads are sometimes also referred to as "Russian threads." After a local anaesthetic has been administered, the specialist inserts the threads into the subcutaneous tissue using a fine cannula (a trocar). The threads are pulled along the direction of the tissue fibres so that the face is smoothed – around the eyes, cheeks, mouth or neck. Additionally, new connective tissue may form on top of the lifting threads during healing, which further tightens the skin. The threads do not cause any pain, but the face will swell initially and haematomas (bruises) may appear. After two or three weeks, the effects of the procedure become visible. Scars and allergies are uncommon.

— If this method is supplemented by facial injections once the swellings have receded, a surgical facelift can be delayed by approximately ten years.

All of the plastic fibres described are suitable for superficial or pronounced nasolabial folds, drooping corners of the mouth, upper lip wrinkles and lip remodelling.

NOTE: A substance called *Derma-Live*, also a combination product, should be avoided as it has a number of undesirable side-effects. Frequently, it causes granulomas, which are solid lumps underneath the skin. These can only be removed surgically.

C) *Fat-dissolving injection*: This method was developed by the Brazilian dermatologist Dr. Patricia Rittes. A medical product called *Lipostabil* is injected directly into the areas containing fat deposits. Lipostabil was first approved as a medical substance in the 50s, when it was used to reduce high cholesterol levels.

NOTE: Neither European nor US authorities have approved *Lipostabil* as a substance for dissolving subcutaneous fat! As yet, there is no long-term evidence to prove its effectiveness.

Application:

— Around three treatment sessions are needed within the space of several weeks to dissolve minor fat deposits (up to three kilograms of weight reduction in total). The results are visible after three to four weeks. The advantage of this treatment is that the fat cells in the treated tissue areas never regenerate. Immediately following the procedure, which employs a local anaesthetic, the injection sites may be reddened or swollen and itchy.

Common aspects of all the injection methods described:
Combinations with cosmetic operations:
The substances described complement a number of aesthetic surgical procedures very well, such as eyelid corrections, brow and face lifting, as well as *laser skin resurfacing* (see next section), which is used to smooth fine static wrinkles of the skin. **NOTE:** Botox should never be injected during a cosmetic operation. A separate appointment should be made for the injection.

Preparing for the treatment:
A few days before the procedure, the patient should be taking neither *Aspirin* nor *Warfarin* or any other blood-thinning agents, as these substances increase the possibility of bruises and haematomas. Alcohol is also to be avoided the day before and after the treatment. Immediately before the procedure, the skin areas to be treated are anaesthetised with a cream.

After the treatment:
For at least four hours after the procedure, the patient should avoid movement, body contact and facial expressions as much as possible, as well as exposure to sunlight.

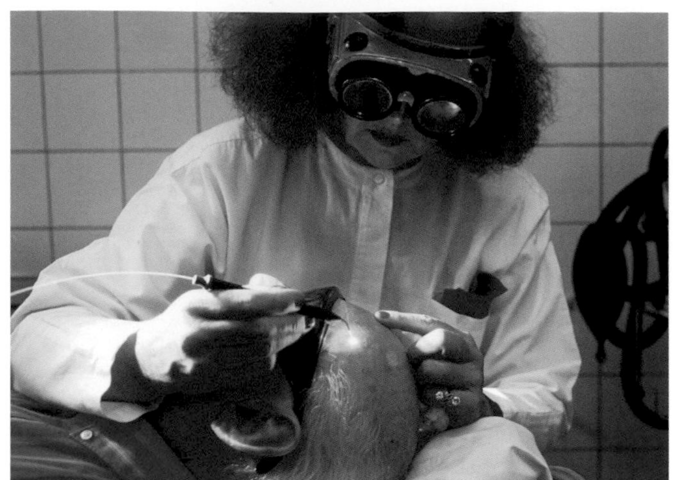
fig. 5

fig. 5

Dermatologists have been using laser beams for treating skin problems since 1961 – e. g. against rosacea, pronounced lachrymal sacks, folds, wrinkles, scars and warts. © *laif*

Talking, laughing and especially grimacing are to be avoided in particular.

Possible risks and complications:
With experienced specialists such as dermatologists and aesthetic/plastic surgeons, the risks are low. However, if the injection is carried out unprofessionally or if the substance isn't injected into exactly the right area, this may result in e. g. skewed or raised eyebrows or drooping eyelids etc. If the dosage is too high, the face may appear asymmetrical or mask-like. In some cases, granulomas (lumps) may form around the injected substance.

Age and gender considerations:
25 years or older; male and female patients are equally eligible. The average patient age ranges from 25 to 50 years. The international share of female patients is still at roughly 60 percent.

Laser

The laser is based on a physical law discovered by Albert Einstein at the beginning of the 20th century. The word "laser" is an acronym for "Light Amplification by Stimulated Emission of Radiation". First used in 1961, this energy beam has proven to be most effective as a surgical tool in the field of dermatology. A variety of laser beams are now in use, each focusing the wavelength of the light differently. A wide range of cosmetic and medical skin treatment applications is available:

— *Ruby laser and Neodymium YAG laser:* Both of these are based on infrared light and deeply penetrate the skin. They are used to treat pigmentation changes in the skin (e. g. freckles) and tattoos. Note that treatment does not work for tanned or bronzed skin.

— *Pulsed dye laser:* This is particularly suitable to treat vascular changes in the skin of the legs or face, e. g. minor hemangiomas or red blood vessels visible on the nose or cheeks. The yellow light of the pulsed dye laser targets the discoloured vessels without damaging the surrounding tissue. The treated area swells and develops a scab that eventually peels off. Facial treatment usually takes no longer than 15 minutes; treating the legs sometimes requires up to five sessions. Sclerosis is still the best way to treat spider veins.

— *Diode laser (LightSheer, Epilight):* These apply bursts of high-energy laser light to the skin and are exclusively directed at the hair roots. For the treatment to be effective, hair growth needs to be at an early stage. Because of this, epilation often takes several hours and requires repeat sessions. It is effective for up to two years. All that can be felt during treatment is a light prickling sensation, and the skin is slightly flushed afterwards. Only very rarely do crusts form.

— *Ultrapulse carbon dioxide laser (CO_2 laser):* This laser beam is mostly used to superficially vaporise the skin, a process also known as "resurfacing." This process tightens the collagen tissue, and therefore the skin. Wrinkles are eliminated without scarring and without any loss of blood. The skin is quite raw for a few days after surgery; to protect it from scarring, a thin film of moisturising ointment is applied. The ultrapulse laser can also be used to remove bags and wrinkles around the eyes, a surgical procedure called *laser blepharoplasty*. Incisions into the skin are not required at all. After surgery, the skin may look reddened for a brief period of time.

— The *CO_2 laser* is also used for the effective treatment of scars, birth marks, warts, crow's feet around the eyes, small wrinkles on the lower eyelid, upper lip wrinkles and stretch marks.

— *Cool Touch laser:* This is used for smoothing wrinkles very gently. The method, developed in the US, is called *subsurfacing*. Immediately before the laser treatment, the uppermost layer of the skin – the epidermis – is exposed to a cooling gas. This lowers the skin temperature to a level that makes the skin

fig. 6

"Laser" is an acronym for "Light Amplification by Stimulated Emission of Radiation". A range of devices is used to focus the light beam's wavelength precisely to match various cosmetic and medical skin irritations.

impervious to heat damage; it remains completely intact. The laser beam only affects the connective tissue, with the result that the worn-out collagen fibres re-contract. This is especially effective for eliminating wrinkles around the eyes, cheeks and lips. However, at least six laser treatments are needed at a monthly interval to achieve the desired effect.

— Total *skin resurfacing*, i. e. the removal of the entire facial skin surface with laser beams, is becoming increasingly unpopular for wrinkle treatment. The cost, pain and postoperative bother are no longer proportionate to the benefits of the procedure. Before the skin is "resurfaced," it is treated with fruit acids and hydroquinone, a bleaching agent. The procedure is carried out while the patient is fully sedated; for the first 24 hours after the operation, the skin feels extremely burnt. The patient cannot go out for two weeks, and the reddened tone of the skin only fades after three months. Interestingly, the best results are achieved on deeply tanned skin. After a laser treatment, sports and sauna sessions need to be abstained from for several weeks. Prolonged exposure to sunlight is only possible after three months, and a highly protective sunblock needs to be used.

— The *Rio Method*, developed by a renowned Brazilian surgeon, is designed to remove stretch lines on the breasts, upper arms, abdomen and upper thighs. The areas to be treated are prepared with a special cream for two weeks before the procedure. During the procedure itself, the stretch lines are highlighted and

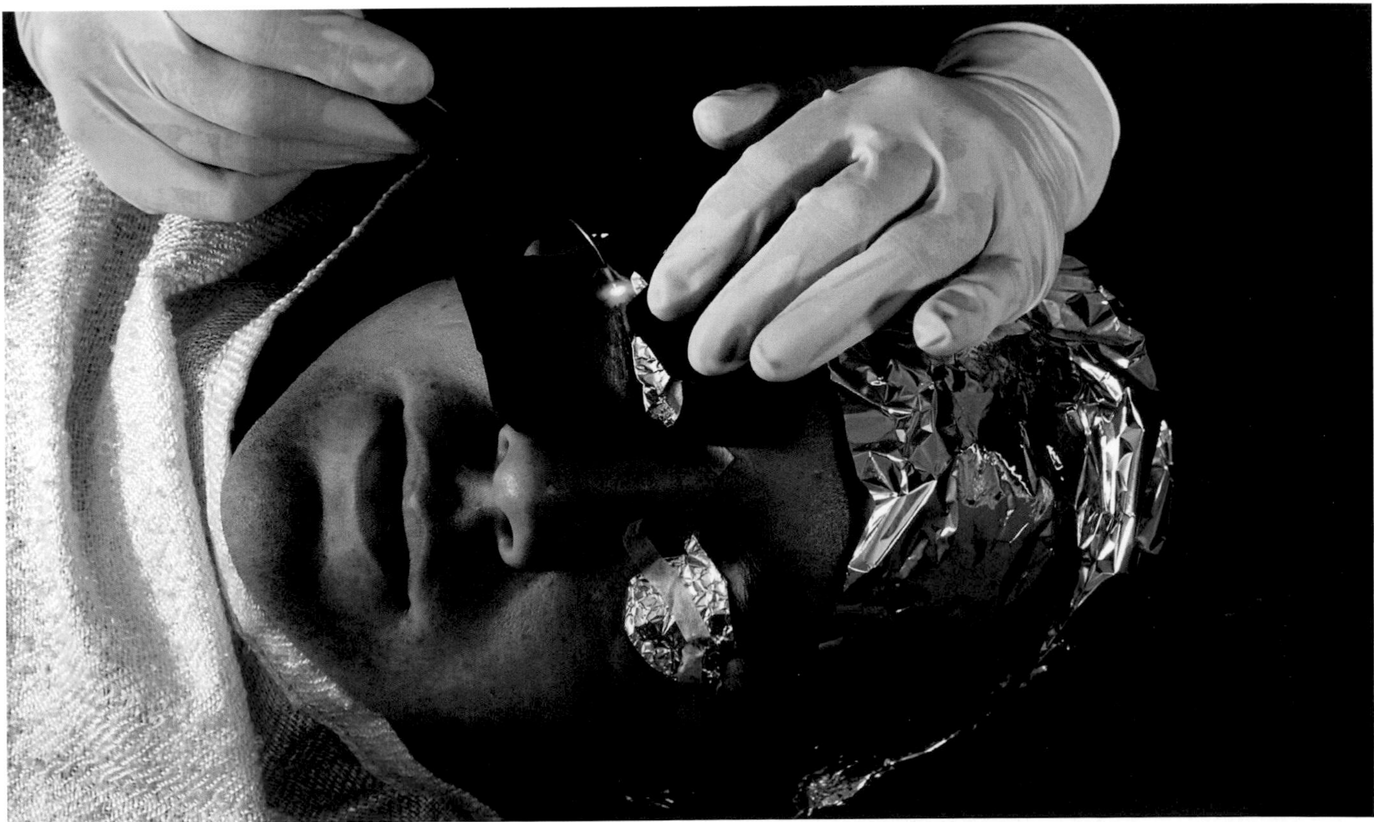

fig. 6

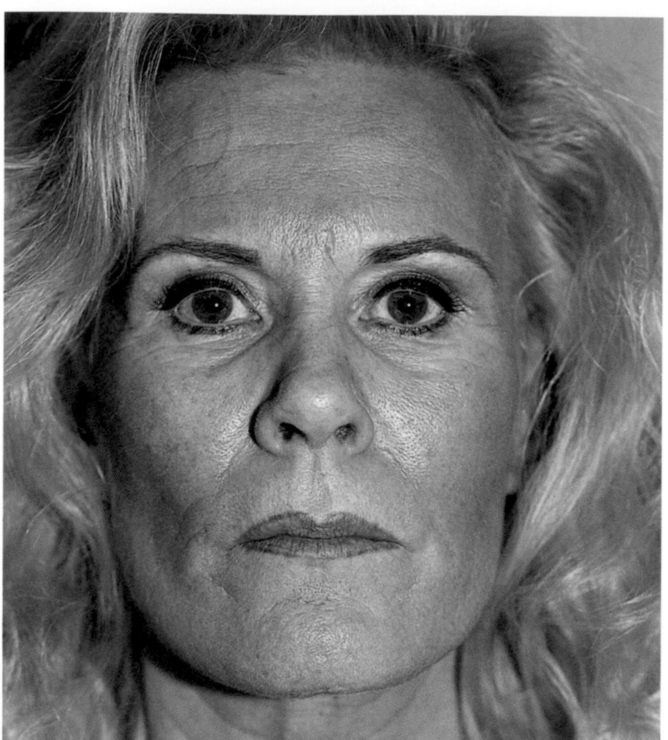

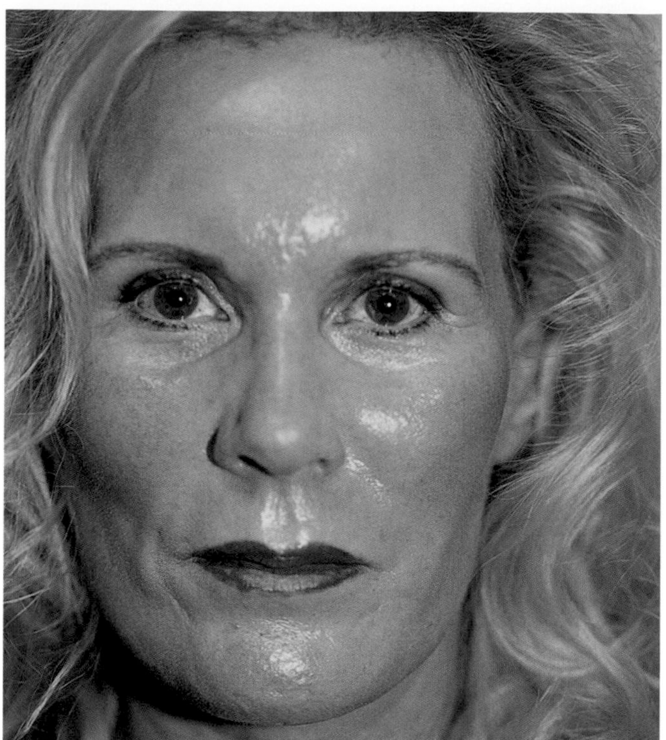

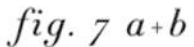

fig. 7 a+b

then punctured with a fine needle underneath the skin along their entire length. The needle is pulled back out of the skin in a "wiping" motion. This is followed by a subsequent treatment using a CO_2 laser and four weeks later a fruit acid peeling. The success rate is at 80–100 percent.

— *erbium: YAG laser:* This is even gentler than the CO_2 laser, as well as being more precise and facilitating greater coverage. It is often used alternatingly with the CO_2 laser (which has a deeper effect) for removing wrinkles. Delicate wrinkles on the lower eyelid are easily removed with this laser after a local anaesthetic has been applied. Following the procedure, the eyelids are reddened for approx. two weeks.

NOTE: People suffering from raised scarring (keloids) should never receive laser treatments!

Peeling

There are three levels of treatment – *soft peelings*, *medium peelings* and *deep peelings*.

Soft peeling: A 10–70 percent dilution of fruit acid is applied to the skin – either glycolic acid obtained from sugar cane or a blend of AHAs (Alpha Hydroxy Acids) that occur in milk, apples, pineapples, citrus fruit and almonds. The acid makes the top skin layer peel off.
In the four weeks preceding the treatment, products containing Vitamin A or highly diluted fruit acid are applied to the skin every day. This prepares the skin for the more intensive fruit acid treatment. During the procedure, the patient's skin may feel inflamed, and it will be slightly flushed for a few days after. In this time, the patient needs to protect his or her skin with special moisturising products. Sunbathing and solariums are strictly out of bounds for two weeks. Even after a single treatment with strong fruit acid, the skin's complexion looks much more consistent. Pigment irregularities and freckles disappear. For a more effective change, the treatment can be spread over several weeks with the fruit acid concentration increasing gradually. The results are visible for 6 -12 months.

Medium peeling: A 20–40 percent dilution of trichloroacetic acid (TCA) is applied to cauterize the entire top skin layer, down to the so-called *reticular dermis*. Deep pigment discolourations, acne scars and minor wrinkles around the eyes and mouth are eliminated, and rough, porous skin becomes significantly smoother. Again, this treatment requires meticulous preparation. Two days before the peeling, preventive medication against herpes blisters needs to be taken. The procedure is quite painful; a local anaesthetic is usually required. When the treatment is finished, the skin is heavily flushed. The complexion soon changes to a dark shade of brown, the skin dries out and flakes off. After around a week, delicate rosy new skin appears. In some cases, the red flushes on the skin are visible for several weeks. In the first few months after the treatment, sunblock should always be applied before exposing the skin to the sun. The treatment is effective for several years.

Deep Peeling: This is the most aggressive skin peeling treatment; it achieves a lifting effect for approx. five years. The procedure takes place while the patient is fully sedated. After the skin has been cleansed of all oils, the practitioner applies two or three layers of a 30–40 percent dilution of trichloroacetic acid. After the procedure, the face is very swollen. The skin stings strongly and weeps. Cool, wet compresses and special ointments alleviate these symptoms, but the skin needs two weeks to recover

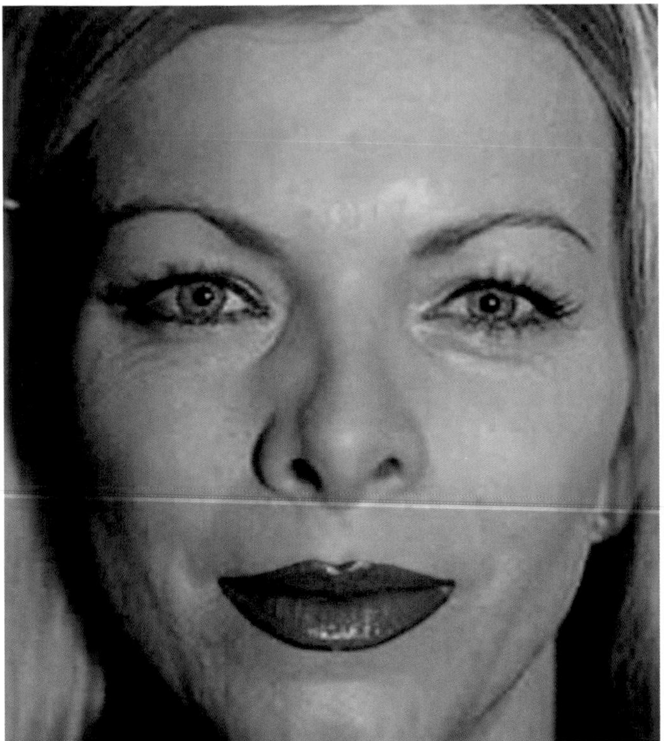
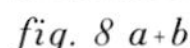
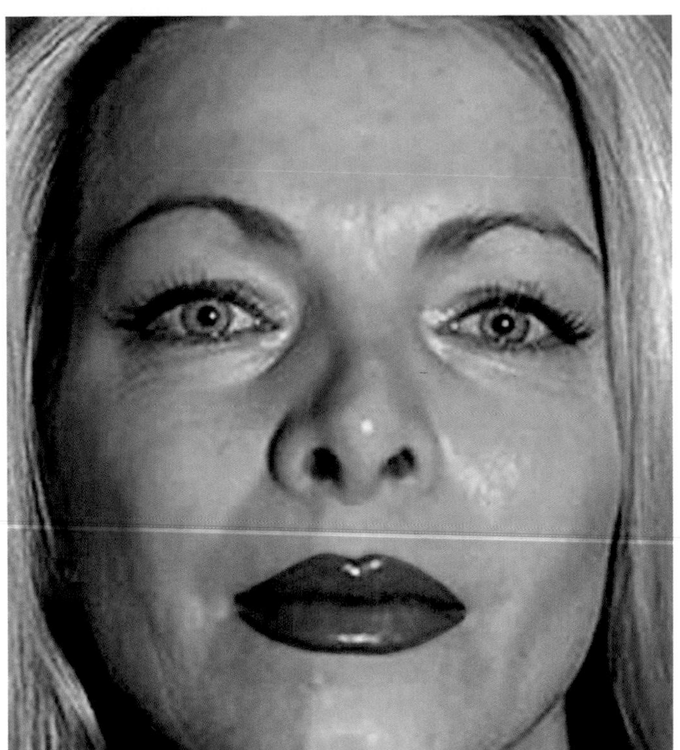

fig. 8 a+b

before the patient can go outside. Even at this point, make-up is needed and sunblock is a must in daylight. The skin takes at least two months to fully regenerate.

NOTE: Especially for the application of peelings, an experienced and meticulous practitioner is essential. If the treatment is not carried out faultlessly, the skin may be damaged irreversibly.

Dermabrasion is a mechanical procedure whereby the uppermost skin layer is "peeled" with a sanding unit. A spinning diamond fraise is used to smooth and reduce upper lip wrinkles, eliminate acne scars and remove pigment discolourations on the face or the hands. The treated skin heals much like a graze. Depending on the intensity of the treatment, the skin fully regenerates after 8–10 days.

Microdermabrasion is a subtle peeling treatment for the skin using a jet spray of microcrystals. It improves and refreshes the skin; redundant keratin cells are exfoliated.

Dermaplaning is a gentle peeling alternative applied in the US. After the skin has been cleansed with alcohol and dried, a special scalpel is used to shave off the topmost, damaged skin layer. The epidermis reacts to this process like to an injury and begins to repair itself. The treatment regenerates the skin cells and stimulates the collagen; it is so gentle that the skin doesn't even redden. Afterwards, a moisturising cream containing sunblock needs to be applied as the skin is as tender and soft as a baby's.

Endermology: This method, also known as the *LPG® technique*, efficiently stimulates the healing of scar tissue. The deeper skin tissue is stretched and made more elastic. Scar pain is reduced, and the patient's quality of life improves significantly.

Mesotherapy: Mesotherapy has been used as a natural remedy in France for over 50 years. Internationally, aesthetic dermatology has discovered it more recently as a treatment against skin aging and skin laxity. When performing a so-called *mesolift*, the practitioner injects minutely-dosed compounds exactly into the areas to be treated.

For the successful application of this technique, developed by Dr. Michel Pistor in 1952, it is paramount that the dosage of the substances injected is precise and low. In a series of 70–80 shots, minute droplets are injected under the skin, specifically into areas that are visibly aged and contain large amounts of blood vessels, e. g. the cheeks or the hands. The result is a long-term increase in the skin's suppleness and moisture-storing capacity.

Before treatment commences, the skin needs to be analysed thoroughly to prevent allergic reactions to the substances used. The injection compound is based on a biosynthetic, non-reticulated form of hyaluronic acid. Other substances are added to accommodate the patient's individual skin composition, e.g. a poly-vitamin complex or immune stimulators such as echinacea. Three 20-minute treatment sessions spaced 14 days apart are recommended, with follow-up treatments taking place 6–12 months later.

fig. 7 a+b & fig. 8 a+b

The most suitable treatment for impure skin, e. g. skin that has been damaged by nicotine or alcohol, is a chemical peeling. Prospective patients should be aware, however, that different types of skin will require different types of peeling. The most universally compatible peeling treatment uses trichloroacetic acid (20-40 percent dilution). This causes a thorough peeling of the upper epithelial cells and a rapid re-epithelisation after approx. eight days. As a result of any chemical peeling, the skin is reddened for approx. two weeks. After this time, makeup can be applied again. The skin also needs to be protected from UV rays for two months (SPF 20 lotion). Chemical peelings are effective for a long time. However, patients need to be aware that they can also cause pigment discolourations, i. e. hyper- or hypo-pigmentation. © Bodenseeklinik Prof. Mang

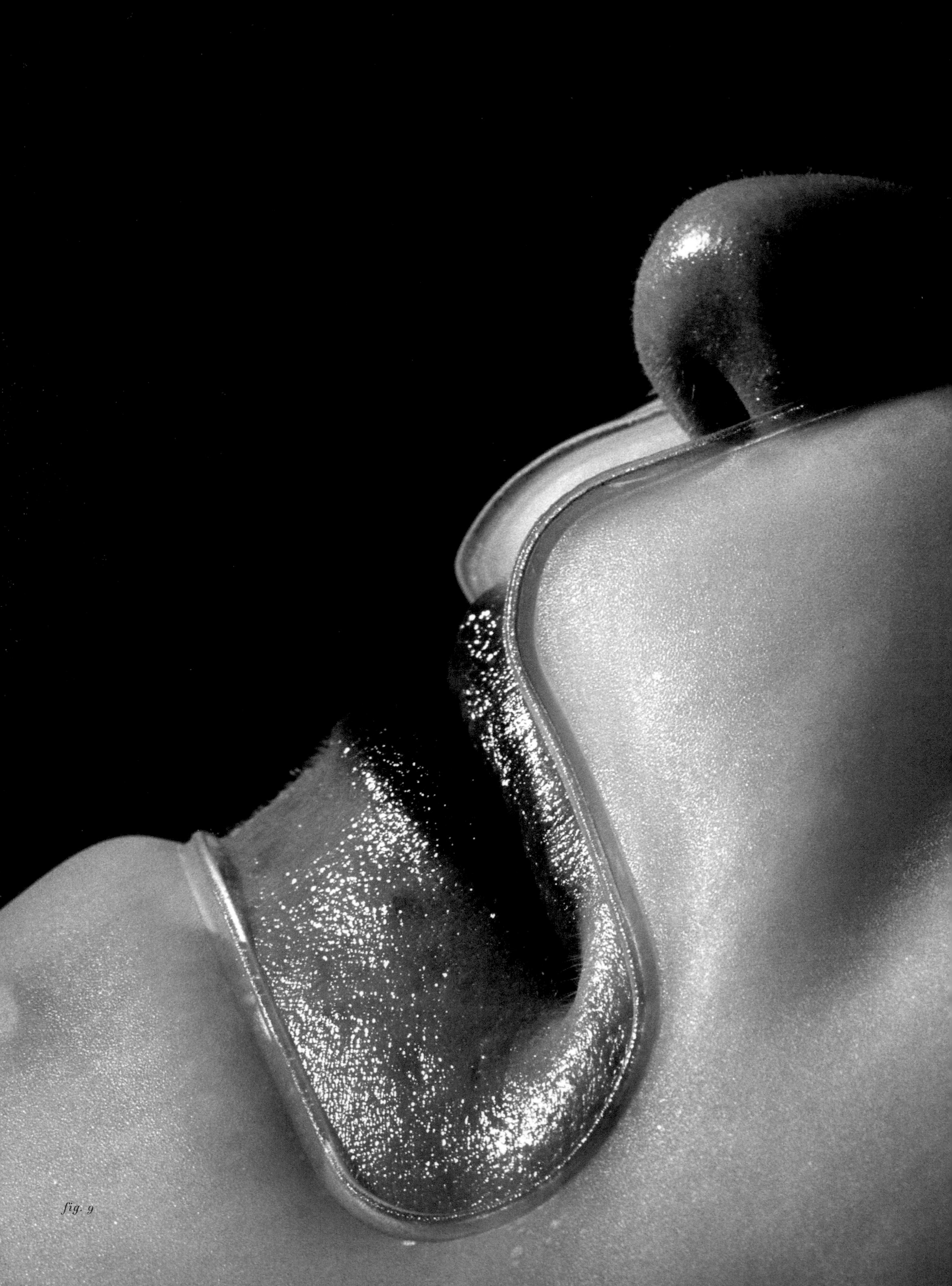

fig. 9

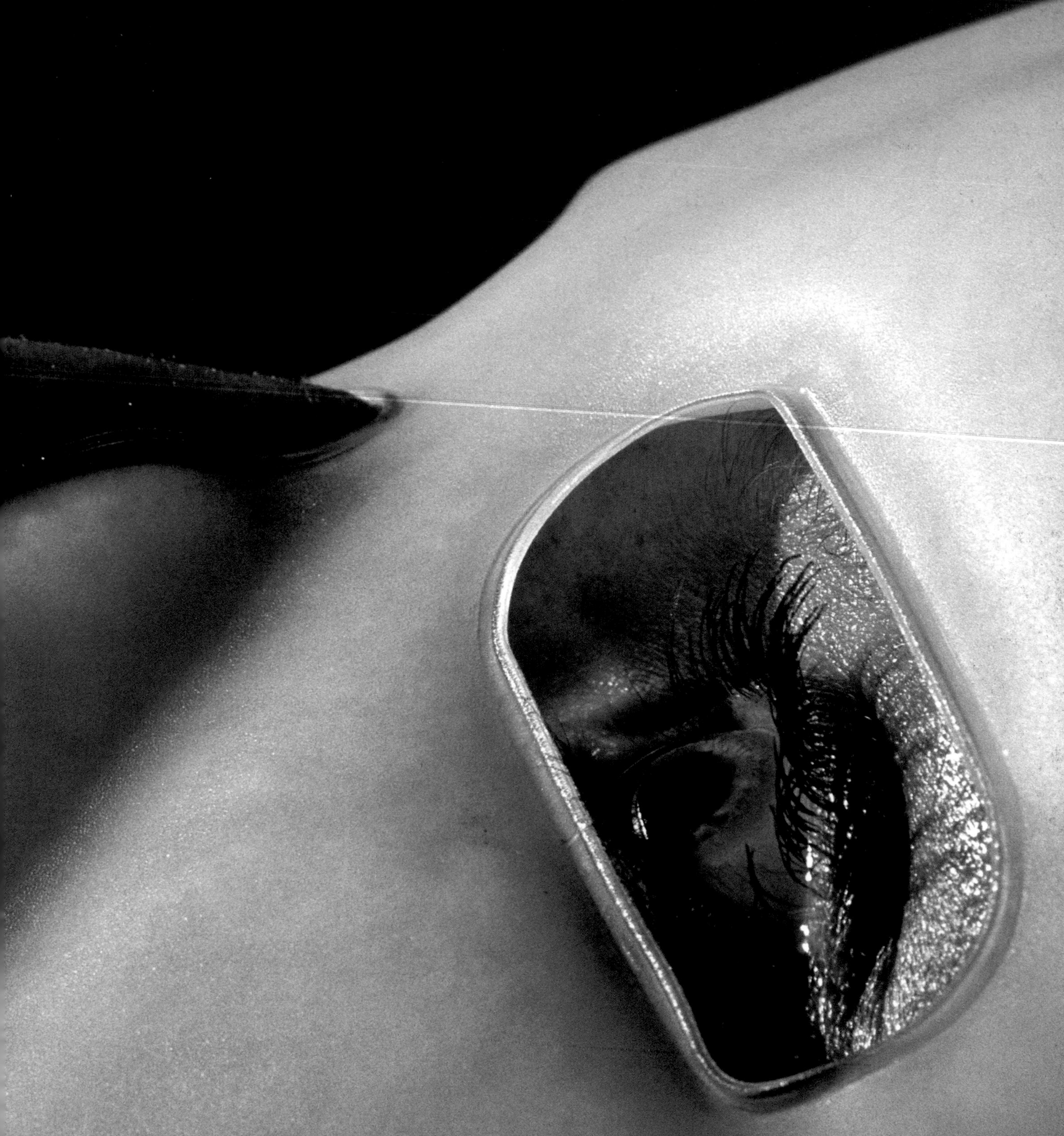

Medicine is like love. It always begins and finds no end.

Juarez Avelar

Surgical Procedures

EVA KARCHER, Munich
in collaboration with
DR. CHRISTOPH WOLFENSBERGER, Zurich
and PROF. DR. DR. WERNER L. MANG, Lindau

FACE
Facelifts

Face-and-neck lifting, also known as face-and-neck contouring. Medical term: Rhytidectomy.

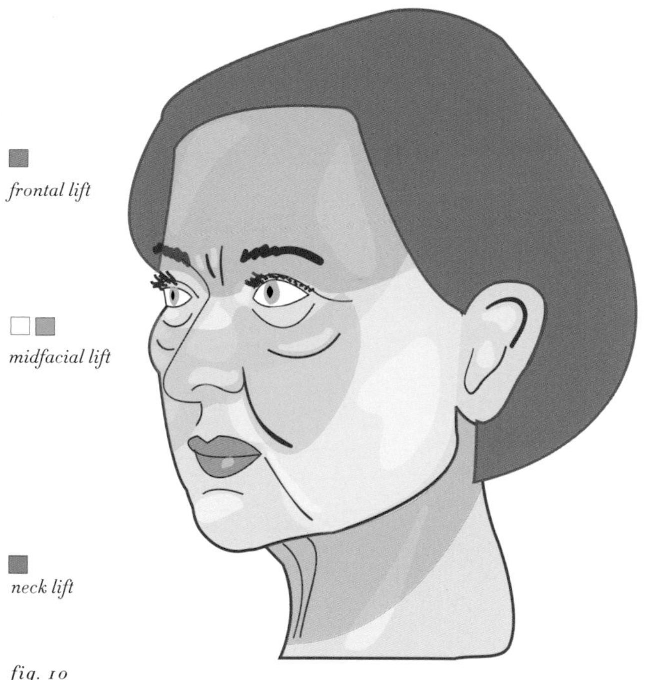

fig. 10

The following types of facelift are available:
SMAS lift: The classic, most popular face-and-neck lift. Its success relies primarily on lifting the cheek/neck contour. The ideal age for this procedure is 45–55. As well as smoothing the skin, the operation also tightens the face's subcutaneous layer of muscles, connective and fatty tissue, the so-called SMAS layer (Superficial Musculo-Aponeurotic System). At the same time, the neck region is corrected, e. g. in case of a so-called "turkey gobbler" neck. This platysmaplasty tightens the neck muscle. Contracted regions are fixed with non-dissolving sutures; the skin is smoothed, then sutured or clamped.

Mini lift: The most basic lifting operation, suitable for women below the age of 40. It is frequently requested by models. The same incisions as for the SMAS lift are used, but only the skin is tightened. This has a rejuvenating effect particularly on the middle and upper regions of the face – the brow and eye areas. The effects of a mini lift are frequently only visible for several months, and it doesn't change the nasolabial folds.

Mid-face lift: This lifts sagging cheek tissue below the lower eyelid, which also corrects pronounced nasolabial folds and drooping corners of the mouth.

Mask lift or *subperiosteal (deep plane) lift:* Based on a special technique where the incision to dislodge the cheek is made from the inside of the mouth. Skin, tissue and muscles are detached from the bone to achieve a long-lasting effect. As this technique can entail many complications and the healing period is lengthy, it has become unpopular.

Tissue glue facelift: When suturing, many surgeons use *Fibrin sealant*, a "glue" for sealing wounds that is made from human blood-clotting proteins. Fibrin sealant eliminates the need for facial bandages and drainage tubes, and decreases the possibility of haematomas. However, it is expensive and can cause infections. It is somewhat misleading to regard this procedure as a facelift in its own right, as it only describes one aspect of the operation.

The **incision line** is essentially the same for all the types of lifting described above: The surgical cut starts near the temple, continues along the hairline, along the ear and around the ear lobe, and ends in the hair-covered neck area behind the ear. As the suture always borders the hairline, it remains invisible. Hair loss and hairline shifts are avoided.

Endoscopic lift: This technique produces the fewest scars and has the most natural-looking results, but not all surgeons are able to perform it as it is also very complex. Starting at the hairline, the surgeon makes very small incisions

fig. 9

The patient's face after a brow lift. Thanks to sophisticated modern surgical techniques, the skin can be smoothed without any visible scars – the incisions are all made behind the hairline. © laif

fig. 10

Medical professionals talk of three different lifting areas: the brow, the face and the neck. The most common technique is the SMAS lift, a standard treatment that focuses on lifting the cheek and neck contour. © Blue Brain Belgium

fig. 11

Werner L. Mang is Germany's most famous cosmetic surgeon. His Bodenseeklinik at Lake Constance, opened in 2003, is Europe's biggest and most sophisticated centre of aesthetic surgery. © Bodenseeklinik Prof. Mang

fig. 12

During a brow lift, the surgeon inserts specialized implements underneath the skin, removes some of the muscle tissue and thus smoothes the folds. The eyebrows can be lifted in the same procedure. © laif

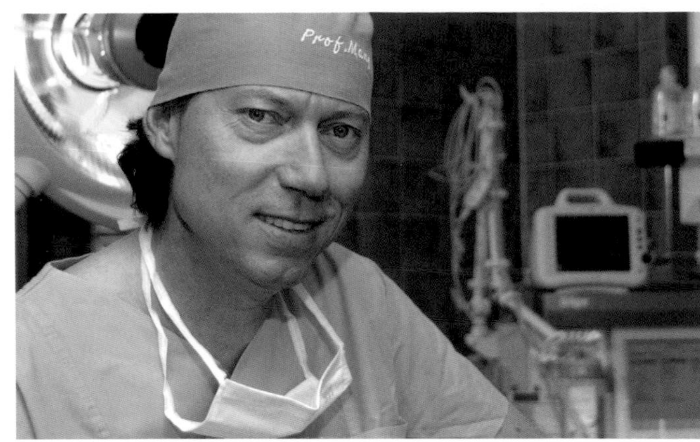

fig. 11

(1–2 centimetres) to feed the endoscope and other miniature instruments beneath the skin. Every movement can then be traced on a video monitor. Sagging tissue is pushed back up and the skin realigns automatically.

NOTE: The surgeon's qualifications are a decisive factor in the success of this procedure. An alternative technique is provided by the MACS lift (Minimal Access Cranial Suspension), developed recently by Dr. Tonnard and Dr. Verpaelen. It only requires a local anaesthetic and produces no scars apart from two tiny incisions at the front of the ear. The healing period is also shorter than for conventional lifting techniques.

Endoscopic brow and eyebrow lift: Brow and eyebrows benefit greatly from a surgical technique that produces no visible scars. Three to six incisions, each approx. one centimetre in length, are made for inserting special surgical instruments under the brow skin. The skin is lifted and some of the brow muscles are removed – which de-emphasises creases. In the same procedure, the eyebrows can be lifted, which improves the field of vision as well as the facial appearance. Excess skin is shifted up behind the hairline, where it is held in position by tiny screws.

Lip lift: If the upper lip and the nose are too far apart, this can be corrected with an invisible cut at the edge of the

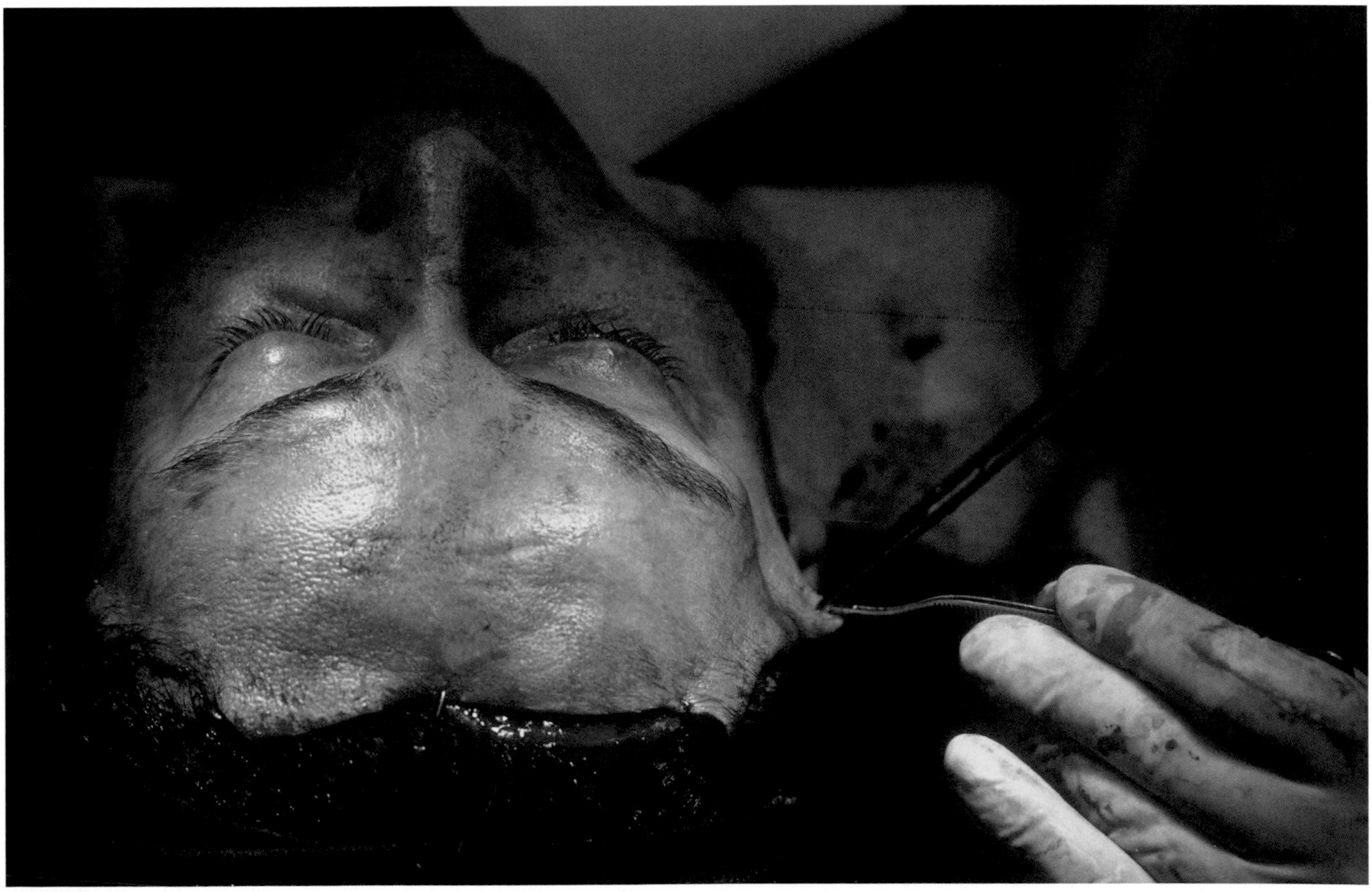

fig. 12

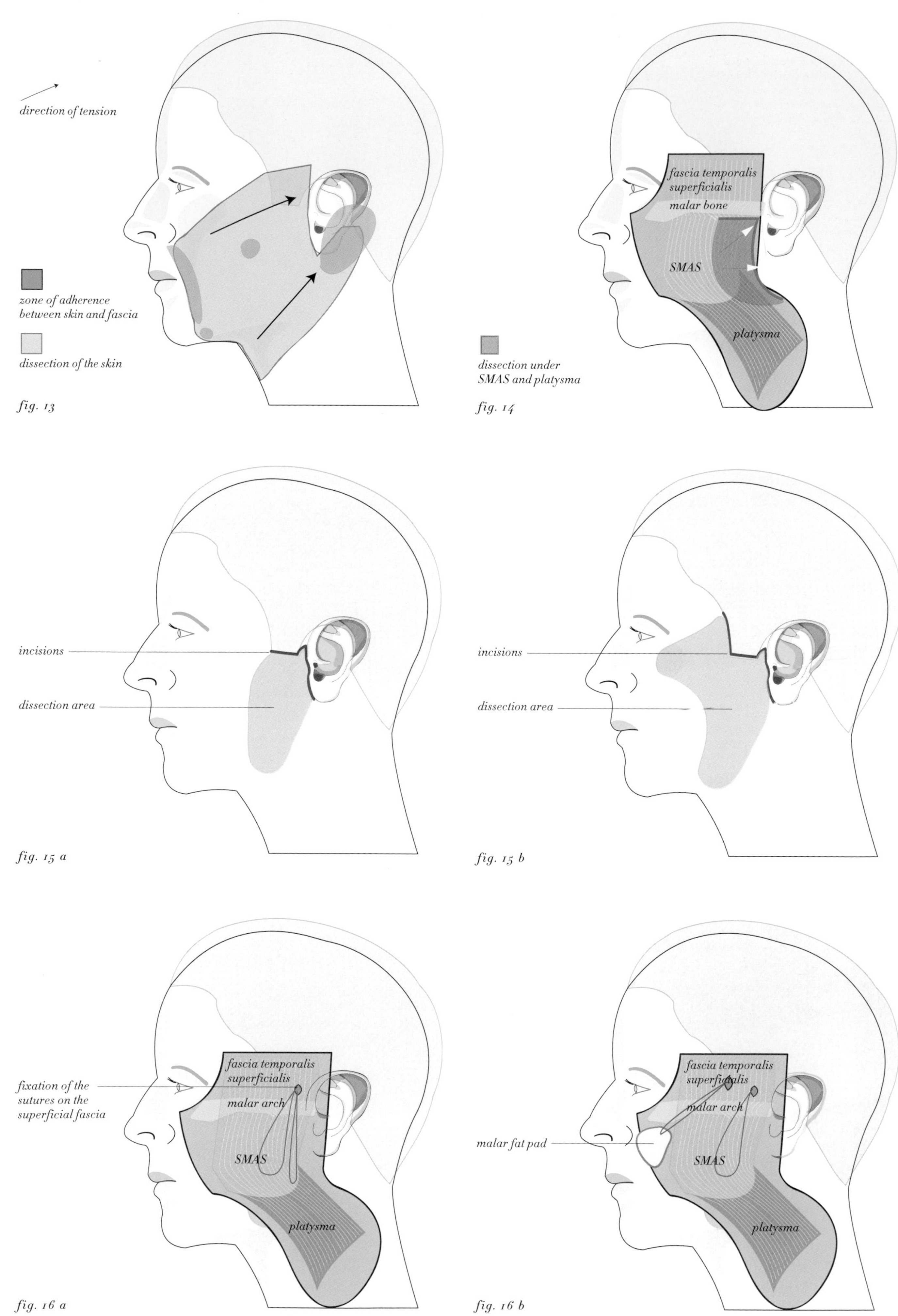

fig. 13

fig. 14

fig. 15 a

fig. 15 b

fig. 16 a

fig. 16 b

fig. 13 & 14

Examples of a cheek/neck lift (13) and a classic SMAS lift in combination with a shortening of the neck muscle – this treatment is also known as platysmaplasty (14). © Blue Brain Belgium

fig. 15 a+b & 16 a+b

The MACS (Minimal Access Cranial Suspension) lift is a recent surgical innovation. It is performed using only a local anaesthetic and produces no scars apart from two or three minor incisions. © Blue Brain Belgium

fig. 17

The lifting of the brow and eyebrows is often combined, as only a few incisions need to be made behind the hairline to access both areas for smoothing. © Blue Brain Belgium

fig. 18

A brow lift: This technique, which involves folding down the brow flap, requires a general anaesthetic. © laif

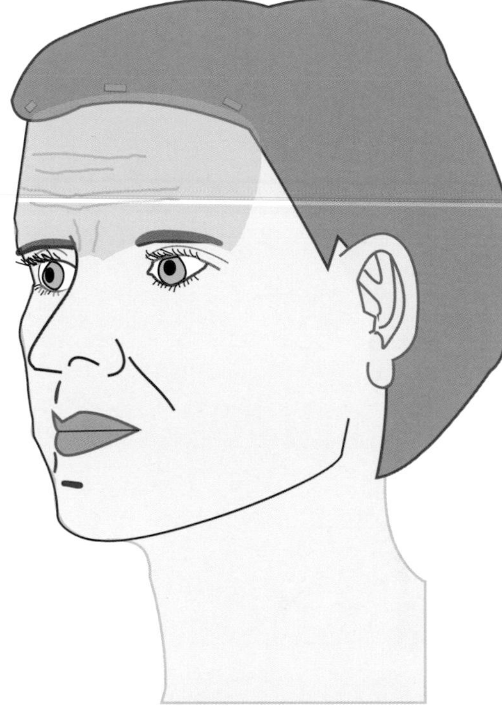

fig. 17

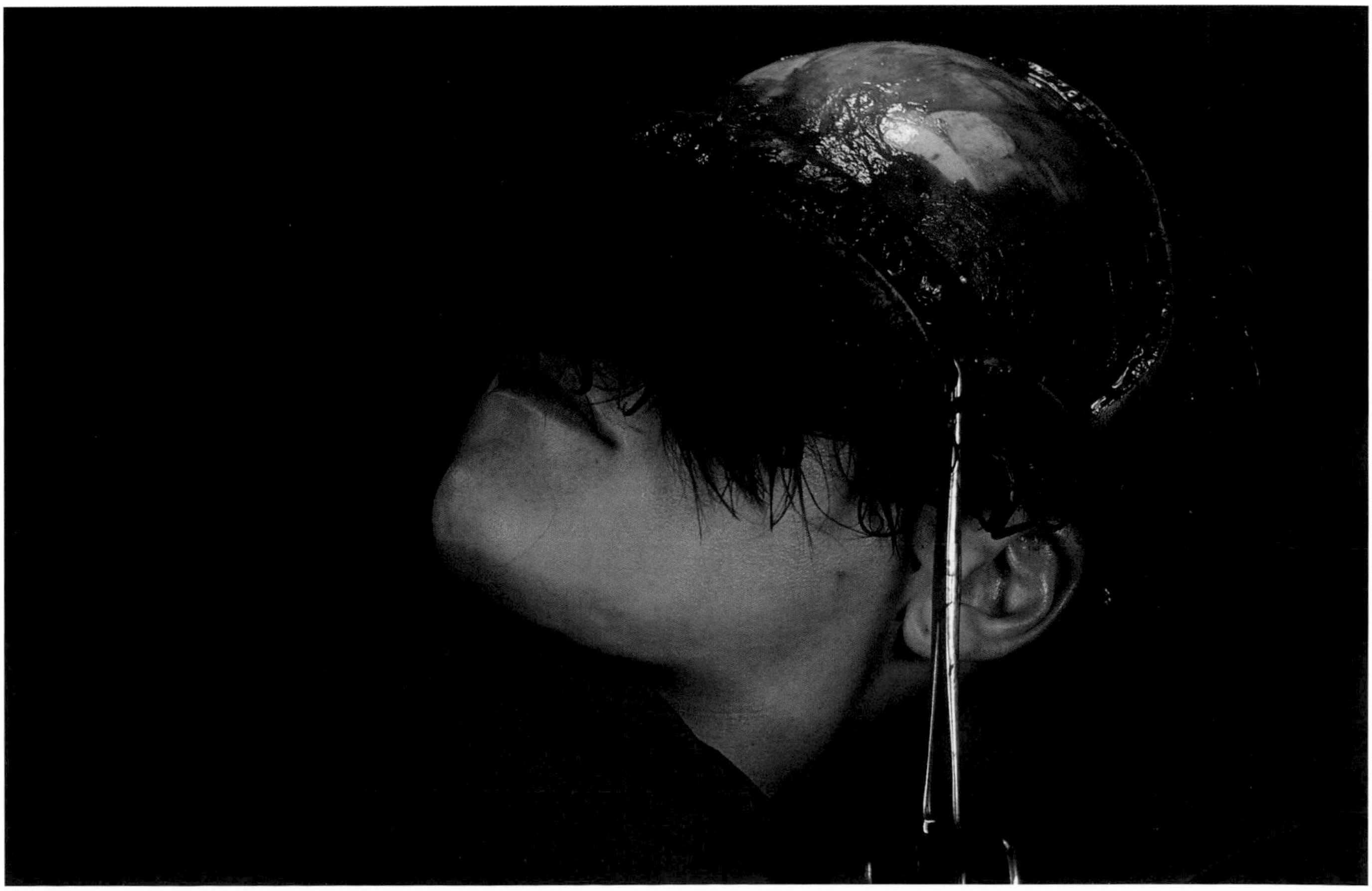

fig. 18

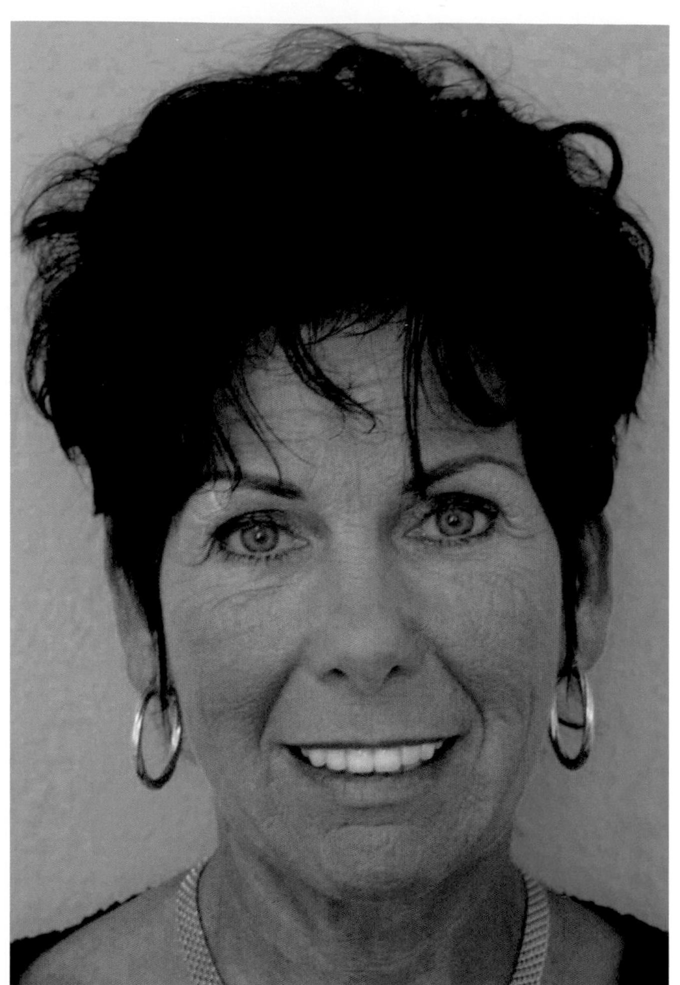

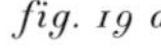

fig. 19 a

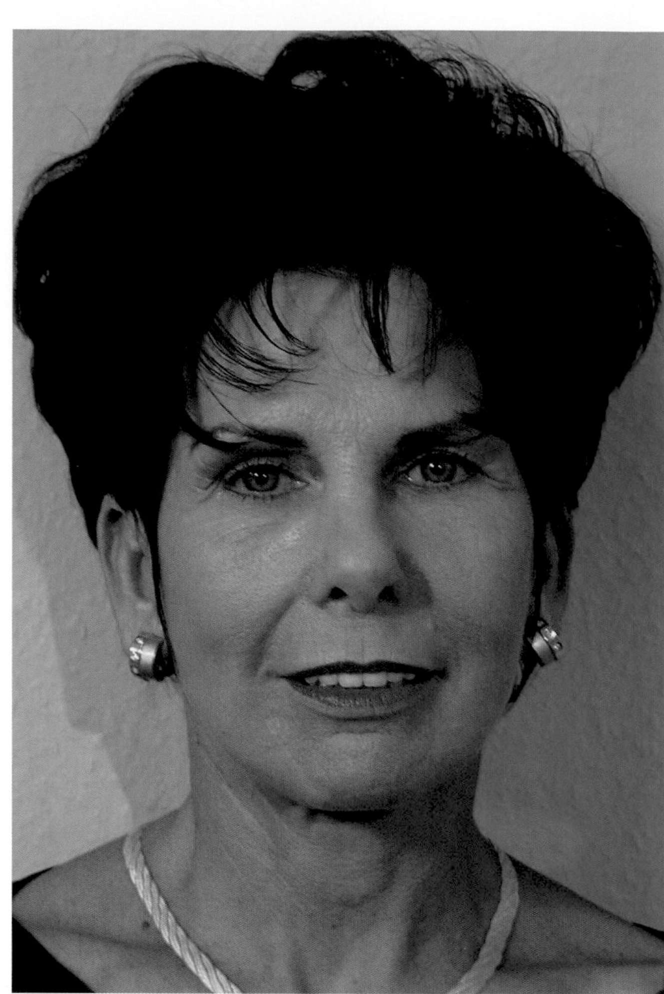

fig. 19 b

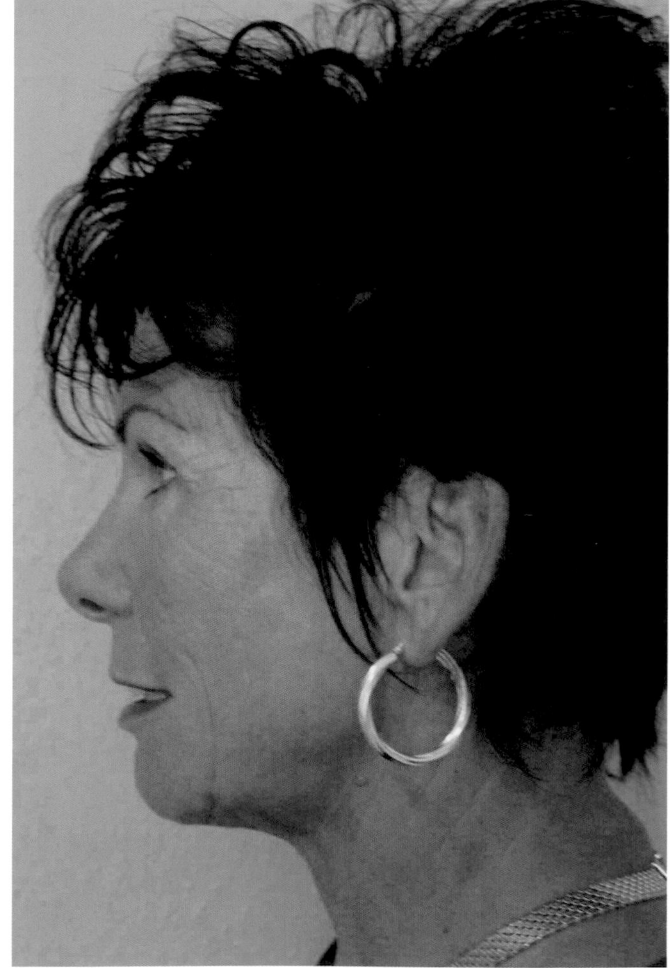

fig. 20 a

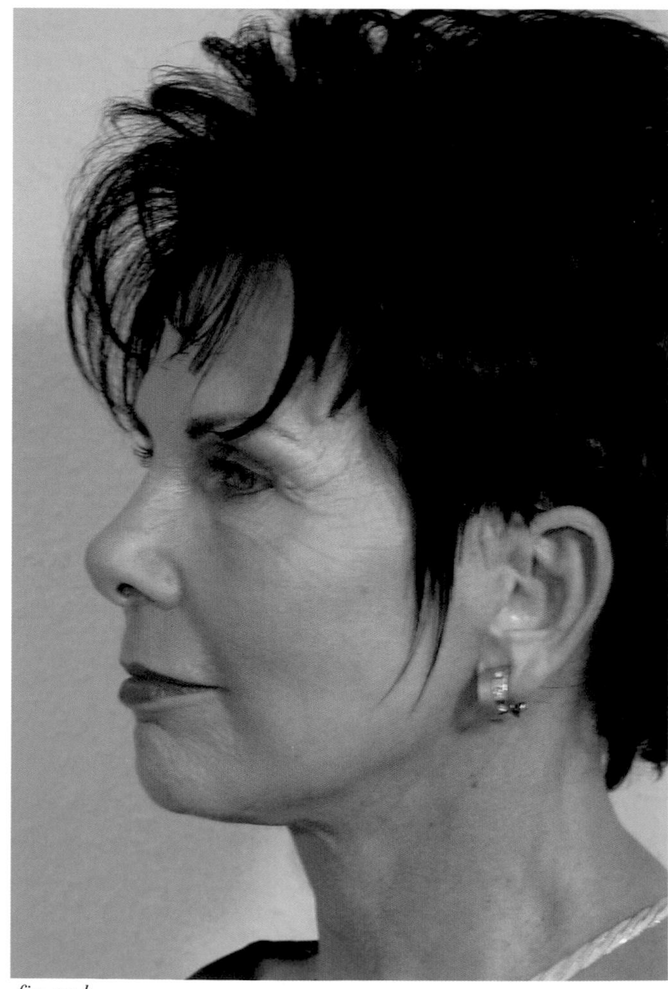

fig. 20 b

fig. 19 a+b & 20 a+b

Two patients, before a facelift and six months later. In both cases, a notable rejuvenation and smoothing of the entire facial and neck area is evident without any artificial-looking side effects. Among women above the age of 45, facelifts are the most popular procedure. An important aspect of this operation is that not only the skin but also the subcutaneous tissue is tightened. The skill required of the surgeon is to achieve a natural-looking rejuvenation, i. e. without giving the face a frozen, mask-like appearance. As well as smoothing the brow and cheek regions, the surgeon also lifts the neck skin; the neck indicates the skin's age more visibly than the facial areas.
© Bodenseeklinik Prof. Mang

fig. 21 a+b

Profileplasty is one of the surgical approaches developed by Prof. Werner L. Mang. On this patient's face, he performed a rhinoplasty and a chin enlargement – the face now looks altogether more feminine. © Bodenseeklinik Prof. Mang

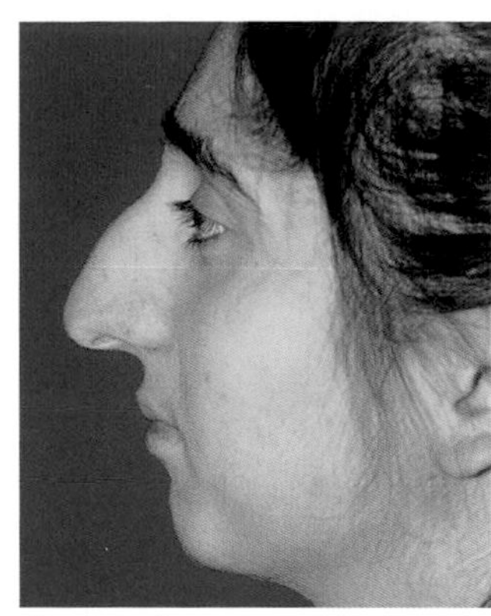

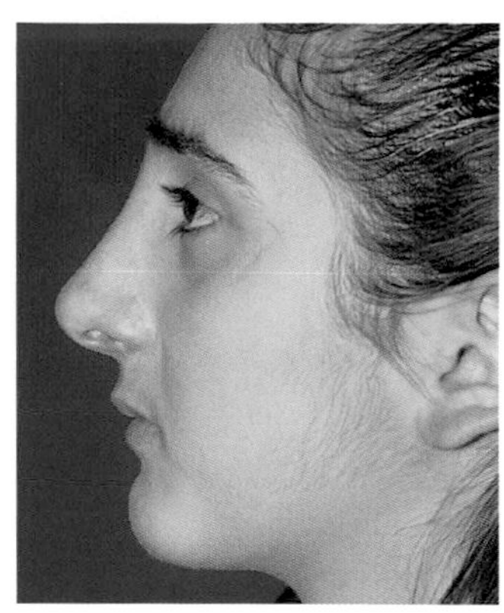

fig. 21 a+b

fig. 22 a+b

A 56-year-old patient with a pronounced double chin in the submental area. A facelift alone could not sufficiently remove these superfluous skin folds. In this case, the most suitable approach is to make a "fish mouth" incision in the neck region and to remove all the excess skin and fatty tissue. It is very important to tighten the platysma so as to avoid later relapses.
The wound is sealed on two intradermal layers using thin skin sutures.
© Bodenseeklinik Prof. Mang

fig. 23 a+b

The photo on the right shows the patient six months after the double chin was removed. If neck liposuction is combined with a minor skin excision, the result will last for several decades. An important postoperative aspect is to treat the skin with special ointments that suppress scar formation; this way, there will be no traces of surgery at all.
© Bodenseeklinik Prof. Mang

upper lip or just underneath the nose. If the problem is a narrow upper lip, one incision is made along the contour of the lip and another several millimetres above it. This second incision defines the new, fuller shape of the lip, and hence needs to be made extremely carefully. The strip of skin between the two incisions is removed, the red of the lip is unfolded from the inside, and the lip is sown onto its new upper edge. If the problem is an oversized lip, the incision is made on the inside of the lip. Again, a flawless technique is decisive for the success of the operation.

NOTE: Following the operation, the mouth is very swollen for approx. one week. There is also an increased risk of infection, raised scarring (keloids) and sustained numbness. Asymmetries may also occur.

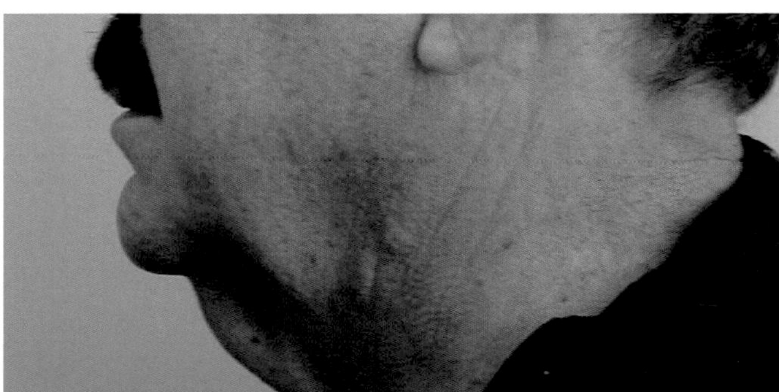

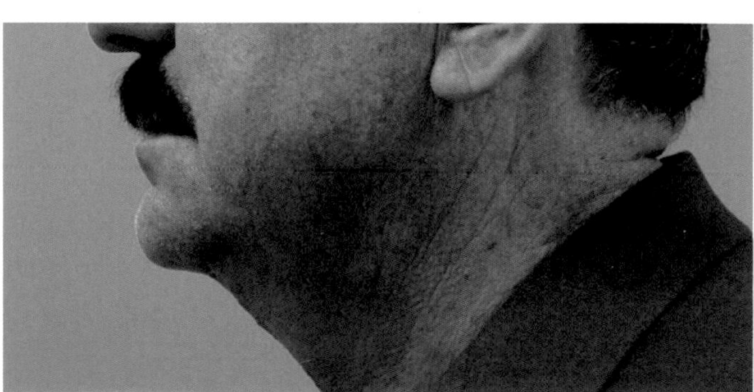

fig. 22 a+b

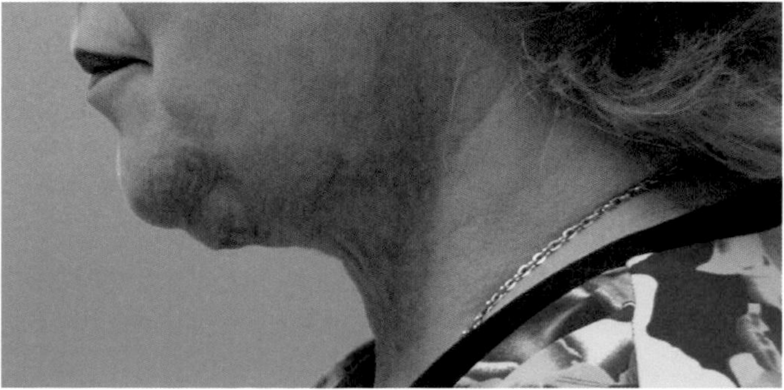

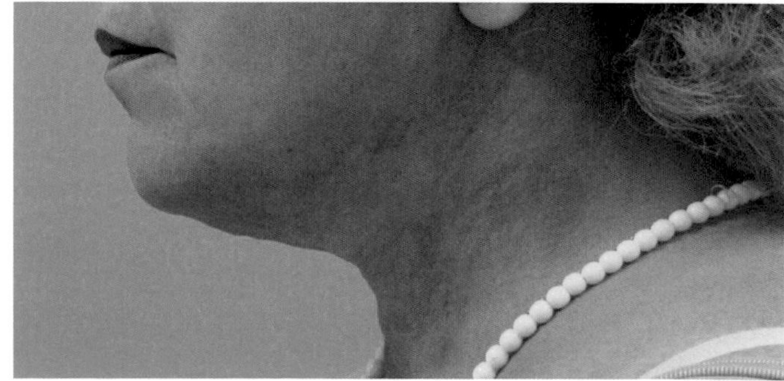

fig. 23 a+b

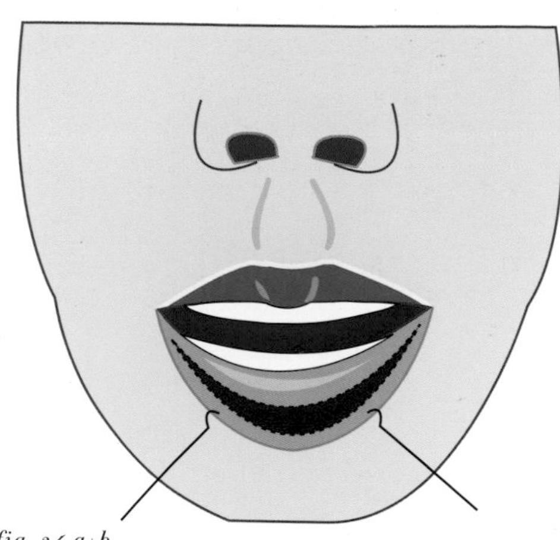

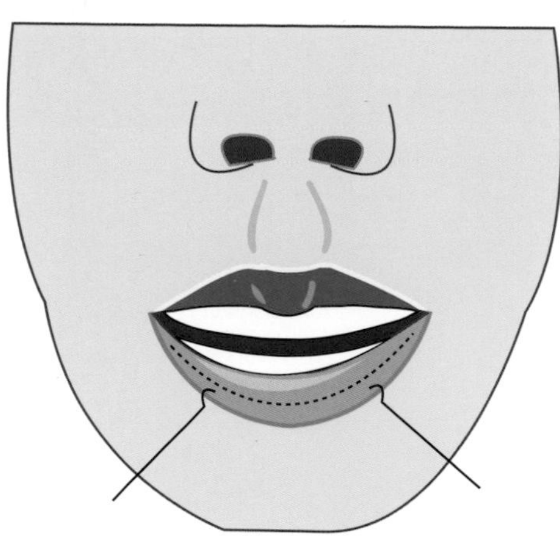

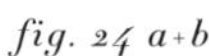

fig. 24 a+b

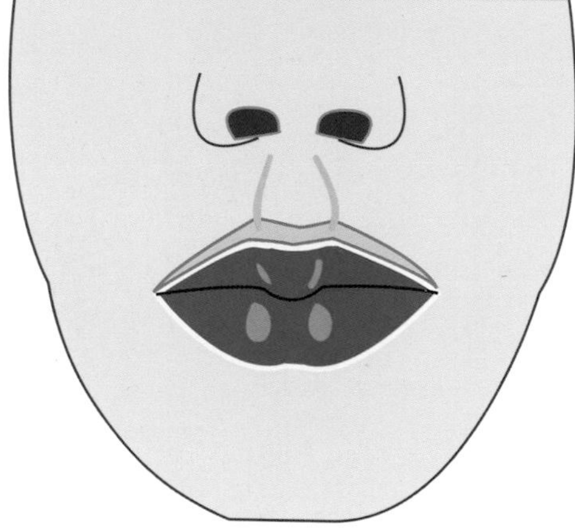

fig. 25 a

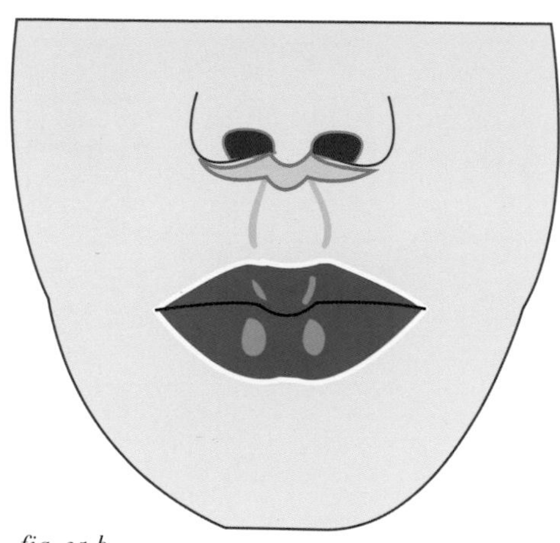

fig. 25 b

fig. 24 a+b & 25 a+b

An oversized lip can be reduced by an excision on the inside of the mouth (24 a+b). If the lip is too small, one cut is made along the lip's contour and another two millimetres above it – this defines the new, fuller outline of the lip (25 a+b). © Blue Brain Belgium

fig. 26 a+b

These photos exemplify that the aging process is indeed most evident in the neck and lower part of the face. After the neck lift, the patient's face also appears to be rejuvenated. This impression is reinforced by the new hairstyle. Fittingly, a good cosmetic surgery clinic has surgeons, cosmeticians and hair stylists working in tandem. Other important aspects of postoperative in-patient care are lymphatic drainage and specialized cosmetic treatment. © Bodenseeklinik Prof. Mang

fig. 27 a+b

A 68-year-old patient with pronounced folds and wrinkles on the sides of her face. The photo on the right depicts the patient six months after the operation, which consisted of the three-step lift developed by Prof. Mang. Both the platysma and the SMAS were lifted so that the subcutaneous tissue and not the surface skin is affected by muscular tension. This approach also eliminates the need for incisions (i. e. scars) in front of and behind the ear. For this level of wrinkling, only a facelift is effective; injection therapies have proven ineffectual. © Bodenseeklinik Prof. Mang

FACELIFT BASICS

Ideal age: Between 45 and 65.
Preparation: You should stop smoking and drinking four weeks before the operation. Stop taking blood-thinning medication (such as *Aspirin*) two weeks before the operation. If possible, stop taking sleep-inducing drugs, as these may adversely affect your sedation. Also, make sure to have a thorough health-check in advance of the operation.
Side effects: After the procedure, the face will be swollen; haematomas and bruises around the cheeks, neck and mouth may appear sporadically, similarly numbness and pain. Sometimes, these symptoms take up to three months to fully disappear. Scars are unobtrusive and usually cannot be seen at all once healing is complete.
Risks / complications: Haematomas are rarely so pronounced that they require further surgical treatment. There may be some temporary hair loss around the temples. Necrosis, i. e. skin cell death due to bad circulation, is predominantly a risk for heavy smokers. Bulging scars (keloids) are a hereditary reaction. If the surgeon is inexperienced, there is a greater risk of facial nerve damage.
Sedation: Usually a general aesthetic.
Length of operation: three to six hours.
Hospital stay: two to five days.
Effectiveness: ten to 15 years.

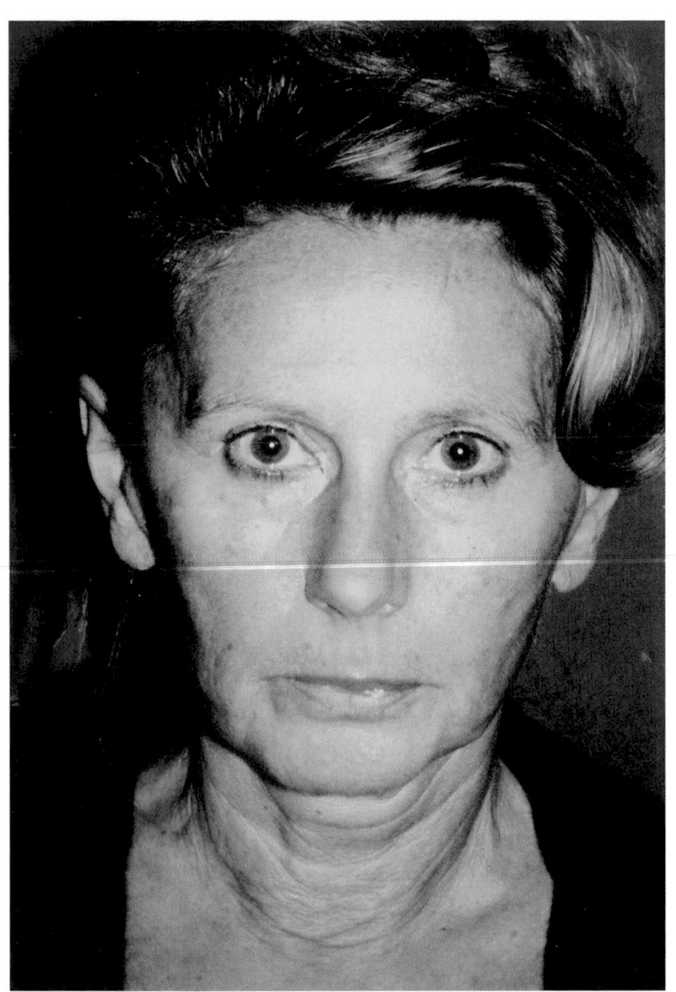

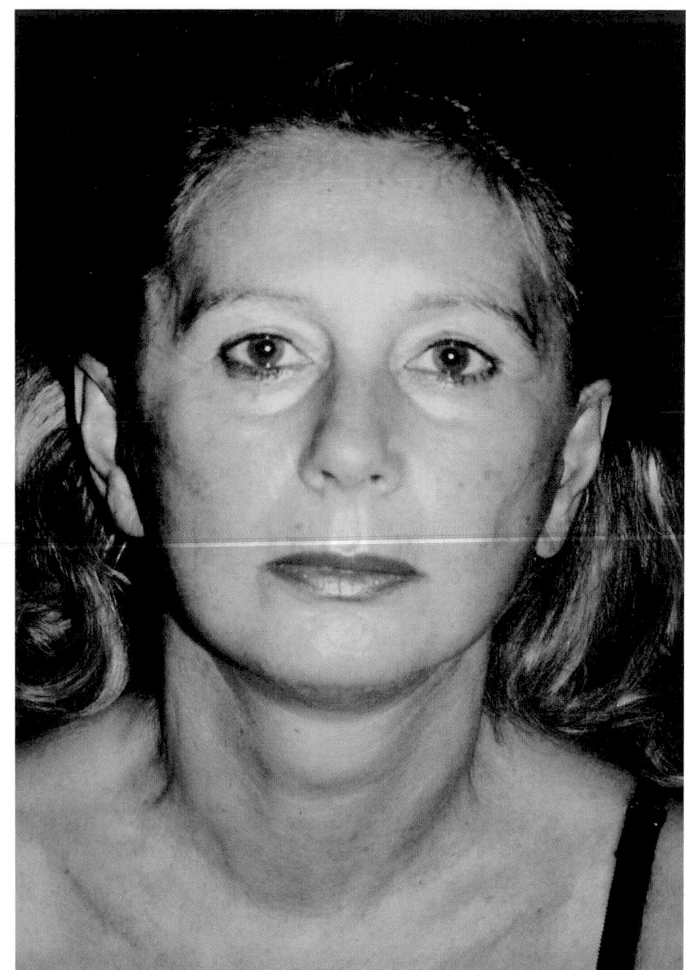

fig. 26 a+b

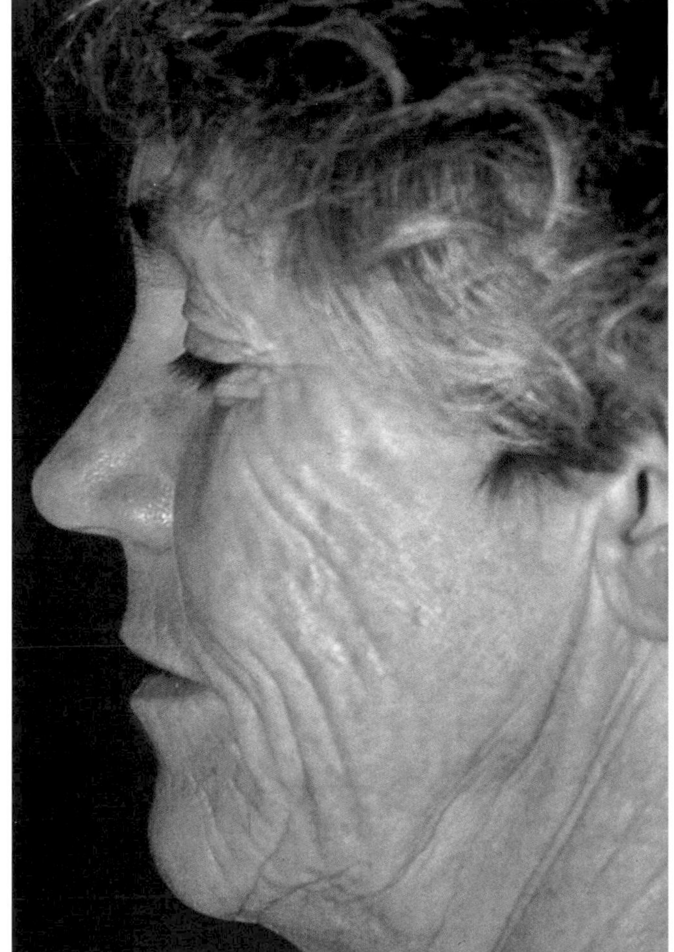

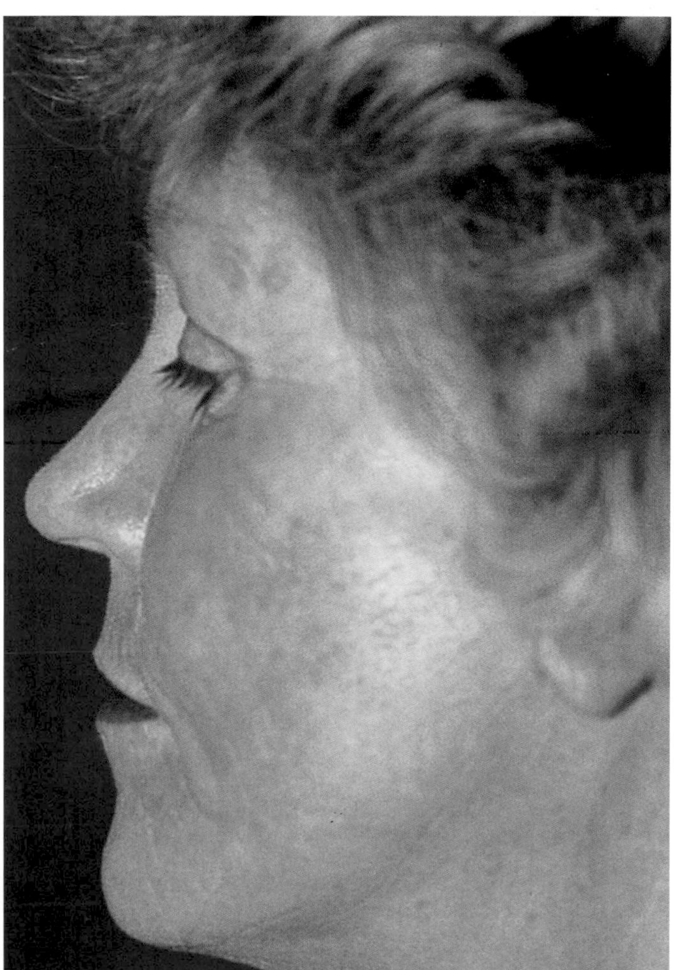

fig. 27 a+b

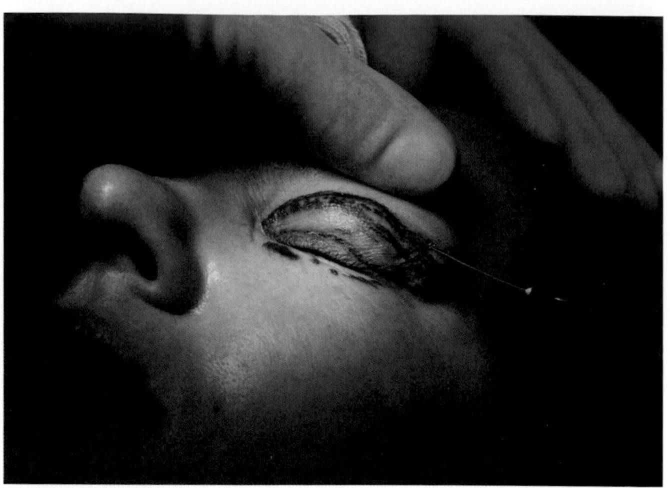

fig. 28

fig. 28

Blepharoplasty (eyelid lifting) is one of the most popular treatments of cosmetic surgery among both men and women. © laif

fig. 30 a–d

With lower eyelid lifts, surgeons are increasingly focusing on redistributing the fatty tissue instead of removing it – this is to reduce risks such as inflammation, dryness and eyes looking "hollow" or even skeletal. © Blue Brain Belgium

fig. 31 a+b

In upper eyelid lifts, the excess skin is removed together with the corresponding muscle strip and the fatty tissue beneath it. Incisions are made with scalpels or laser beams. © Blue Brain Belgium

Eyes

Eyelid correction / blepharoplasty: Blepharoplasty, the medical term for lifting the upper or lower eyelid or removing the lachrymal sacs, is one of the most popular aesthetic procedures with both men and women. Requiring comparatively little surgical work, tired or sad-looking eyes can be given a radiant, youthful appearance. Corrections are mostly performed on upper and lower eyelids with festoons ("hoods" or "bags" respectively), and crow's feet around the eyes. Festoons often appear when the delicate skin surrounding the eyes loses its strength, usually around the age of 40 or 50. Similarly, the eyebrows may droop with age.

Upper eyelid lift: After a local anaesthetic has been administered, a scalpel or CO_2 laser is used to cut along the fold of the eyelid. This removes the excess skin as well as the muscle and fatty tissue underneath it. The wound is closed with a tiny suture inside the skin, a subcuticular suture. If a laser beam is used, the wound takes longer to heal, whereas a scalpel operation requires additional haemostasis. Swellings are soothed with cooling pads. The stitches are removed after five days.

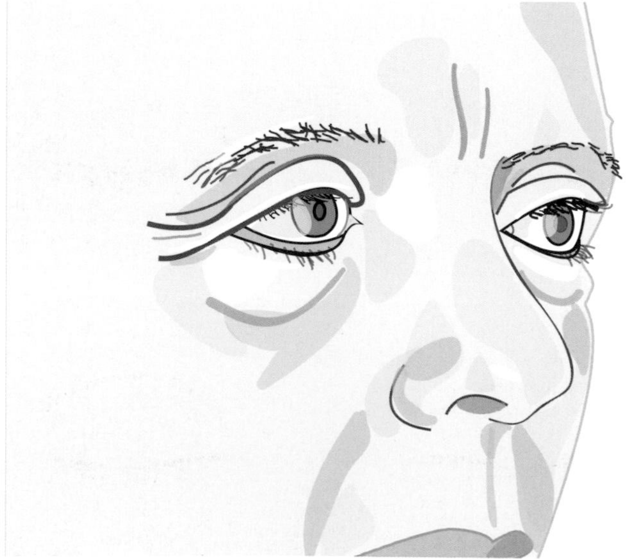

fig. 29

Lower eyelid lift: This procedure is comparatively risky. If too much skin is removed from the eyelid, the cornea may get inflamed or too dry. If too much subcutaneous fat is removed, the eye may look hollow or skeletal. For this reason, recent techniques have focused on redistributing the fatty tissue instead of removing it, a method known as the "SOOF"(Sub-Orbicularis Oculi Fat) lift.

Despite its inherent risks, this is the only effective procedure for treating skin laxity and deposits of fat or fluid in the skin. The incision line is cut 1–2 millimetres below the edge of the lower eyelid. Using a laser is especially advantageous when operating on the lower eyelid — the fatty tissue is easier to access and remove from the conjunctiva located below the eyeball. The laser beam's heat also seals the blood vessels, so sutures aren't needed. A disadvantage of this method is the prolonged wound-healing period. The skin may be reddened for up to six weeks after the procedure. If the festoon is very pronounced, the only way to operate is still with a scalpel.

Hospital stay: No more than one day per procedure.
Social contacts: After one week.

NOTE:
Before the procedure takes place, you should ascertain that you indeed require a correction of the upper eyelid — in many cases, a brow or eyebrow lift will be more successful! Sometimes, both procedures are necessary. In the first couple of days after eyelid surgery, you should always sleep on your back with a raised pillow. Make-up and contact lenses should not be used for eight days. For the first two weeks after the operation, sunglasses should be worn when outside.

fig. 29

Surgical treatments around the eye are comparatively uncomplicated while achieving considerable results. Festoons, lachrymal sacs and crow's feet can easily be eliminated, and tired-looking eyes will look fresh and radiant again. © Blue Brain Belgium

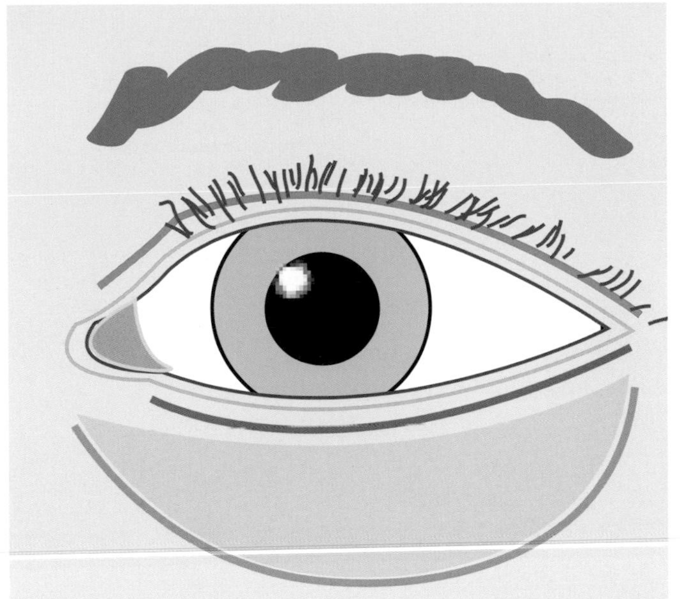

fig. 30 a

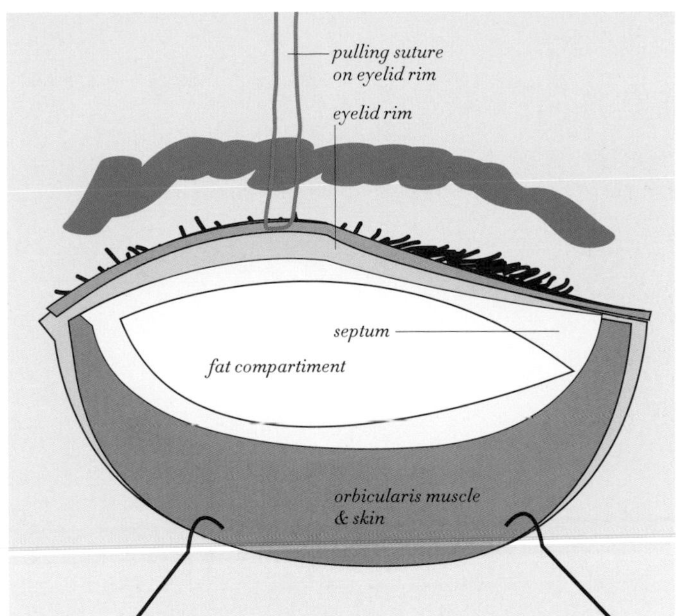

fig. 30 b

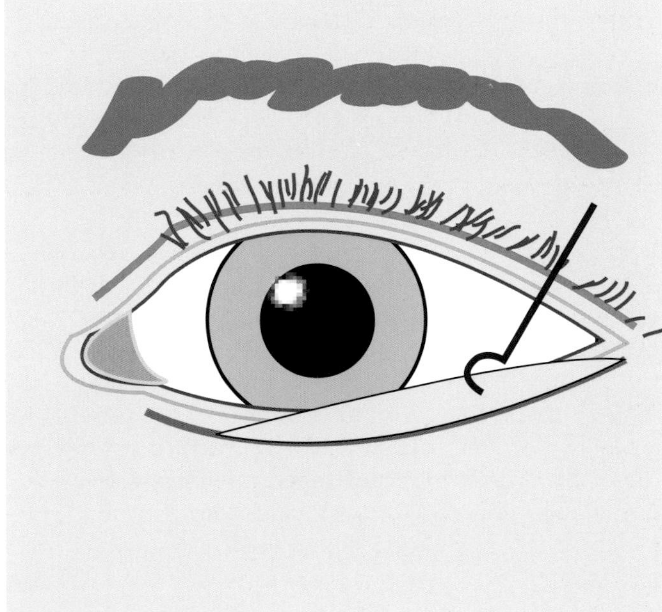

fig. 30 c

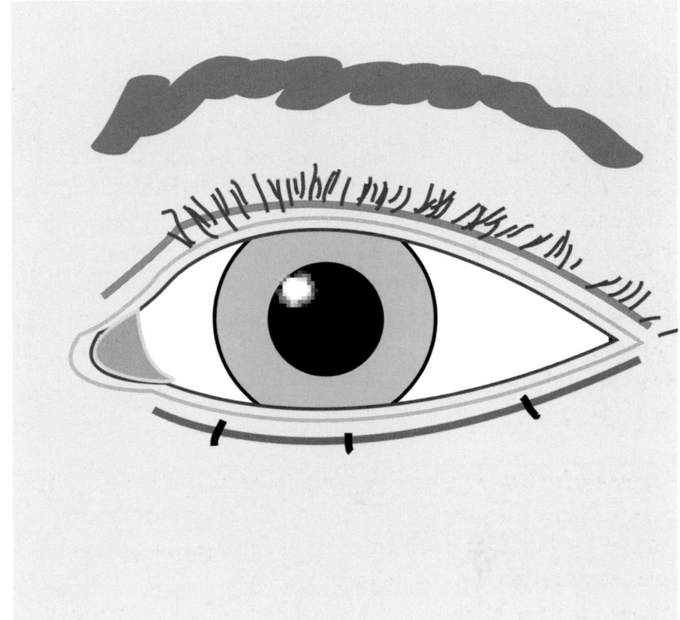

fig. 30 d

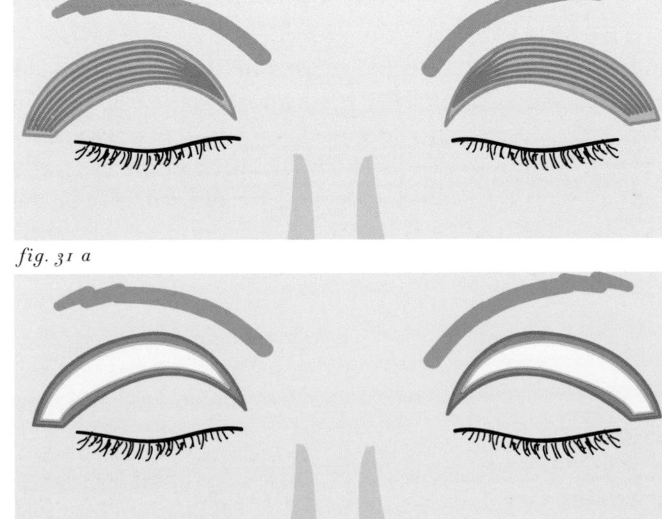

fig. 31 a

fig. 31 c

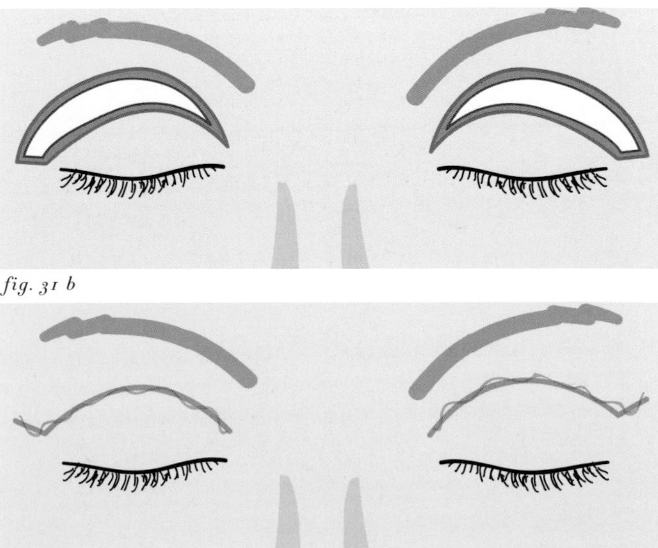

fig. 31 b

fig. 31 d

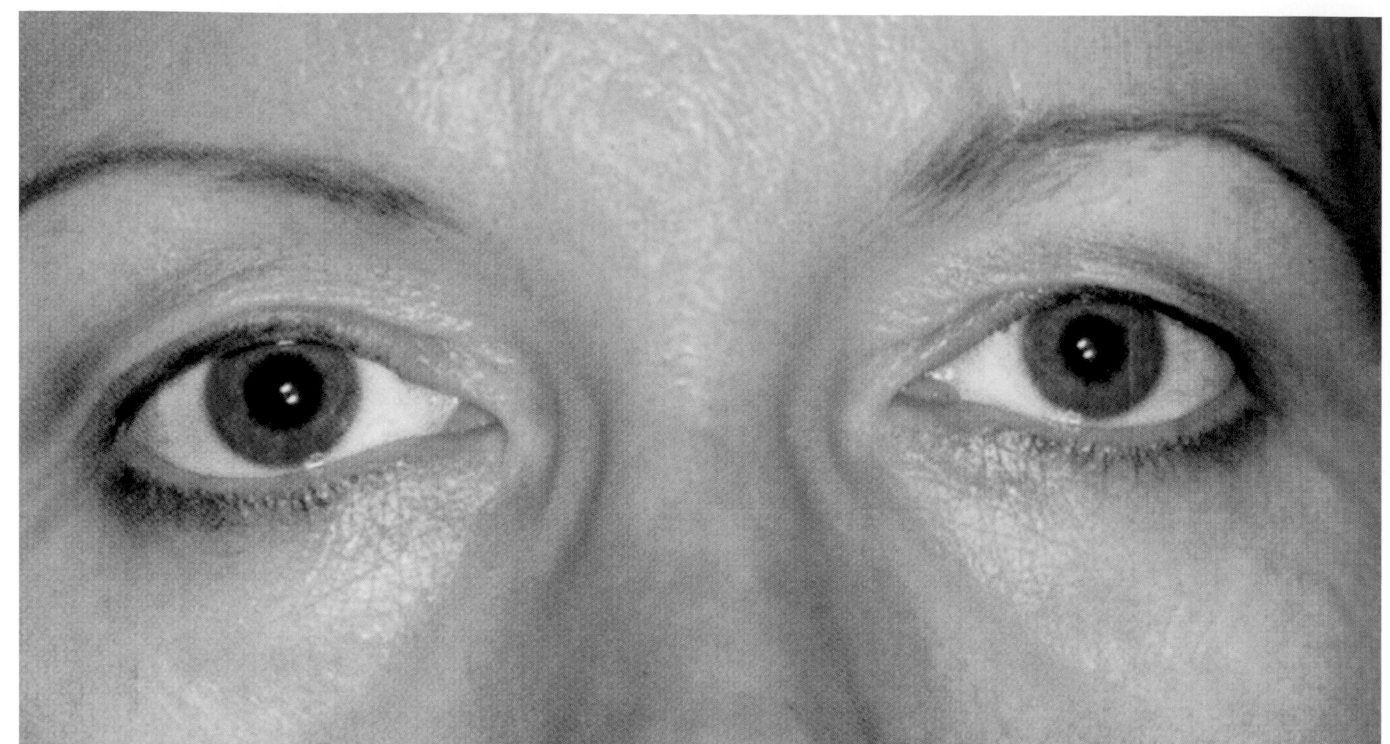

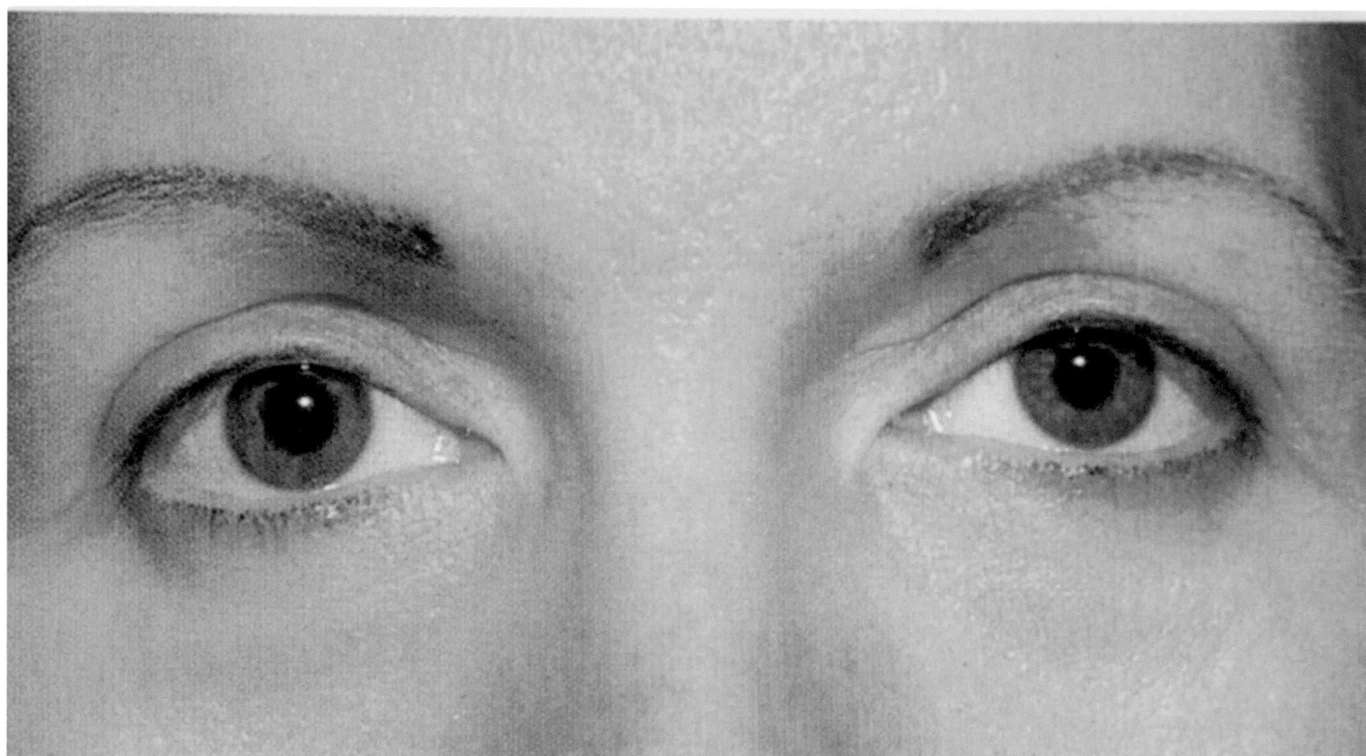

fig. 32 a+b

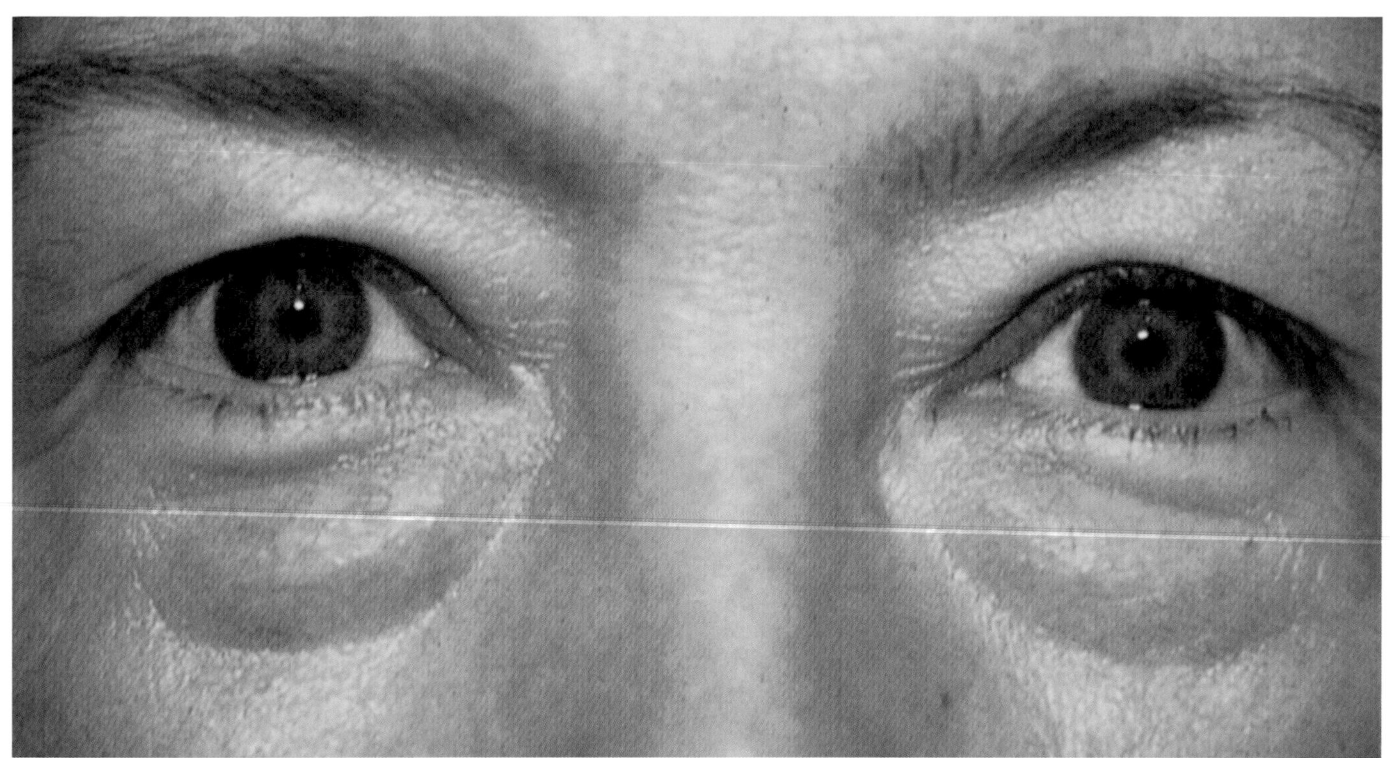

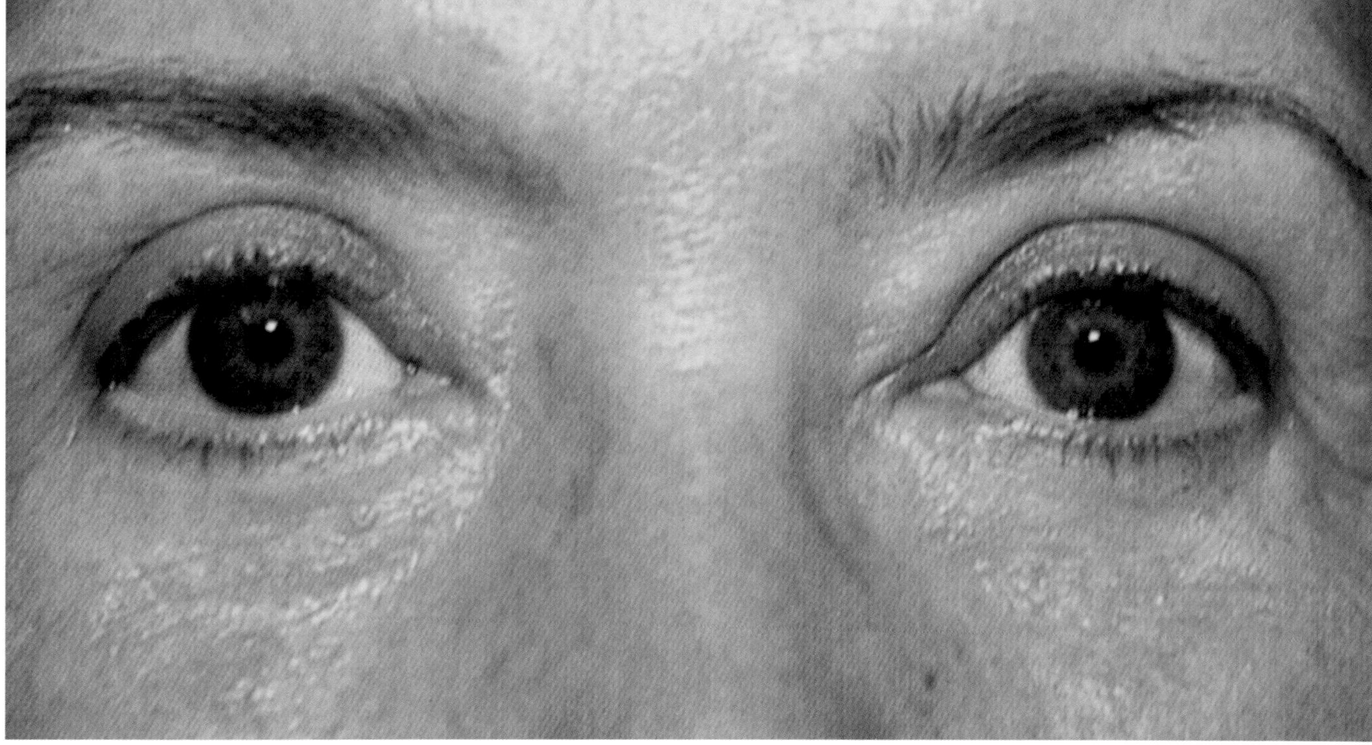

fig. 33 a+b

fig. 32 a+b & 33 a+b

The photos on the left show an upper eyelid correction, the photos on the right a lower eyelid correction. The upper eyelid correction, which removes so-called festoons, is a quick surgical procedure that achieves an effective and long-lasting change. After the excess skin is carefully excised, previously having been outlined on the skin surface, the eye looks much more "awake." Even greater care needs to be exercised with lower eyelid corrections (lachrymal sac operations) so that the eyelid will not droop after the procedure. A tiny incision is made exactly along the border of the eyelash line and the problematic excess tissue is removed – this tissue is filled with lymph and needs to be excised completely to achieve a satisfactory result. After the fatty tissue is removed, the excess skin is carefully shortened so that the lid is not wrinkled. Both treatments are outpatient procedures that only require a local anaesthetic – per eye, the operation usually only takes around 15 minutes. After a week, the swellings recede. The changes should be effective for several years. © Bodenseeklinik Prof. Mang

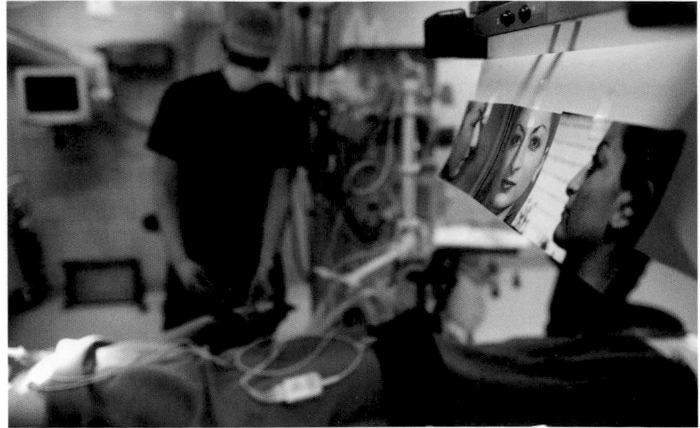

fig. 34

fig. 34

Rhinoplasties (nose operations) should not be performed on women under the age of 16 or men under the age of 19 – the nose is still growing.
© laif

Nose

Rhinoplasty is the medical term for a "nose job." In contrast to the ears, which are already quite close to their final size by the time a person has reached the age of five, the nose only begins to grow significantly at the age of 13 or 14. Girls' noses stop growing around the age of 16, boys' noses around 19. An operation should never be considered before the natural growth spurt has ended.

Rhinoplasties are among the most popular but also the most challenging operations. Basically, the nose can be reduced, augmented, widened, narrowed, straightened and reshaped by correcting the bones and the cartilage. Similarly, different parts of the nose, tip of the nose and nostrils can be altered with surgical and minimally invasive procedures, as can the angles between the brow and the root of the nose and between the upper lip and the tip of the nose. In any case, the procedure is highly demanding of the surgeon's technical skills, and extensive practical experience is needed if a follow-up procedure is to be avoided. Before the operation, the surgeon analyses all parts of the nose and their proportions to each other and the other facial features. A nose operation, after all, has to fulfil aesthetic as well as functional criteria.

Geometrically, the ideal shape of the nose supposedly has a 110-degree-angle between the nose and the lips and a 35-degree-angle between the nose and the face. However, a beautiful nose depends just as much on its proportions to the face, the head and the body. As part of the preoperative consultations, medical professionals often use a portrait photo to produce a computer-simulated mock-up featuring the desired nose. Alternatively, they may project a profile view of the patient's head onto the wall and draw in the modifications, or draw them directly onto an X-ray print of the patient's nose and jaw. In addition, the doctor needs to test if the nasal mucous membrane and the breathing function are fully intact.

Most operations last for one or two hours; the patient is fully sedated. Tiny incisions are made in the mucous membrane directly behind the nostrils, avoiding any visible scars. The surgeon inserts his tools through these — a miniature hammer, chisel and scalpel. He can then

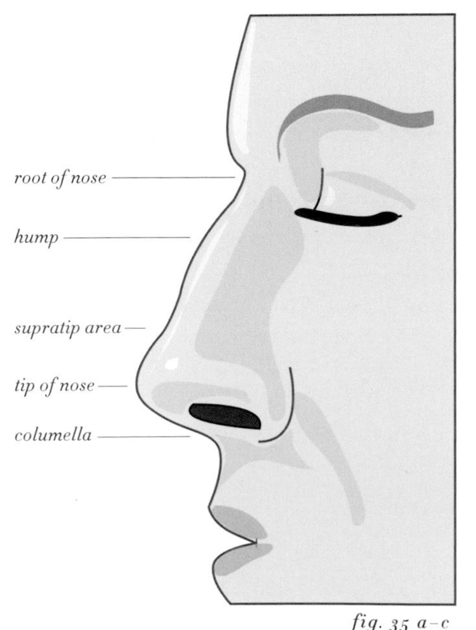

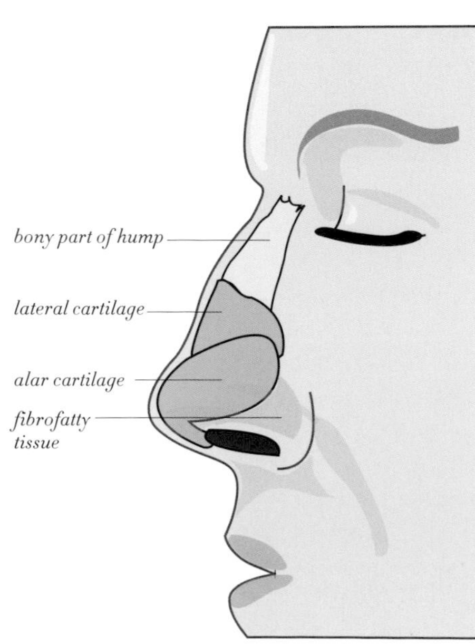

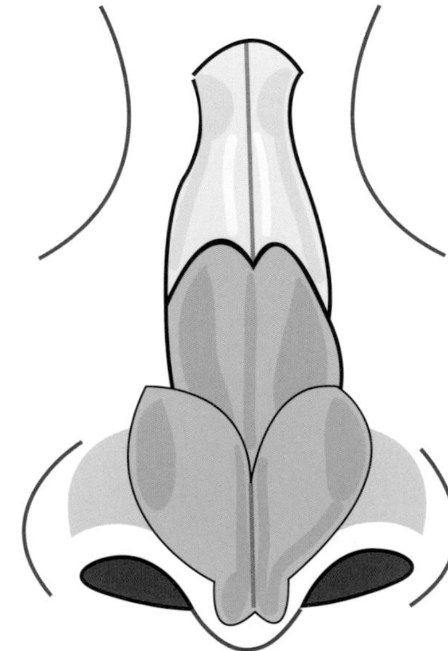

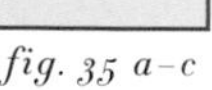

fig. 35 a–c

fig. 35 a–c

Anatomy of the nose. This area of the face purportedly looks best if the angle between the nose and lips is 110 degrees, and the angle between nose and face is 35 degrees. © Blue Brain Belgium

fig. 36 a–c

Many rhinoplasties are minimally invasive procedures. These photos show a nostril reduction, which only requires a few tiny incisions. © Blue Brain Belgium

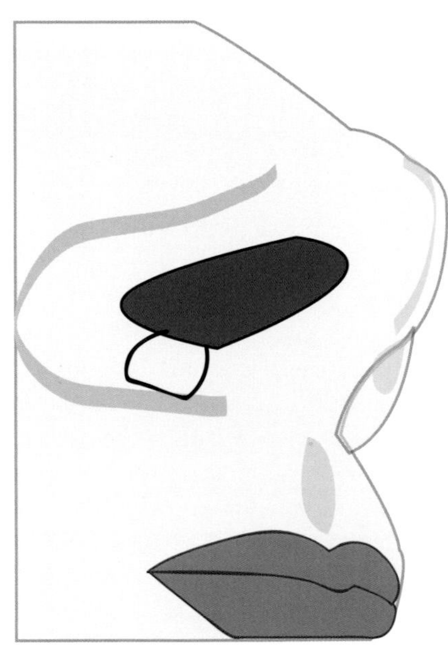

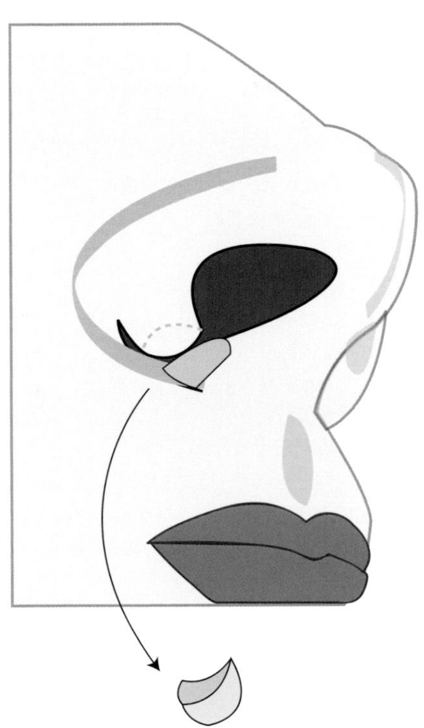

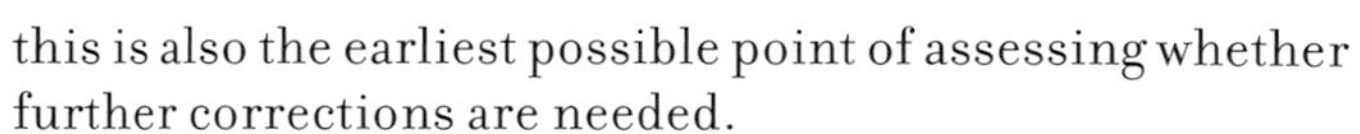

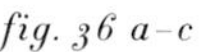

fig. 36 a–c

reduce nose bumps, correct unsightly nose tips or enlarge a saddle nose with bone and cartilage material. The skin naturally realigns to the new shape of the nose. After the incisions have been sutured, tamponades are placed in the nostrils for 24 hours to prevent seeping haemorrhages. An adhesive dressing is placed on the ridge of the nose to minimise and prevent haematomas and swellings. A plaster bandage is placed on top of the dressing, which in turn is protected by a plastic pressure pad. After 6–8 days, the doctor changes the dressing. Up to this point, the patient should move about as little as possible, not lie down or sleep with the head in a horizontal position, avoid talking and laughing, never rub or massage the nose, and only ingest liquid or soft food. For the first 14 days, kissing is not allowed, nor are hot baths. Hairdressers may initially only wash the hair with the head tilted to the back. Sports, sunbathing and heavy spectacle frames are not allowed for 6–8 weeks. The last swellings disappear no earlier than six months after the operation. After this point, the nose is as sturdy as it was originally. Unfortunately, this is also the earliest possible point of assessing whether further corrections are needed.

Risks: The operative risks are not to be underestimated! In the first two weeks after the operation, breathing difficulties may be experienced. Nosebleeds, dry mucous membranes, nasal fluid secretion, decreased sensitivity in the tip of the nose and in the upper lip are complications that usually disappear after some time. Bone or cartilage growths are extremely rare, as are injuries to the tear duct, skull or nasal septum. Delicate skin, incidentally, makes the operation more difficult.

Hospital stay: One day.
Fit for work: After one to two weeks.

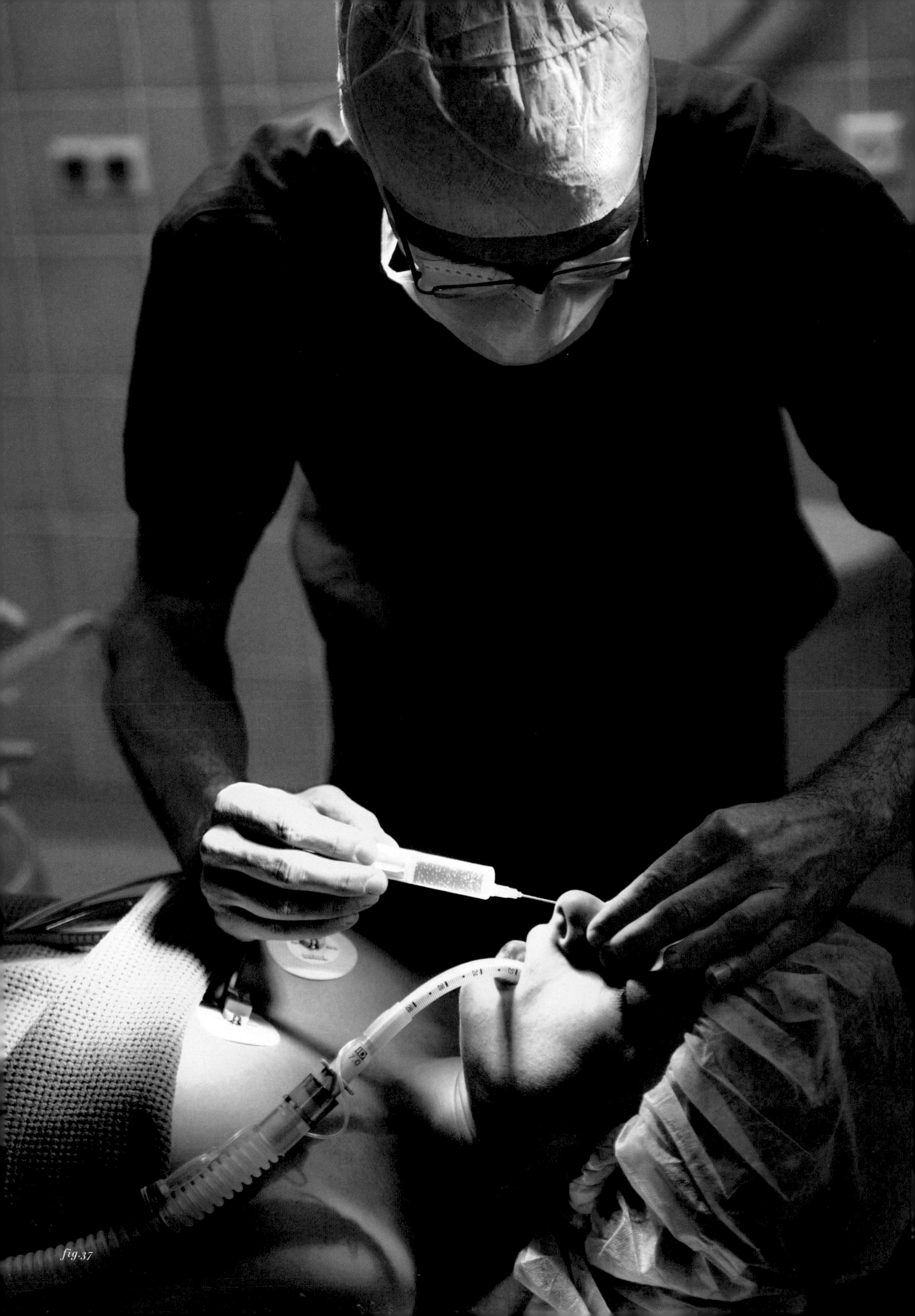

fig.37

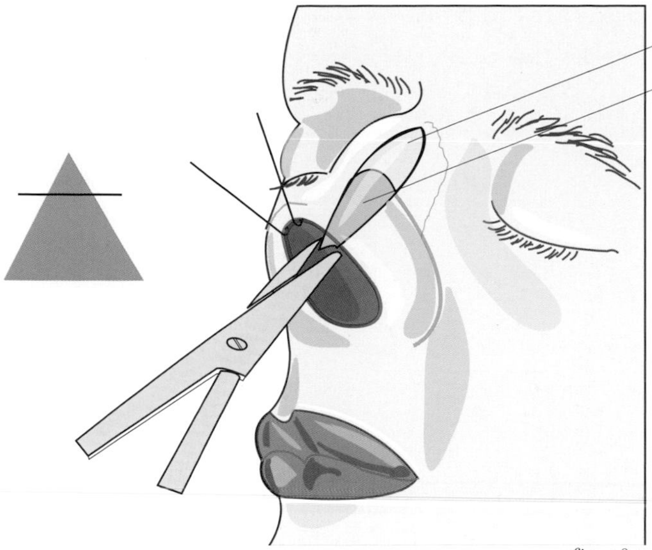

bone

cartilage

fig. 38 a

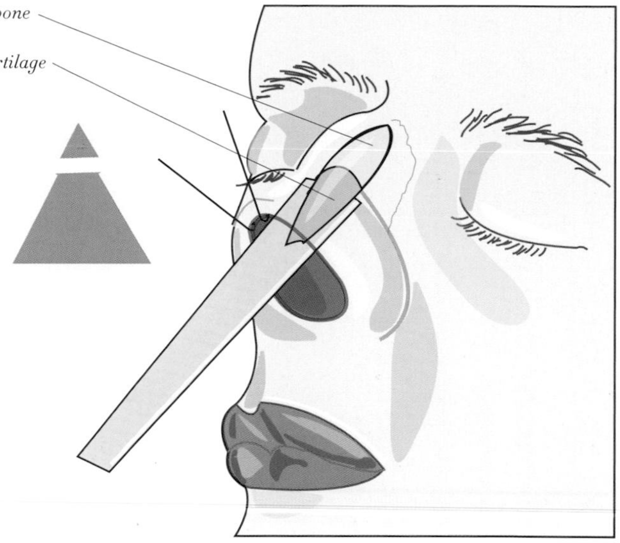

fig. 38 b

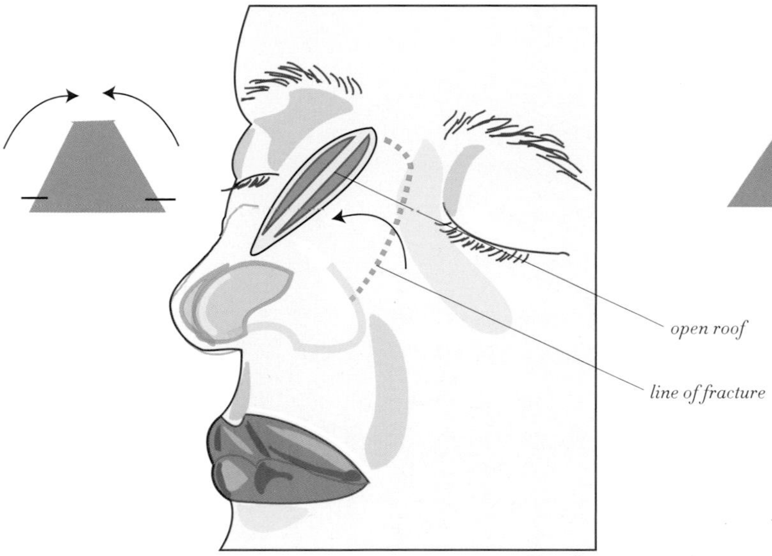

open roof

line of fracture

fig. 38 c

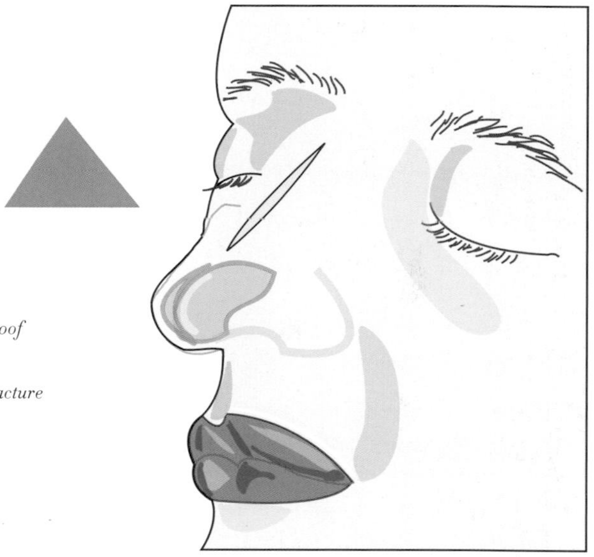

fig. 38 d

fig. 37

Most rhinoplasties take 1–2 hours and require a general anaesthetic. © laif

fig. 38 a–d

Drawings of a hump nose correction where cartilage and bone is shaved off. The surgeon inserts all implements through the nostrils so there are no visible scars. © Blue Brain Belgium

fig. 39

Among plastic surgeons, rhinoplasties are known as extremely difficult procedures, as they require great technical skill as well as aesthetic sensibilities – every nose needs to be sculpted differently. © laif

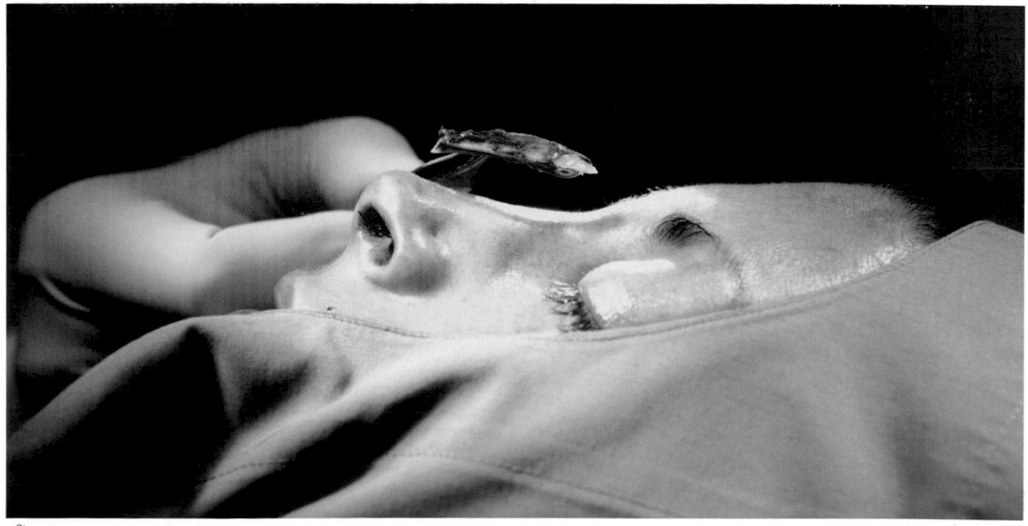

fig. 39

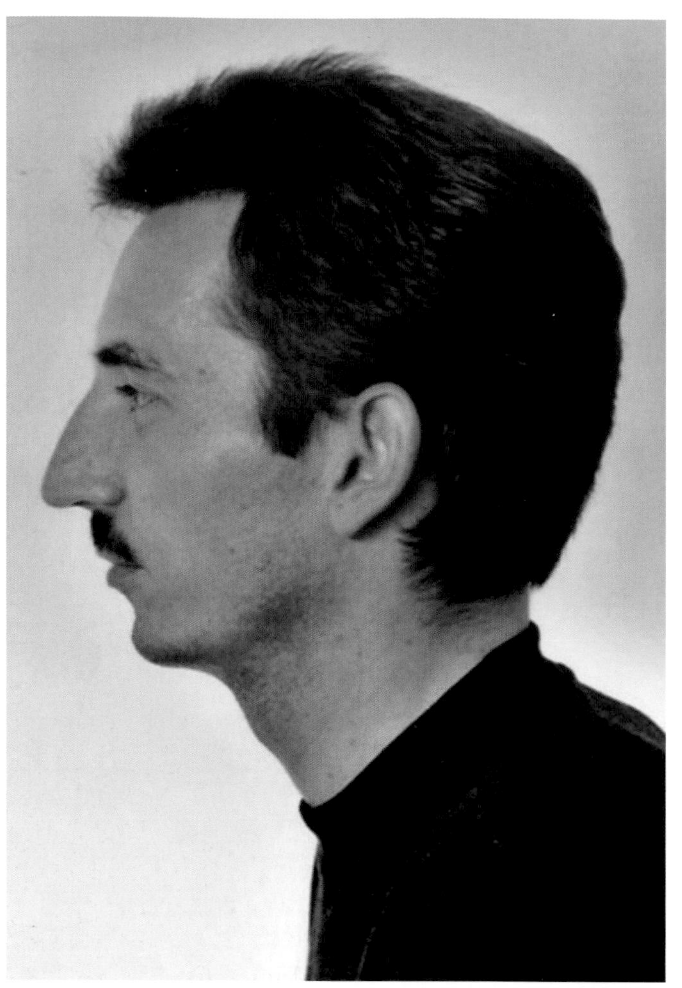

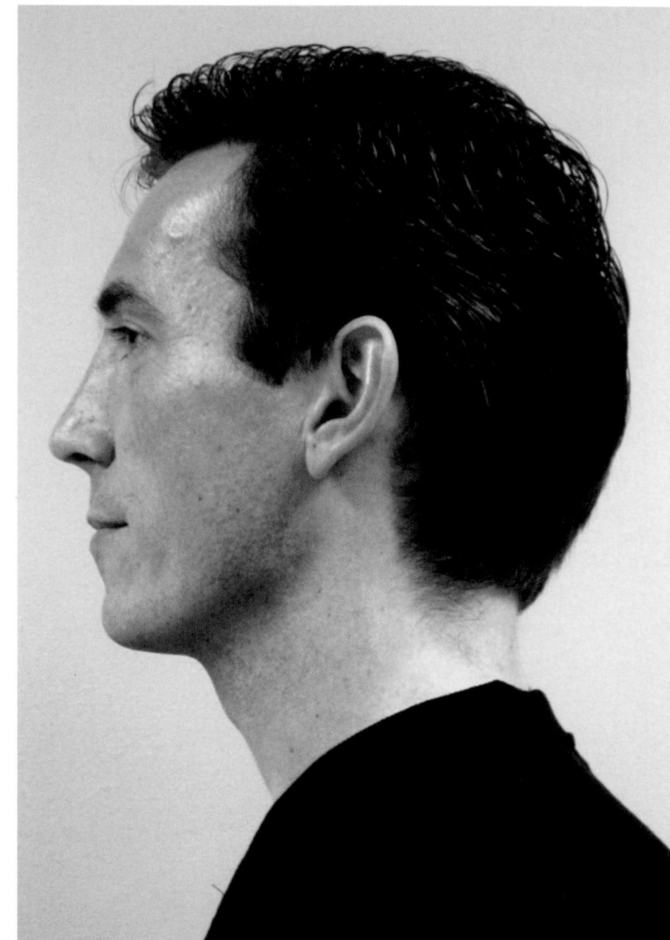

fig. 40 a+b

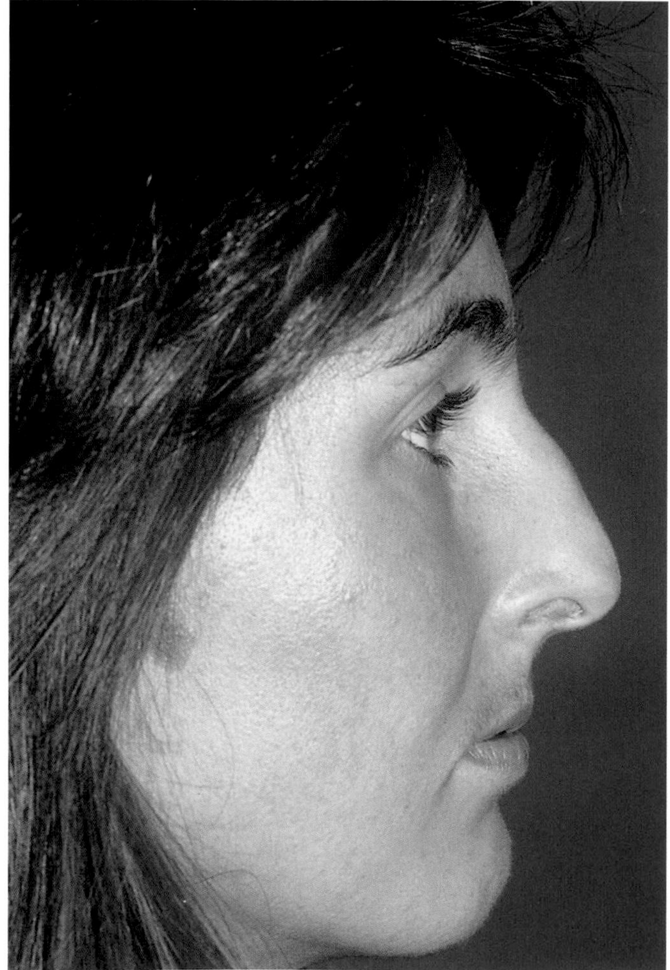

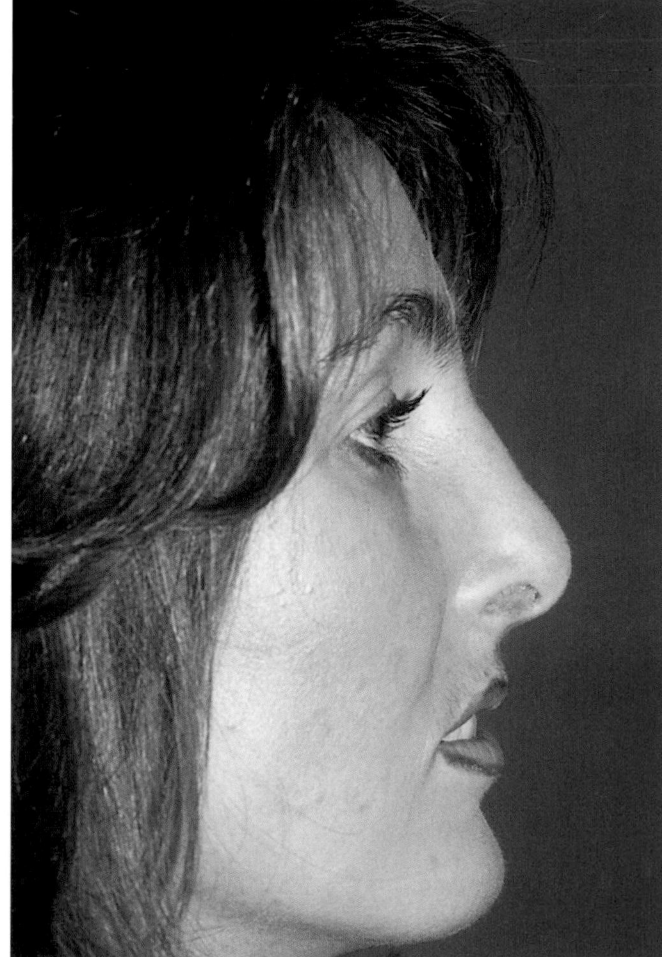

fig. 41 a+b

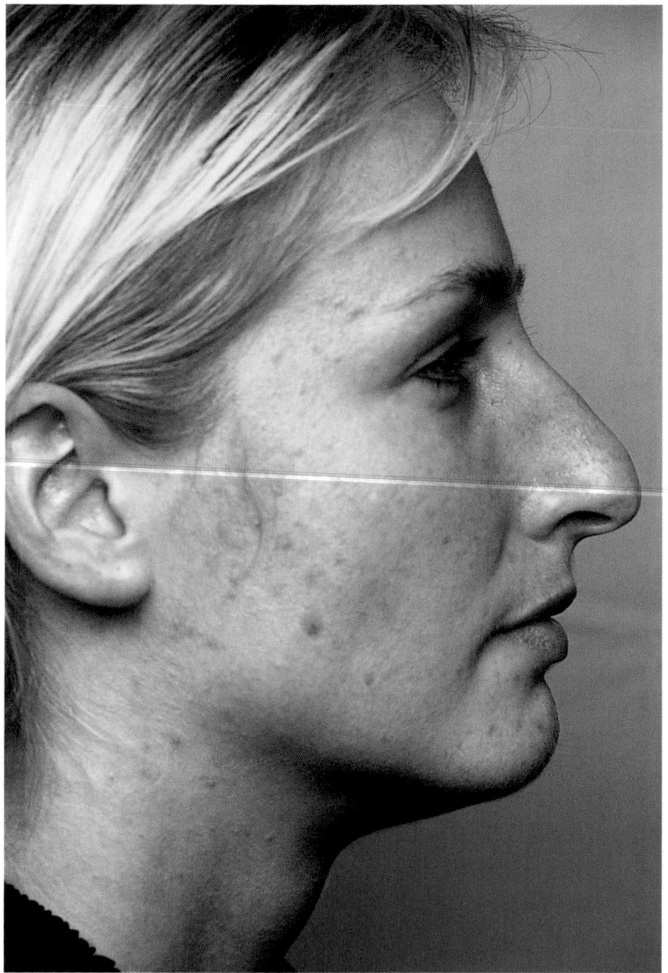

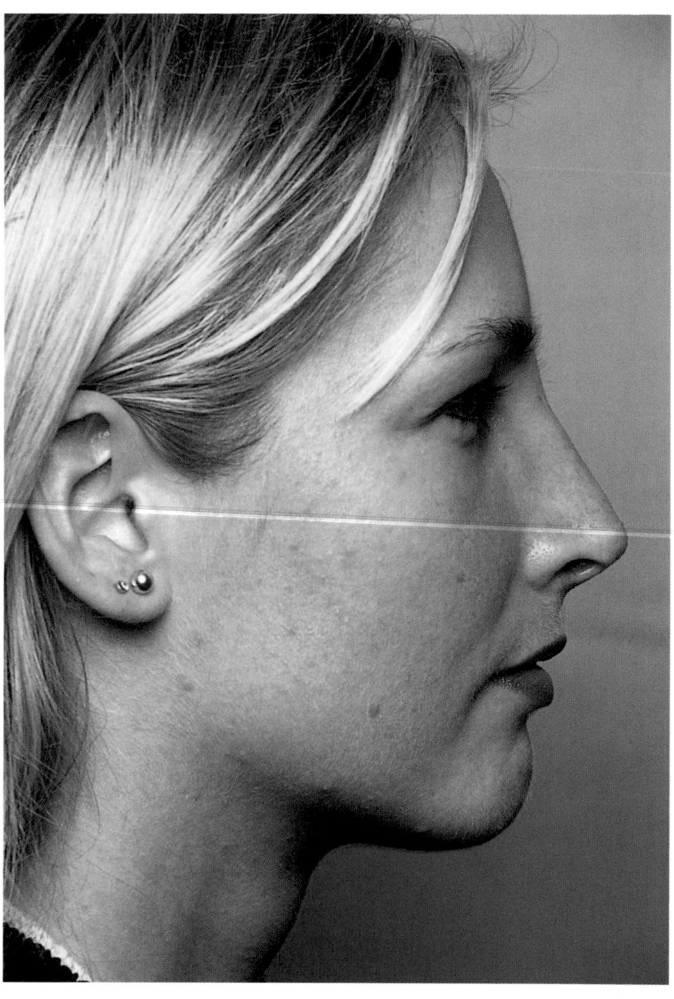

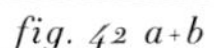

fig. 42 a+b

fig. 40 a+b to 42 a+b

The photos depict three different persons, one man and two women. Rhinoplasties are frequently combined with chin and/or cheek contouring procedures. In case of the man, a profileplasty was also performed – since the operation, he claims to have attained a new quality of life. Most commonly, however, rhinoplasties are performed to correct long hump noses for women. The goal is to make the facial features look more harmonious with each other. The women typically claim that their pronounced noses make them appear too masculine, and after the operation they usually feel much more feminine. Prof. Mang has operated on more than 10,000 noses and developed his own surgical technique. The nose is resculpted endoscopically, i.e. without incisions on the skin surface. Mang's approach aims to harmonise the entire face, and the angle between the nose and the upper lip is ideally centred around 110 degrees. © Bodenseeklinik Prof. Mang

fig. 43 a–c

Examples of unshapely noses: hump nose (left, centre) and a pronounced nose tip (right). © Blue Brain Belgium

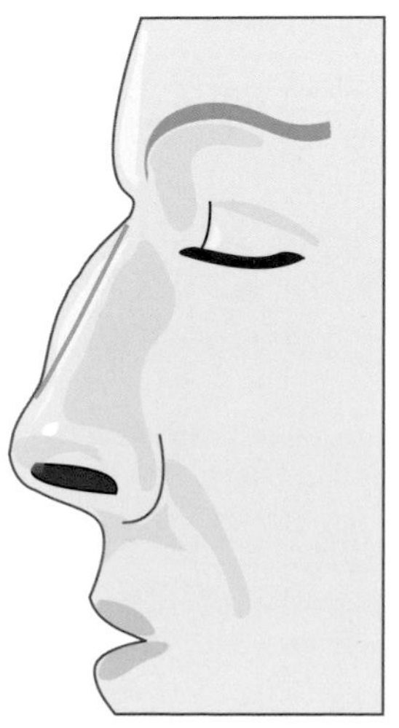

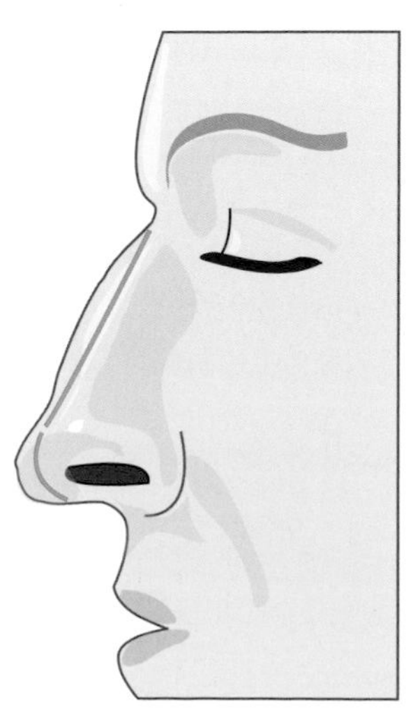

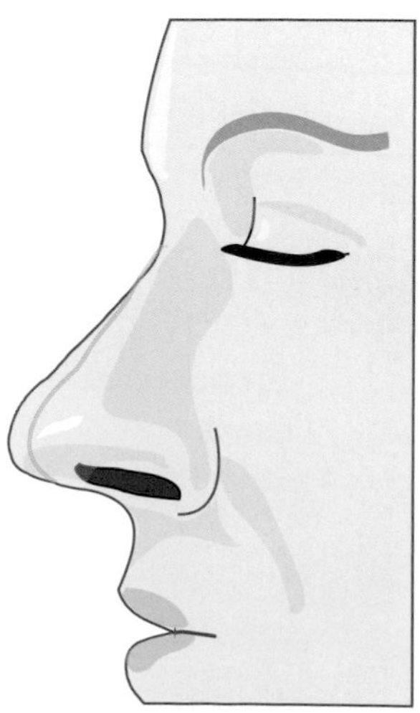

fig. 43 a–c

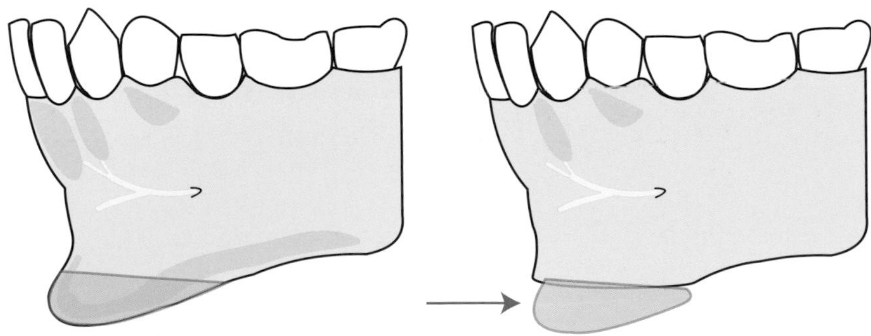

fig. 44 a+b

fig. 44 a+b

In a chin reduction, the protruding bone is filed down or shortened. The incision into the skin can be made from the inside or the outside. © Blue Brain Belgium

fig. 45 a+b

If the chin is too small or if it is receding, it can be augmented with a hard implant (silicone etc.). Alternatively, bone or cartilage fragments can be transplanted. © Blue Brain Belgium

fig. 46 a–c

When an ear is pinned back, the incision is usually made on the back of the ear. The cartilage is then thinned and resculpted. Procedures like these can also be performed on children, as the ear reaches its final size very early in life. © Blue Brain Belgium

fig. 47 a+b

Pinning an ear back requires highly sterile surgical conditions, as the cartilage will deform when inflamed. The procedure can be performed for patients six years of age or older. The cartilage is taken out and resculpted so that it cannot shift at any later point. Ears are perceived to look ideal at an angle of 30 degrees. © Bodenseeklinik Prof. Mang

Genioplasty / chin corrections

A protruding or receding chin is often corrected in conjunction with a rhinoplasty.

Chin augmentation: A receding or diminutive chin is frequently augmented using a pre-modelled implant, e. g. made of silicone. Alternatively, if the operation is performed alongside another correction such as a rhinoplasty, the cartilage removed can be used to augment the chin. Bones from the pelvis or the skullcap and cartilage from the ears or the ribs are also suitable materials. These heal very well, but the aesthetic success isn't as high as with synthetic materials or artificial bone (hydroxyapatite).
For the operation, a general anaesthetic is usually employed. To avoid visible scars, a 2–4 centimetre incision is made on the inside of the lower lip. The implant is inserted through this opening and attached to the existing bone using sutures – or screws, if it is a cartilage implant. The advantages of having an external incision, on the other hand, are lower risks of infection and implant rejection.

Chin reduction: The bone is filed down or shortened. The inside wound is closed with a dissolving suture; if an external incision is used, the stitches are removed after a week.

Risks: Swellings, pain and numbness disappear after around three weeks.
Risks of infection, allergic reaction or of the implant slipping are comparatively low.

Hospital stay: One to three days.
Fit for work: After one week.

Osteotomy: In this complex procedure, the surgeon shifts the chin bone forward and sets it in place using metal plates and screws. These are removed after 6–12 months. The healing period is lengthy, but aesthetically, this method has the most convincing results.

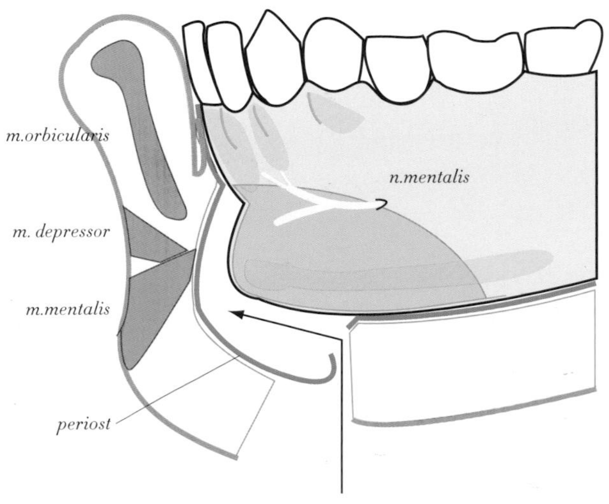

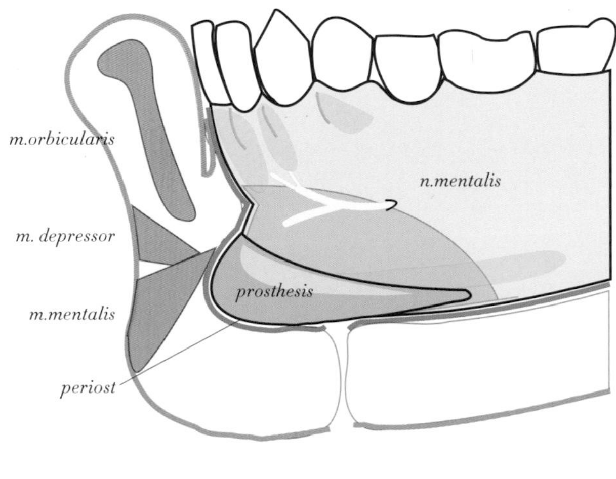

fig. 45 a+b

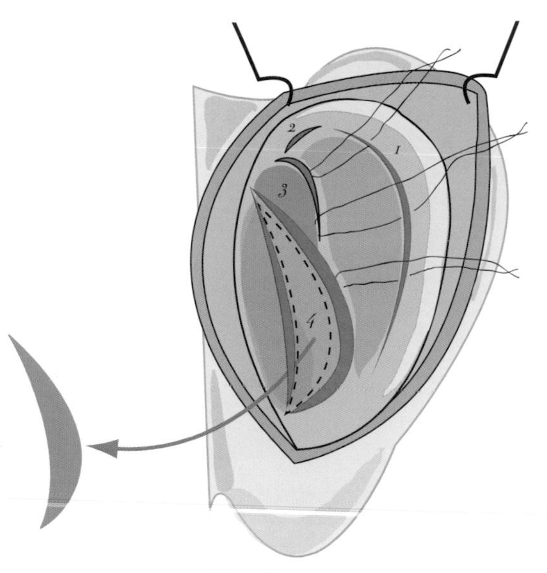

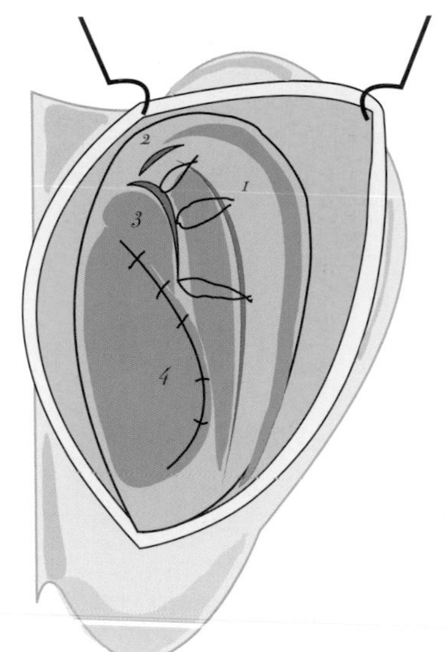

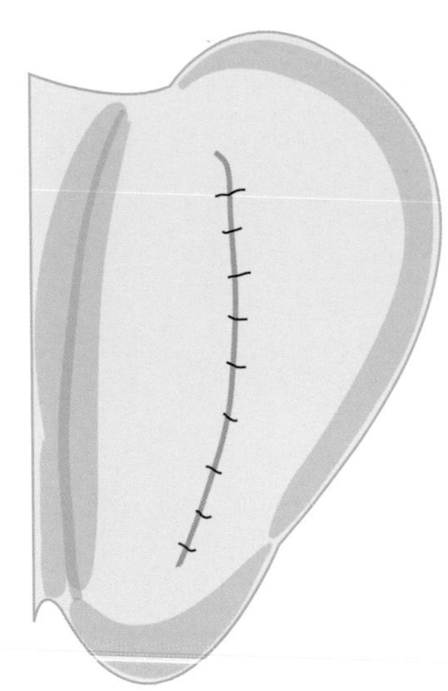

fig. 46 a–c

Ears

Ear correction or *otoplasty*: This is the only aesthetic procedure regularly performed on children (aged six to 14), as the ear of a four-year-old has already reached eighty percent of its final size. In most cases, the ears are either reduced (e.g. for elderly patients whose ears have grown disproportionately large), remodelled if asymmetrical or pinned back if they protrude noticeably. 90 percent of all ears are corrected because of this latter symptom. The surgical cut is made on the back of the ear or on the inside of the concha; the cartilage is shortened with a file or diamond fraise and then remodelled. Finally, the cartilage is fastened in its new position with three or four sutures. After the procedure, the ears need to be protected with a dressing and a bandage. After approx. ten days, the stitches and the bandage are removed. Minor swellings and heightened sensitivity may be experienced for approx. one month. After one further month, the ear has fully adjusted to its new shape.

Risks: Very rarely, the blood flow may be impaired after the procedure. If there are scarring complications, a further operation may be required.

Hospital stay: One day maximum.
Fit for work/school: After two to four days.

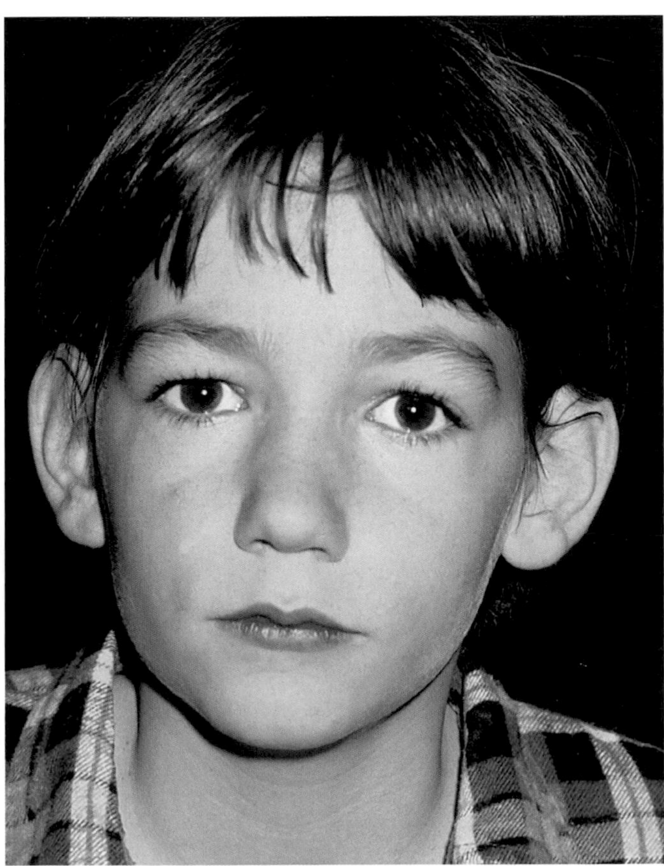
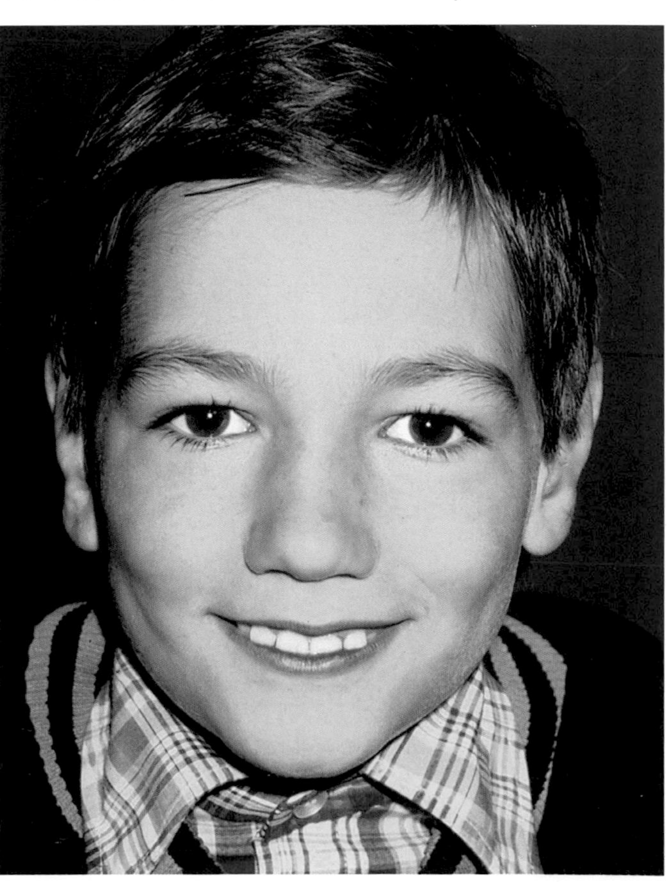

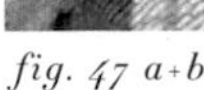
fig. 47 a+b

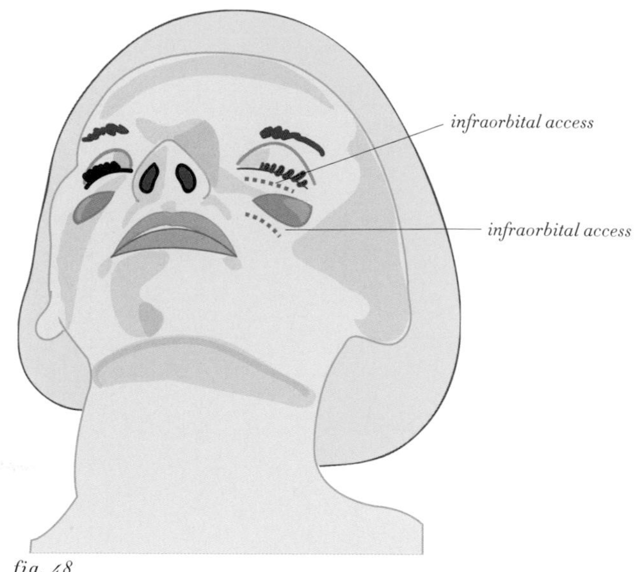

fig. 48

fig. 48

For the cheekbones to appear raised, the zygomatic arch can be corrected, e. g. with a silicone implant. © Blue Brain Belgium

fig. 49 a+b

The face can also be changed by injecting vital fat cells into the zygomatic region and the cheek/chin area. This not only rejuvenates the face but also emphasises the facial features. The same clinical effect can be achieved with the injection of newer generation fillers, a procedure which takes 5 minutes, requires no anaesthesia and has virtually no downtime. © Dr. Woffles Wu

fig. 50 a+b

Men in particular suffer from hair loss. They can opt for autologous hair transplants – with the micrografting technique shown here, the surgeon transplants tiny strips of skin containing hair follicles into the subcutaneous tissue. © laif

fig. 51

During the first stage of the operation, the surgeon harvests a skin section containing donor hair – e. g. from the back of the patient's head – and slices it into thin strips. The strips, each containing 1–4 hair follicles, are then transplanted onto the bald spots. These implants are called micrografts. *© Blue Brain Belgium*

Cheeks

Correction of the zygomatic arch: A procedure that is usually carried out to produce higher cheekbones. To achieve this effect, the surgeon implants autologous material or a silicone pad. The operation requires local or general anaesthesia. The surgical cut is made either on the inside, i. e. from the lip fold above the upper teeth, or below the lower eyelid on the outside. To create space for the implant, the skin and the subcutaneous tissue are detached from the bone temporarily, and sown on again after the implant has been placed. Very rarely, the opposite result is desired – a reduction of an over-sized zygomatic bone. In this case, the bone is shortened surgically and filed down for added roundness. Cheekbone operations are predominantly performed on Asian patients. In Europe, it is more common for the rim of the eye socket to be augmented or reduced, respectively by screw-mounting a prosthesis or by filing down the bone.

Swellings or haematomas may occur for one or two weeks. Visible sutures are removed after five days, sutures on the inside of the mouth are self-dissolving.

Risks: In some instances, the implant may shift.

Hospital stay: Outpatient.
Fit for work: After one week.

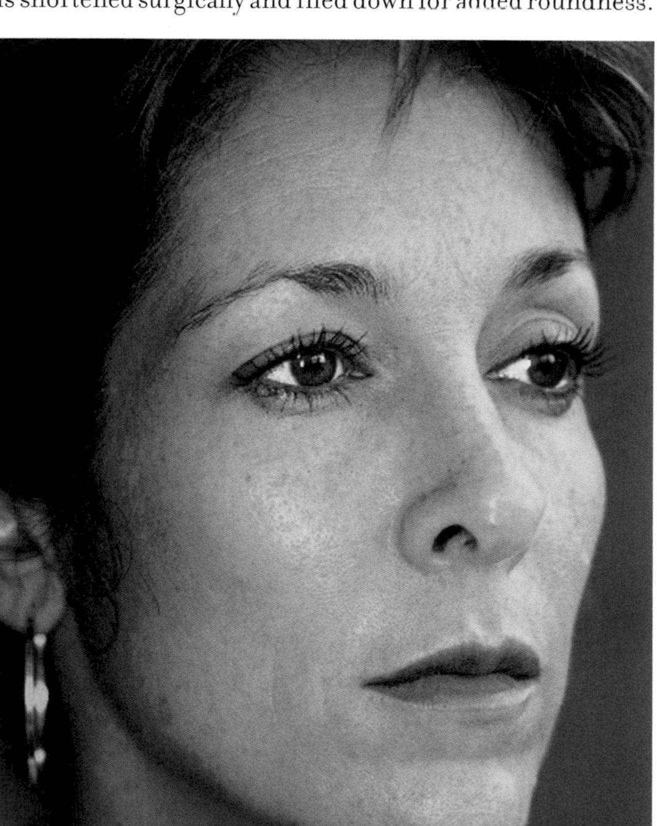

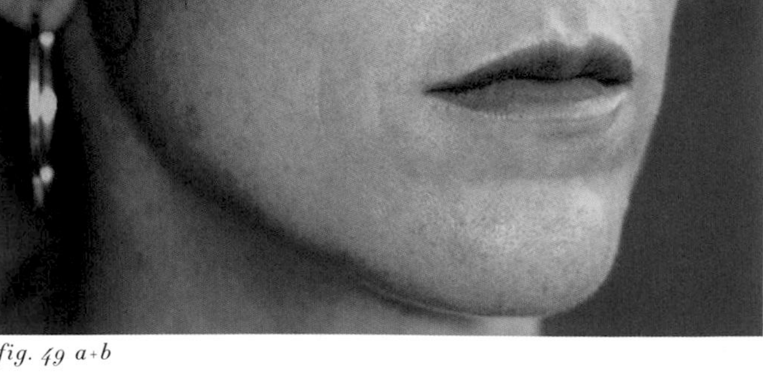

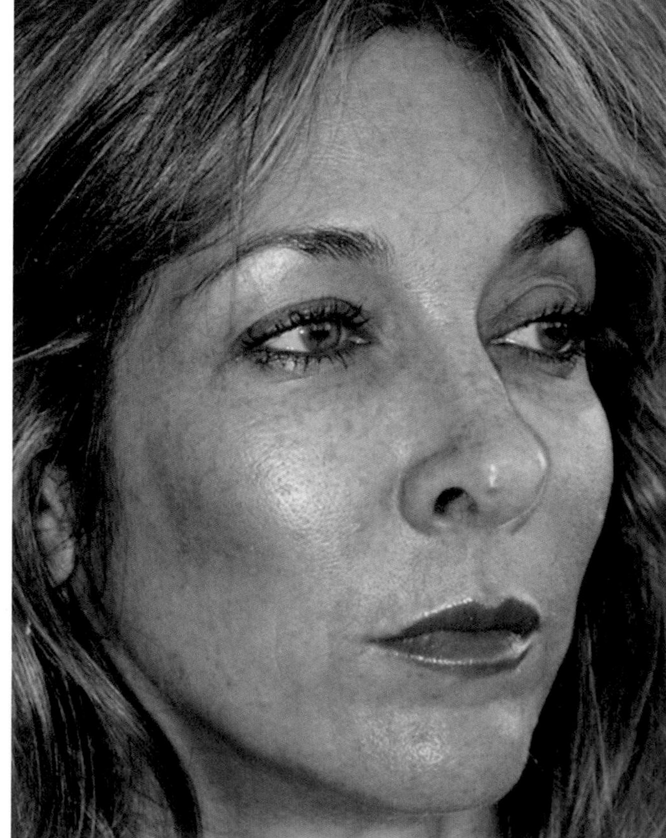

fig. 49 a+b

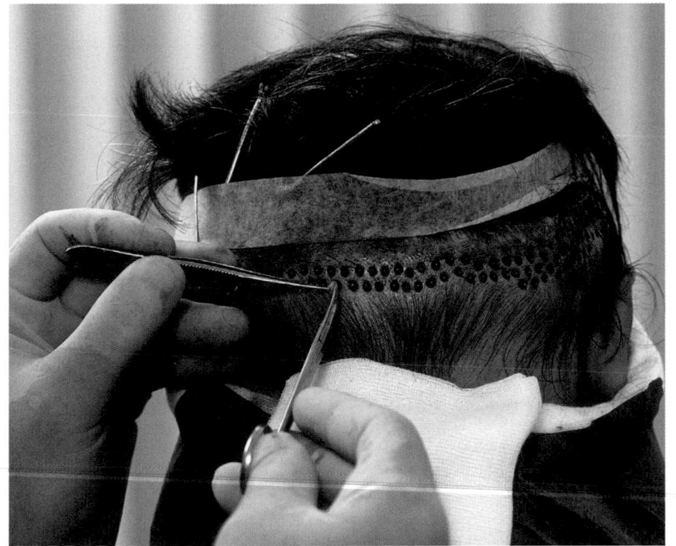

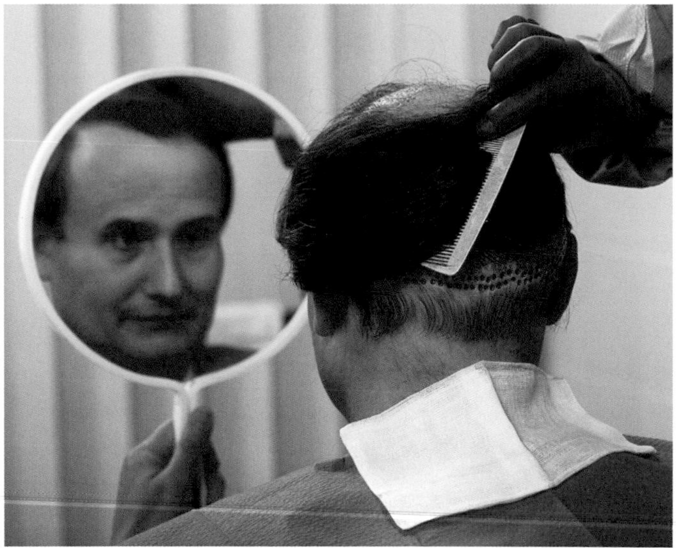

fig. 50 a+b

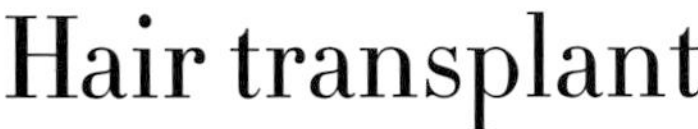

Hair transplant

Hair loss and *baldness* are age-related problems predominantly encountered by men. If products such as *Rogaine* (*Minoxidil*) or *Finasteride* don't work, hair replacement may be a feasible option.

Receding hairlines and bald spots can be repopulated with hair using so-called micro-hair transplants. The surgeon uses the patient's own side and neck hairs, as these remain largely unaffected by hormone-induced hair loss. Firstly, a suitable skin strip of donor hair, approx. 10–12 centimetres long and 2–5 centimetres wide, is selected and shaved. A local anaesthetic is administered; this is mixed with adrenalin to minimise bleeding. The selected strip of skin is cut out with a scalpel and the wound is closed with sutures. Next, the transplant is sliced into narrow strips – *micrografts*, each containing 2–5 hair follicles to be added to the brow hairline or top/back of the head.

During the actual transplantation, the micrografts are embedded in the subcutaneous tissue with a pincer, after the tissue has been punctured with a laser or scalpel. It is crucial that the implants face in the right direction, as otherwise the hair will grow at random angles and look artificial.

This method can be used to transplant thousands of hairs; the body's autologous fibrin secures them in their new locations. To minimise bleeding as much as possible, a compression bandage is usually applied at the end of a session. This is removed 48 hours later. The scabs that have formed around each transplanted hair follicle should never be scratched off! After 15–20 days, they fall out with many of the transplanted hairs, which then regrow.

For a few days after the operation, minor swellings may appear on the brow, and skin tension may be felt.

The biggest operative risk is that the transplanted follicles don't grow into the skin. Several operations are needed to achieve natural-looking hair. Be aware, however, that transplants are not designed to return normal hair growth to a bald head – the main objective is to disguise hair loss.

NOTE: Although micrografting is still regarded as a standard technique, the so-called *FUT* (Follicular Unit Transplantation) method is becoming increasingly popular. In this technique, naturally-occurring follicle groups are transplanted individually, each containing 1–4 hairs.

Tissue expansion is a lengthy, expensive and painful procedure mostly required by patients with severe burns or other injuries. The tissue is expanded so that the skin still containing hair can be used to cover as much of the head as possible. After the patient is given a local anaesthetic, silicone balloons are inserted underneath the undamaged skin. Over a period of three months, the balloons are injected with a saline solution once a week to inflate them. Like in pregnancy, the skin gradually stretches; unfortunately, the outline of the head also inflates very unnaturally. Sometimes, the balloon shapes may be seen through the skin, which progressively thins out. There is also a heightened risk of infection. During this time, the patient should not be working or frequenting public places.
A local anaesthetic is again administered before the balloons are removed. The bald skin is excised and replaced by the stretched skin still containing hair. In this procedure, it is of decisive importance to maintain the blood flow supplying the stretched skin strips.

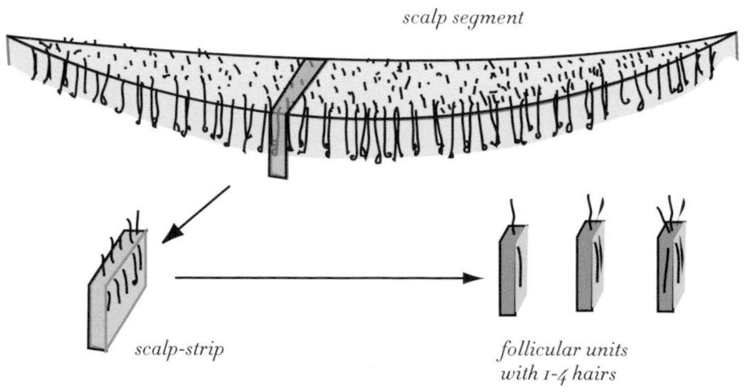

fig. 51

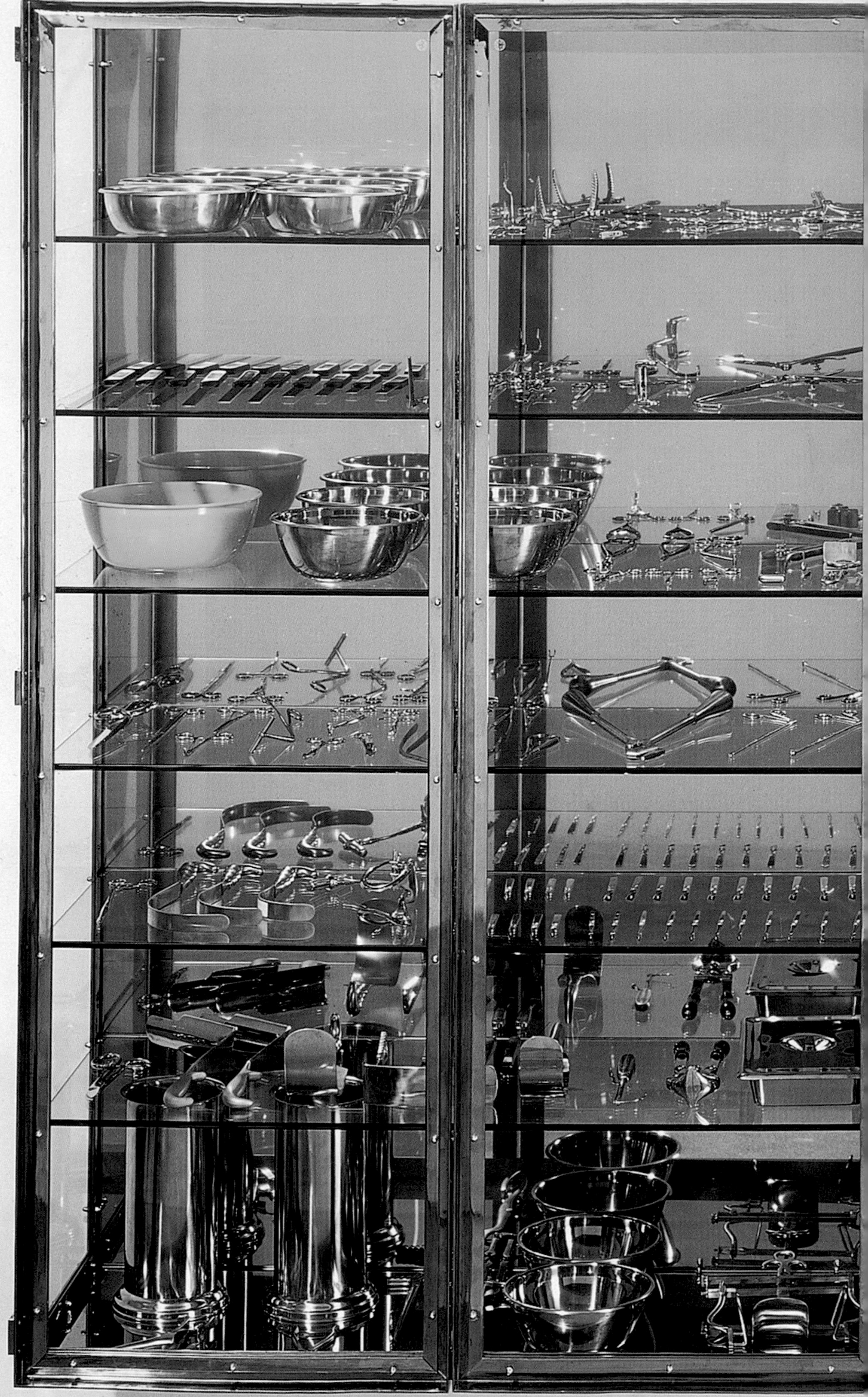

fig. 52

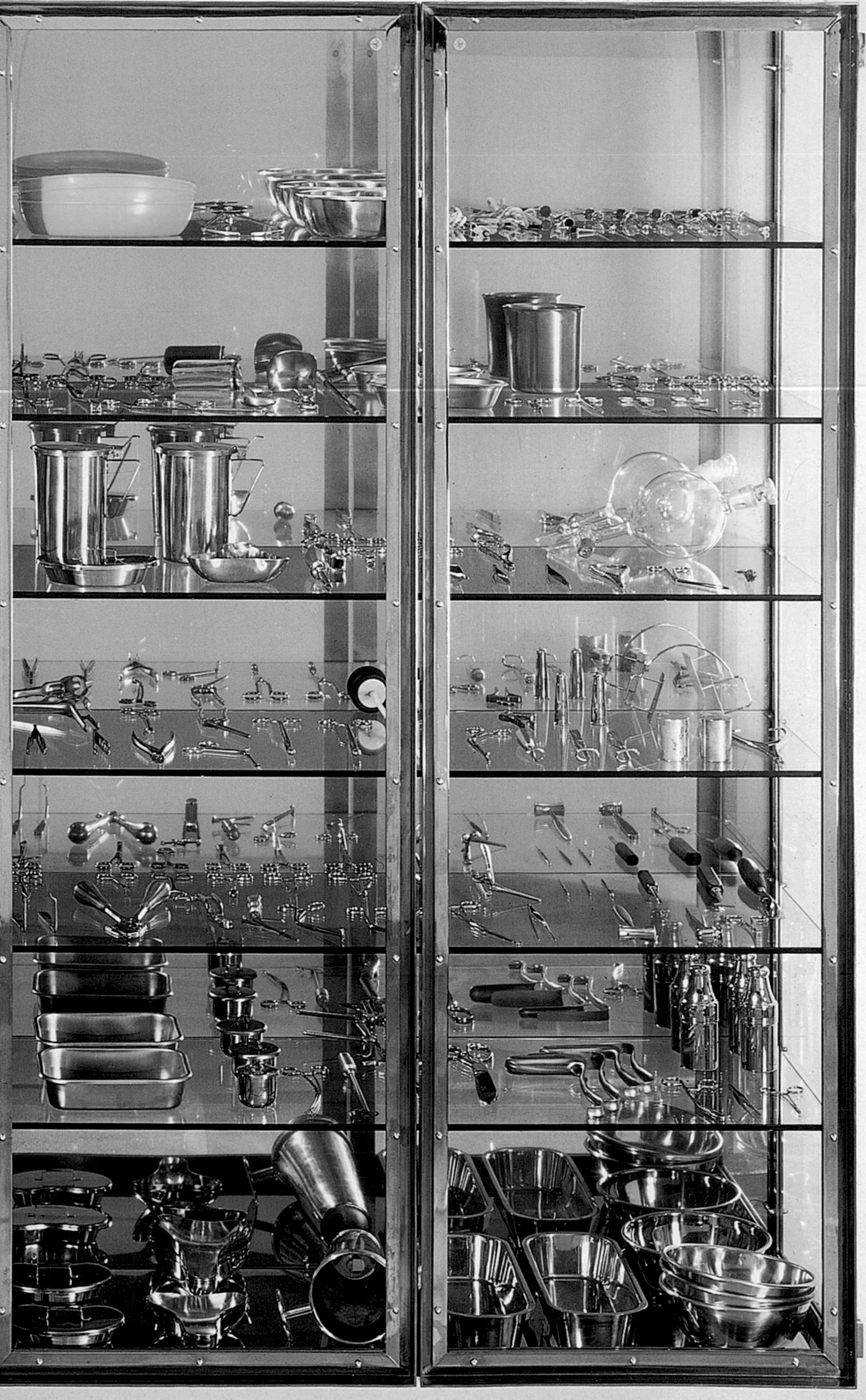

fig. 52

Damien Hirst (U.K.): Still, 1994. Glass, stainless steel, surgical equipment 196 x 251 x 51 cm © The artist Courtesy Jay Jopling/White Cube, London. Photo: Stephen White

fig. 53

For breast operations, the surgical incision can be made in the armpit or around the nipple – most commonly, however, it is made in the submammary fold, i. e. the fold below the breast. This technique also has the lowest risks. © Blue Brain Belgium

fig. 54 a+b

Breast enlargements always employ implants. The drawing on the left shows an inlay placed in front of the muscle; the drawing on the right shows an inlay placed behind the muscle. © Blue Brain Belgium

fig. 55 a+b

The Singapore-based cosmetic surgeon Woffles Wu has developed his own zigzag technique for breast augmentations. The Invisible WW Stealth Technique *produces hardly any discernible scars. © Private archive Dr. Woffles*

fig. 56

The most common complication associated with breast operations is capsular fibrosis, a painful thickening and hardening of the connective tissue around the implant. It is most effectively avoided by rinsing the operative site with a saline solution. © Blue Brain Belgium

fig. 57 a+b

The photo on the left shows a patient with pronounced capsular fibrosis after the inlay was placed on top of the muscle. The photo on the right shows the woman a year later and without any problems – the inlay has been repositioned underneath the muscle. Thanks to modern surgical techniques and recent implant developments, the risk of capsular fibrosis is less than five percent for gentle techniques. © Bodenseeklinik Prof. Mang

BODY CONTOURING
Breasts

Breast enlargement or *augmentation mammaplasty:* This procedure is always performed using *implants*. Without fail, the implants are made of a silicone shell, which can be filled with silicone gel, a physiological saline solution or hydrogel.

Most *implants* contain *silicone gel*, as this substance provides the best durability and malleability. The reputation of silicone gel has been fully restored – contrary to some claims, it has been proven not to cause rheumatism, and implants do not rupture at high altitudes. However, silicone does block X-rays, which is why breast cancer checks should always be done with nuclear magnetic resonance imaging (NRMI) instead of mammography.

Saline solution is filled into the implant during the operation – the amount of saline is adapted to the breast size. If the implant ruptures, the solution breaks down completely. However, saline implants do not feel as natural as silicone gel implants.

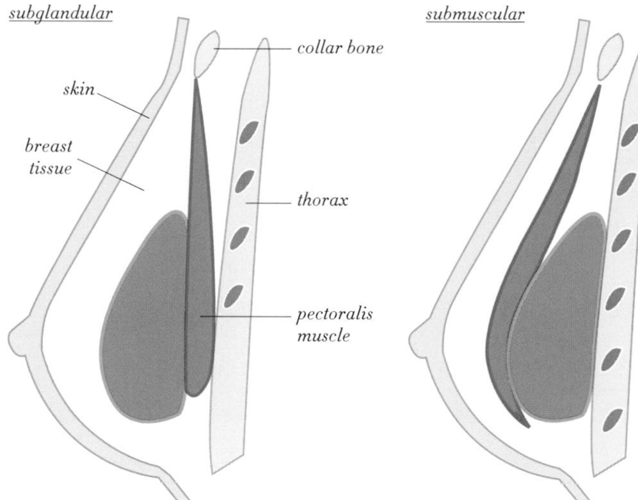

fig. 54 a+b

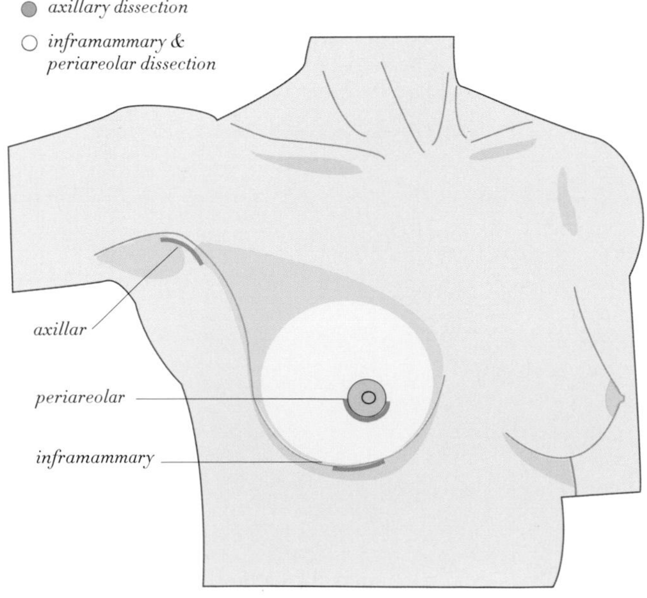

fig. 53

Hydrogel is a solution consisting of water and polysaccharides (sugars). The implants feel very natural, but tissue compatibility has not been proven as yet.

A roughened, texturised surface on the silicone shell is preferable to a smooth surface, as it will cause less capsular fibrosis. There are round, oval and drop-shaped implants. The latter correspond most to the natural female anatomy and also look natural in a horizontal position. Standard implant sizes range from 60 to 600 cubic centimetres. The most popular implant type is a silicone gel inlay with a size of 200 cubic centimetres.

The operation, which takes two to three hours, is carried out while the patient is fully anaesthetised or a "twilight" anaesthesia has been administered. An incision approx. four centimetres in length is made in the skin, usually either in the armpit (axilla), below the nipple (mammilla) or in the fold under the breast. The risks associated with an axillar point of entry are keloids (raised scarring) and

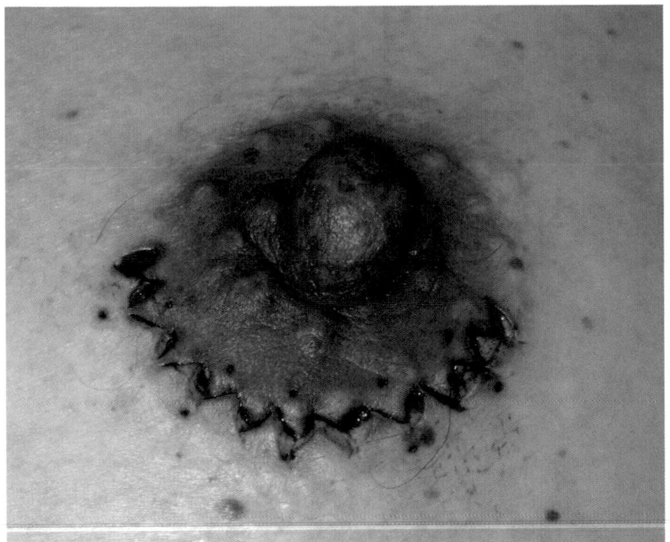

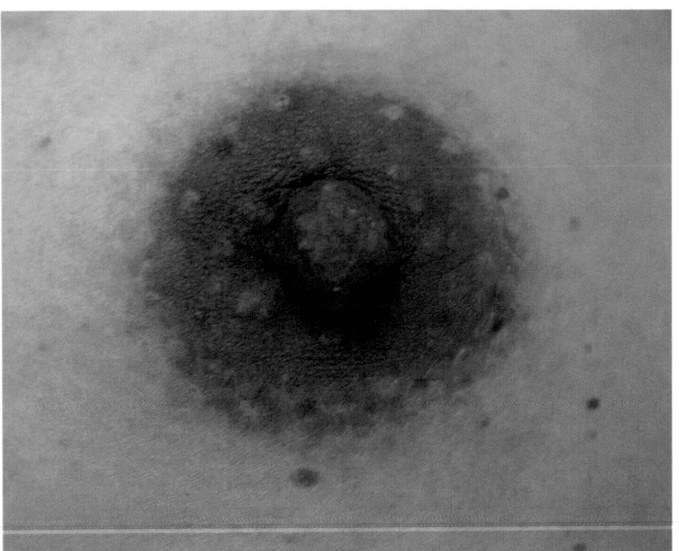

fig. 55 a+b

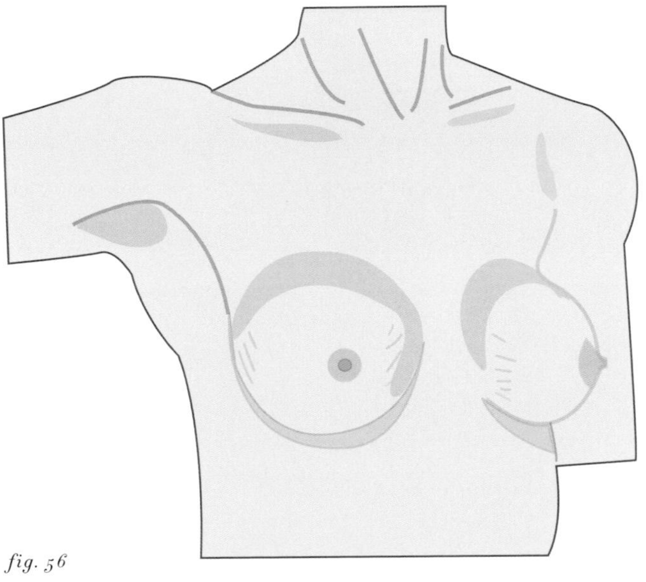

fig. 56

The cavity for the implant is prepared through the incision; the implant can be placed either behind the mammary gland (subglandular position) or behind the pectoral muscle (submuscular or subpectoral position). The latter is opted for by 80 percent of surgeons, despite a lengthier healing period – the muscle conceals the implant very well, and the result is very natural-looking. After the implant has been placed, the incisions are sutured and sealed with a sterilised dressing.

Risks: The most frequent risk is capsular fibrosis, the thickening and hardening of the connective tissue around the implant. This can be very painful. It occurs when there is stray blood in the implant cavity; this can cause exaggerated scarring. If the cavity is thoroughly rinsed with a saline solution, capsular fibrosis is unlikely. Other risks are stretch lines and circulatory difficulties. Furthermore, oversized implants an a subglandular position can have a visible outline. In the breasts of very thin women, inlays filled with saline can crease the skin. With all implants, there is a risk of asymmetry. In most cases, the only solution is to re-operate. Implants should be replaced after approx. 15 years.

inhibited haemostasis. If the incision is made at the nipple, a deflated inlay is implanted, and the inlay is filled once in place. The most common practice is to make the surgical cut in the submammary fold under the breast. The only disadvantage of this approach is that it leaves a hairline scar – which eventually becomes imperceptible.

Hospital stay: One to two days.
Fit for work: After one week.

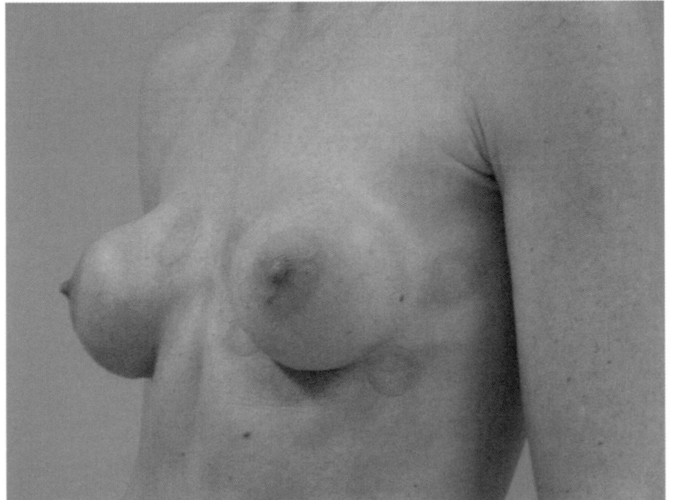

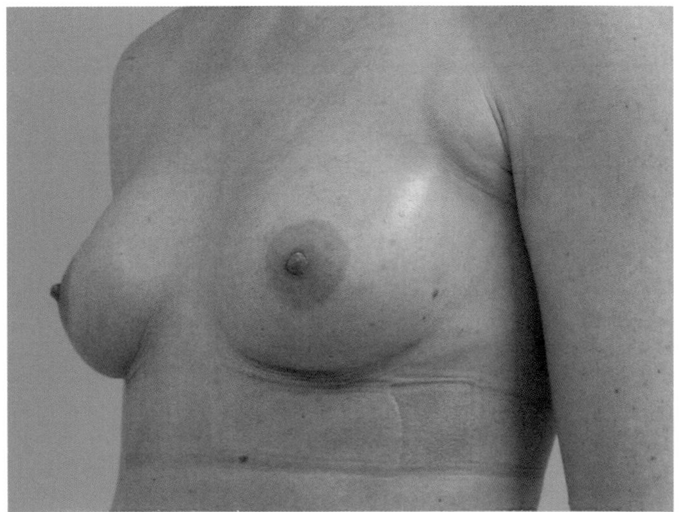

fig. 57 a+b

fig. 58 a–g

The different stages of breast augmentation surgery. Breast augmentation takes two to three hours and requires general anaesthesia. Today, implants are most commonly made of silicone gel; silicone inlays are very durable and are available in many different shapes and sizes. The only disadvantage is that the substance blocks X-rays – for breast cancer checks, women with silicone gel implants should therefore undergo nuclear magnetic resonance imaging (NRMI) instead of a mammography. © laif

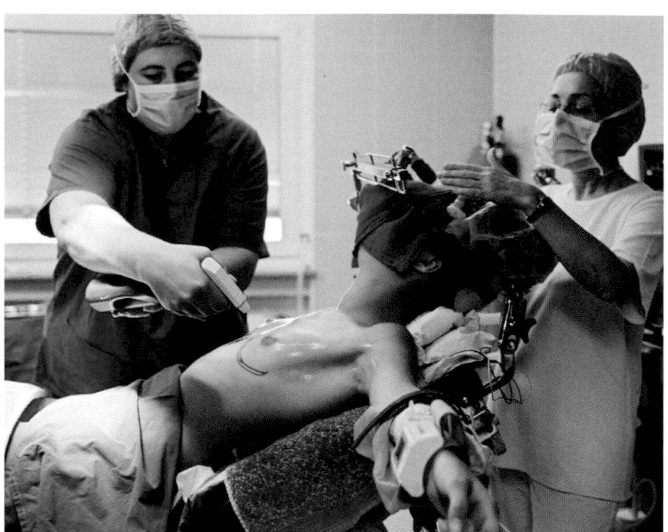

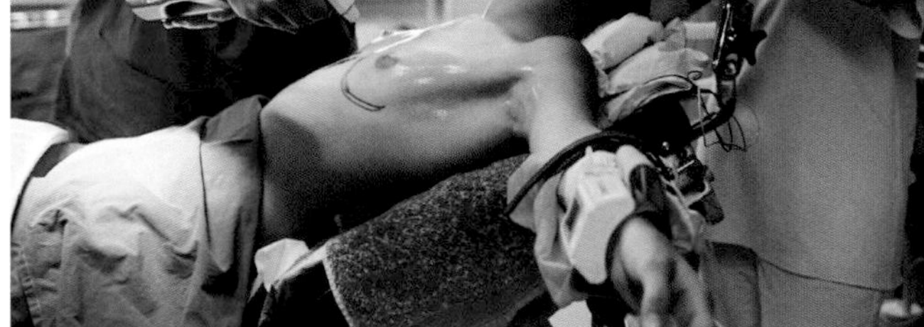

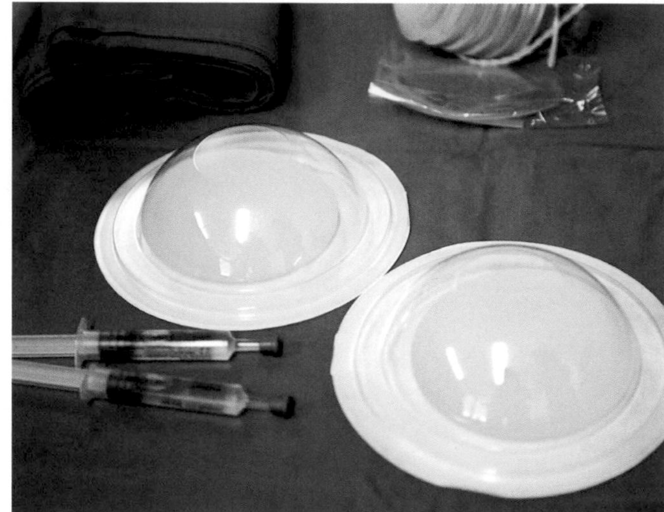

fig. 58 a+b

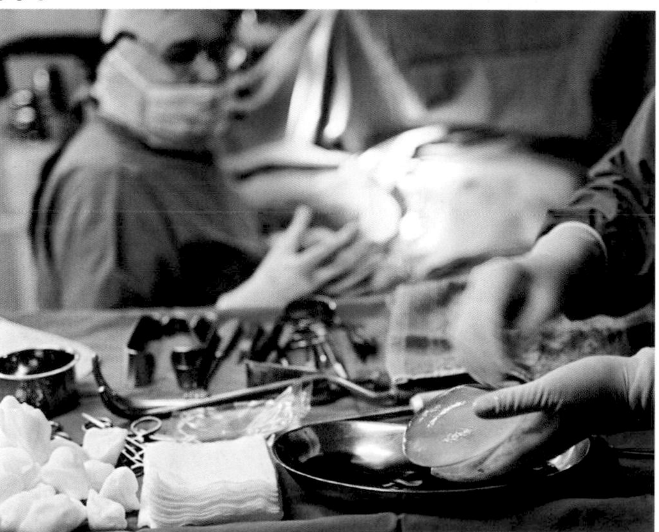

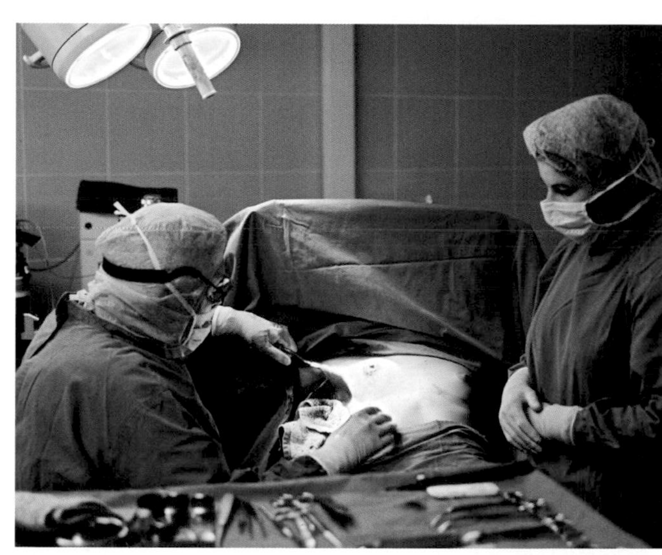

fig. 58 c+d

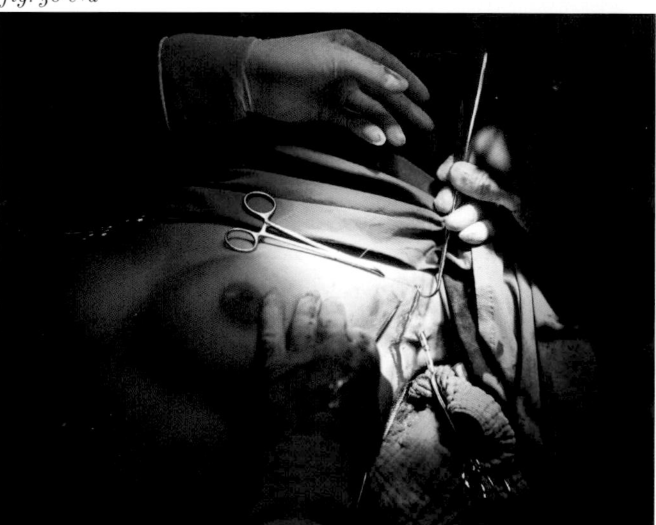

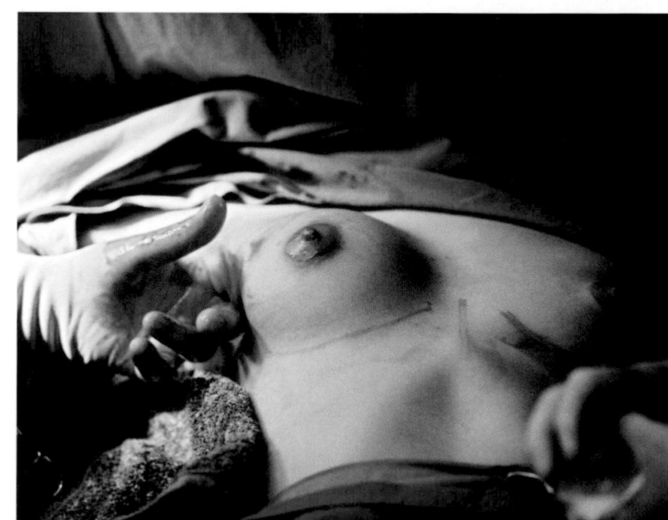

fig. 58 e+f

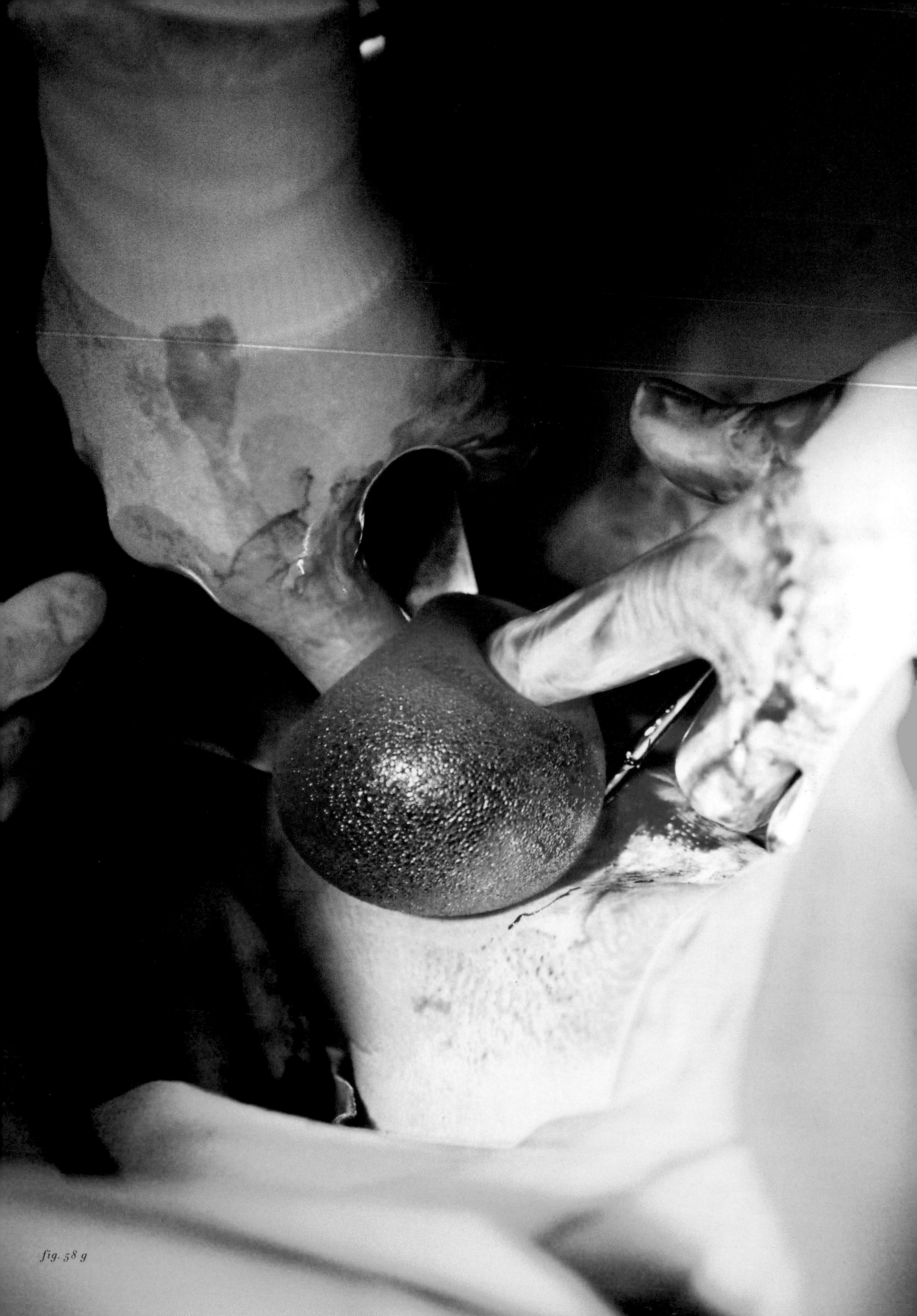

fig. 58 g

fig. 59 a+b to 64 a+b

The best method for breast augmentations with silicone implants is to position the pad underneath the pectoral muscle (submuscular implantation). This achieves a more natural appearance, reduces capsular fibrosis and prevents striation lines. Most women want a cup size of B or C; caution is advised for implants larger than 400 ml, as these may not only cause an unnatural appearance but can also make the breast sag more quickly. © Bodenseeklinik Prof. Mang

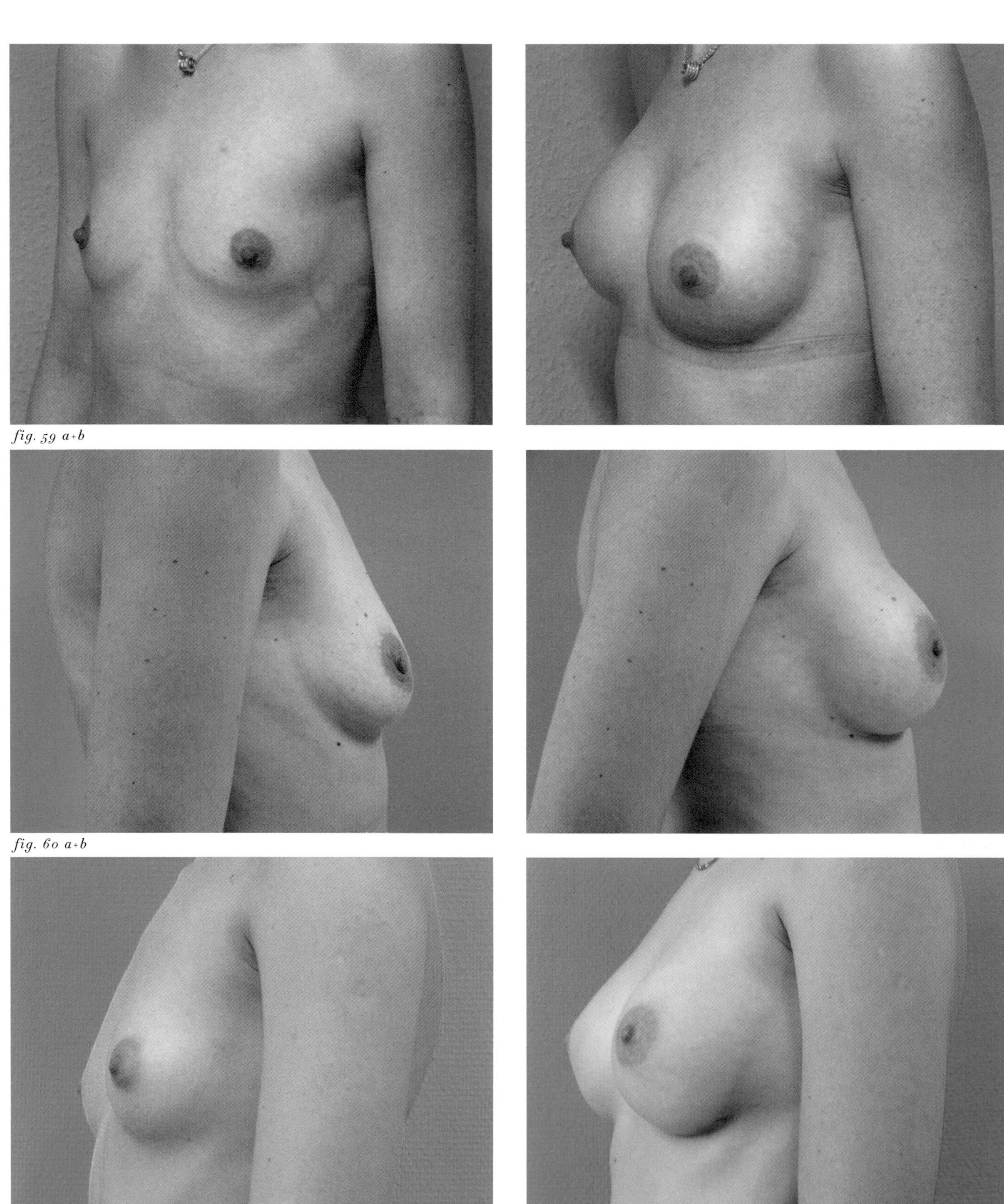

fig. 59 a+b

fig. 60 a+b

fig. 61 a+b

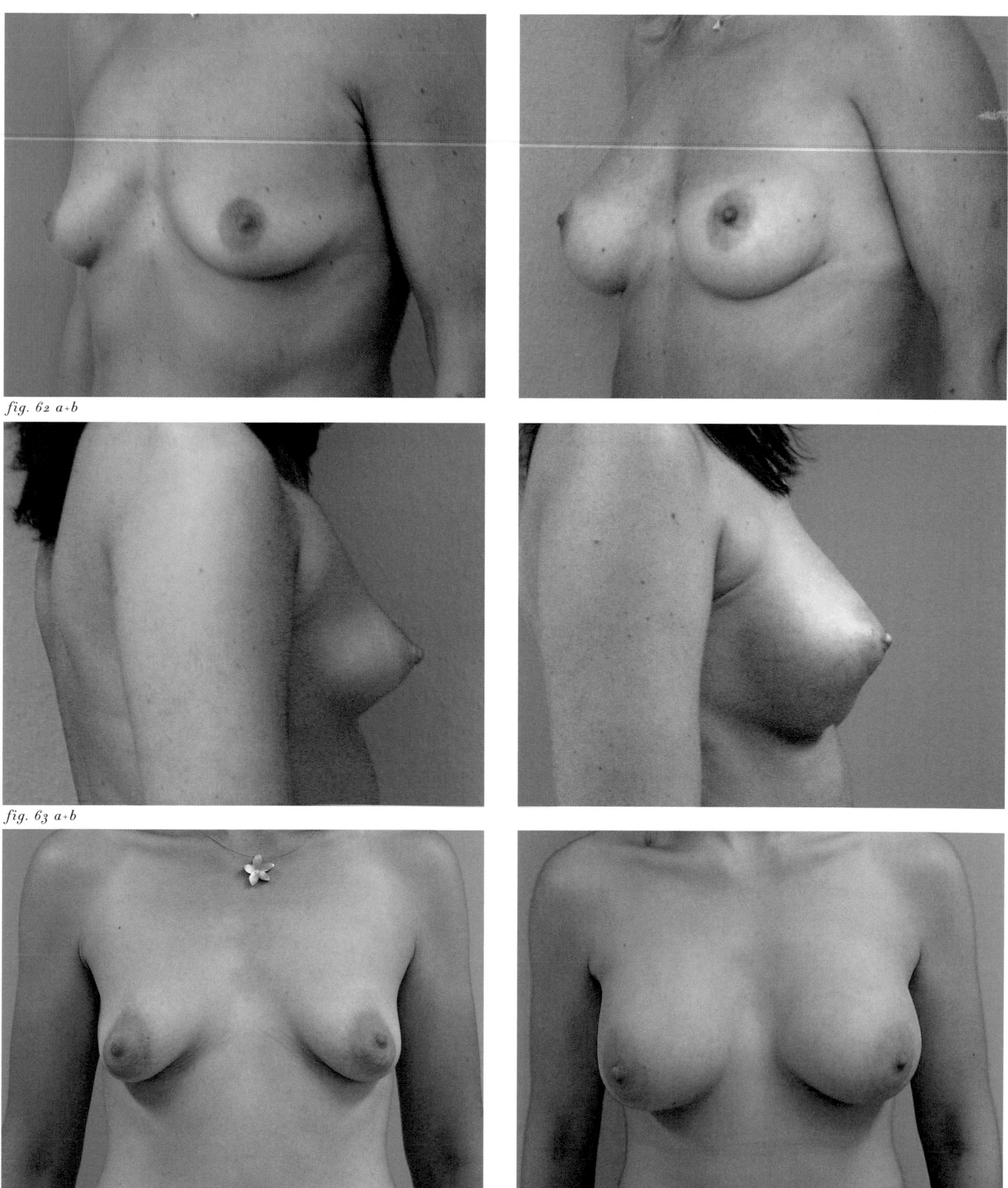

fig. 62 a+b

fig. 63 a+b

fig. 64 a+b

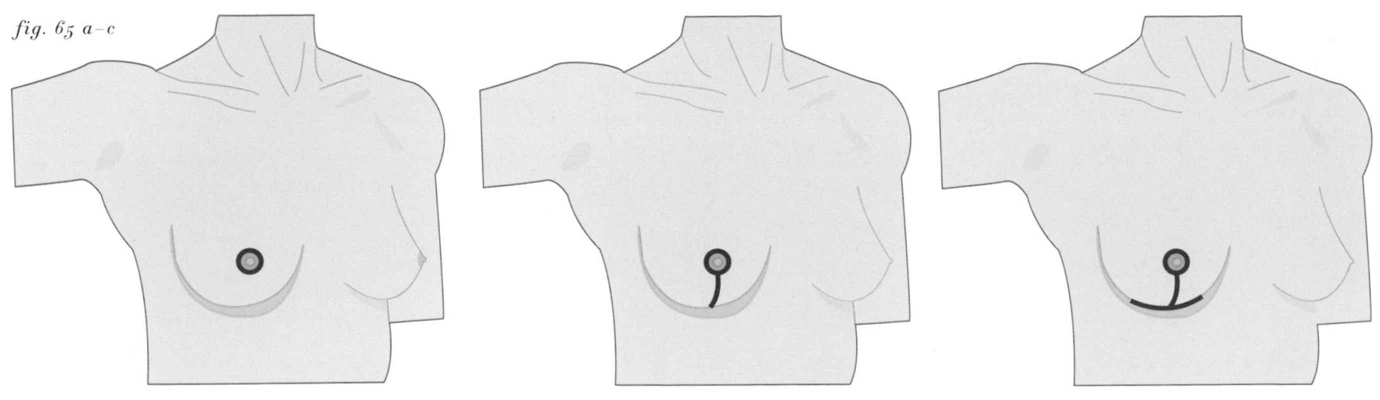

fig. 65 a–c

The incision required for breast reductions can be made around the nipple areola (a), around the nipple areola and vertically down to the submammary fold (b) or around the nipple, vertically down and horizontally along the submammary fold (c). © Blue Brain Belgium

fig. 66 a–f

These figures show different breast reduction techniques. The procedures are more complicated than breast augmentations but are frequently advisable from a medical perspective – for example when overly heavy breasts cause neck or back pain. © Blue Brain Belgium

Breast reduction or *reduction mammaplasty*: This procedure is more complicated than a breast enlargement. Often, there is a medical necessity to operate; breasts weighing more than 400 grams can cause neck and back pain, overtax the spine and even lead to osteoporosis. Very young women and women beyond menopause are affected the most.

The operation takes approx. three hours. The patient is fully sedated during the procedure and stays in the clinic for 2–10 days. The aim of the operation is to reduce skin, subcutaneous fat and gland tissue, to lift up the nipple's mammillary and areolar tissue and to thereby reshape the breast.

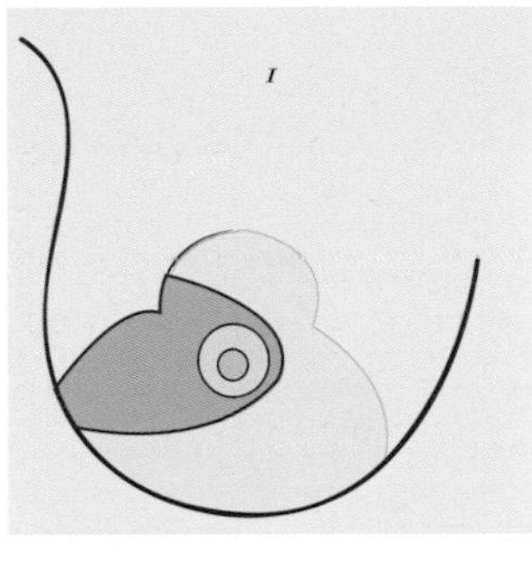

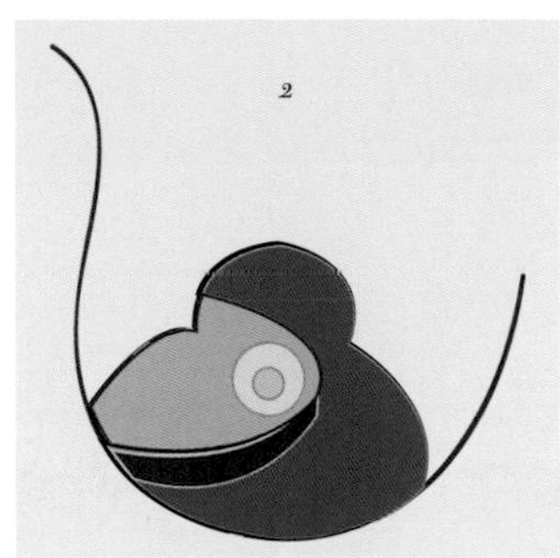

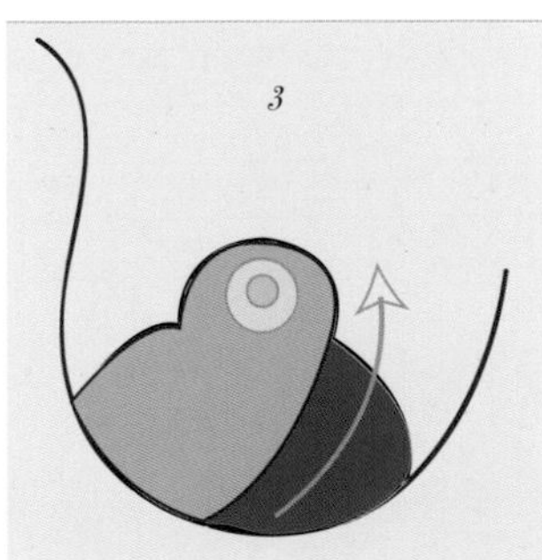

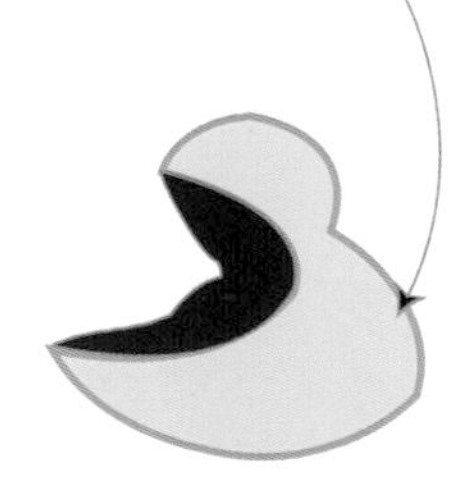

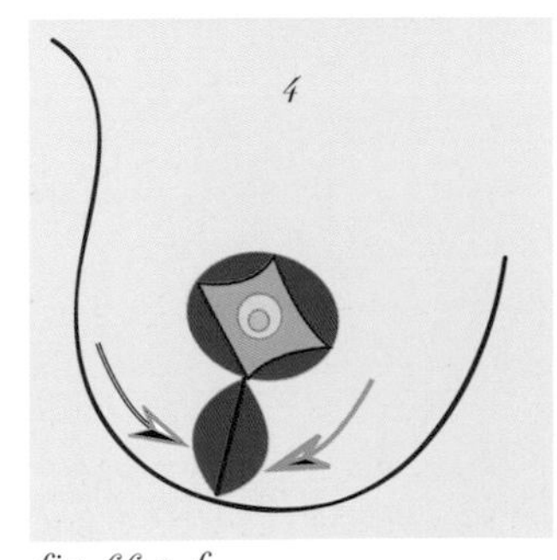

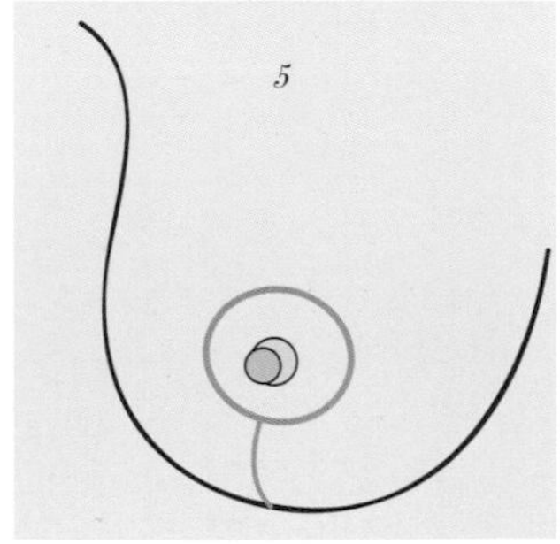

fig. 66 a–f

To shift the nipple upwards, the envisioned position is marked on the skin while the patient is sitting upright. Except in very extreme operations, the mammilla is never detached completely from the gland system. The connections to the gland and to the underlying tissue layer are preserved so that the breast's sensitivity and ability to produce milk are maintained after the operation.

The following surgical techniques may be used:

— *Classic "T-incision" technique*, as developed by McKissock, Pitanguy, Ribeiro etc.: The scar runs around the nipple areola, down to the submammary fold and horizontally along it – describing the shape of an inverted "T". The horizontal incision is kept as short as possible so as to avoid thickening and keloid formation.

— *Vertical reduction mammaplasty (Lassus-Lejour):* The Belgian surgeon Dr. Madeleine Lejour developed this technique with minimised scarring. Again, the scar runs around the areola and vertically down to the submammary fold, but there is no horizontal incision along the fold. The skin is "frilled" by the vertical scar, but within three months after the operation, it is smooth again.

— *Periareolar reduction mammaplasty:* The scar only runs around the areola. This method is successfully used for minor procedures. Small creases may initially appear on the skin, but again these smooth out within several months.

After an augmentation or reduction procedure, drainage tubes are installed and a firm bandage is applied. The drains, situated on either side of the breast, transport wound fluids and excess blood. The surgeon removes them after 24–48 hours. After the dressing is changed for the first time, a support bra is fitted over the bandage for added stability. The breast is initially quite swollen. Wound pain, tension and skin discolouration may be ex-

fig. 67 a+b

After cancerous tumours have been amputated from a breast, the breast can be reconstructed using tissue expansion. After the surface skin is stretched, an empty synthetic pouch is placed under the pectoral muscle. This is regularly pumped full of saline water for up to two months; after six months, the expander can be replaced by a silicone inlay. © Blue Brain Belgium

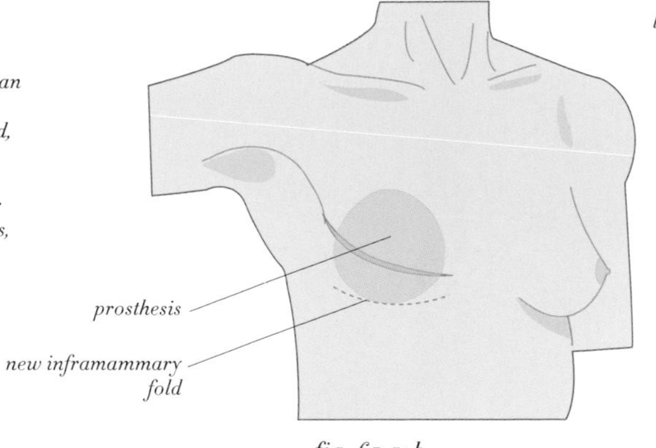

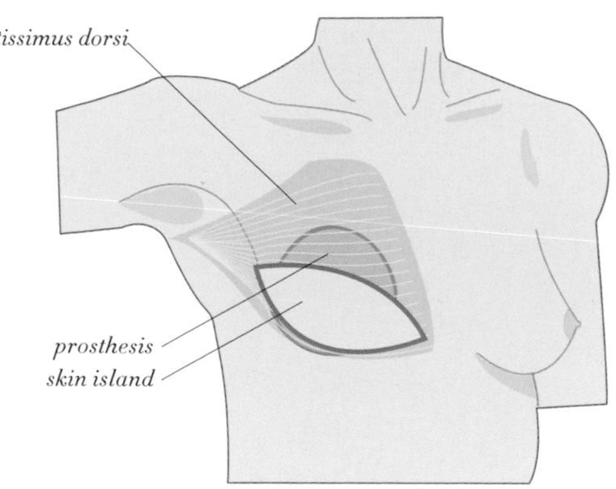

fig. 67 a+b

fig. 68 a–d

A Lassus-Lejour breast augmentation: The Belgian surgeon Dr. Madeleine Lejour developed this technique where the scar runs along the nipple and vertically down to the submammary fold. There is no horizontal incision, and the skin smoothens out after three months. © Blue Brain Belgium

perienced. Frequently, the breast seems to be very tight and raised too high; these symptoms are gradually alleviated by gravity as part of the healing process.

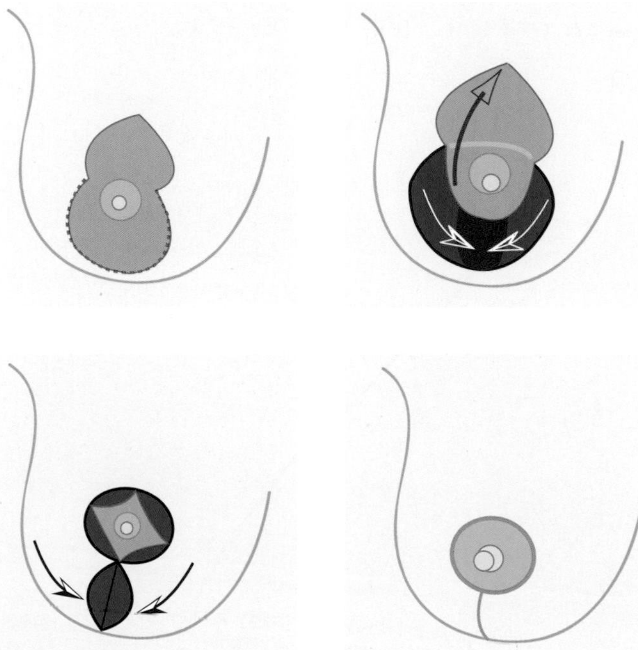

fig. 68 a–d

After 8–14 days, the stitches are removed. The suture scar is protected by a bandage for the following month. For approx. three months, a support bra needs to be worn at all times so that the healing process of the interior wounds is not interfered with. After a week, the patient can resume floor exercises and leg training; swimming is permitted after a month, fitness training after two months, tennis, golf and horse riding after three.

Risks: Asymmetrical breasts, i. e. uneven nipples. This usually requires surgical correction.
Fit for work: After 1–2 weeks.

Breast lift or *mastopexy:* Breasts that have sagged, due to significant weight loss or one or more pregnancies and subsequent breastfeeding periods, can be lifted using the methods described for reduction mammaplasty above. Instead of reducing the size, however, the operation focuses on lifting the mammilla and the breast – only the skin is reduced. In individual cases, the breast lift can be combined with an implant for added breast volume.

Breast reconstruction after cancer or *reconstructive mammaplasty:* If a woman suffers from breast cancer, the foremost medical aim is to preserve the breast. However, if an amputation (mastectomy) is unavoidable, there are two ways of reconstructing the breast:

— Silicone implant following tissue expansion: The skin above the removed breast tissue is expanded. The surgeon places an empty synthetic pouch under the pectoral muscle, and over a period of one to two months, this is pumped full of saline solution several times a week. When the desired size is reached (usually after six months), the surgeon replaces it with a prosthesis, e. g. a texturised silicone inlay.
— The breast is remodelled from autologous tissue. A model technique for this procedure has been developed by Professor Dr. Axel-Mario Feller (Munich): The breast is reconstructed with an autologous tissue flap harvested from the buttocks or lower abdomen (Transversus Rectus Abdominis Muscular or *TRAM* flap). Firstly, the surgeon cuts the blood vessels that supply the abdominal skin and fatty tissue using a microscope. He then takes out the tissue flap containing the blood vessels. Again using the microscope, he sews the harvested vessels onto the blood vessels that run along the thoracic wall, and finally sculpts the new breast from the tissue flap. A significant advantage of this technique is that the stomach muscles remain completely intact. Harvesting the tissue from the abdomen also has the added benefit of a tummy tuck!
In cases without any excess abdominal tissue, fatty tissue can also be harvested from the back muscles – the so-called "Latissimus flap". This method is well suitable for young patients and patients who have had radiation therapy. It heals well, and the result is permanent. However, the surgical technique is very complex and demanding, the team needs perfect coordination.

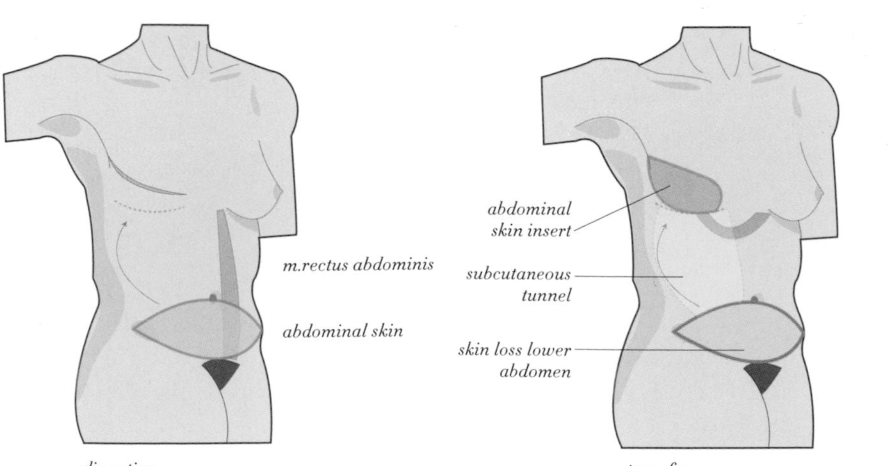

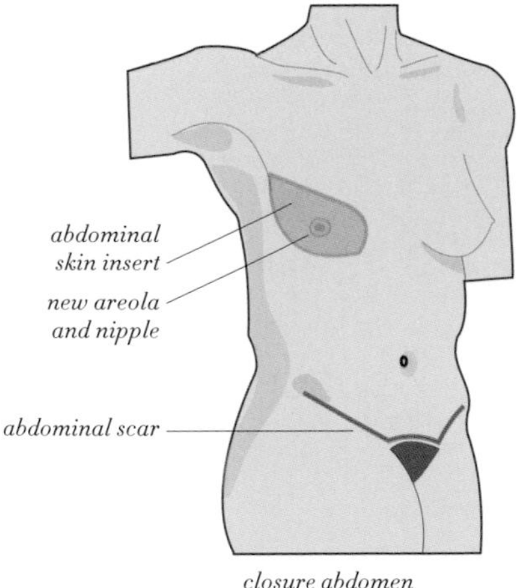

fig. 69 a–c

fig. 69 a–c

Reconstructing a breast using the TRAM (Transversus Rectus Abdominis Muscular) flap method – a tissue flap harvested from the abdomen or buttocks is transplanted to the breast. The abdominal muscles remain fully functional, and for the patient, the operation has the added benefit of a cosmetic tummy tuck. © Blue Brain Belgium

Breast reconstruction procedures always require general anaesthesia. A hospital stay of 2–5 days is required for any reconstructive method, for the Feller method up to two weeks are needed.

Risks: The implant may stiffen. In rare cases involving circulatory problems, autologous tissue can be rejected by the body.

NOTE: The nipple is only reconstructed once the breast healing process is complete. It is usually sculpted from the skin covering the transplanted tissue; the areola is tattooed on. This procedure only requires local anaesthesia and no hospital stay.

Special case I: *Breast enlargements for men:* Body builders, but also men with sunken-in, small or asymmetrical chests may desire breast augmentation. 1–5 centimetre-wide silicone implants are inserted under the pectoral

fig. 70

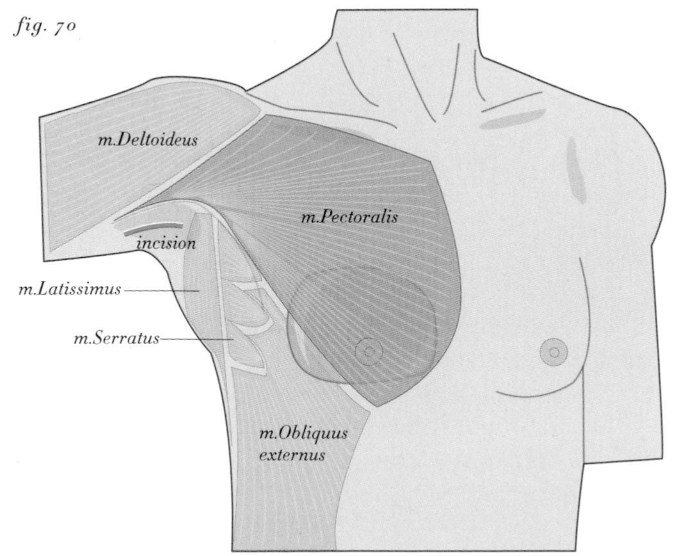

muscle via an axillary incision. A hospital stay of one day is required; the risks are the same as for a woman's breast enlargement. The result is permanent, i. e. the inlays do not need to be replaced.

Special case II: *Enlarged male breast* or *gynecomastia:* Hormone imbalances are a common cause for fat deposits in the male breast. If there is an excess of subcutaneous fat, this can be addressed by liposuction using thin, specially-designed cannulas. (See following section –

fig. 71

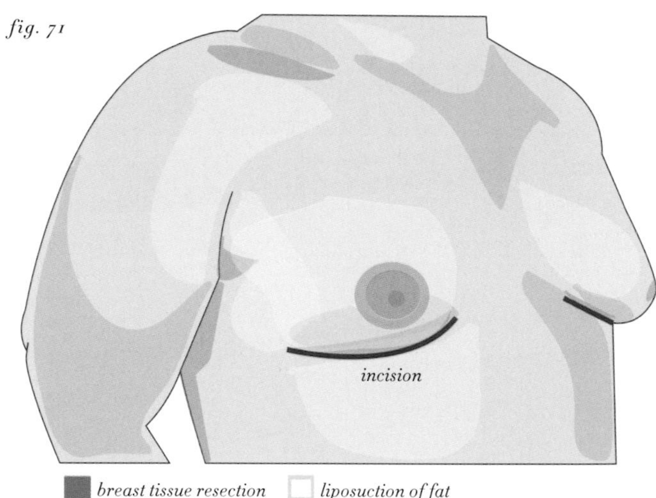

Liposuction.) The surgical risk for this procedure is very low.

If the enlarged breast is caused by excessive glandular tissue, a surgical procedure with general anaesthesia or twilight anaesthesia plus a local anaesthetic is required. The surgeon cuts along the lower border of the nipple areola, removes the excess tissue, sutures the wound and applies a firm dressing. After approx. two weeks, the stitches are removed. Sports can be recommenced after three weeks. Complications are rare.

fig. 70

Body builders, but also men with diminutive breasts, sometimes desire breast augmentation. The incision for this procedure is made in the armpit, and the inlay — up to five centimetres deep – is placed underneath the pectoral muscle. © Blue Brain Belgium

fig. 71

Hormonal imbalances can cause enlarged male breasts. In simple cases, the fatty tissue is removed using cannulas; if there is too much glandular tissue, the surgeon needs to perform an operation to remove it (requiring a local or general anaesthetic). © Blue Brain Belgium

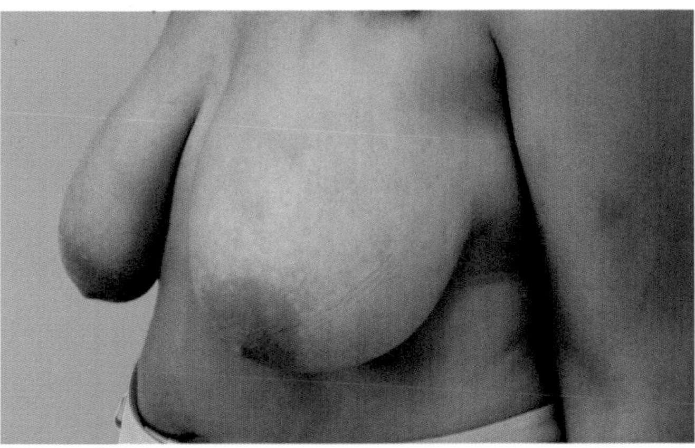
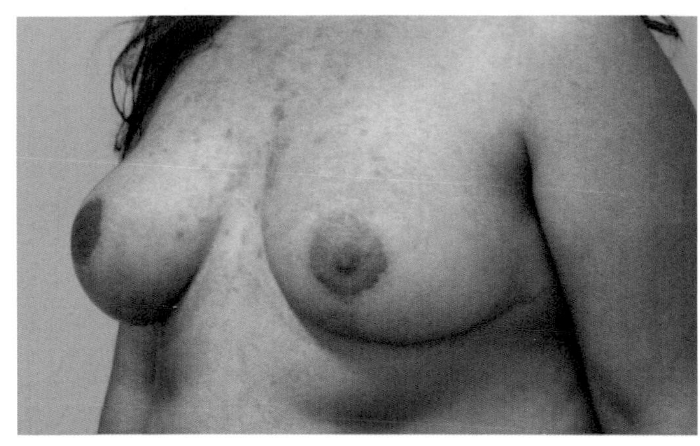

fig. 72 a+b

fig. 72 a+b to 74 a+b

The most common problem encountered as a result of standard breast reductions is pronounced scarring. The visible traces of the operation can only be de-emphasised by intensive wound care for up to three months. © Bodenseeklinik Prof. Mang

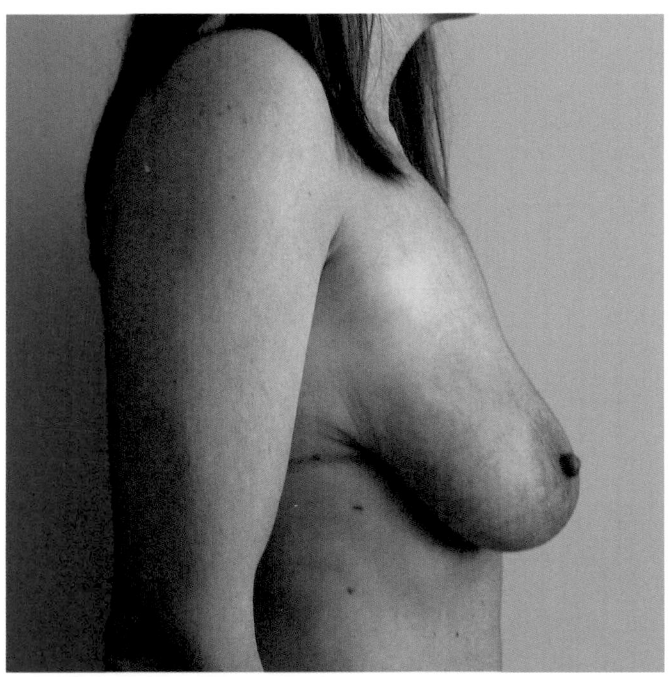
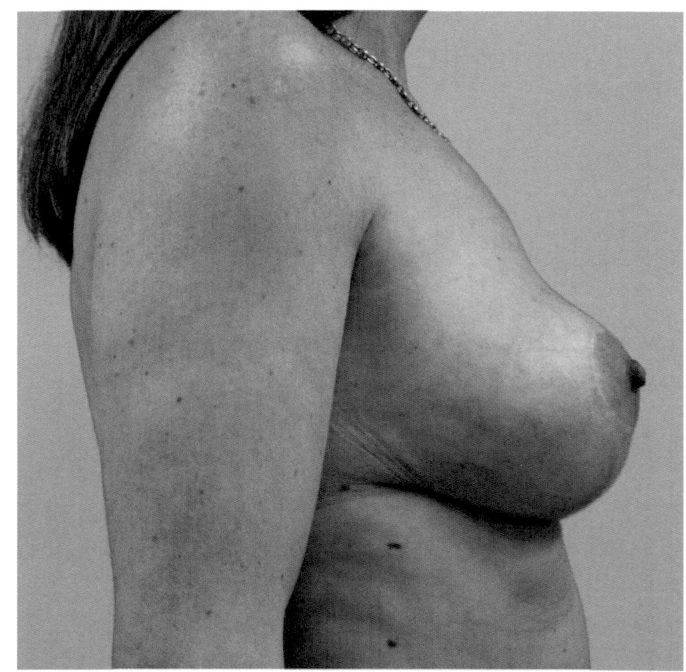

fig. 73 a+b

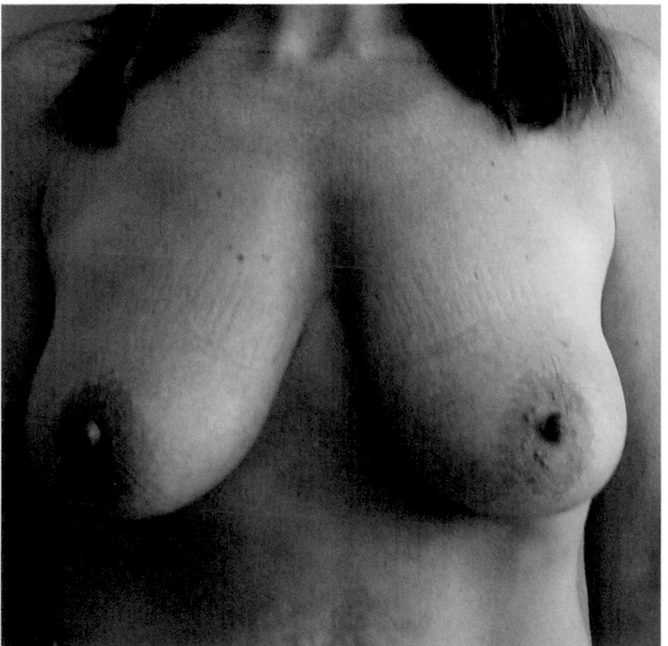
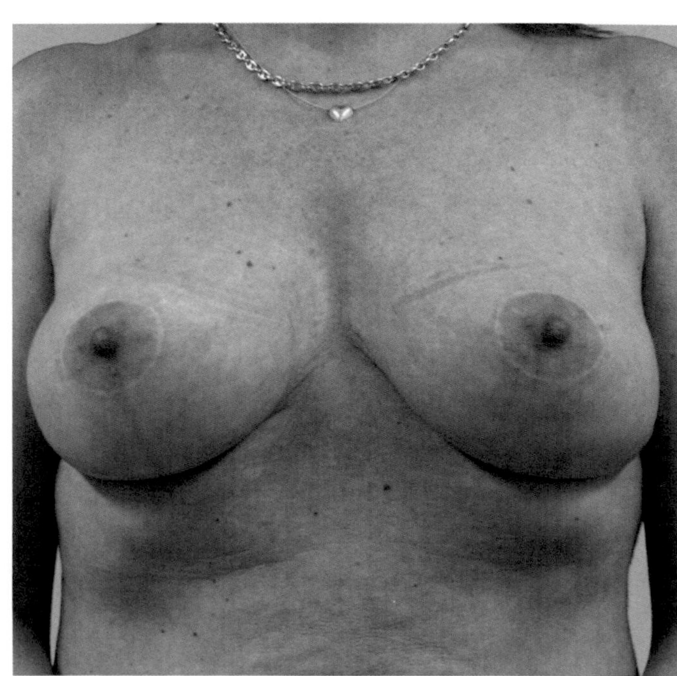

fig. 74 a+b

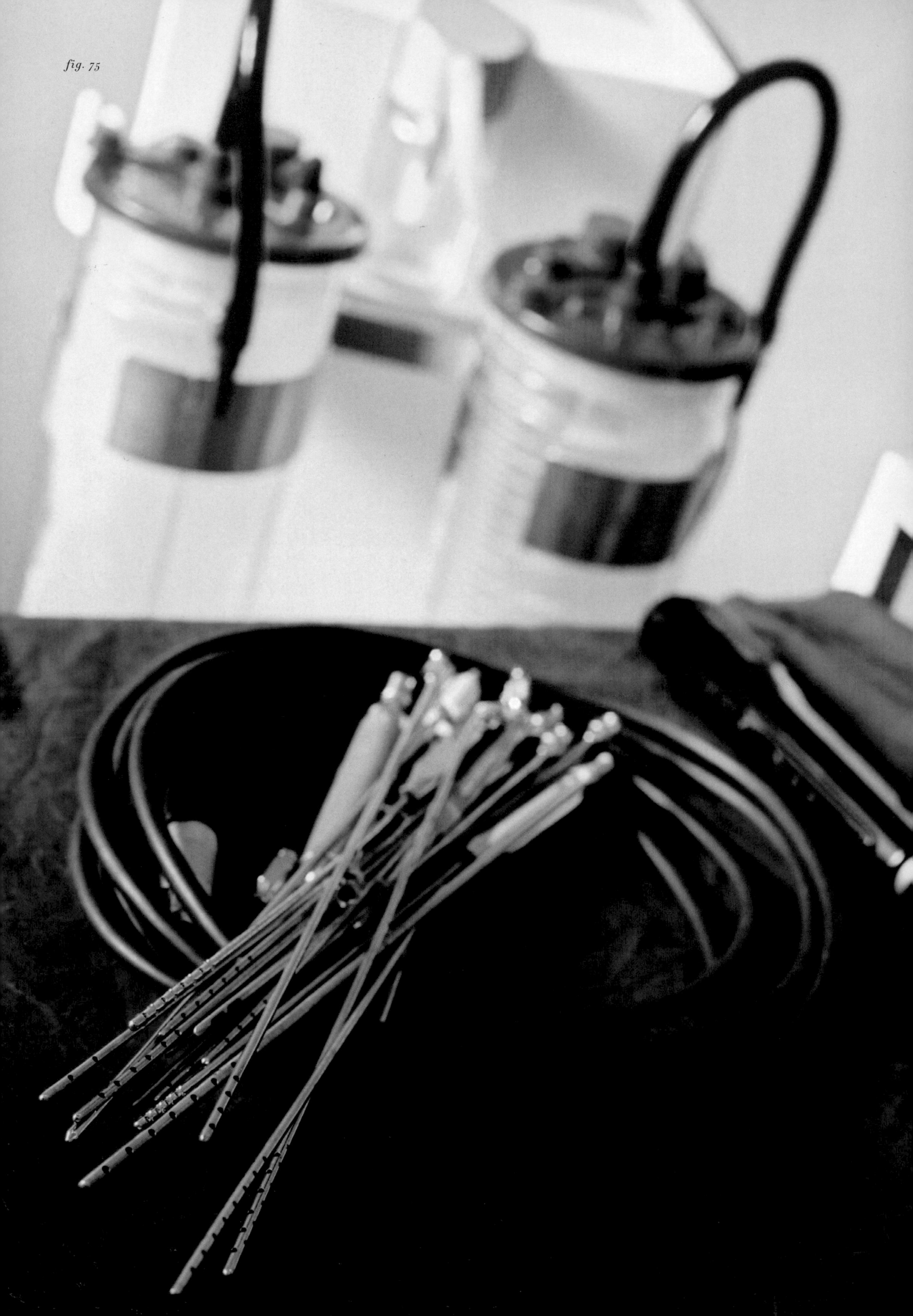

fig. 75

fig. 75

Liposuction cannulas. Liposuction, which is used to improve body contours, is one of the most popular cosmetic surgical procedures around the world. © laif

fig. 76

Liposuction on the buttocks and the upper thigh. Up to three litres of pure fat can be removed in a single operation – the patient may not be overly obese, however, and his/her connective tissue needs to be adequately flexible. © laif

fig. 77

The classic liposuction unit. Up to six litres of saline solution are pumped into the tissue; the soaked fat cells are then sucked off using a cannula. © Blue Brain Belgium

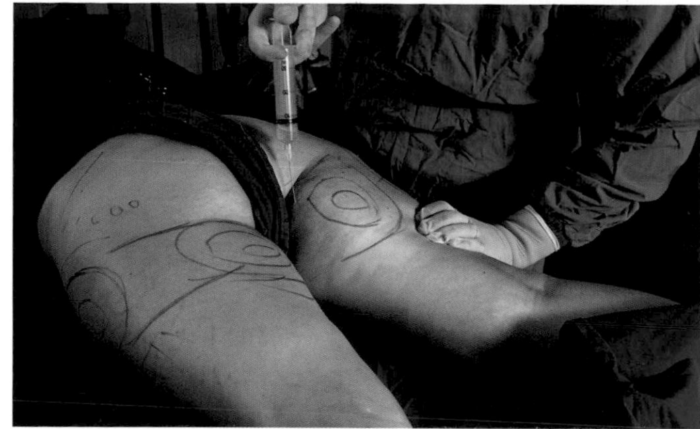

fig. 76

Liposuction / body contouring / lipoaspiration

In collaboration with Dr. Ulrich K. Kesselring and Prof. Dr. Dr. Werner L. Mang

Liposuction is used to improve the body's contours, a technique used on its own or in conjunction with other procedures. It has been practiced since the late 60s, and with more than 400,000 treatments a year, it is one of the most popular cosmetic procedures. Liposuction is an operation, which is why it should only be performed by an experienced surgeon. The technical skill and aesthetic judgement required are considerable. Patients eligible for liposuction should not be overly obese, as no more than three litres of fat (in total around six litres of fluid) can be removed. Also, the patient's connective tissue needs to be fairly flexible. Patients should have tried out weight loss approaches such as dieting and sports previously – with the conclusion that their problematic areas remain unaffected by low-calorie food and fitness training.

Techniques

Tumescent technique (lat. *tumescere* = to swell): This is the most commonly used method. Tiny incisions are made in the skin on top of the fatty tissue, and approx. three litres of saline solution are pumped into the tissue through these holes. The fat cells absorb the liquid and swell up, which makes it easier to dislodge them. The saline solution ocontains a local anaesthetic, as well as adrenalin to minimise blood loss. Already during the one-hour soaking stage, the fat cells begin to detach from the connective tissue, nerves, blood vessels and lymphatic vessels surrounding them.

The surgeon removes the loosened fat cells using a thin suction cannula, covering the tissue in a rapid, powerful wiping motion. With his other hand, he controls the suction. The procedure can last up to three hours and requires substantial physical stamina on the part of the surgeon. In large-scale operations, a general anaesthetic is used.

Power assisted liposuction (lipolysis by vibration): This is an enhanced variation of the tumescent technique, in large parts developed by Dr. Gerhard Sattler german surgeon. An electrically powered cannula containing 24 suction holes, the "Sattler cannula," is used to agitate the fat cells up to 4,000 times per minute and literally shake them out of the connective tissue. With this method, it is impossible to damage any blood vessels or nerves, and difficult areas containing a large amount of connective tissue (e. g. calves or ankles) can also be lifted and contoured. Another advantage of this technique is that the patient only needs a local anaesthetic; together with the surgeon, he or she can control the cannula's suction path.

fig. 77

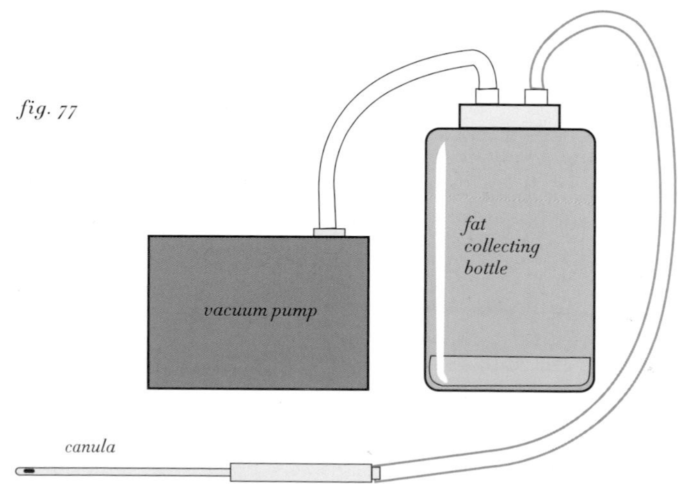

Ultrasonic liposuction (also known as *"Ultrasound-Assisted Lipoplasty"* or *UAL*): This method complements the tumescent technique, employing special cannulas that project ultrasound waves into the fatty tissue. This sonic treatment explodes and liquefies the fat cells without damaging the connective tissue. UAL is used predominantly for areas with a significant amount of connective tissue, e. g.

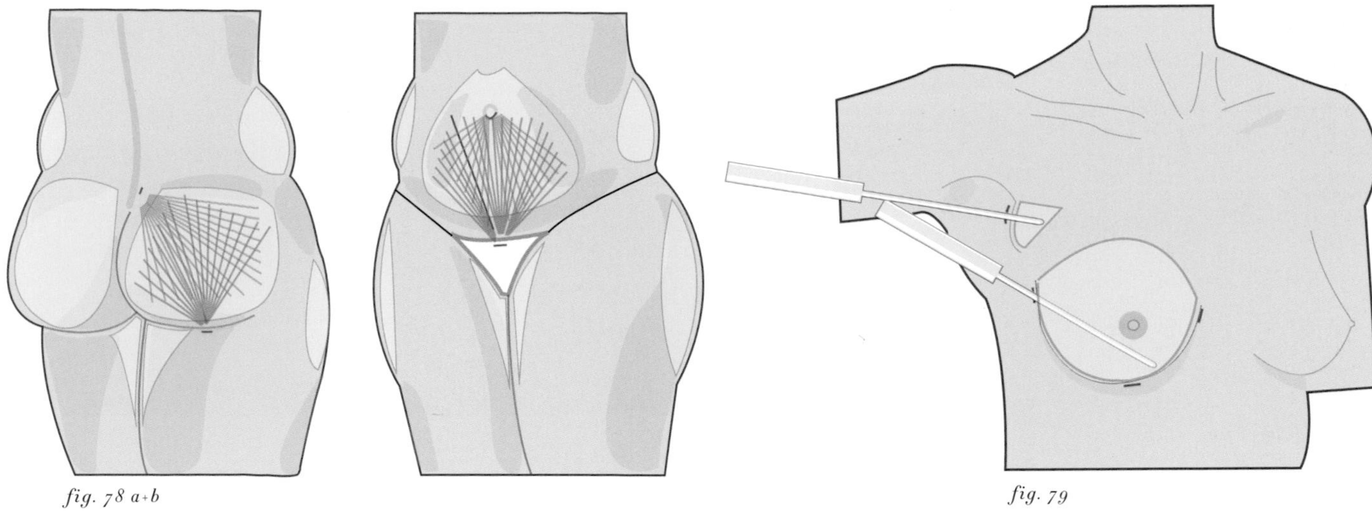

fig. 78 a+b

fig. 79

the male breast or the upper back, but also for follow-up operations. The technique is more elaborate, requires a longer period of sedation and contains the risk of burning the skin or subcutaneous tissue.

Electrolipolysis: This technique is normally employed in conjunction with a hormone therapy for treating cellulite. (See Section A – Anti-Aging.) The practitioner inserts a fine acupuncture needle into the fatty tissue and induces an electrical current. The fat cells become porous and the fatty acids drain out. The procedure usually takes no longer than an hour. After 8–12 sessions, the orange-peel skin on the thighs should be gone.

Liposuction offers varying degrees of success for different problem areas:

- Suction works well on fat deposits on the
  - hips and upper thighs (also known as "saddlebags")
  - waist
  - inner knees,
- less well on the
  - tummy (after the operation, the patient should sit upright as little as possible as permanent folds may appear in the tissue)
  - neck, back of the neck
  - double chin, nasolabial folds (the tissue can be reduced by up to ten percent without the risk of later creasing; see also Section Facelifts)
  - cheeks,
- with partial success on the
  - back
  - inner thighs
  - buttock folds (sitting down should be avoided in the weeks after the operation as much as possible, as there is a possibility that the skin around the fold will bulge inwards; if too much fatty tissue is removed, the buttocks may soon sag again)
  - ankles (the flow of lymphatic fluids and venous blood may be impaired for several months and the ankle may swell up considerably; haematomas may result in skin discolouration),
- and with little success on the
  - back and front of the upper thighs
  - calves
  - lower arms.

Once fatty tissue is removed, it is eliminated permanently – at least from the areas treated. Unfortunately, weight may still be gained in other parts of the body. If liposuction was performed on the upper thighs, for example, new fat pads may form on the hip or the lower abdomen. Some surgeons don't remove all the fatty tissue in one session but choose to remove only e. g. 70 percent; in subsequent sessions, they again remove 70 percent (of the remaining 30 percent) and continue in this manner until the desired result is achieved. This spread-out approach gives the surgeon greater aesthetic control over contouring the body.

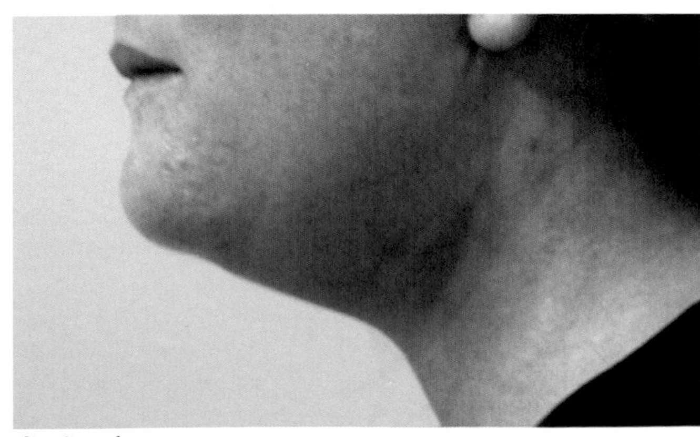

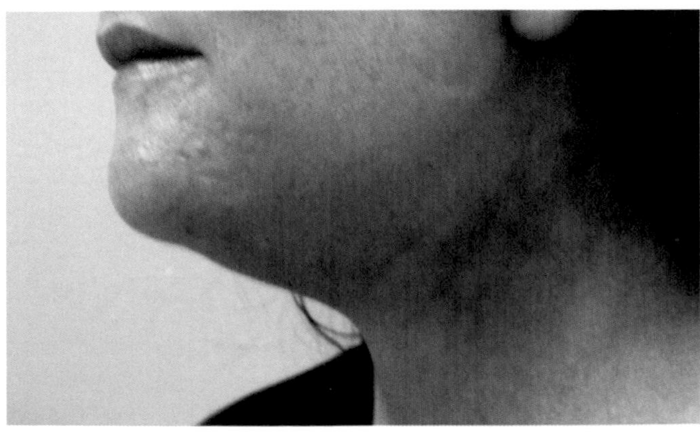

fig. 80 a+b

fig. 78 a+b & 79

The most common problem areas include the upper thighs, buttocks, hip, tummy and breasts. Not all of these are easy to treat – sometimes the surgeon cannot remove all the fat in a single session; two or more sessions may be required to contour the problem areas with sufficient precision. © Blue Brain Belgium

fig. 80 a+b

Even without a neck lift, a double chin can be diminished significantly – using tumescent liposuction. The problem area is soaked with 250 ml of saline solution, and the fat cells are subsequently removed using thin cannulas (2–3 mm in diameter). © Bodensee-klinik Prof. Mang

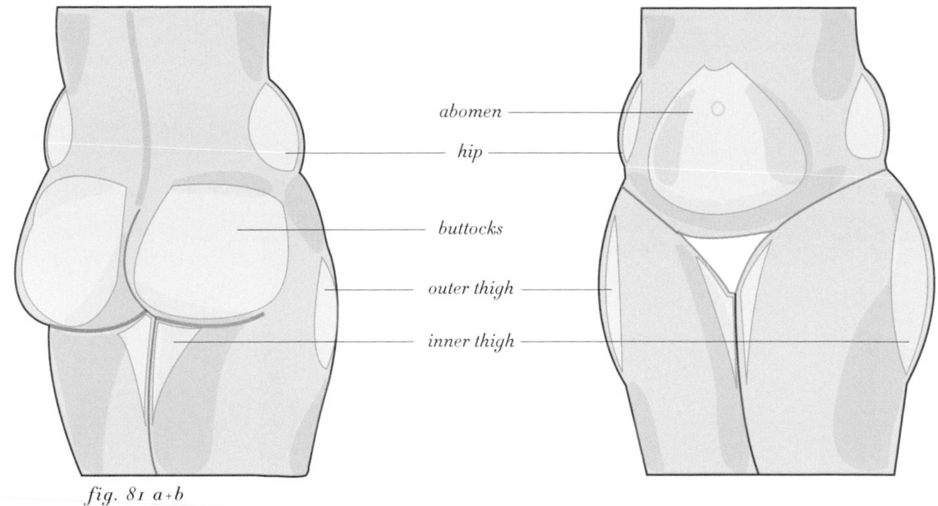

fig. 81 a+b

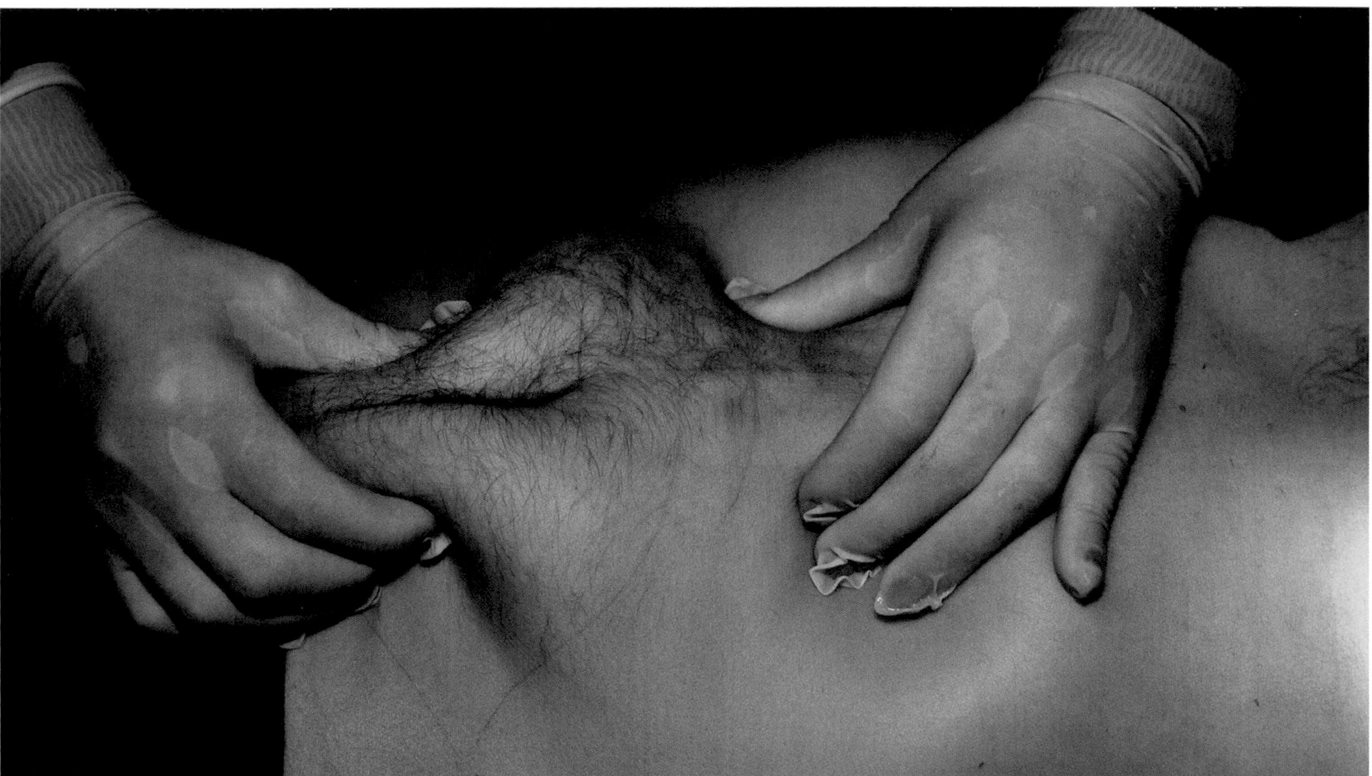

fig. 82

Before the operation:
- The surgeon outlines and shades the skin areas to be treated with coloured marker pens.
- Depending on the extent of the operation, general or local anaesthesia is administered.

After the operation:
- Immediately after the procedure and for the following six weeks, the patient needs to wear elastic support garments. These are essential for relieving swellings and haematomas and help the skin adjust to the new contours.
- 7–10 days after the operation, the stitches are removed.
- At the earliest, the new body contours become visible six weeks after the operation.
- The patient is ready for work or social life after one week.

Risks:
- Pronounced swellings which may persist for three to six months or longer, particularly on the face or ankles
- Small scars (these are soon indistinguishable from normal skin)
- Stinging or numbness of the skin in the wound area – may last for a week or up to two months
- Intense pain, especially where fatty tissue is located next to muscle tissue (e. g. back, upper hip, waist)
- Sensory nerve damage.
- An asymmetrical body outline, bumps or dents in the skin surface; surgical corrections may be performed after six months

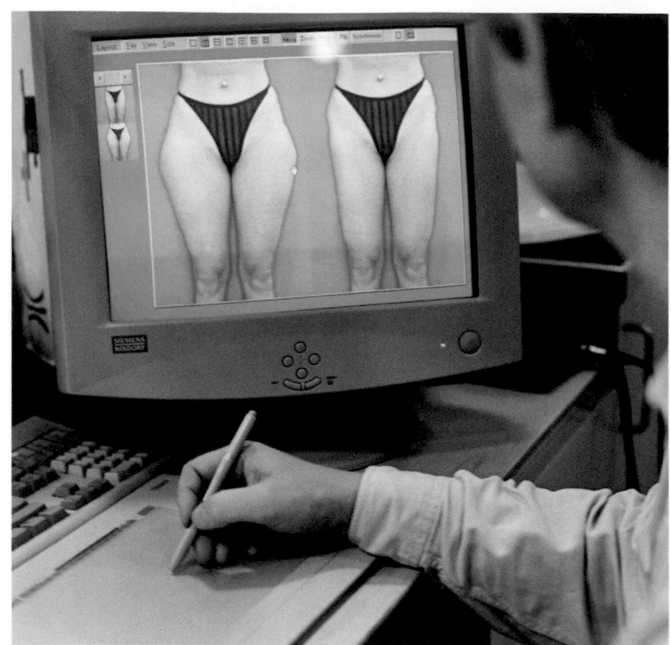

fig. 83

fig. 81 a+b

The most popular body areas eligible for liposuction. Modern surgery employs more than just a pump and a cannula – some surgeons use electrically powered cannulas that "shake" the fat cells out of the connective tissue. Other cannula-based devices emit ultrasound frequencies that liquefy the cells. © Blue Brain Belgium

fig. 82

Following a liposuction treatment, the patient is unable to work or socialise for a week. The patient also needs to wear support garments for approx. six weeks – to reduce swellings and for the skin to align to the new body contours. © laif

fig. 83

Computer-aided diagnosis: The possibilities and limitations of liposuction for a particular patient can be precisely mapped and displayed on screen. © laif

fig. 84 a+b to 86 a+b

The photos highlight problem areas around the buttocks, abdomen, hips and upper thighs (inside, outside). Tumescent liposuction can be employed to remove large amounts of fatty tissue, achieving a noticeable recontouring of the body. The patient should not, however, rely on cosmetic surgery alone for this renewed body shape – just as important for the ideal figure are a balanced nutrition, ample physical activity and sports. © Bodenseeklinik Prof. Mang

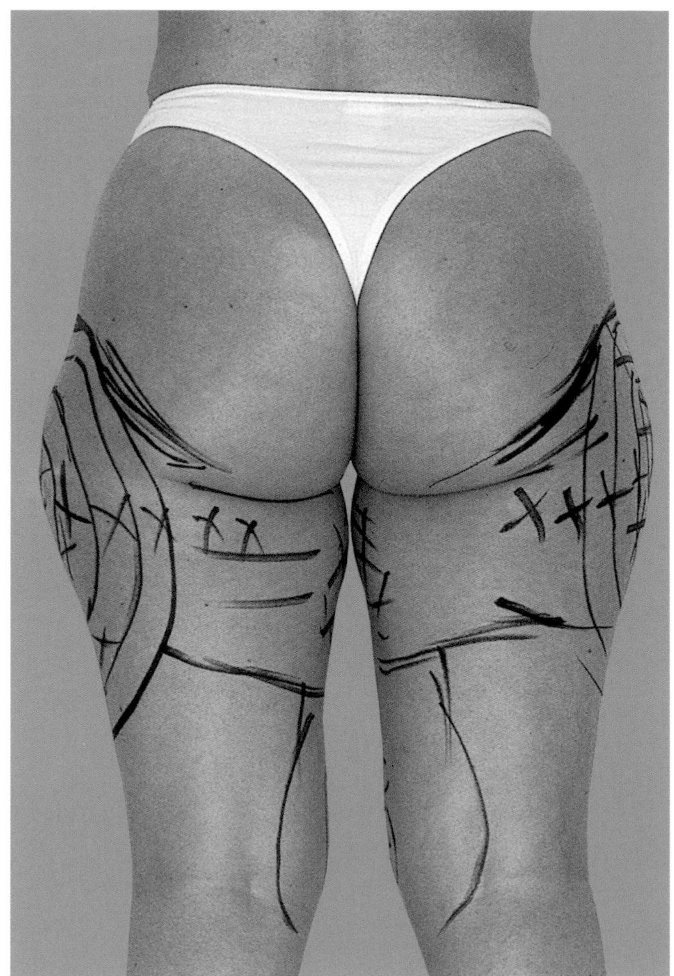

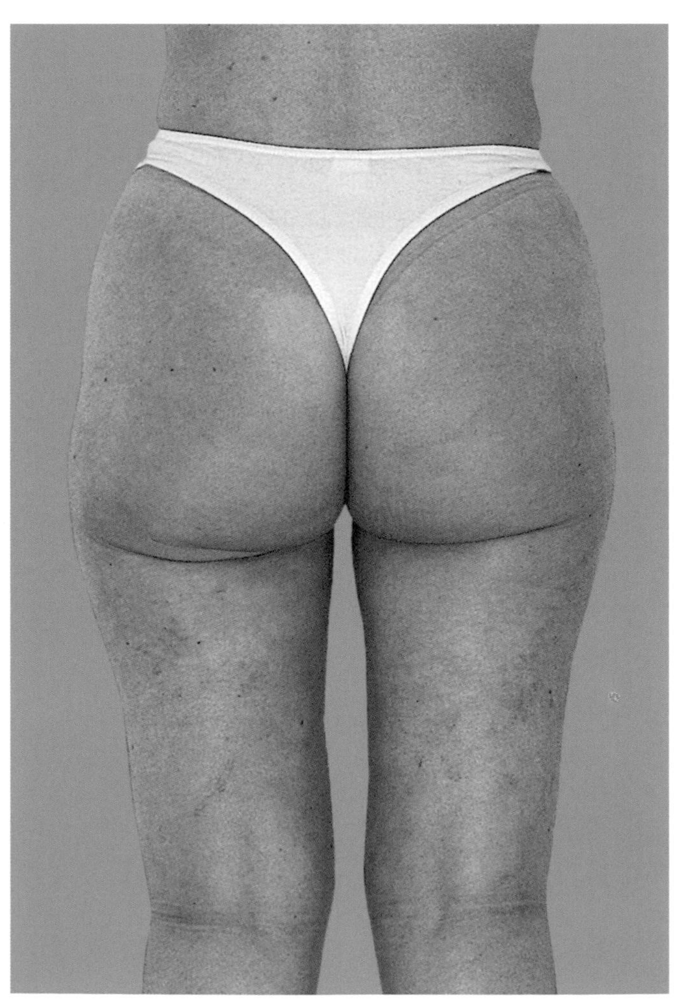

fig. 84 a+b

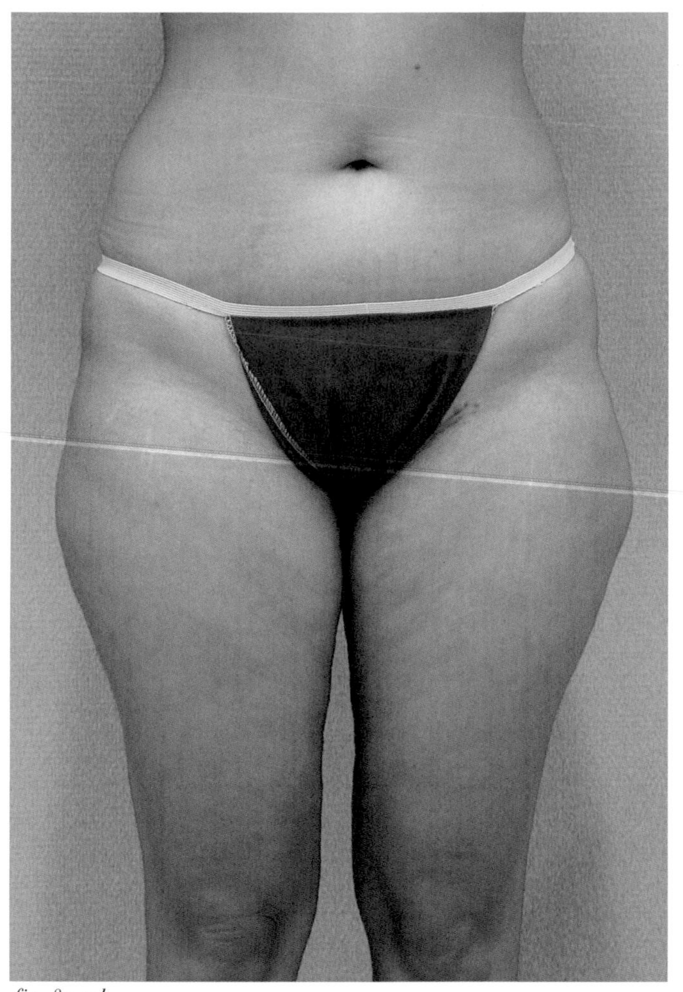

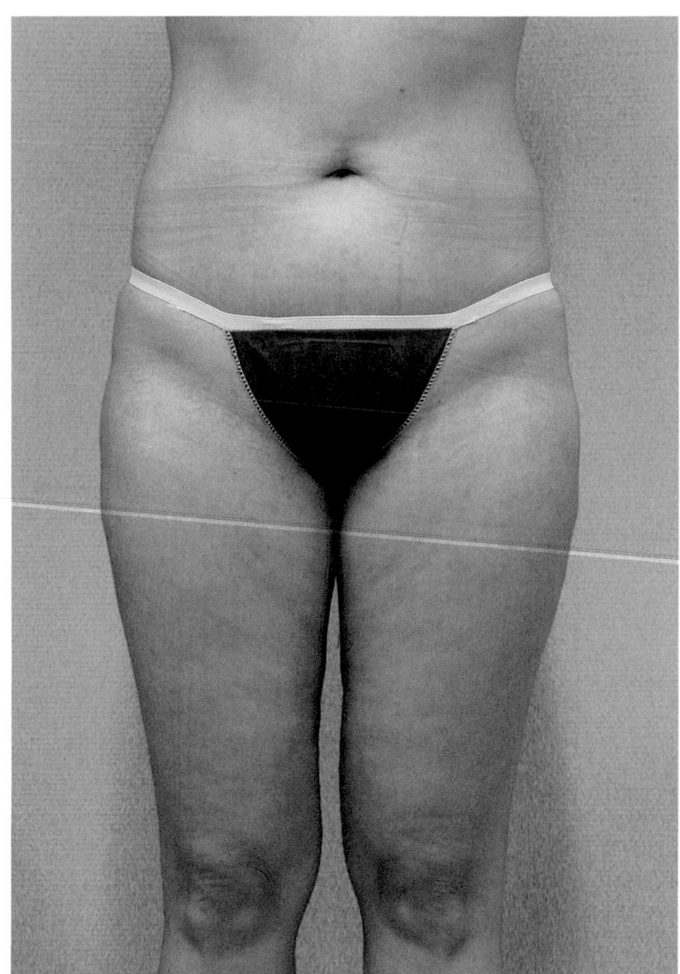

fig. 85 a+b

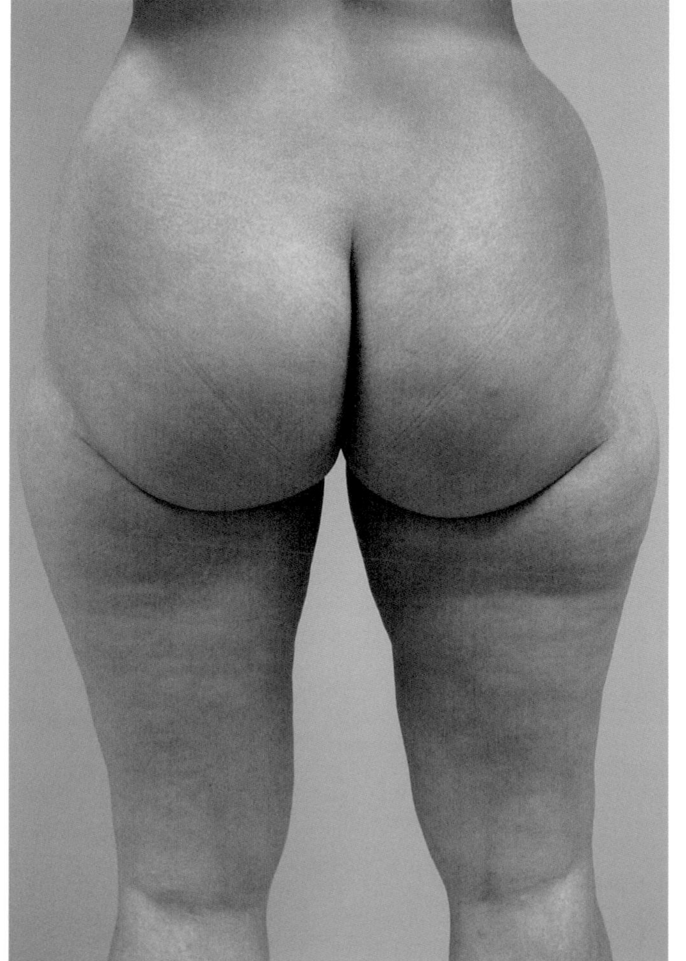

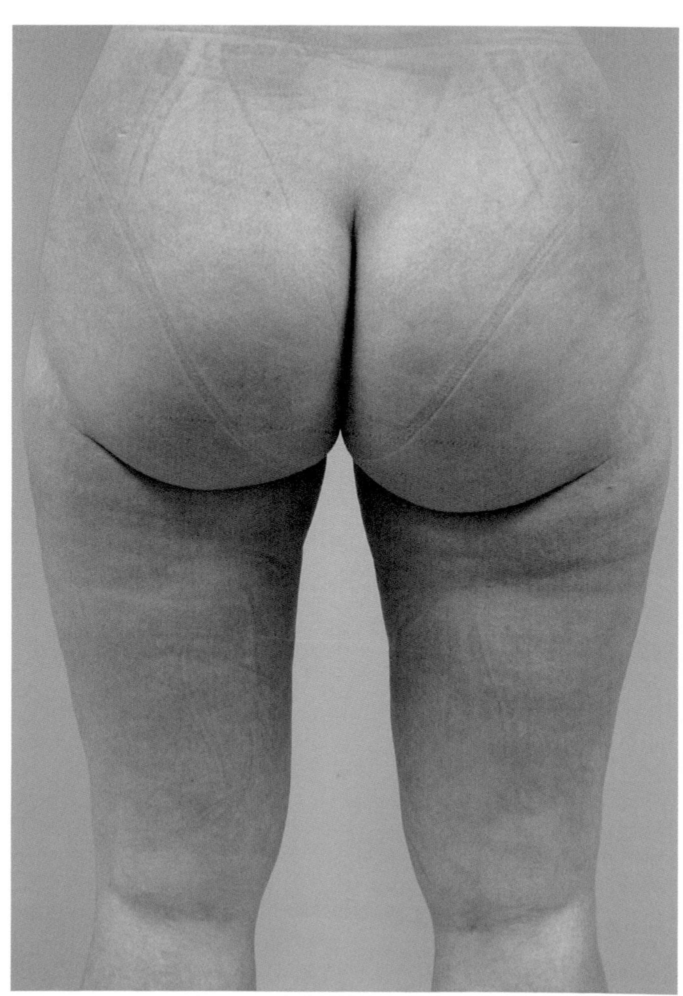

fig. 86 a+b

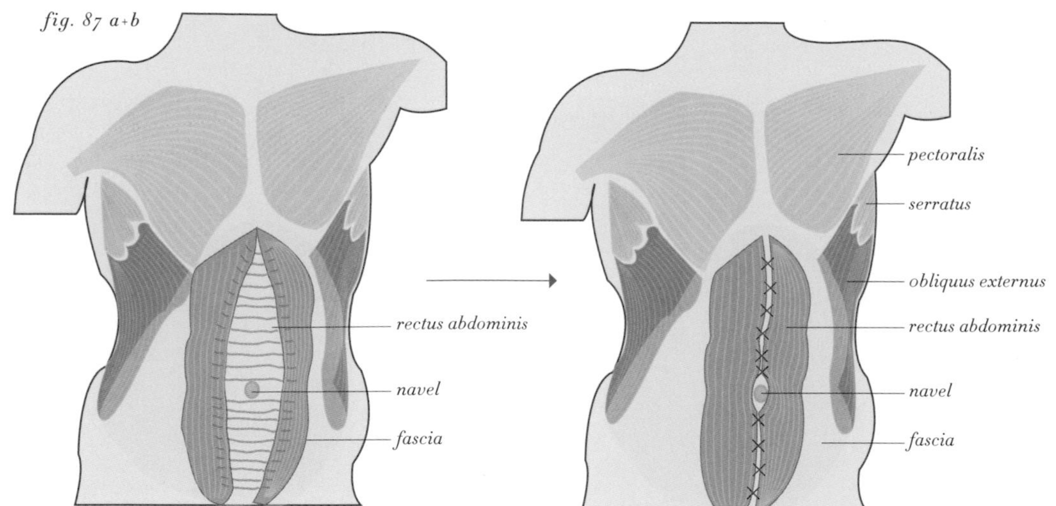

fig. 87 a+b

The abdominal muscles can be tightened using conventional methods or an endoscopic technique. For this, the surgical implements are inserted into the abdominal cavity through several small incisions. Using a tiny camera for guidance, the surgeon then shortens the two slackened muscle cords. *© Blue Brain Belgium*

fig. 88 a+b & 90 a+b

When excess skin needs to be removed, a "tummy tuck" can be combined with liposuction. Alternatively, the surgeon may opt for abdominoplasty. The finer points of this procedure include the resculpting of the navel, which is crucial to the aesthetics of the abdominal region. © Bodenseeklinik Prof. Mang

Body contouring with the scalpel

If a patient's skin is no longer sufficiently flexible to contract around reduced tissue (e. g. after liposuction), a surgical procedure may be needed to contour the body aesthetically. However, there is a substantial risk of large, visible scars.

Abdominoplasty or "tummy tuck:" This is often performed after several pregnancies, when the abdominal muscles have been overstretched, or after extreme weight loss – which can lead to a so-called "spare tyre" flab of skin hanging over the lower abdomen.

An abdominoplasty is a major procedure involving a large loss of blood. It requires general anaesthesia and lasts for approx. two hours. Two long, arching incisions are made along the bikini line, just above the pubic hair.

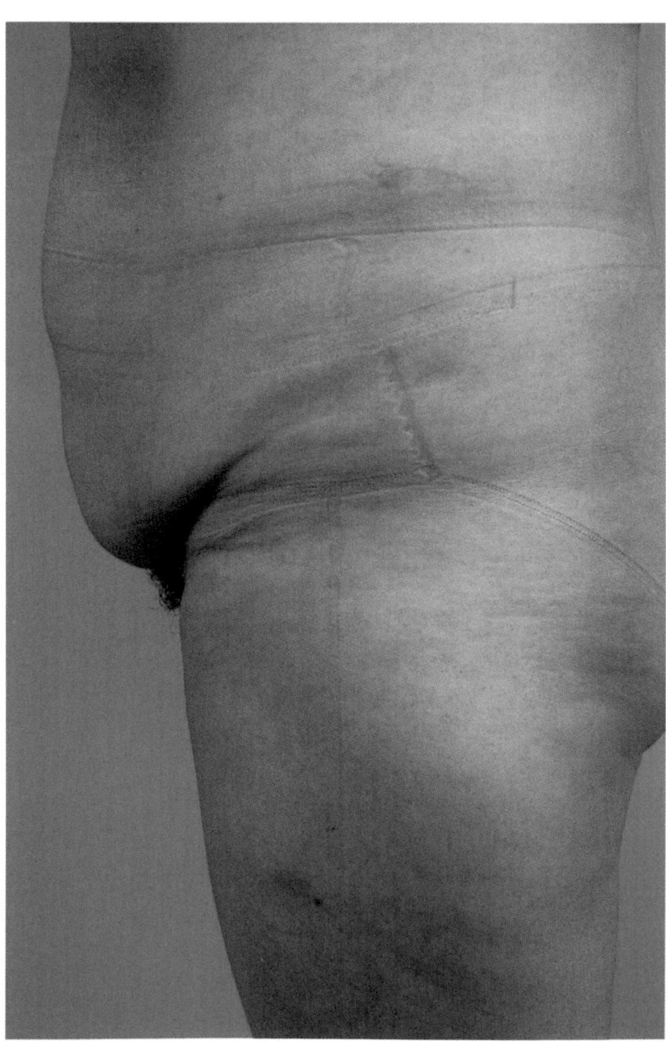

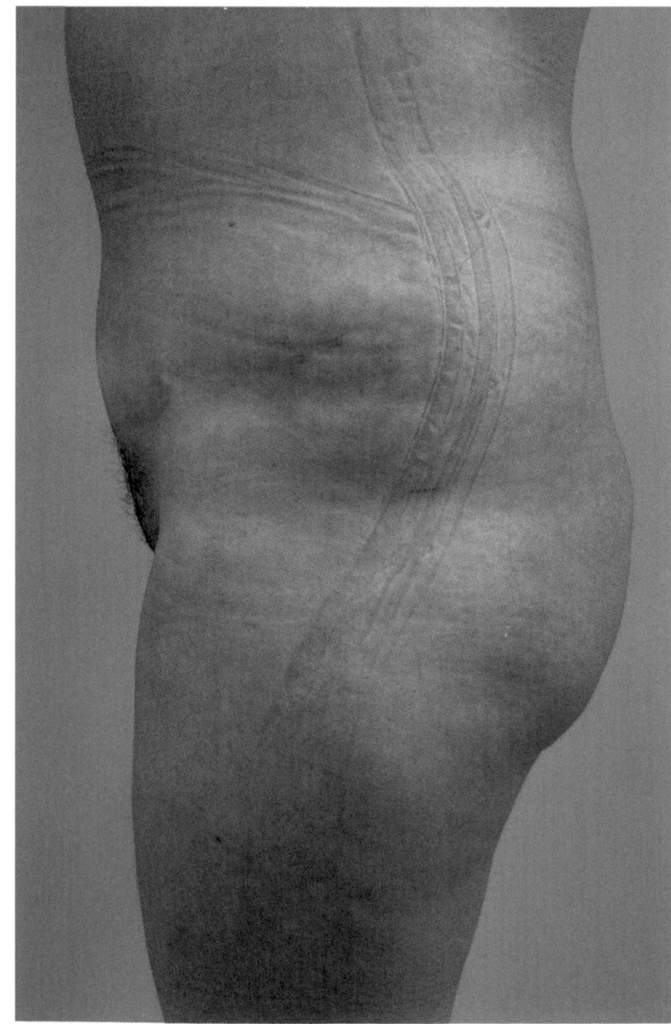

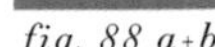
fig. 88 a+b

fig. 89 a+b

For an abdominoplasty, the surgical incisions are made inside the "bikini" zone – the resultant scars are hardly noticeable. © *Blue Brain Belgium*

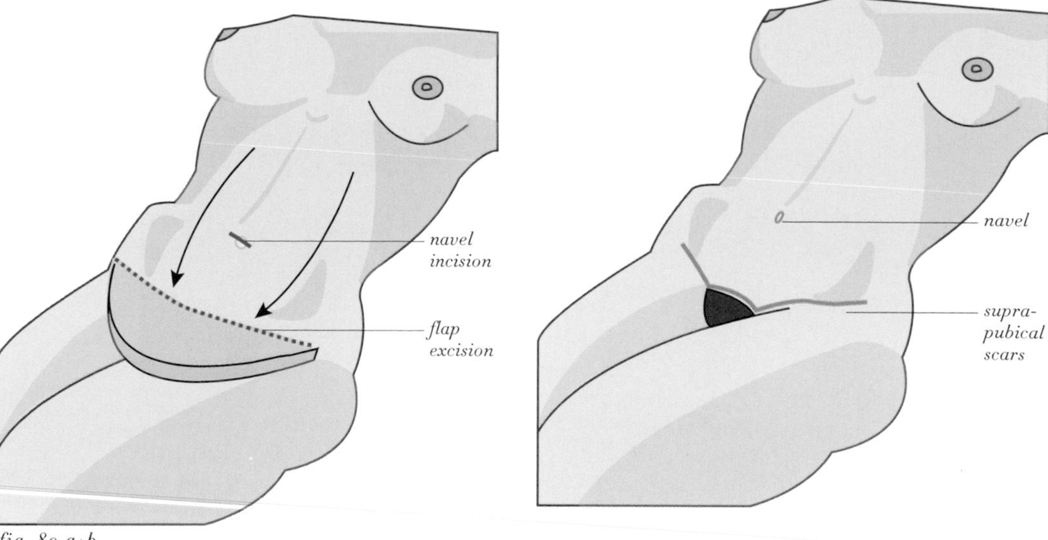

fig. 89 a+b

The skin is cut right up to the lowest ribs, sparing out only the navel. Like in a facelift, the surgeon then pulls the undamaged skin downward and removes the excess skin. The fatty tissue excised can weigh up to ten kilograms. Secondary haemorrhaging may occur. The risk of embolisms and thrombosis is minimised by physical exercise, anti-thrombosis support garments and heparin injections. Three to ten days of hospital stay are common.

In contrast to conventional abdominoplasty, the *endoscopic technique* only requires several small incisions above the pubic hair area, each measuring up to five centimetres. This is especially recommended for men or women with a "potbelly," i. e. a round, tight belly that has pushed the excess fatty tissue and lax muscles downwards. The endoscope and other surgical instruments are fed through the incisions. Long barbs with a miniature camera at the tip are used to sever the abdominal skin and tighten the muscles.

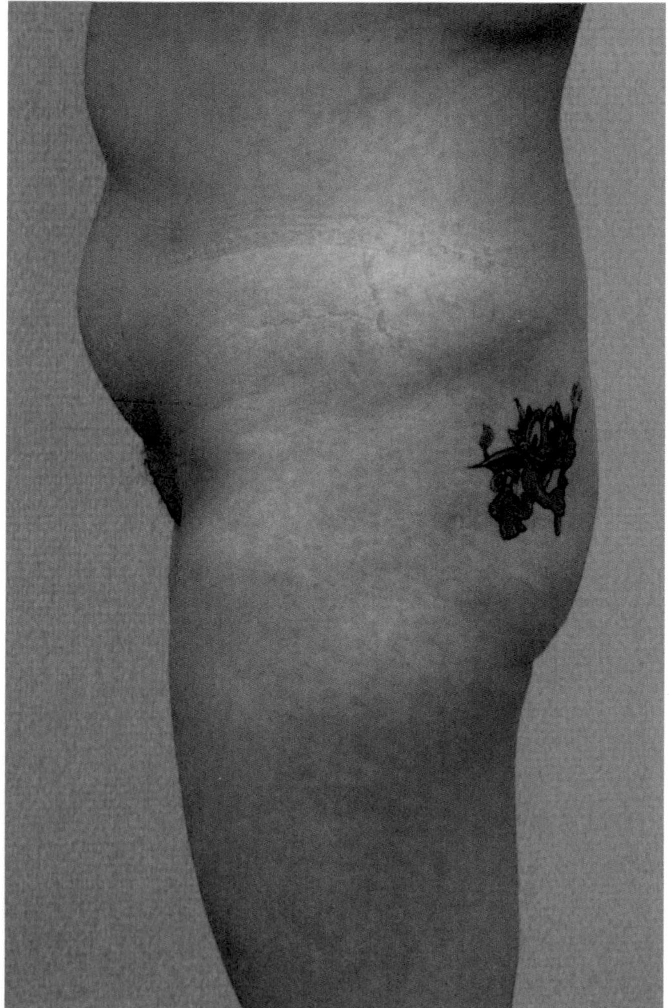

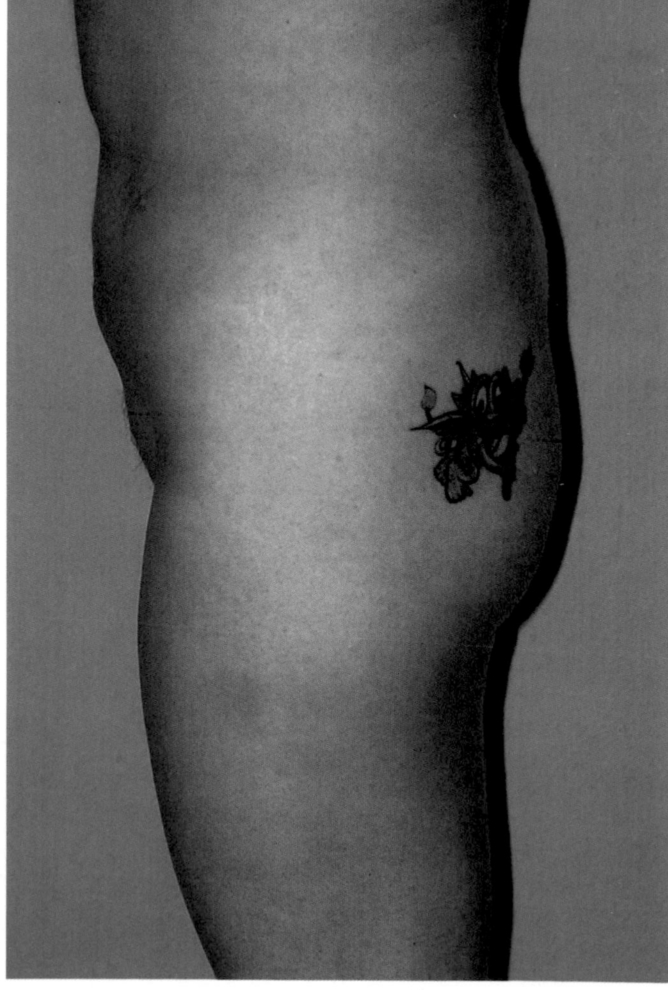

fig. 90 a+b

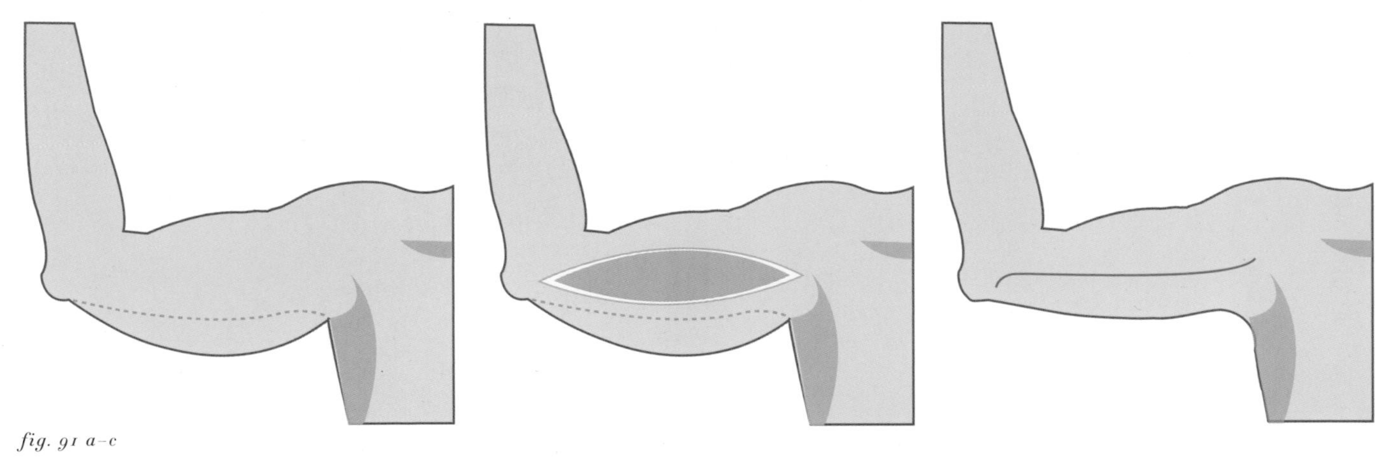

fig. 91 a–c

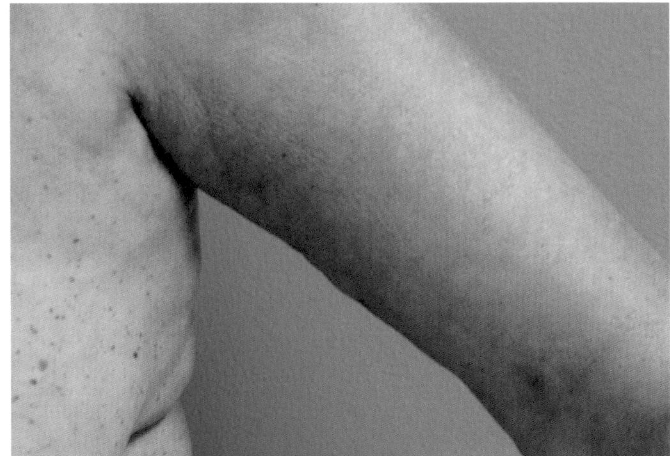

fig. 92 a+b

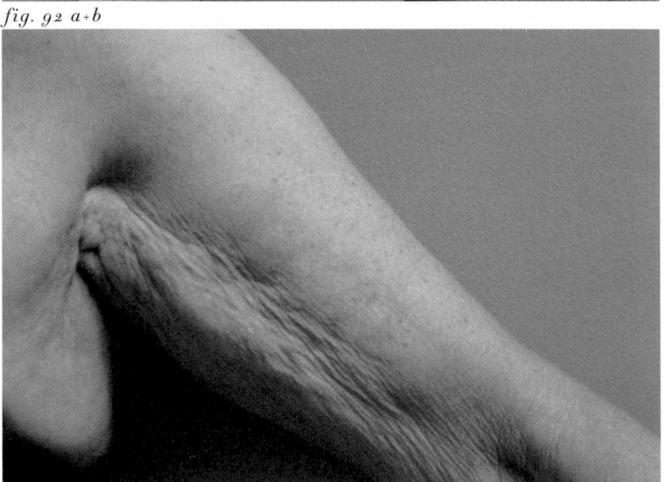

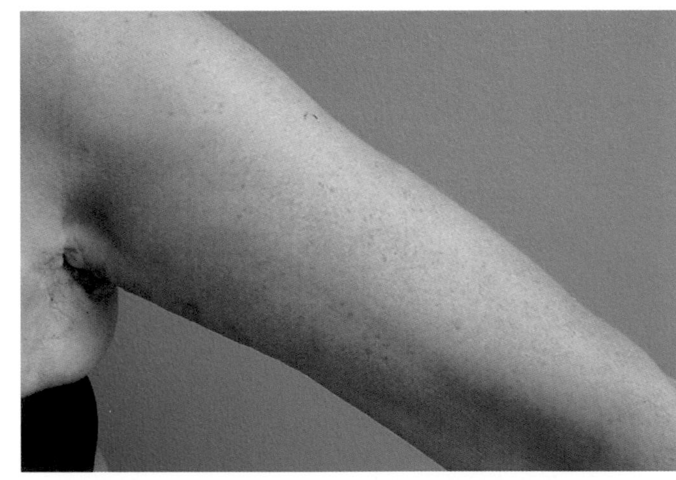

fig. 93 a+b

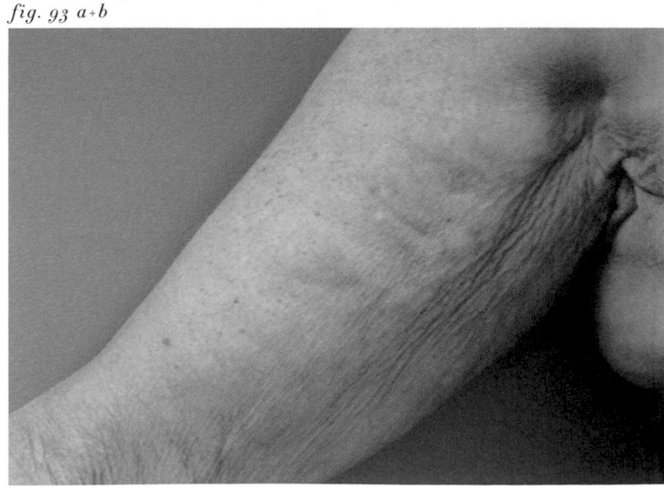

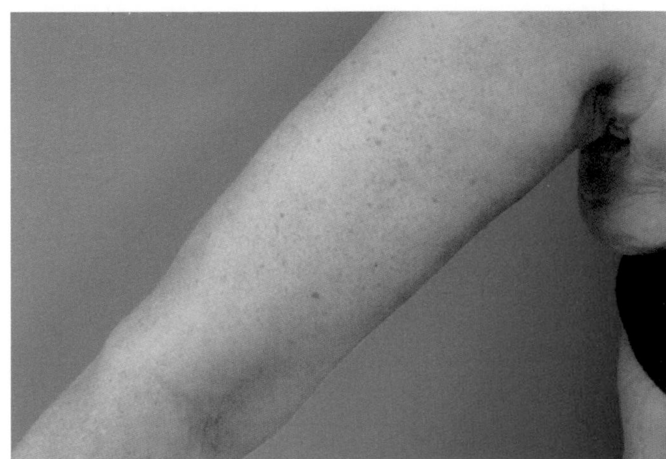

fig. 94 a+b

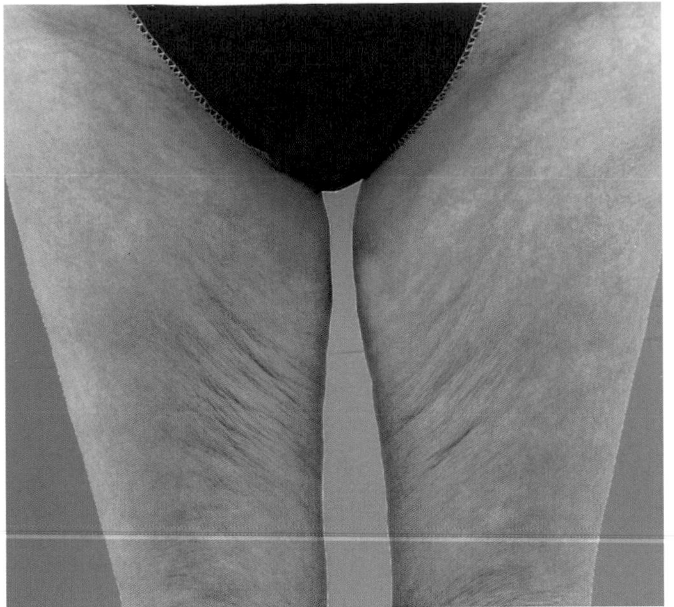

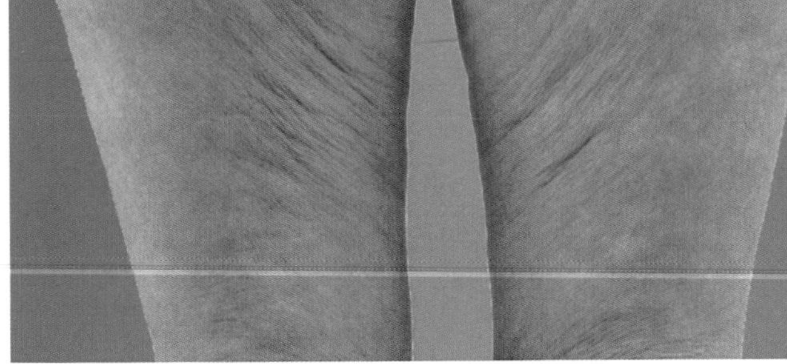

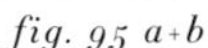

fig. 95 a+b

fig. 91 a–c

Illustrations of a brachioplasty (upper arm lift): here both skin and fatty tissue were removed. The disadvantages of this procedure: it isn't permanent, and it leaves a long scar on the inside of the arm. © Blue Brain Belgium

fig. 92 a+b to 94 a+b

After a certain age, the skin on the upper arms begins to sag and wrinkle, especially on the visible front side of the arm. With well-placed incisions in the armpit and on the inside of the upper arm, both the wrinkles and the amount of fatty tissue can be reduced. Having received a brachioplasty, many patients also want the skin on their hands to be lifted a procedure that has become quite successful. The wrinkles are either filled with autologous fat, or the skin on the fingers is tightened. © Bodenseeklinik Prof. Mang

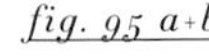

fig. 95 a+b

The inner thighs are one of the main age-related problem areas for women; physical exercise is ineffective for tightening the lax skin. For a thigh lift, the incision is made from the buttocks to the groin. The skin is cut, tightened and fastened to the inguinal ligament so there isn't too much stress on the scar. If the folds are very pronounced, a long incision along the inner thigh can be used to achieve the desired lifting effect. © Bodenseeklinik Prof. Mang

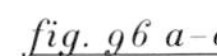

fig. 96 a–c

A thighplasty can be used to lift just the inner thighs, the inner and outer thighs, or also the buttocks. One of the risks associated with this procedure is that the skin may be stretched too much, which can have an unpleasant effect on the outer labia: these may no longer close completely. © Blue Brain Belgium

Upper arm lift (brachioplasty): This is sensible for women and men with pronounced cellulite or where the skin around the arm is "baggy" and sags when the arm is stretched out. Long scars on the inside of the upper arm stay permanently, and the effect wears off with time. The surgical cut runs from the armpit down to the elbow joint.

Thigh lift (thigh dermolipectomy or *thighplasty):* With age, the skin becomes especially lax and wrinkled around the inner thighs. A thigh lift can be performed on just the inner thighs, on the inner and outer thighs, or also on the buttocks. The surgical incisions run along the left and right side of the pelvic bone down to the groin and around the inner thighs towards the buttocks. On the back of the torso, the cut runs along the buttocks' horizontal folds, ending at the gluteal furrow. If the inner thighs are to be lifted along their entire length, the cut runs from the groin down to the inside knees.

Risk: Lifting the inner thighs too significantly can have a very unpleasant effect on the outer labia, as these may no longer close fully.

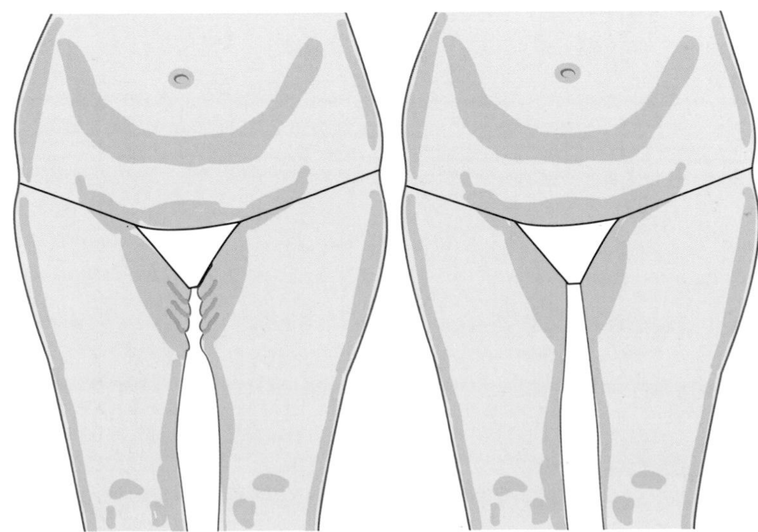

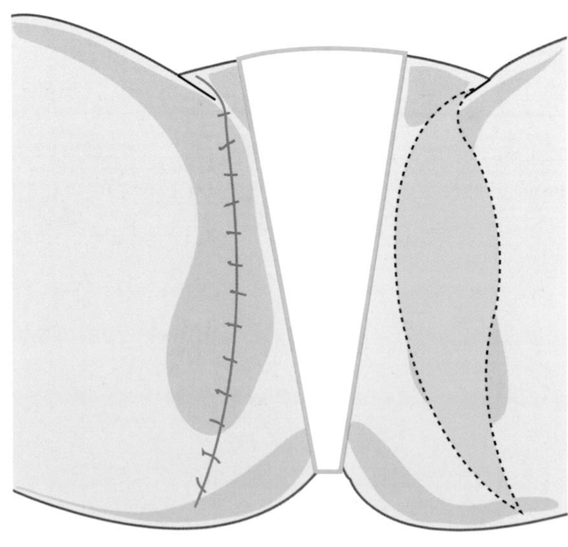

fig. 96 a–c

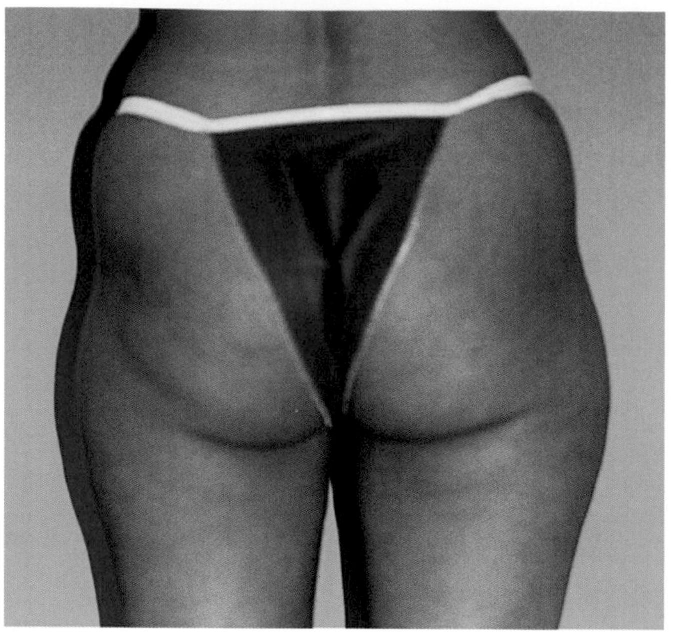

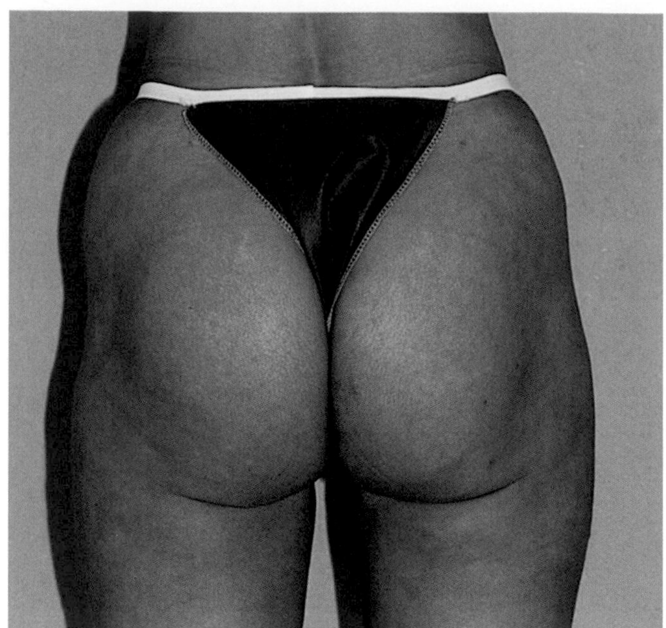

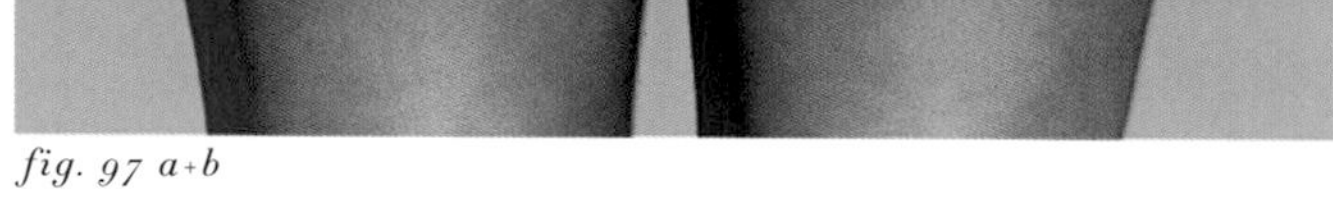

fig. 97 a+b

Calf augmentation: Overly narrow calves, a problem predominantly encountered by men, and calves that are dissimilar may be caused by a congenital muscular weakness or by complex bone fractures. To counter this, the calves can be enlarged with hard or soft silicone gel implants. While the patient is fully sedated, the surgeon cuts two pockets between the lower thigh muscles and tissue, and the implants are inserted. The operative risks are low; in rare cases, fluid may gather in the tissue pockets which needs to be drained – surgically, if necessary.

Buttocks augmentation: Predominantly men, but also some women get their flat buttocks rounded out with butt implants. The silicone gel-filled inlays are round or drop-shaped. The operation requires general anaesthesia. The incision is made between the two buttocks, creating a right and left tissue pocket between the buttock muscles. The implants are placed between the gluteus muscles.

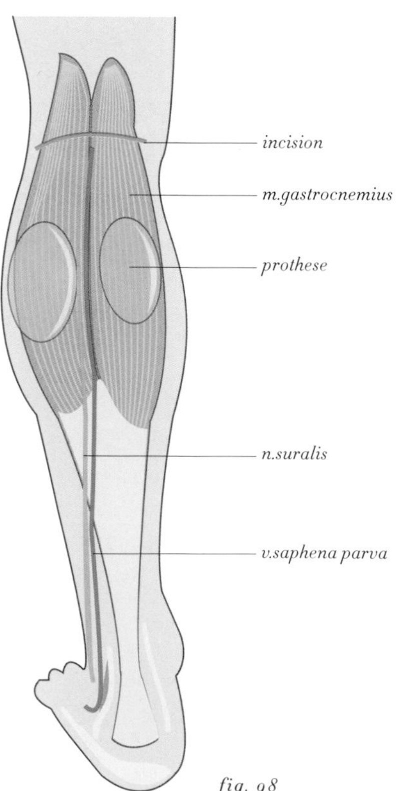

fig. 98

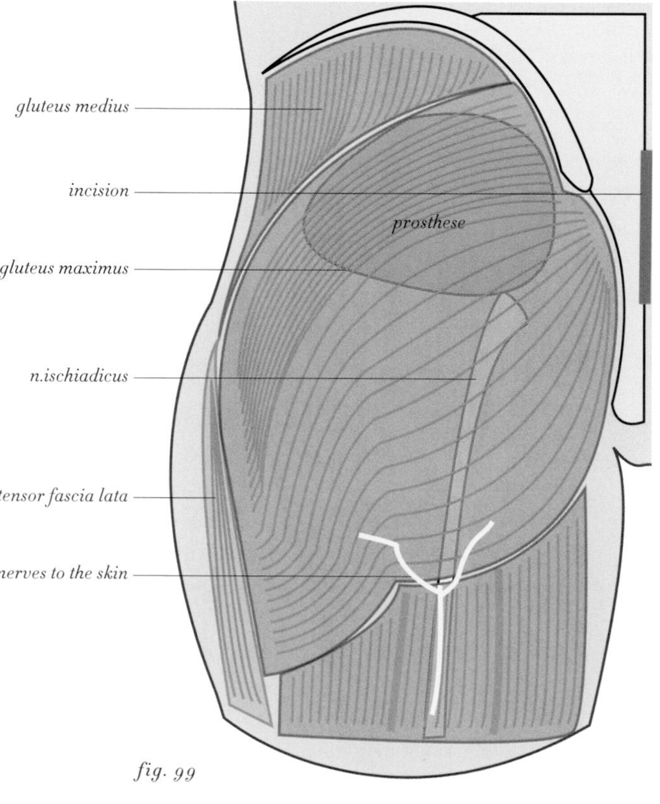

fig. 99

fig. 97 a+b

Calf and buttocks implants are to be used with caution. The surgical technique to place them is comparatively simple, but the patient needs to be aware that the implant may shift as a result of extreme physical activity. This can cause inflammations and pain. Because of this, augmentations in these areas should only be performed after extensive consultation with a practitioner. © Bodenseeklinik Prof. Mang

fig. 98 & 99

Implants made of silicone gel can be used to bolster flat buttocks and overly narrow calves. The drawings show the incision areas and the positions for the implants. © Blue Brain Belgium

fig. 100 a+b

For a penis extension, a crescent-shaped incision is made at the root of the penis. This severs the ligaments that suspend the penis from the pubic bone. As a result, the penis slides outwards by several centimetres. © Blue Brain Belgium

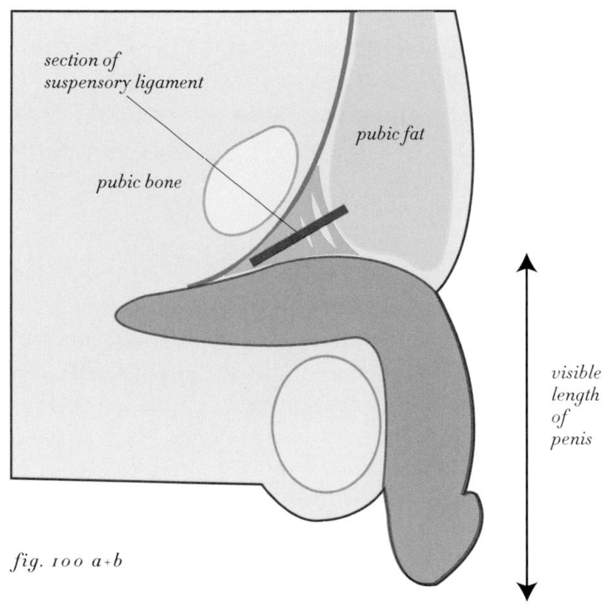

fig. 100 a+b

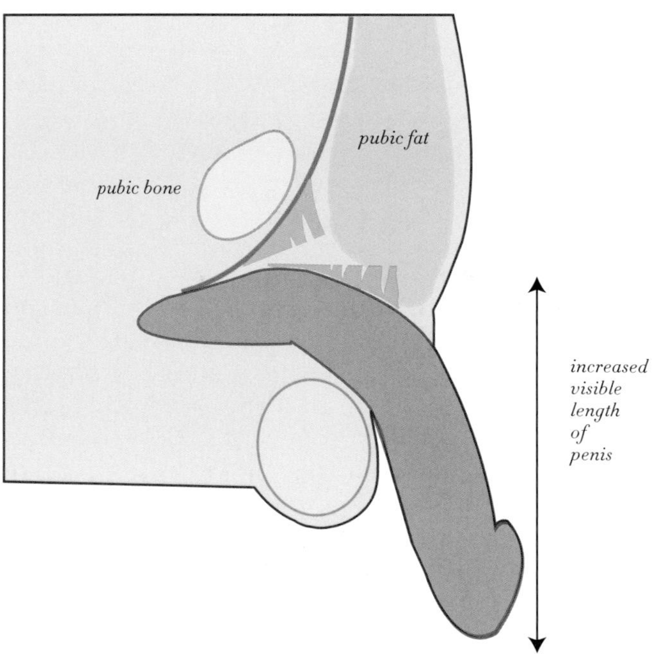

Genitals

Penis enlargement (phalloplasty): For European men, the average length of the erect penis is assumed to be 13 centimetres. Although the length of the penis is not a crucial factor for sexual pleasure, an extension of up to five centimetres can increase the man's self-confidence and libido. Similarly, a narrow penis (standard circumference ca. 12 centimetres when erect) can be widened by approx. two centimetres. Both procedures, extension and widening, require full sedation and an advance urological examination. The pubic hair is shaved off. A hospital stay of three to four days should be planned for. After the operation, the wound is initially quite sore, and urinating may be difficult. In this case, a catheter can be inserted. The patient should refrain from sexual activities for eight weeks.

Extension: A small, crescent-shaped cut is made in the root of the penis. This severs the ligaments that suspend the penis from the pubic bone inside the abdominal cavity. As a result, it slides several centimetres outwards. The incision is sutured and sealed with a sterilised bandage. In the first six months, the penis needs to be stretched for thirty minutes every day with weights ranging from 500 to 3,000 grams.

Widening: This procedure utilises autologous skin strips (5 cm x 15 cm), harvested from the groin or the buttocks fold. Using small incisions, they are placed underneath the penis skin starting at the glans – sometimes with the help of an endoscope.

— Risks: Wound pain persisting for weeks, secondary haemorrhages, infections, unsightly scars, erection problems, lack of sensation. If a nerve tract is damaged during the procedure, this may cause impotence. If the nerve tracts are fully severed, a penis prosthesis will be necessary.

NOTE: Unfortunately, both the extension and the widening of the penis are very challenging procedures. An intense period of preoperative consultation is essential to address all possible outcomes.

fig. 102 a+b and 103 a+b

These photos show the enlarged outer labia of a 28-year-old patient. The entire operative site is shown at the top (102 a+b); before and after photos of the labia are shown at the bottom (103 a+b). © Gary J. Alter M.D.

fig. 101 a-d

After a woman has given birth to one or more children, experienced menopause or had cervical cancer, her vagina may be enlarged significantly. By removing a wedge-shaped flap from the back of the vagina, it can be narrowed. Note that this operation can be very painful. © Blue Brain Belgium

Vaginoplasty: Some women's vaginas are significantly enlarged by giving birth. A vagina reduction may also be desired after menopause or after cervical cancer, as it will increase both partners' sexual enjoyment.

The operation requires general anaesthesia and a hospital stay of one day. The surgeon removes a small, wedge-shaped flap from the back of the vagina and then sutures together the gap between muscle and skin. For the first few days after the operation, strong pain may be experienced. After approx. ten days, the wound has largely healed. Sexual intercourse should only be undertaken with great care in the first weeks.

Risk: If the surgeon makes the vagina too narrow, sex will be painful until the scar has stretched sufficiently. This takes approx. four weeks.

Labiaplasty: Sometimes, the inner labia extend beyond the outer labia. Discomfort can be caused by sexual intercourse or contact with garments.
The labia can be reduced or reshaped according to the patient's wishes. This only requires a local anaesthetic and usually entails no complications. The healing processis complete after approx. one month.

Hymen restoration: Virginity is a prerequisite for marriage in some cultures, particularly for religious reasons.
The patient is sedated and the hymen is restored using approx. six sutures. Operative complications are unknown; healing is completed after one week.

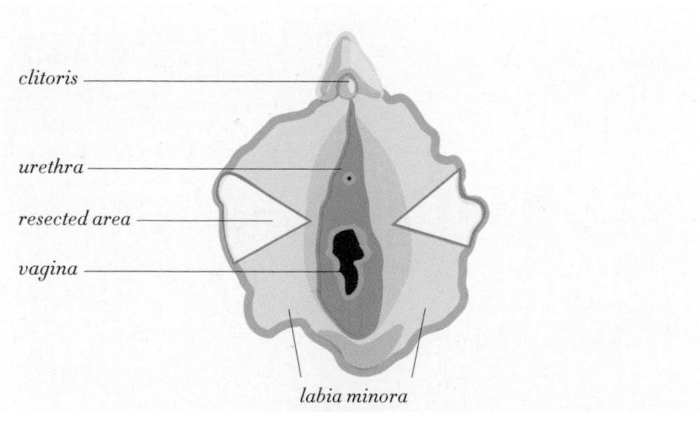

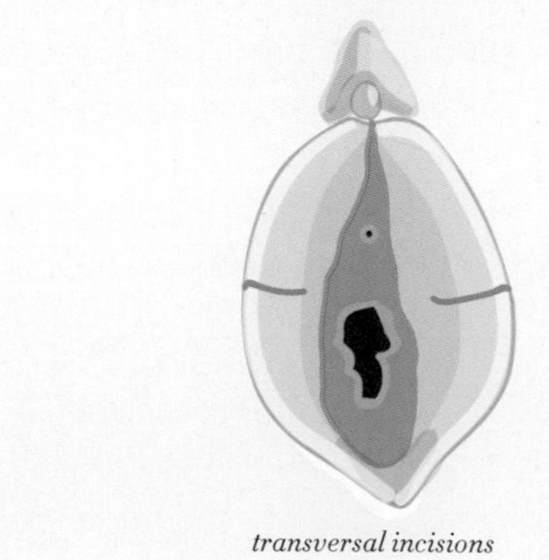

before

labia majora

labia minora

after

labia majora

labia minora

fig. 101 a–d

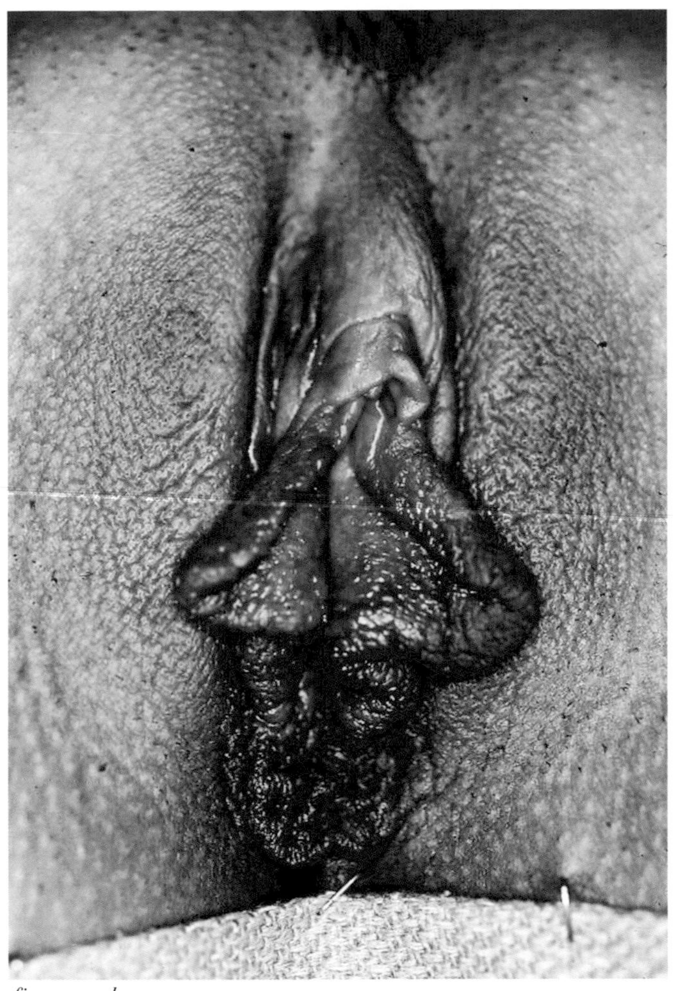

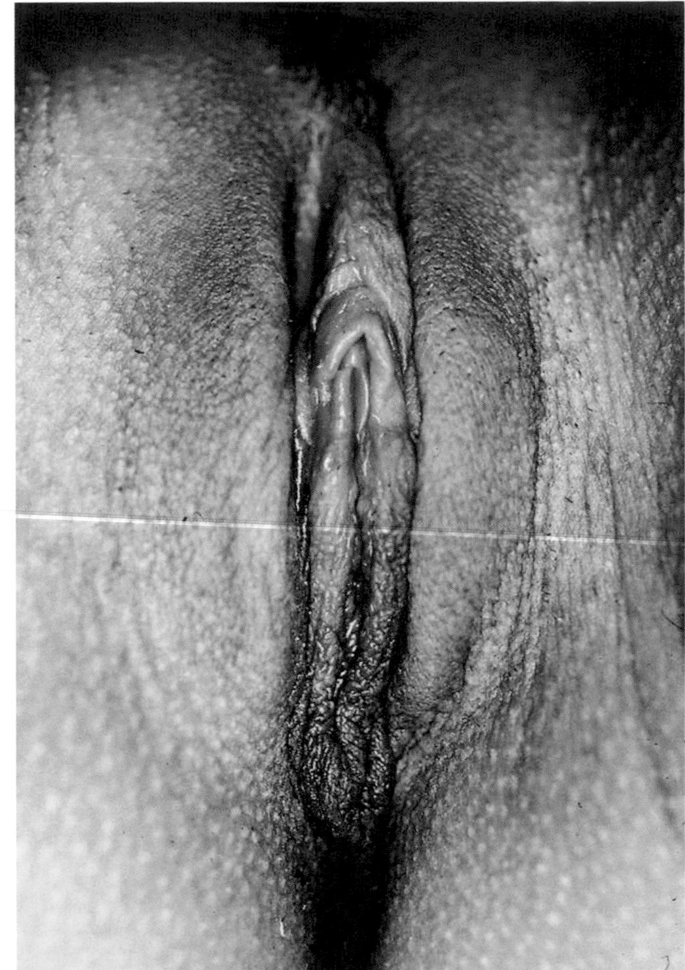

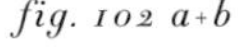

fig. 102 a+b

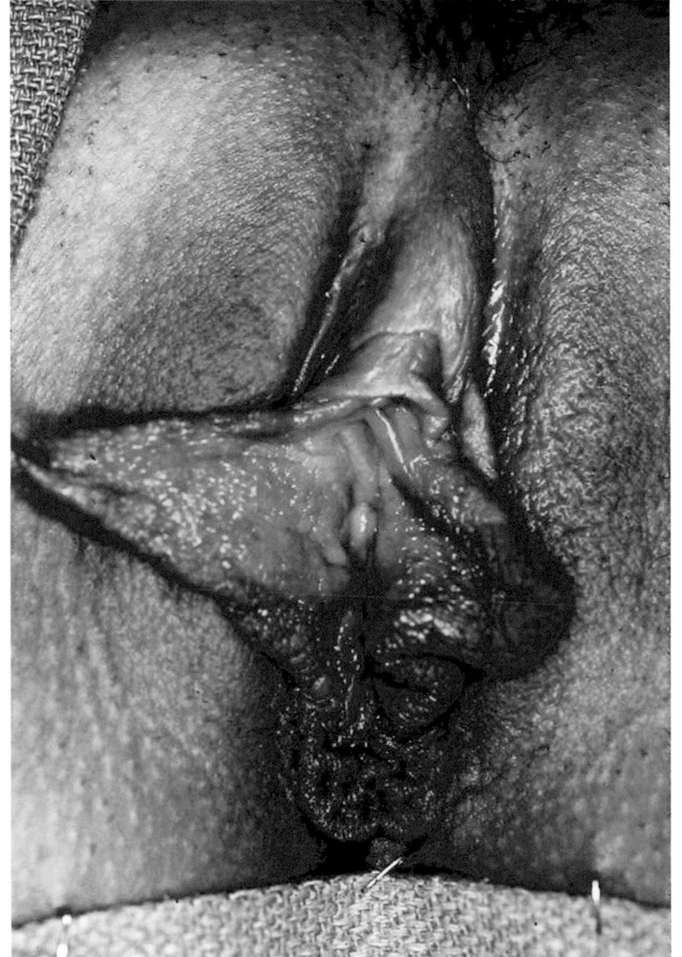

fig. 103 a+b

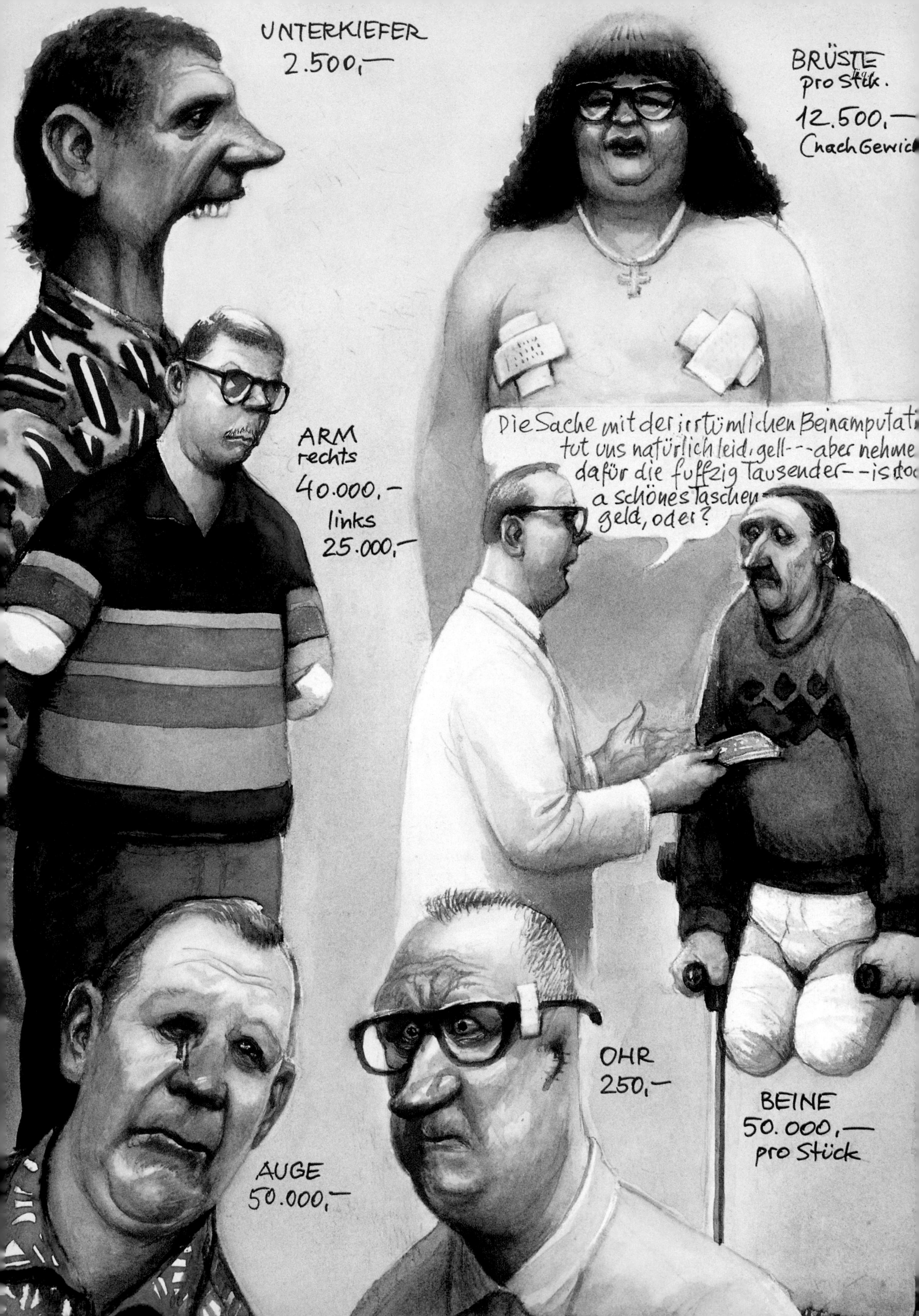
UNTERKIEFER
2.500,–
BRÜSTE
pro Stück.
12.500,–
(nach Gewic
ARM
rechts
40.000,–
links
25.000,–
Die Sache mit der irrtümlichen Beinamputati
tut uns natürlich leid, gell---aber nehme
dafür die fuffzig Tausender--is doc
a schönes Taschen
geld, oder?
OHR
250,–
BEINE
50.000,–
pro Stück
AUGE
50.000,–

X.

JOKES AND CARICATURES

compiled by

NANNETTE BUEHL

Jokes and Caricatures

NANNETTE BUEHL, Paris

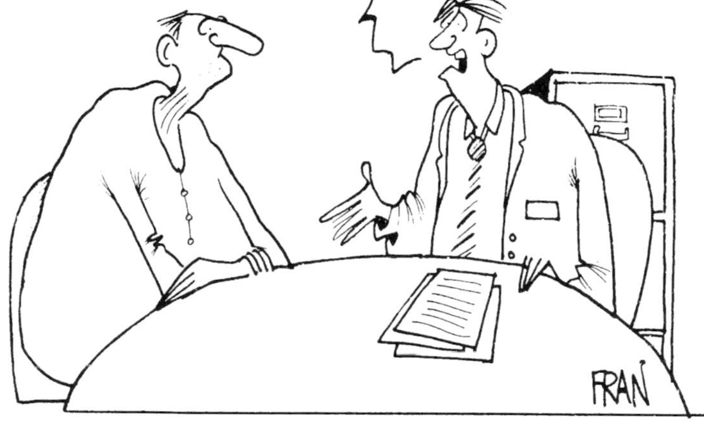

fig. 1

The plastic surgeon and his wife
are walking on the beach when they
find an old oil lamp.
As they brush the sand from the lamp,
a genie appears.
"You each may have one wish."
the genie says.
"Well, I'm 45 and it's time I had
what's due to me." says the wife.
"I wish I lived in a ten-million-dollar
mansion overlooking this beach."
And – poof – she disappears,
and a huge ornate building suddenly
appears on the bluff.

In her court testimony, Anna Nicole Smith said she and her 90-year-old husband were like 'two peas in a pod.' More like two melons and a prune. It turns out the old billionaire's last mistress died during plastic surgery — or as they call it in L.A., natural causes.

The Tonight Show with JAY LENO

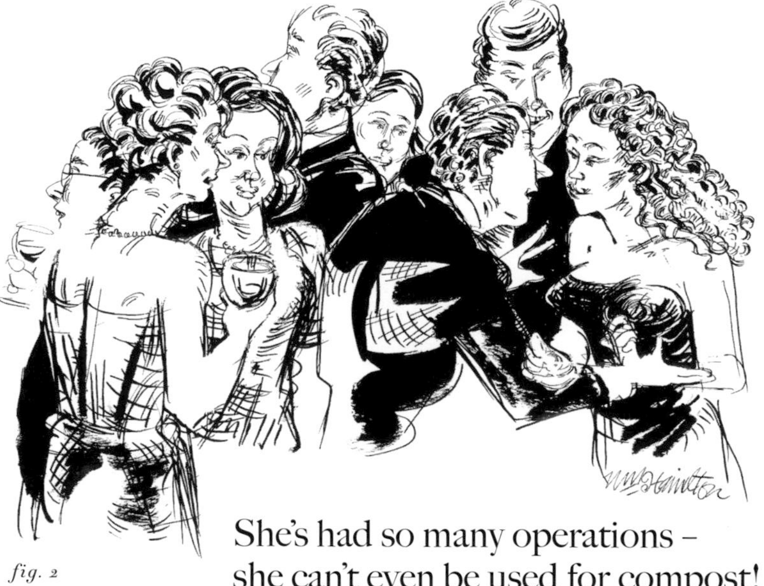

fig. 2

She's had so many operations –
she can't even be used for compost!

fig. previous pages

(from top left): lower jaws – 2.500,–; breasts, per piece – 12.500,– (depending on weight); right arm – 40.000,–; left arm – 25.000,–; "Of course we're sorry about mistakenly amputating the leg ... what would you say about the fifty grand – that's a nice tip, isn't it?"; eye – 50.000,–; ear – 250,–; legs, per piece – 50.000,–. © Manfred Deix

I was going to have cosmetic surgery until I noticed that the doctor's office was full of portraits by Picasso.

RITA RUDNER, show mistress, comedienne

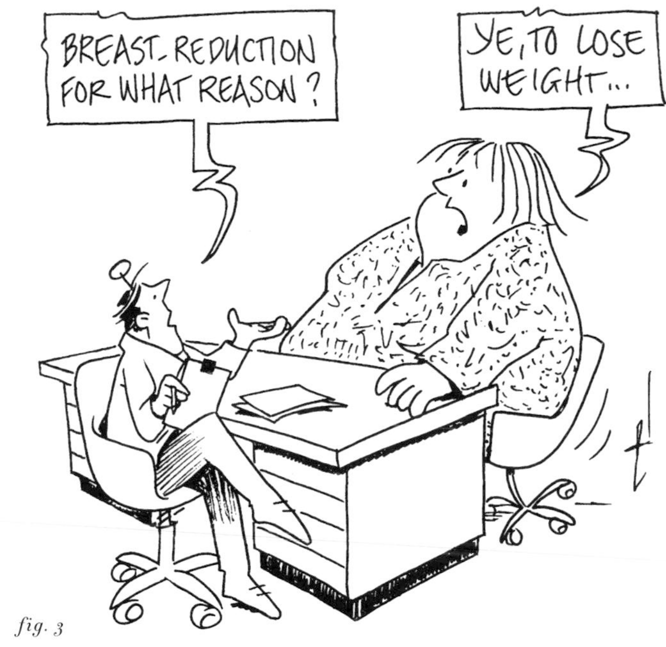

fig. 3

Miss Winterbottom, go have a tummy tuck, get some breast implants, have a session on the sun bed, and then come back to take a dictation!

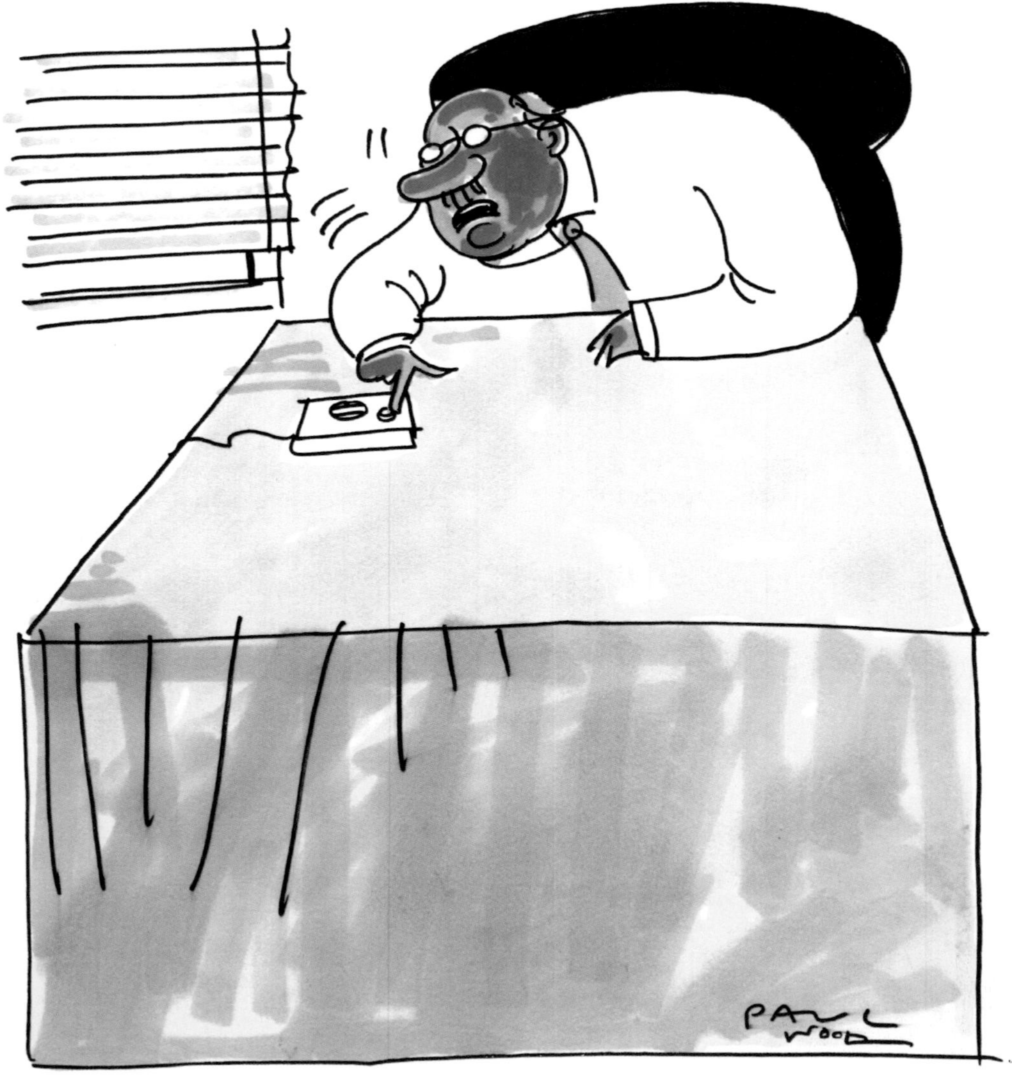

fig. 4

They can take the fat from your rear and use it to bang out the dents in your face. Now that's what I call recycling. It gives a whole new meaning to dancing cheek to cheek.

ANITA WISE, comedienne

fig. 5 © www.CartoonStock.com
fig. 6 © www.CartoonStock.com

Monica Lewinsky says she's thinking of having plastic surgery on her forehead. She's having a cup holder put in.

The Tonight Show with JAY LENO

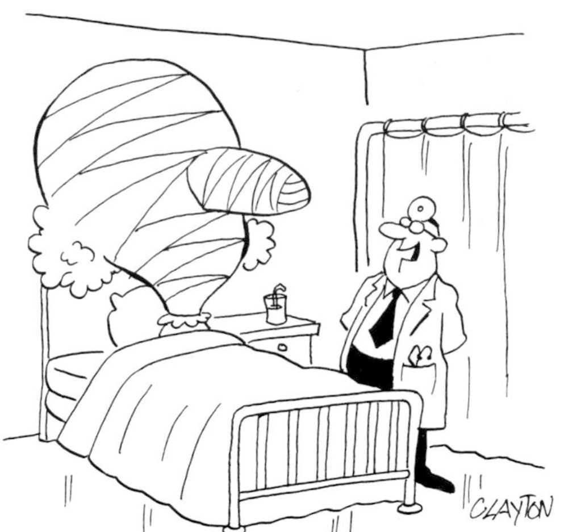

"NO NEED TO WORRY, MRS. JOHNSON— — A LITTLE SWELLING IS PERFECTLY NORMAL AFTER A FACE-LIFT."

fig. 5

There was a married couple who were in a terrible accident. The woman's face was burned severely. The doctor told the husband they couldn't graft any skin from her body because she was so skinny. The husband then donated some of his skin ... However, the only place suitable to the doctor was from his buttocks. The husband requested that no one be told of this, because after all this was a very delicate matter! After the surgery was completed, everyone was astounded at the woman's new beauty. She looked more beautiful than she ever did before! All her friends and relatives just ranted and raved at her youthful beauty! She was alone with her husband one day and she wanted to thank him for what he did. She said, "Dear, I just want to thank you for everything you did for me! There is no way I could ever repay you!!!" He replied, "Oh don't worry, Honey. I get plenty thanks enough every time your mother comes over and kisses you on your cheek!!"

You'd think if he was THAT successful, he could have got a different nose.

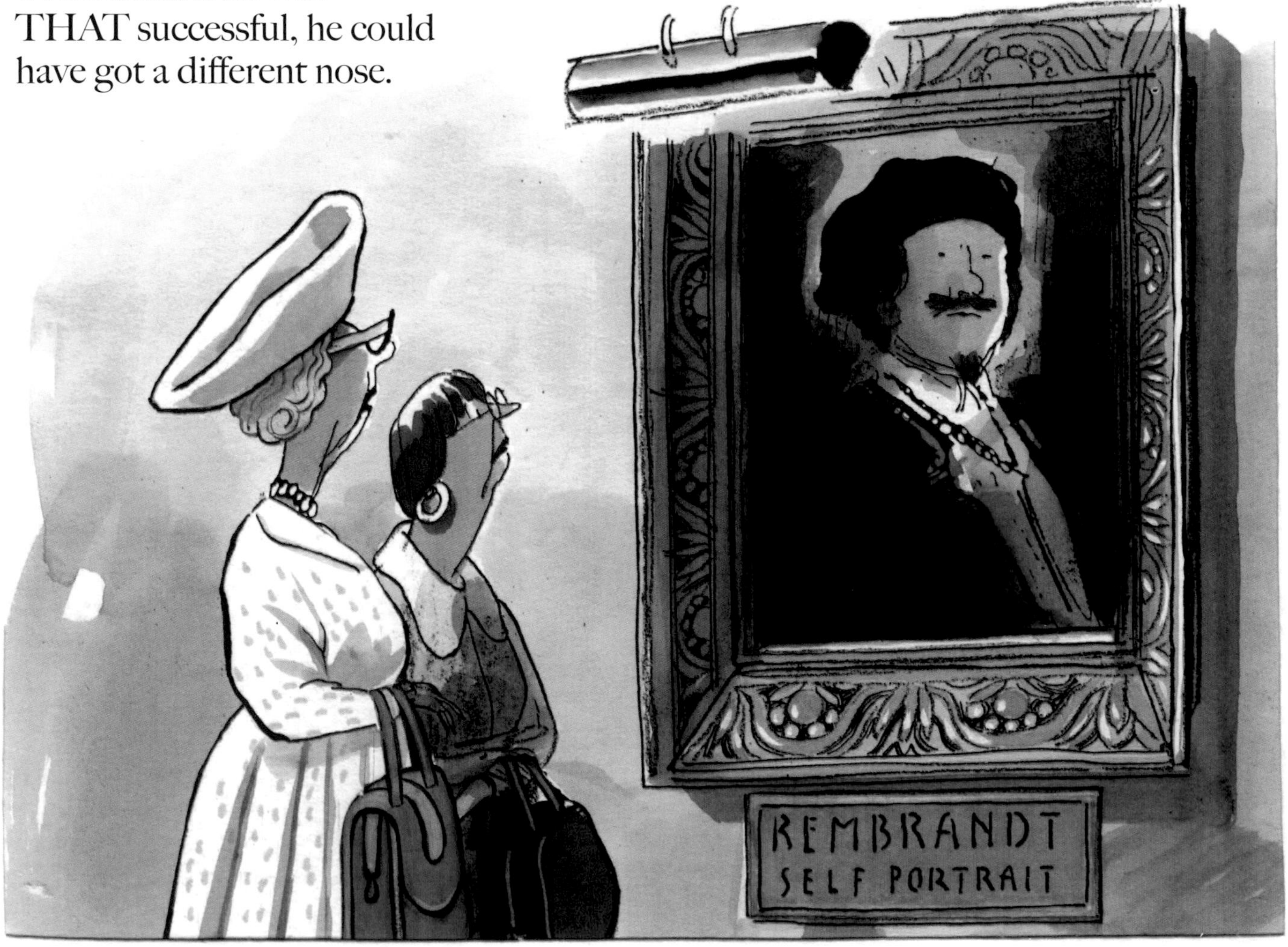

fig. 6

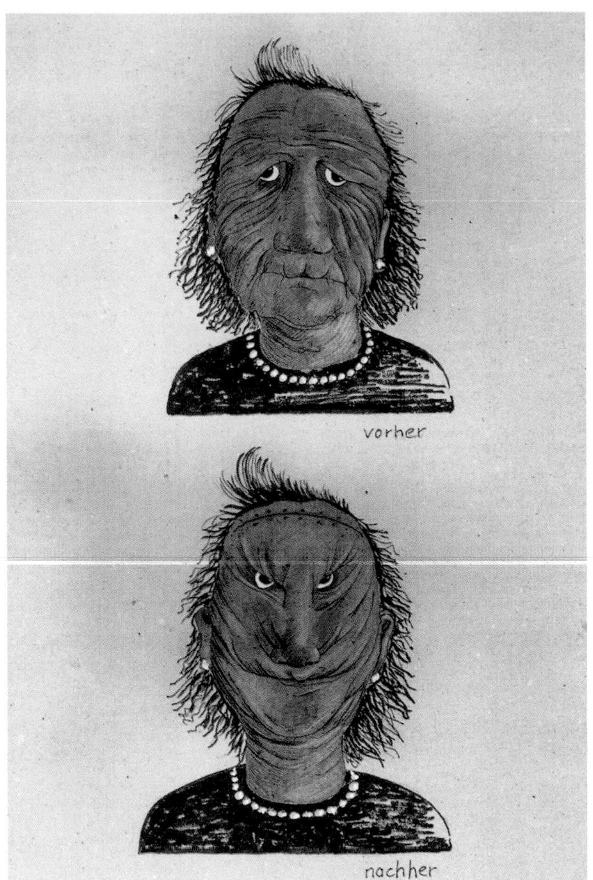

fig. 7 *before … after*

I don't mind to undergo plastic surgery. The only problem is that you end up looking following your dumb doctor's idea of beauty.

ANA VON REBEUR, comedy writer, cartoonist

A Beverly Hills plastic surgeon is being accused of fondling celebrities' breasts while they were under anesthesia. In response the doctor said, "I had to fondle their breasts, I was installing them."

CONAN O'BRIEN, show master, comedy writer

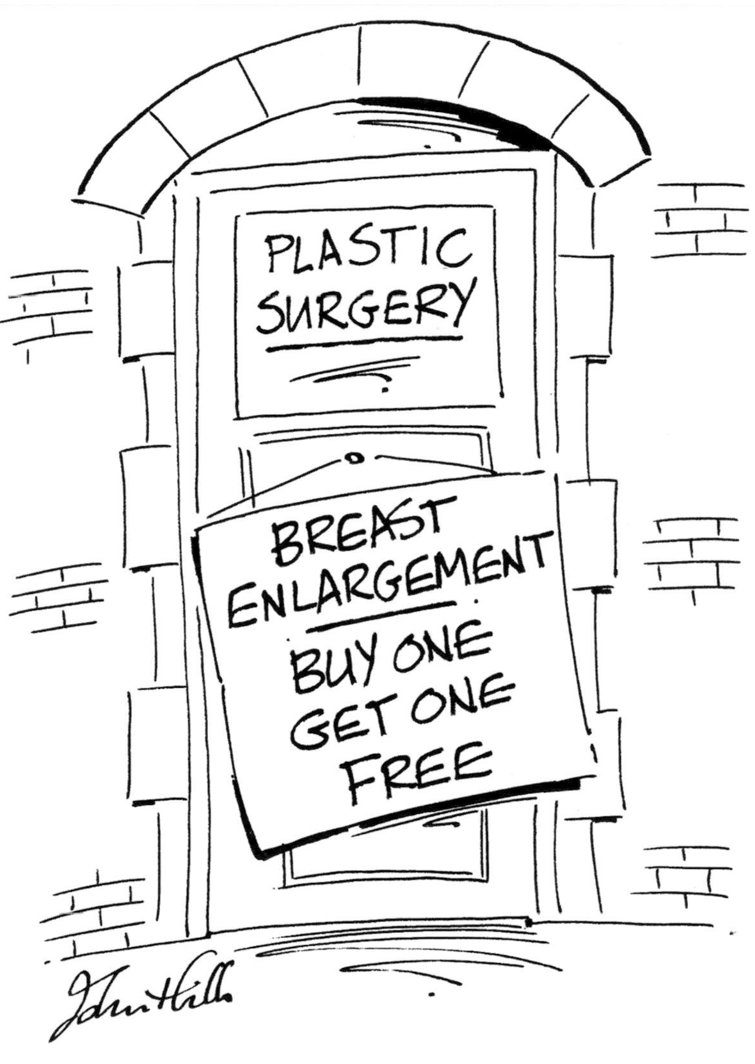

fig. 8

The only parts left of my original body are my elbows.

PHYLLIS DILLER, stand-up comedian

fig. 9

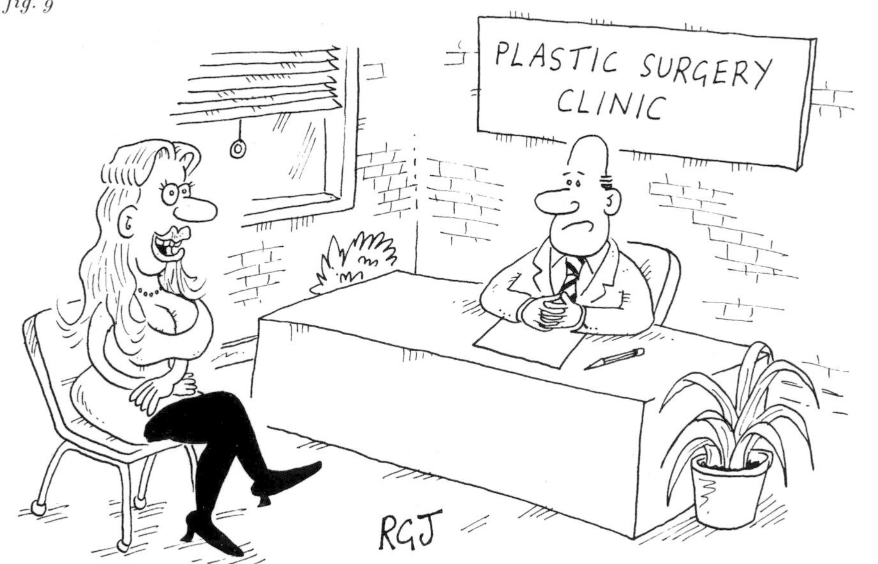

"Do you also do brain enlargements?"

The latest report is that Osama bin Laden has shaved his beard, is wearing Western clothes and has had plastic surgery. Isn't that amazing? The guy has made just two videos and he's already gone Hollywood.

The Tonight Show with JAY LENO

– Doctor, the new nose you made is too small! It doesn't match with my face!
– Don't worry, Madam: it matches with your brain!

ANA VON REBEUR, comedy writer, cartoonist

– Tell me the truth, doctor. After my silicon implant operation, will I be able to play the violin?
– Of course, madam. Perfectly!
– How marvellous! Because I don't know how!

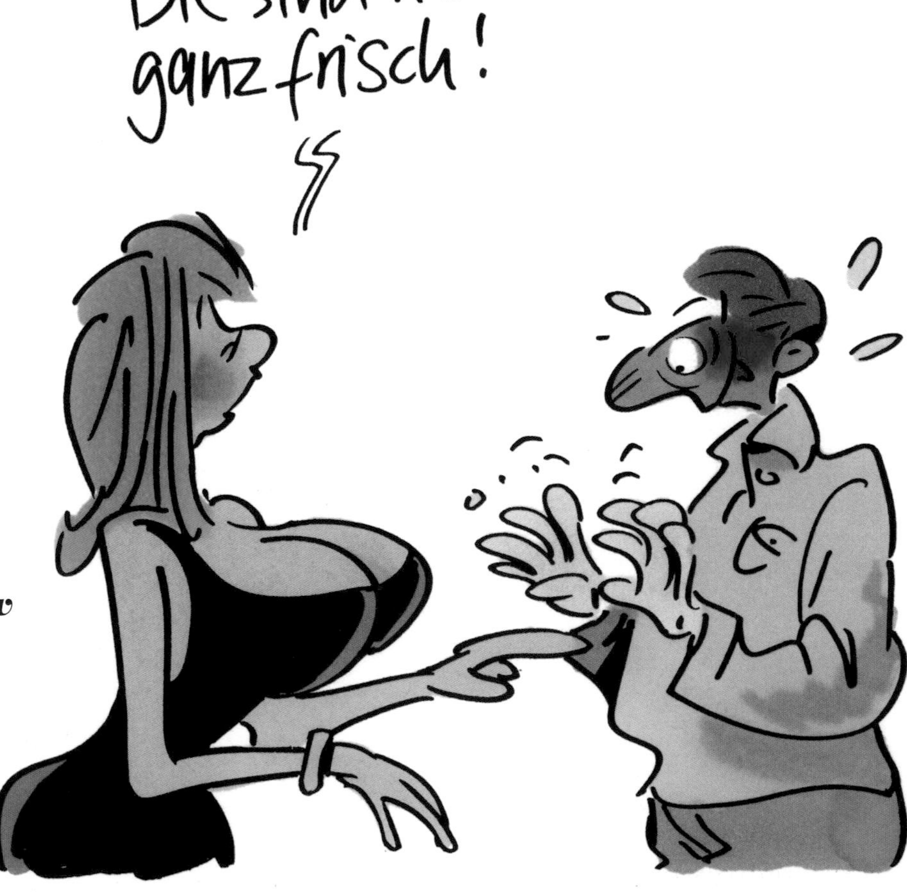

fig. 10 *"Careful! They're brand-new!"*

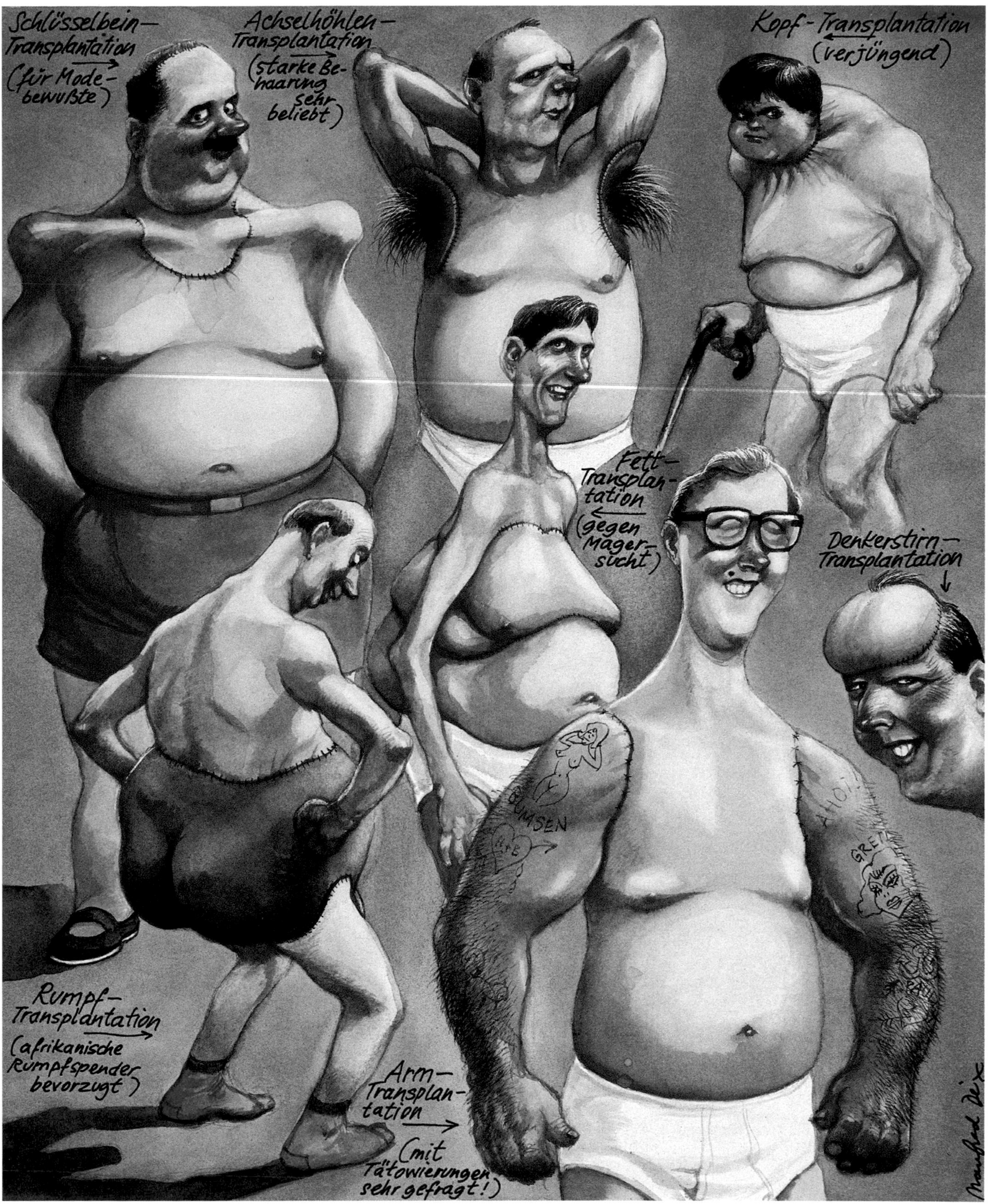

fig. 11

fig. 11

(from top left): clavicle transplant (for the fashion conscious); armpit transplant (dense hair growth, very popular); head transplant (rejuvenating); transplant of fatty tissue (against anorexia); transplant of lofty brow (African rump donors preferred); arm transplant (including tattoos, in high demand!).
© Manfred DeixDeix

I lent my friend $10,000 to pay for plastic surgery. I can't get my money back because I don't know what he looks like now.

Top 10 reasons for being US-American

1. You can claim your country is the best, and really believe it.
2. You can think that American Football is a sport for tough men, while the rest of the world laughs its head off over the monkey suits, panties and shoulderpads taken out of big women's bras.
3. You can claim being the the best democracy while screwing up your own elections.
4. You can assert you are an international super power and elect a president who has been abroad for as much as two times. Or was an actor in B-films.
5. You get to classify McDonalds and Coca Cola as culture.
6. You can criticise China, Turkey and Iran for violating human rights but still legally have capital punishment.
7. You can think that Pharaos ruled over France and nobody will think you are a nitwit.
8. You can be extremely fat or extremely thin, spend 25% of your income on plastic surgery, have two shrinks, do Landmark and be a Scientology fanatic and people will still consider you sane.
9. You can go to Europe for a holiday.
10. Be hysterical about a woman's naked breasts on TV and enjoy live killing on CNN.

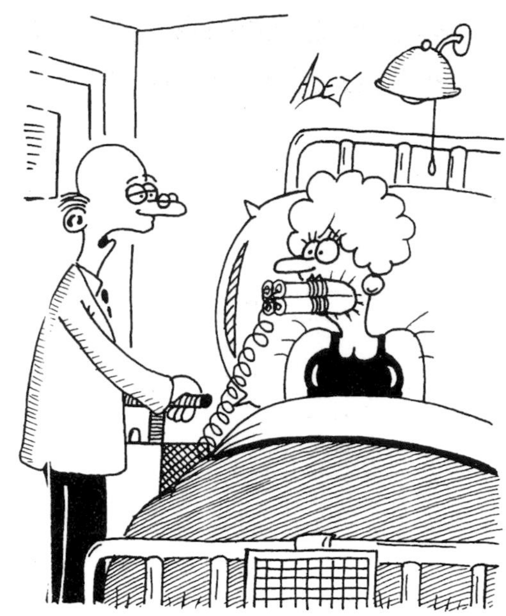

fig. 12

Before we lift your face, we'll have to take off the old one first.

fig. 13

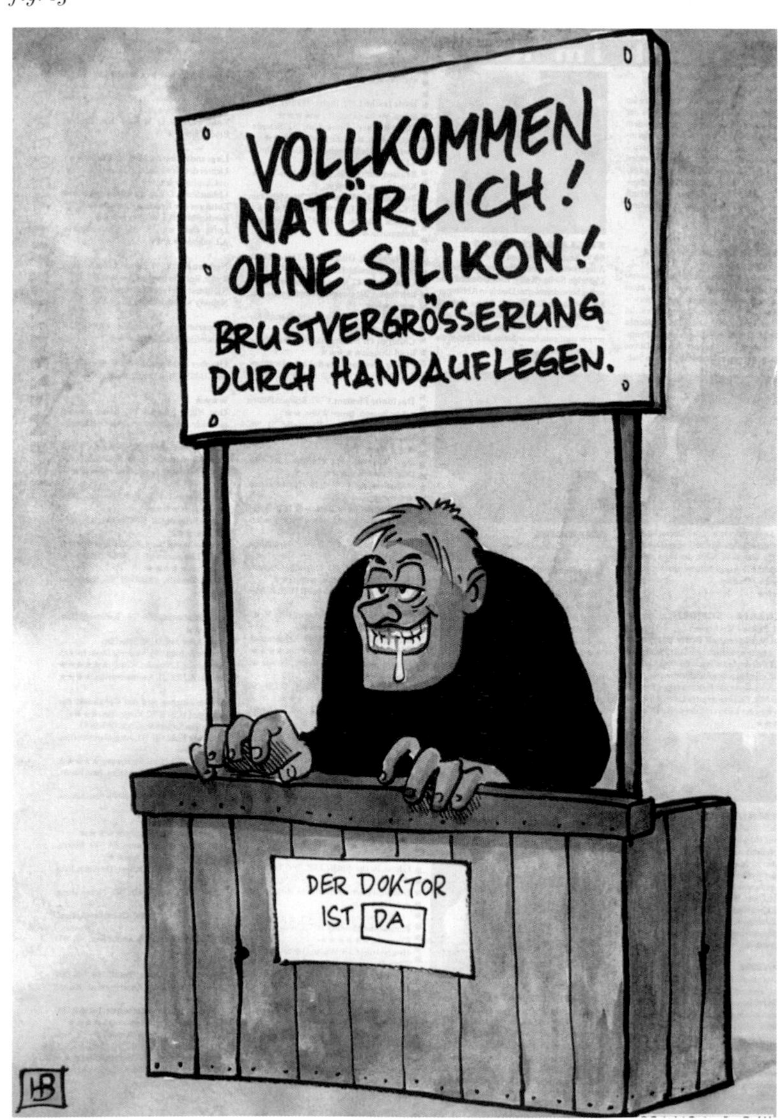

Man: "I'm a photographer. I've been looking for a face like yours!"
Woman: "I'm a plastic surgeon. I've been looking for a face like yours!!!"

*"Men's Health" says men spent as much money on plastic surgery as women did last year. It's epidemic in California. *Hannibal Lector refuses to eat people from L.A. because they contain too many artificial ingredients.*

ARGUS HAMILTON, comedian, joke writer

Totally natural! No silicone! Hands-on breast enlargement! (The doctor is "IN".)

**One plastic surgeon to another:
"My daughter gets her good looks from me."**

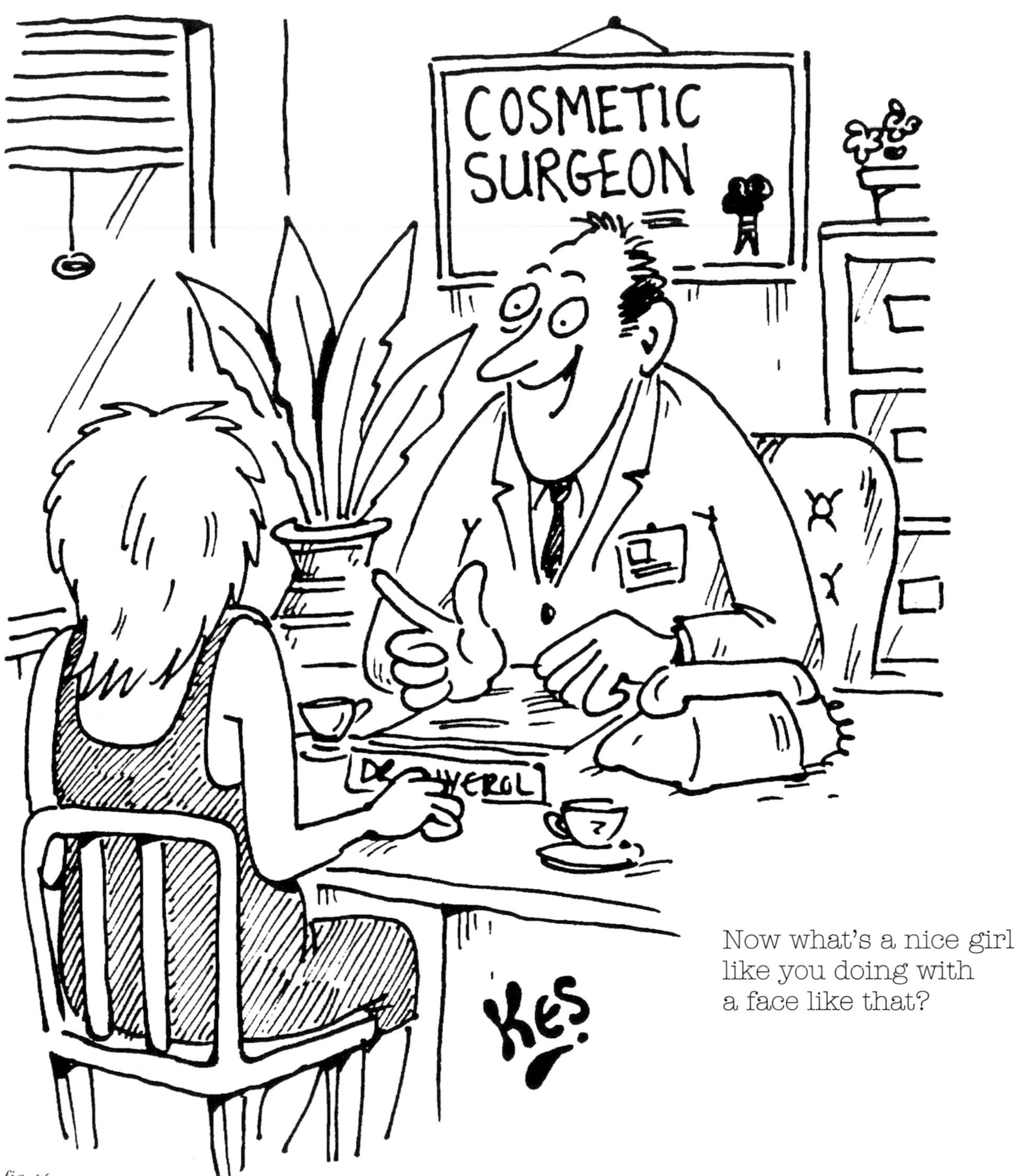

Now what's a nice girl like you doing with a face like that?

fig. 14

I have heard men say that they don't mind the idea of breast implants in a woman because, after all, big breasts are big breasts. On the other hand, I have never met a woman who would rather be with a man in a toupee then a bold man.

MERRILL MARKOE, Stand-up comedian, comedy writer

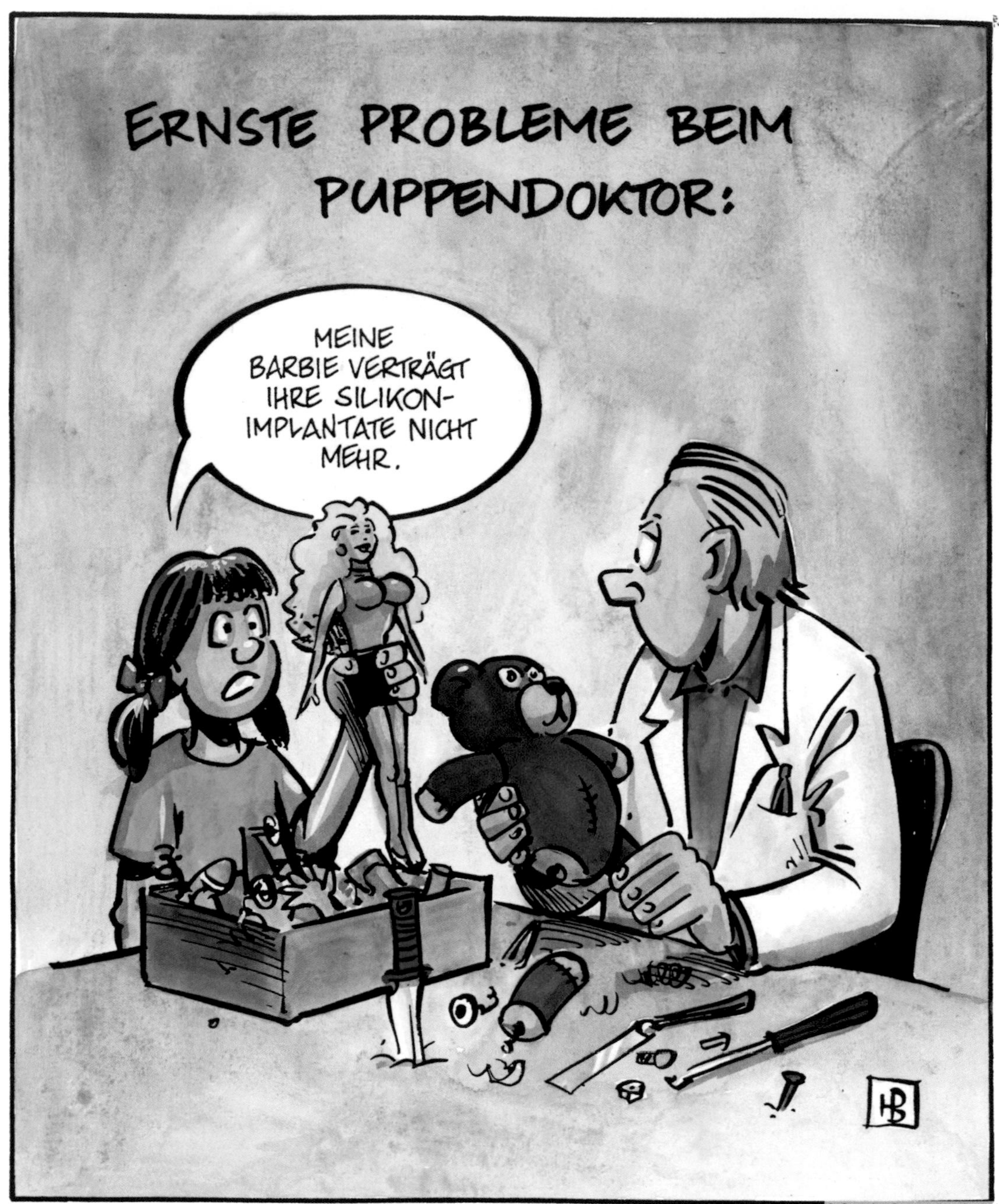

fig. 15

An emergency at the toy doctor's:
"My Barbie doll needs to get her breast implants removed!"

A man is dating three women and wants to decide which to marry. He decides to give them a test.
He gives each woman a present of 5 000 Dollar and watches to see what they do with the money.
The first does a total makeover. She goes to a fancy beauty salon, gets her hair done, new make up and buys several new outfits and dresses up very nicely for the man. She tells him that she has done this to be more attractive for him because she loves him so much. The man is impressed.
The second goes shopping to buy the man gifts. She gets him a new set of golf clubs, some new gizmos for his computer and some expensive clothes. As she presents these gifts, she tells him that she has spent all the money on him because she loves him so much. Again, the man is impressed.
The third invests the money in the stock market. She earns several times the 5 000 Dollar. She gives him back his 5 000 Dollar and reinvests the remainder in a joint account. She tells him that she wants to save for their future because she loves him so much. Obviously, the man is impressed.

The man thinks for a long time about what each woman has done with the money, and then ...
he marries the one with the largest breasts!

How does a woman show she's planning for the future? With plastic Surgery.

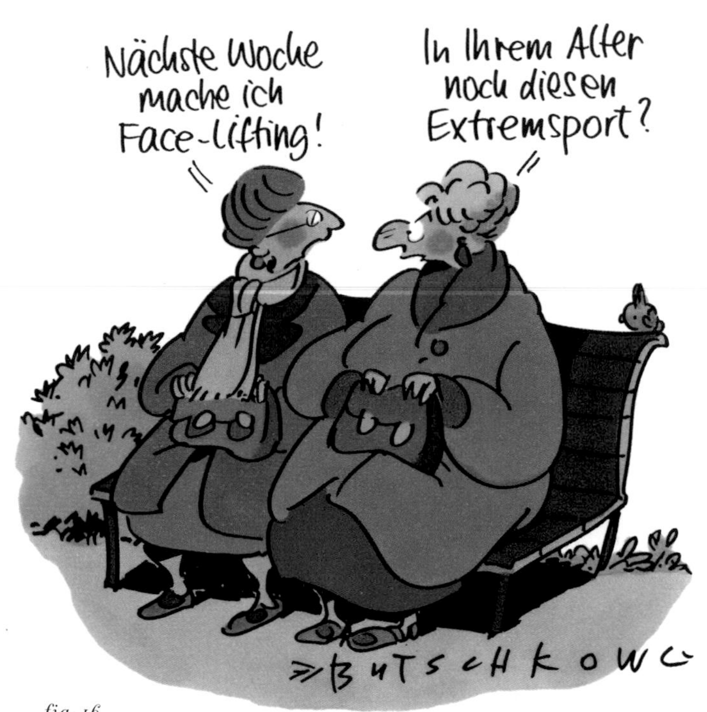

fig. 16

"I've got a face-lifting session next week!" — "You're still doing sports at your age?"

A man lost both ears in an accident. No plastic surgeon could offer him a solution. He heard of a very good one in Sweden, and went to him. The new surgeon examined him, thought a while and said, "yes, I can put you right."
After the operation, bandages off, stitches out, he goes to his hotel. The morning after, in a rage, he calls his surgeon and yells, "You swine, you gave me a woman's ears."
"Well, an ear is an ear, what's wrong? Can't you hear?"
"You're wrong, I hear everything, but I don't understand a thing!"

The wife complains to her husband that her boobs are too small and wants to get a boob job!
Husband replies "Honey, where we gonna get the money for that?" "You know we are strapped for money with the new house and new pool. Do you think money grows on trees?"
Wife says, "but honey, It will make you real happy and help me with my self esteem!!! Don't you want to have a pretty woman with large breasts on your arm when we go out, not to mention the joys of playing with them?"
Husband, "Well yes, honey, I would like that. But we really can't afford it! Tell you what hon, how about if I help you."
Wife, "Okay sweety, what do you have in mind??"
Husband, "How about if I take some tissue paper and rub it on each breast everyday for about a year. That ought to do it!"
Wife: "How the hell will that help them grow ???"
Husband: "I'm not sure, honey, but it certainly worked for your butt!!!"

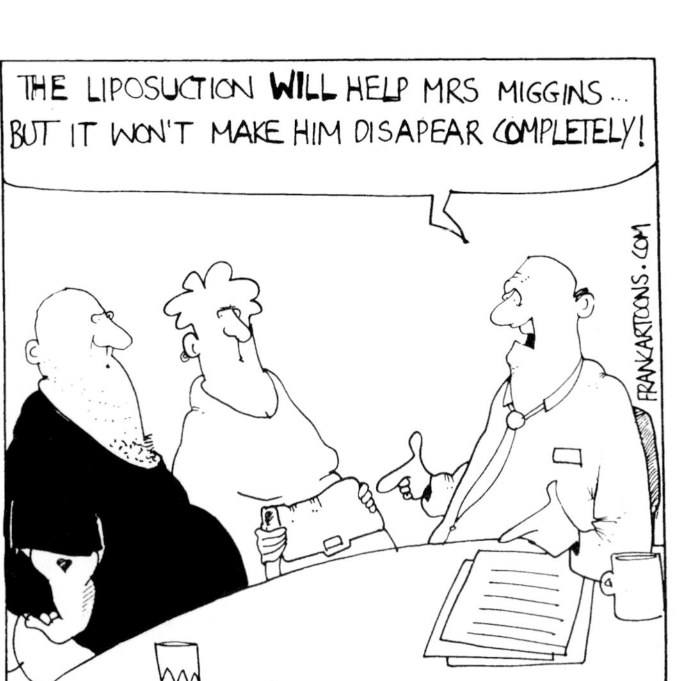

fig. 17

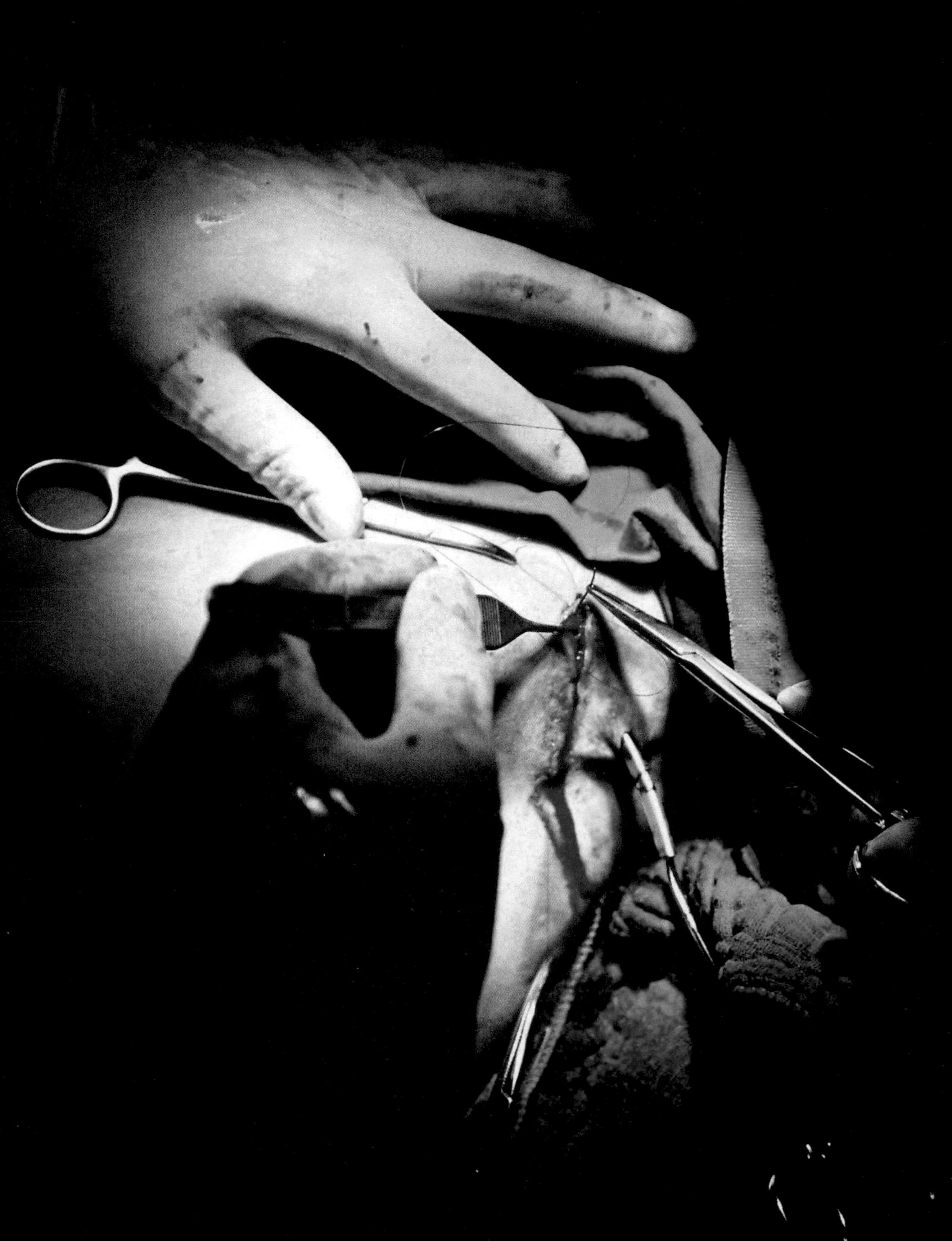

XI.

APPENDIX

XI.1
BIBLIOGRAPHY ON
AESTHETIC SURGERY

XI.2
WEBSITES FOR
PLASTIC SURGERY

XI.3
AESTHETIC SURGEONS'
BIOGRAPHIES AND ADDRESSES

Bibliography on Aesthetic Surgery

Historical Medical Books

- "**B. L.**" *A Curious Chirurgical Operation – in: The Gentleman's Magazine*, October 1794, Vol. 64, Part II (London: John Nichols, 1794)
- **Bankoff, George** *The Story of Plastic Surgery* (London, 1952)
- **Bigelow, Henry Jacob** *Insensiblity during surgical operations produced by inhalation – in: Boston Medical and Surgical Journal*, Vol. XXXV, No. 16 (Boston: David Clapp, 1847)
- **Bigelow, Henry Jacob** *Ether and Chloroform. Their Discovery and Physiological Effects* (Boston: David Clapp, 1848)
- **Carpuc, Joseph Constantine** *An Account of Two Successful Operations for restoring a Lost Nose* (London: Longman, Hurst, Rees, Orme & Brown, 1816)
- **Celsus, Aulus Cornelius** *De medicina* transl. & introd. by W. G. Spence. 3 vol. (London: W. Heinemann; Cambridge MA: Harvard University, 1935–38)
- **Dieffenbach, Johann Friedrich** *Chirurgische Erfahrungen, besonders über die Wiederherstellung zerstörter Theile des menschlichen Körpers nach neuen Methoden.* 4 vols. in 3 und Atlas (Berlin: Enslin, 1829–34)
- **Dieffenbach, Johann Friedrich** *Die Operative Chirurgie*, 2 vols. (Leipzig: Brockhaus 1845–48)
- **Fritze, Hermann Eduard; Reich, O. F. G.** *Die Plastische Chirurgie in ihrem weitesten Umfange dargestellt* (Berlin: Hirschwald, 1845)
- **Frühwald, Victor** *Korrektiv-Kosmetische Chirurgie der Nase, der Ohren und des Gesichts* (Wien: W. Maudrich, 1932)
- **Gnudi, Martha Teach; Webster, Jerome Pierce** *The Life and Times of Gaspare Tagliacozzi, Surgeon of Bologna 1545–1599* (Mailand: U. Hoepli; New York NY: H. Reichner, 1950)
- **Gurlt, Ernst** *Geschichte der Chirurgie und ihrer Ausübung: Volkschirurgie, Alterthum, Mittelalter, Renaissance* 3 vols. (Berlin: Hirschwald, 1898)
- **Hildebrand, Otto** *Die Entwicklung der plastischen Chirugie* (Berlin: Hirschwald, 1909)
- **Hughes, Wendell L.** *Reconstructive Surgery of the Eyelids* (St. Louis MO, 1943)
- **Imre, Josef** *Lidplastik und Plastische Operationen anderer Weichteile des Gesichts* (Budapest: n. d., ca. 1940)
- **Joseph, Jacques** *Nasenplastik und sonstige Gesichtsplastik, nebst einem Anhang über Mammaplastik und einige weitere Operationen aus dem Gebiete der äußeren Körperplastik: ein Atlas und Lehrbuch* (Leipzig: C. Kabitzsch, 1931; limitierter reprographischer Nachdruck der Luxusausgabe: Heidelberg: Kaden, 2004)
- **Joseph, Jacques** *Eine Nasenplastik, ausgeführt in Lokalanaesthesie* (Berlin: G. Stilke, 1927)
- **Joseph, Max** *Handbuch der Kosmetik* (Leipzig, 1912)
- **Kassel, Karl** *Geschichte der Nasenheilkunde von ihren Anfängen bis zum 19. Jahrhundert* (1914; Hildesheim: Olms, 1967)
- **Keegan, D. F.** *Rhinoplastic Operations with a discription of Recent Improvements in the Indian Method* (London, 1900)
- **Kolle, Frederik Stange** *Plastic and Cosmetic Surgery* (New York, 1911)
- **Lampe, Richard** *Dieffenbach* (Leipzig: J. A. Barth, 1934)
- **Lexer, Erich** *Die gesamte Wiederherstellungschirurgie.* 2 vols. (Leipzig: J. A. Barth, 1931)
- **Maltz, Maxwell** *Evolution of Plastic Surgery* (New York: Froben Press, 1946)
- **Margetson, Elizabeth** *Living Canvas. A Romance of Cosmetic Surgery* (London, 1936)
- **McDowell, Frank** *The Source Book of Plastic Surgery* (Baltimore MD, 1977)
- **McDowell, Frank; Brown, James B.; Fryer, Minot P. (ed.)** *Surgery of Face, Mouth and Jaws* (St. Louis MO, 1942)
- **Miller, Charles Conrad** *Cannula Implants and Review of Implantation Technics in Esthetic Surgery* (Chicago IL, 1926)
- **Miller, Charles Conrad** *Cosmetic Surgery. The Correction of Featural Imperfections* (Philadelphia PA, 1924)
- **Noël, A.** *La chirurgie esthétique* (Paris: Masson, 1926)
- **Pancoast, Joseph** *A Treatise on Operative Surgery* (Philadelphia: Carey & Hart, 1844)
- **Pohl, Leander** *Chirurgische und konservative Kosmetik des Gesichts* (Berlin, 1934)

fig. previous pages

Breast augmentation.
© Huber H.-B. / Laif

- **Roberts, John Bingham** *The Cure of Crokked and Otherwise Deformed Noses* (Philadelphia PA, 1889)
- **Sanvenero-Rosselli, Gustavo** *Chirurgia plastica del naso* (Rom: Pozzi, 1931)
- **Schireson, Henry J.** *As Others See You: The Story of Plastic Surgery* (New York NY: Macaulay, 1938)
- **Schönberg, Jorgen Johann Albrecht von** *Sulla restituzione del naso* (Napoli: Tipografia della Guerra, 1819)
- **Seiffert, A.** *Die Operationen an Nase, Mund und Hals*, 2 vols. (Leipzig, 1936)
- **Stotter, James** *Beauty Unmasked* (New York: The Raymond Press, 1936)
- **Strange Kolle, Frederick** *Plastic and Cosmetic Surgery* (New York NY; London: D. Appleton, 1911)
- **Tagliacozzi, Gaspare** *De Curtorum Chirurgia per insitionem* (Venezia: Gasparo Bindoni giov., 1597)
- **Trendelenburg, Friedrich** *Die ersten 25 Jahre der Deutschen Gesellschaft für Chirurgie: Ein Beitrag zur Geschichte der Chirurgie* (Berlin: Julius Springer, 1923)
- **Von Graefe, Carl Ferdinand** *Rhinoplastik oder die Kunst den Verlust der Nase organisch zu ersetzen* (Berlin: Realschulbuch, 1818)
- **Willi, Charles H.** *The Face and its Improvement by Aesthetic Plastic Surgery* (London, 1949)
- **Willi, Charles H.** *Facial Rejuvenation: How to Idealise the Features and the Skin of the Face by the Latest Scientific Methods* (London: Cecil Palmer, 1926)
- **Zeis, Eduard** *Handbuch der plastischen Chirurgie (900 v. Chr. – 1863 n. Chr.)* (Berlin: G. Reimer, 1838)

Contemporary Medical Books

- **Alter, Gary J.; Ehrlich, Richard M. (ed.)** *Reconstructive and Plastic Surgery of the External Genitalia: Adult and Pediatric* (Philadelphia PA: W. B. Saunders, 1999)
- **Aiach, Gilbert; Levignac, Jacques** *La rinoplastia estética* (Barcelona: Masson, 1989)
- **Aiach, Gilbert** *Atlas de rinoplastia y de la vía de abordaje externo* (Barcelona: Masson, 1994)
- **Alfaro Fernández Antonio** *Cirugía plástica y reparadora* (Madrid: Consejo General de Colegios Oficiales Médicos, 1990)
- **Arnold, David** *Colonizing the Body: State Medicine and Epidemic Disease in Nineteenth-Century India* (Berkeley CA: University of California, 1993).
- **Asami, Yoshiyasu** *Saishin Biyou Seikei De Anatamo Kirei-ni Nareru - The latest plastic surgery* (Tokyo: Gendai Shorin, 2004)
- **Avelar, J. M.; Malbec, E. F.** *Cirugía plástica y estética.* (São Paulo: Ed. Hipócrates, 1990)
- **Baker, Shan R.** *Principles of Aesthetic Nasal Reconstruction* (St. Louis MO: C. V. Mosby, 2002)
- **Bankoff, George** *The Story of Plastic Surgery* (London: Faber and Faber, 1952)
- **Banzet, Pierre** *Chirurgie plastique reconstructrice et esthétique* (Paris : Flammarion Médicine, 1993)
- **Barron, J. N.; Saad, M. N. (ed.)** *Operative Plastic and Reconstructive Surgery* (Edinburgh: Churchill Livingstone, 1980)
- **Bazán Álvarez, Antonio; Elejabeitia González, Javier; Puertas Ruiz, Amaya** *Fundamentos de cirugía plástica reparadora, estética* (Aizoain: Gráficas Barañain, 1999)
- **Behrbohm, Hans; Tardy, M. E.** *Funktionell-ästhetische Chirurgie der Nase* (Stuttgart: Thieme, 2003)
- **Benatar, Daniel** *La chirurgie esthétique au masculin* (Montreal: Isabelle Quentin, 2003)
- **Benatar, Daniel** *La chirurgie esthétique du corps* (Montreal: Isabelle Quentin, 2003)
- **Benatar, Daniel** *La chirurgie esthétique du visage* (Montreal: Isabelle Quentin, 2003)
- **Benatar, Daniel** *Tout sur la chirurgie esthétique* (Montreal: Isabelle Quentin, 2002)
- **Benito, Javier de** *El gran libro de la cirugía estética* (Barcelona: RBA Libros, 2001)
- **Benito, Javier** *Estética y cirugía* (El Masnou: Manuel Salvat Vilá Editor, 1992)
- **Berman, W. E.** *Rhinoplastic Surgery* (St. Louis MO: C. V. Mosby, 1989)
- **Bernklau, M.** *Über die historische Entwicklung der rekonstruktiven Gesichtschirurgie in der Zeit von 1800 bis 1950* (Diss.; Giessen, 1992)

- **Brown, J. B.; McDowell, F.** *Plastic Surgery of the Nose* (St. Louis MO: C. V. Mosby, 1965)
- **Bruck, Johannes C.; Müller, Friedrich E.; Stehen, Michael (ed.)** *Verbrennungstherapie* (Heidelberg: Ecomed – Hüthig Jehle Rehm, 2002)
- **Brunner, Peter Paul** *Die Entwicklung der Knochenplastik am Unterkiefer im Ersten Weltkrieg* (Zürich: Juris, 1996)
- **Camp, John** *Plastic Surgery: The Kindest Cut* (New York NY: Henry Holt, 1989)
- **Caslav Covino, Deborah** *Amending the Abject Body: Aesthetic Makeovers in Medicine and Culture* (New York NY: State University of New York Press, 2004)
- **Cerasano, S. S.; Wynne-Davies, Marion (ed.)** *Gloriana's Face: Women, Public and Private, in the English Renaissance* (New York NY: Harvester Wheatsheaf, 1992)
- **Châtelet, Noëlle** *Trompe-d'œil: voyage au pays de la chirurgie esthétique* (Paris: Belfond, 1993)
- **Coiffman, Felipe** *Cirugía plástica, reconstructiva y estética* (Barcelona: Masson, 1994)
- **Conley, J.; Dickinson, J. T. (ed.)** *Plastic and Reconstructive Surgery of the Face and the Neck* (New York NY: Grune and Stratton, 1972)
- **Converse, J. M. (ed.)** *Reconstructive Plastic Surgery, Vol 2* (Philadelphia PA: W. B. Saunders, 1977)
- **Crestinu, Jacques** *Du bout du nez au bout des seins* (Paris : Résidence, 2000)
- **Daniel, R. (ed.)** *Aesthetic Rhinoplasty* (St. Louis MO: C. V. Mosby, 1993)
- **de Moulin, Daniel** *A History of Surgery, with Emphasis on the Netherlands* (Dordrecht: Nighoff, 1988)
- **Depani, Sarita** *"The Pursuit of Beauty" The Rise of Cosmetic Surgery in Britain in the Twentieth Century*, (Diss.; Wellcome Trust Centre for the History of Medicine at University College, London, 2001)
- **Dirschka, Thomas; Sommer, Boris; Usmiani, Jerko (ed.)** *Klinikleitfaden Ästhetische Medizin* (München: Urban & Fischer, 2002)
- **Duke, Martin** *The Development of Medical Techniques and Treatments: From Leeches to Heart Surgery Madison* (Madison CT: International Universities Press, 1991)
- **Earle, Scott (ed.)** *Surgery in America: From the Colonial Era to the 20th Century* (2nd edition; New York NY: Praeger, 1983)
- **Eberle, M.** *Die Geschichte der Lippenplastik* (Diss.; Freiburg im Br., 1982)
- **Engler, Alan M.** *BodySculpture: Plastic Surgery of the Body for Men & Women* (New York NY: Hudson, 1998; 2nd edition revised and expanded 2000)
- **Fernández de la Fuente, Pedro** *Cirugía estética de párpados y cejas* (Madrid: Sociedad Española de Oftalmología, 1998)
- **Fomon, Samuel** *Cosmetic Surgery. Principles and Practice* (Philadelphia PA, 1960)
- **Fox, Sidney A.** *Ophtalmic Plastic Surgery* (New York, 1952)
- **Franklyn, Robert Alan** *Beauty Surgeon* (Long Beach, CA: Whitehorn Pub. Co., 1960)
- **Franklyn, Robert Alan** *The Art of Staying Young* (New York NY, 1968)
- **Fraser, Suzanne** *Cosmetic Surgery, Gender and Culture* (Basingstoke; New York NY: Palgrave Macmillan, 2003)
- **Gabka, Joachim; Vaubel, Ekkehard** *Plastic Surgery, Past and Present: Origin and History of Modern Lines of Incision* (Basel: S. Karger, 1983)
- **Genschorek, Wolfgang** *Wegbereiter der Chirurgie: Johann Friedrich Dieffenbach, Theodor Billroth* (Leipzig: S. Hirzel, 1982)
- **Georgiade, Nicolas G.; Georgiade, Gregory S.; Riefkohl, Ronald (ed.)** *Aesthetic Surgery of the Breast* (Philadelphia PA: W. B. Saunders, 1990)
- **Gert H. Brieger (ed.)**, *Medical America in the Nineteenth Century: Readings from the Literature* (Baltimore MD: The Johns Hopkins University Press, 1972)
- **Gillies, Harold; Millard, D. Ralph** *The Principles and Art of Plastic Surgery.* 2 vols. (Boston MA: Little, Brown and Co., 1957)
- **Glicenstein, Julien** *La chirurgie esthétique* (Paris: Hermann, 1993)
- **Goin, John M.; Kraft Goin, Marcia** *Changing the Body: Psychological Effects of Plastic Surgery* (Baltimore MD; London: Williams & Wilkins, 1981)
- **Gola, Raymond** *Chirurgie esthétique et fonctionnelle de la face* (Berlin, Heidelberg, New York NY: Springer, 2004)
- **Goldwyn, Robert M. (ed.)** *Long-term Results in Plastic and Reconstructive Surgery* (Boston MA: Little, Brown, and Co., 1980)
- **Goldwyn, Robert M.** *The Patient and the Plastic Surgeon* (Boston MA: Little, Brown and Co., 1991)
- **Goldwyn, Robert M. (ed.)** *The Unfavorable Result in Plastic Surgery: Avoidance and Treatment* (Boston MA: Little, Brown, and Co., 1972)
- **González-Ulloa, Mario (ed.)** *The Creation of Aesthetic Plastic Surgery* (New York NY: Springer, 1985)
- **González-Ulloa, Mario et al.** *Aesthetic Plastic Surgery: Advances in Aesthetic Plastic Surgery: 6* (Padova: Piccin Nuova Libraria, 2001)
- **Grabb, William C.; Smith, James W. (ed.)** *Plastic Surgery: A Concise Guide to Clinical Practice, 4th ed.* (Boston MA: Little, Brown and Co., 1991)
- **Greer, Steven; Benhaim, Prosper, et al. (ed.)** *Handbook of Plastic Surgery* (New York, NY: M. Dekker, 2004)
- **Grigaut, Pierre-François** *La chirurgie esthétique et plastique* (Paris: Presses Universitaires de France, 1962)
- **Haas, Erwin** *Plastische Gesichtschirurgie* (Stuttgart, New York NY: Thieme 1991)
- **Haiken, Elizabeth G.** *Body and Soul: Plastic Surgery in the United States, 1914–1990* (Diss.; University of California, Berkeley, 1994)
- **Haiken, Elizabeth G.** *Venus Envy: A History of Cosmetic Surgery* (Baltimore MD: Johns Hopkins University Press, 1997)
- **Hetter, Gregory S. (ed.)** *Lipoplasty: The Theory and Practice of Blunt Suction Lipectomy* (Boston MA: Little, Brown, and Co., 1990)

- **Hildebrand, Otto** *Die Entwicklung der plastischen Chirurgie* (Berlin: Hirschwald, 1909)
- **Hirose, Shinji** *Medical Bust Up* (Tokyo: Gendai Shorin, 2000)
- **Hoefflin, Steven M.** *Ethnic Rhinoplasty* (New York NY: Springer, 1998)
- **Hoffmann-Axthelm, Walter et al.** *Die Geschichte der Mund-, Kiefer- und Gesichtschirurgie* (Berlin: Quintessenz, 1995)
- **Hönig, Johannes F.** *Ästhetische Chirurgie* (Berlin, Heidelberg: Springer, 2000)
- **Horay, Pascal (coord.) et Chavoin, Jean-Pierre (préface)** *Chirurgie plastique du sein* (New York NY: Elsevier, 2003)
- **Horay, Pascal (coord.) et Jost, Guy (préface)** *Chirurgie plastique du nez* (New York NY: Elsevier, 2003)
- **Ichikawa, Rino** *Bijo No Mahousho – Kin No Ito Biyoujutsu – Magic book for beauty: gold string* (Tokyo: Gendai Shorin, 2004)
- **Jacquemin, Jeannine** *Suzanne Noël* (Paris: Soroptomist International, 1988)
- **Jaeckel, Gerhard** *Die Charité: Die Geschichte eines Weltzentrums der Medizin* (Bayreuth: Hestia, 1963)
- **Jost, G.** *Cirugía, plástica y estética* (Barcelona: Masson, 1992)
- **Kastenbauer, Ernst R.; Tardy, M. E.** *Ästhetische und Plastische Chirurgie an Nase, Gesicht und Ohrmuschel* (Stuttgart: Thieme, 2004)
- **Kawakita, Yoshio; Sakai, Shizu; Otsuka, Yasuo (ed.)** *History of Therapy. Proceedings of the 10th International Symposium on the Comparative History of Medicine – East and West* (Tokio: Tanaguchi Foundation, 1990)
- **Klingbeil, Jerome R.** *Body Image: A Surgical Perspective* (St. Louis MO: The C. V. Mosby Company, 1980)
- **Kotler, Robert (ed.)** *Chemical Rejuvenation of the Face* (St. Louis MT: Mosby Year Book, 1992)
- **La Trenta, G.** *Atlas of Aesthetic Face and Neck Surgery* (Philadelphia PA: W. B. Saunders, 2003)
- **Lawrence, Christopher (ed.)** *Medical Theory, Surgical Practice* (London: Routledge, 1992)
Levy-Lenz, Ludwig *Praxis der kosmetischen Chirurgie, Fortschritte und Gefahren* (Stuttgart: Hippokrates, 1954)
- **Lewis, John R. Jr. (ed.)** *The Art of Aesthetic Plastic Surgery. 2 vols.* (Boston MA: Little, Brown and Co., 1989)
- **Maloney, W. H. (ed.)** *Otolaryngology* (New York NY: Harper & Row, 1971)
- **Maltz, Maxwell** *Doctor Pygmalion: The Autobiography of a Plastic Surgeon* (New York: Crowell, 1953)
- **Mang, Werner L.; Kokoschka, Eva-Maria (ed.)** *Ästhetische Chirurgie, Band II: Laserchirurgie, Plastiken, Implantate* (Reinbek: Einhorn-Presse, 1998)
- **Mang, Werner L.; Bull, Heinz-Gerhard** *Ästhetische Chirurgie* (Reinbek: Einhorn-Presse, 2002)
- **Mang, Werner L.** *Manual of Aesthetic Surgery 1: Rhinoplasty; Rhytidectomy; Eyelid Surgery; Otoplasty; Adjuvant Therapies* (New York NY, Berlin, Heidelberg: Springer, 2002); *Manual de cirugía estética* (Barcelona: Masson, 2004)
- **Mang, Werner L.** *Manual of Aesthetic Surgery, w. DVD-Video* (Berlin: Springer, 2004)
- **Mang, Werner L.** *Manual of Aesthetic Surgery 2: Breast Augmentation; Brachioplasty; Abdominoplasty; Thigh and Buttock Lift; Liposuction; Hair Transplantation; Adjuvant Therapies* (New York NY, Berlin, Heidelberg: Springer, 2005)
- **Mathes, Stephen J.; Hentz, Vincent R. (ed.)** *Plastic Surgery*, 2nd ed; here: Gary J. Alter *Aesthetic Genital Surgery* (Philadelphia, PA: WB Saunders, 2005)
- **Matory, W. Earle, Jr. (ed.)** *Ethnic Considerations in Facial Aesthetic Surgery* (Illustrator: Kim Hogatt; Philadelphia PA: Lippincott-Raven, 1997)
- **McDowell, Frank (ed.)** *The Source Book of Plastic Surgery* (Baltimore MD: The Williams & Wilkins Company, 1977)
- **Meyer, R.** *Secondary and Functional Rhinoplasty* (Orlando Fla: Grune and Stratton, 1988)
- **Millard, D. R., Jr. (ed.)** *Symposium on Corrective Rhinoplasty* (St. Louis MO: C. V. Mosby, 1976)
- **Miller, M. D. et al.** *2004 Yearbook of Plastic and Aesthetic Surgery* (St. Louis MO: C. V. Mosby, 2004)
- **Millikan, Larry; Parish, Lawrence Charles (ed.)** *Global Dermatology* (New York NY: Springer, 1994)
- **Minagawa, Hiroshi** *Honmono No Men's Biyou Seikei – Plastic surgery for men* (Tokyo: Kowa Kikaku, 2004)
- **Mir y Mir, Lorenzo** *Cirugía del rejuvenecimiento facial: ritidoplastias, blefaroplastias. Técnicas auxiliares* (Barcelona: Editorial Jims, 1994)
- **Mitz, Vladimir** *La chirurgie esthétique* (Paris: Flammarion, 2002)
- **Mitz, Vladimir** *Manuel de chirurgie plastique et esthétique du sein* (Paris: Frison-Roche, 1995)
- **Morselli, Paolo G.; Spinetta, Jean (ed.)** *Mieux dans sa peau : Les métamorphoses de la chirurgie esthétique, Causes et effets morpho-psychologiques* (Paris: Holoconcept, 2004)
- **Murray, Joseph E.** *Surgery of the Soul: Reflections on a Curious Career* (New York NY: Science History Publications, 2001)
- **Natvig, Paul** *Jacques Joseph: Surgical Sculptor* (Philadelphia PA: W. B. Saunders, 1982)
- **Nesi, Frank A.; Gladstone, Goeffrey J.; Brazzo, Brian G.; Myint, Shoib (ed.)** *Ophthalmic and Facial Plastic Surgery: A Compendium of Reconstructive and Aesthetic Techniques* (London: Slack Incorporated, 2000)
- **Oliveri, Neven** *Praktische Plastische Chirurgie* (Heidelberg: Kaden, 2004)
- **Ortiz-Monasterio, Fernando** *Rinoplastia* (Madrid: Editorial Médica Panamericana, 1996)
- **Ostermaier, Rudolf** *Liposkulptur (Tumeszenzliposkulptur)* (Stuttgart: Hirzel, 2003)
- **Panfilov, Dimitri** *Moderne Schönheitschirurgie*, with CD-ROM (Stuttgart: Trias, 2003)
- **Paparella, Shumrick (ed.)** *Otolaryngology* (Philadelphia PA: W. B. Saunders, 1973)

- **Peck, G. C.** *Techniques in Aesthetic Rhinoplasty* (New York NY: Gower Medical, 1984)
- **Pitanguy, Ivo** *Aesthetic Plastic Surgery of Head and Body* (Berlin, Heidelberg, New York NY: Springer, 1981)
- **Pitman, G. H.**, *Foundation face lift*, in **Nahai, F. (ed.)** *Aesthetic Plastic Surgery* (St. Louis: Quality Medical Publishing, 2005)
- **Pitman, G. H.; Giese, S. Y.** *Liposuction*, in **Mathes, S. (ed.)** *Plastic Surgery* (Philadelphia, PA: Elsevier, 2005).
- **Pitman, G. H.; Stoker, D.; Stevens, G.**. *Liposuction and Body-contouring*, in **McCarthy, Galiano, Boutros (ed.)** *Current Therapy in Plastic Surgery* (Philadelphia, PA: Elsevier, 2005)
- **Pouchelle, Marie-Christine** *Corps et chirurgie à l'apogée du Moyen Age* (Paris: Flammarion, 1983)
- **Preuss, Julius** *Biblical and Talmudic Medicine* transl. by Fred Rosner (New York NY: Sanhedrin, 1978)
- **Raffalli, Cristina** *Debo operarme?: verdades, ventajas y riesgos de la cirugía plástica* (Caracas: Los Libros de El Nacional, 1999)
- **Ragnell, Allan** *The Development of Plastic Surgery in Stockholm in the Last Decennium* (Stockholm: Acta chirurgica Scandinavica. Supplementum 348, 1965)
- **Raulin, Christian et al.** *Laser und IPL-Technologie in der Dermatologie und Ästhetischen Medizin* (New York NY: Schattauer, 2003)
- **Ravitch, Mark** *A Century of Surgery: The History of the American Surgical Association* (Philadelphia PA: Lippincott, 1981)
- **Rees, T. D. (ed.)** *Aesthetic Plastic Surgery* (Philadelphia PA: W. B. Saunders, 1980)
- **Regnault, P.; Daniel, R. K. (ed.)** *Aesthetic Plastic Surgery* (Boston MA: Little, Brown, and Co., 1984)
- **Reifler, David M. (ed.)** *The American Society of Ophthalmic Plastic and Reconstructive Surgeons (ASOPRS): The First Twenty-Five Years: 1969–1994; History of Ophthalmic Plastic Surgery: 2500 BC-AD 1994* (Winter Park FL: American Society of Ophthalmic Plastic and Reconstructive Surgery, 1994)
- **Romo, T.; Millman, A. L. (ed.)** *Aesthetic Facial Plastic Surgery: A Multidisciplinary Approach* (New York NY: Thieme, 1999)
- **Rosen, H. M.** *Aesthetic Perspectives in Jaw Surgery* (New York NY: Springer, 1999)
- **Rothman, Sheila and David** *The Pursuit of Perfection: The Promise and Perils of Medical Enhancement* (New York NY: Vintage, 2004)
- **Sava, George** *Surgery and Crime* (London: Faber and Faber, 1957)
- **Scheer, Robert** *The Cosmetic Surgery Revolution: An Objective Guide to Understanding your Cosmetic Surgery Choices* (Los Angeles CA: Summit Pines Press, 1992)
- **Schiefer, U.; Wilhelm, H.; Zirenner, E.; Burk, A. (ed.)** *Praktische Neuroophthalmologie* (Heidelberg: Kaden, o. J.)
- **Schmiedebach, Heinz-Peter; Winau, Rolf; Häring, Rudolf (ed.)** *Erste Operationen Berliner Chirurgen 1817–1931* (Berlin: De Gruyter, 1990)
- **Serra Renom, José María; Vila Rovira, Ramón** *Endoscopia en cirugía plástica y estética* (Barcelona: Masson, 1995)
- **Sheen, J. H.** *Aesthetic Rhinoplasty* (St. Louis MO: C. V. Mosby, 1978)
- **Sommer, Boris; Sattler, Gerhard** *Botulinumtoxin in der ästhetischen Medizin* (Stuttgart: Thieme, 2001)
- **Spinelli, Henry** *Atlas of Aesthetic Eyelid Surgery* (Philadelphia PA: W. B. Saunders, 2002)
- **Stoler, Ann** *Laura Race and the Education of Desire: Foucault's History of Sexuality and the Colonial Order of Things* (Durham NC: Duke University, 1995)
- **Sullivan, Deborah A.** *Cosmetic Surgery: The Cutting Edge of Commercial Medicine in America* (New Brunswick NJ: Rutgers University Press, 2001)
- **Tagliacozzi, Gaspare** *La Chirurgia Plastica per Innesto* trad. and ed.: Werner Vallieri. Bologna Università. Cattedra di storia della medicina. Vita e opere di medici e naturalisti, vol. 3 (Bologna: 1964)
- **Takano, Kunio** *Saishin Biyou Geka Kanzen File - Perfect guide of the latest plastic surgery* (Tokyo: Gendai Shorin, 2002)
- **Tytgat, Hubert Van** *Top tot Teen – Alles over plastische chirurgie* (Antwerpen: Standaard Uitgeverij, 2004)
- **Utsugi, Ryuichi** *Bijin Enmei - All about plastic surgery at Kitazato Kenkyujo Hospital* (Tokyo: Shufu No Tomo Sha, 2004)
- **Valentin, Bruno** *Geschichte der Orthopädie* (Stuttgart: Thieme, 1961)
- **Vila Rovira, Ramón; Serra Renom, José M.** *Liposucción en cirugía plástica y estética* (Barcelona: Salvat Editores, 1987)
- **Wallace, Antony F.** *The Progress of Plastic Surgery: An Introductory History* (Oxford: Willem A. Meeuws, 1982)
- **Wangensteen, Owen and Sarah** *The Rise of Surgery: from Empiric Craft to Scientific Discipline* (Minneapolis MN: University of Minnesota Press, 1978)
- **Webb, Mary Sharon** *Beyond Beauty: Philosophy, Ethics and Plastic Surgery* (Diss.; Yale University, 1984)
- **Wilkinson, Tolbert S.** *Practical Procedures in Aesthetic Plastic Surgery: Tips and Traps* (New York NY: Springer, 1994)

Books on Cultural History of the Body

- **Adams, Gerald R.; Crossman, Sharyn M.** *Physical Attractiveness: A Cultural Imperative* (Roslyn Heights NY: Libra, 1978)
- **Albi Parra, Almudena**. *Tu cuerpo es tuyo* (Madrid: Aguilar, 1997)
- **Anderson, Lenore Wright** *Synthetic Beauty: American Women and Cosmetic Surgery* (Diss.; Rice University, 1989)

- **Armstrong, Tim** *Modernism, Technology and the Body: A Cultural Study* (Cambridge MS: Cambridge University Press, 1998)
- **Balsamo, Anne Marie** *Reading the Gendered Body In Contemporary Culture, 1980-1990* (Diss.; University of Illinois at Urbana-Champaign, 1991)
- **Balsamo, Anne Marie** *Technologies of the Gendered Body: Reading Cyborg Women* (Durham NC: Duke University Press, 1996)
- **Banner, Lois W.** *American Beauty* (Chicago IL: University of Chicago Press, 1983)
- **Blum, Virginia L.** *Flesh Wounds: The Culture of Cosmetic Surgery* (Berkeley CA; London: University of California Press, 2003)
- **Braun, Christina v.** *Die schamlose Schönheit des Vergangenen: Zur Geschichte des Geschlechts* (Frankfurt: Neue Kritik, 1999)
- **Bravo, Ángela** *Femenino singular: la belleza a través de la historia* (Madrid: Alianza Editorial, 1996)
- **Brook, Barbara** *Feminist Perspective on the Body* (New York NY: Longman, 1999)
- **Burkhart, Gregor** *Die Kinder Omulús: der Einfluß afro-brasilianischer Kultur auf die Wahrnehmung von Körper und Krankheit* (Frankfurt am Main, New York NY: S. Lang, 1994)
- **Chapkis, Wendy** *Beauty Secrets: Women and the Politics of Appearance* (Boston MA: South End Press, 1986)
- **Comelli, Albino** *Da narciso al narcisismo: storia e psicologia del corpo: costume, medicina, estetica* (Trento: Reverdito, 1993)
- **Cox, June Thurber** *Cultural Images of the Body: An Inquiry into the History of Human Engineering* (Diss, University of California, Berkeley, 1990)
- **Davis, Kathy** *Dubious Equalities and Embodied Differences: Cultural Studies on Cosmetic Surgery* (Lanham; Oxford: Rowman & Littlefield, 2003)
- **Davis, Kathy** *Embodied Practices: Feminist Perspectives on the Body* (London: SAGE, 1997)
- **Davis, Kathy** *Reshaping The Female Body: The Dilemma Of Cosmetic Surgery* (New York NY: Routledge & Kegan, 1995)
- **Domes, Josef et al. (ed.)** *Licht der Natur: Medizin in Fachliteratur und Dichtung* (Göppingen: Kümmerle, 1994)
- **Erb, Rainer; Bergmann, Werner** *Die Nachtseite der Judenemanzipation: Der Widerstand gegen die Integration der Juden in Deutschland 1780–1860* (Berlin: Metropol, 1989).
- **Furman, Frida Kerner** *Facing the Mirror: Older Women and Beauty Shop Culture* (New York NY: Routledge & Kegan, 1997)
- **Gilman, Sander L.** *Creating Beauty to Cure the Soul: Race and Psychology in the Shaping of Aesthetic Surgery* (Durham NC: Duke University, 1998)
- **Gilman, Sander L.** *Making the Body Beautiful: A Cultural History of Aesthetic Surgery* (Princeton PA: Princeton University, 2000)
- **Giménez-Barlett González,** *Alicia La deuda de Eva. Del pecado de ser feas y el deber de ser hermosas* (Barcelona; Editorial Lumen, 2002)
- **Günther, Hans F. K.** *Rassenkunde des jüdischen Volkes* (München: J. F. Lehmann, 1930)
- **Hanchard, Michael** *George Orpheus and Power: The Movimento Negro of Rio De Janeiro and São Paulo, Brazil, 1945–1988* (Princeton: Princeton University Press, 1994)
- **Katz, Jacob** *Out of the Ghetto: The Social Background of Jewish Emancipation 1770–1870* (Cambridge MA: Harvard University Press, 1973)
- **Lakoff, Tolmach; Robin, Scherr; Raquel L. (ed.)** *Face Value: The Politics of Beauty* (New York NY: Routledge & Kegan, 1984)
- **Marwick, Arthur** *Beauty in History: Society, Politics, and Personal Appearance* (London: Thames and Hudson, 1988)
- **Ohnuki-Tierney, Emiko** *Illness and Culture in Contemporary Japan: An Anthropological View* (Cambridge: Cambridge University Press, 1984)
- **Paquet, Dominique** *La historia de la belleza* (Barcelona: Ediciones B, 1998)
- **Parens, Erik (ed.)** *Enhancing Human Traits: Ethical and Social Implications* (Washington DC: Georgetown University Press, 1998)
- **Perry Curtis, Lewis** *Apes and Angels: The Irishman in Victorian Caricature* (Washington DC: Smithsonian Institution Press, 1971)
- **Pitanguy, Ivo** *El arte de la belleza* (Barcelona: Grijalbo, 1984)
- **Rodin, Judith** *Las trampas del cuerpo. Cómo dejar de preocuparse por la propia apariencia física* (Barcelona: Ediciones Paidós Ibérica, 1993)
- **Romm, Sharon** *The Changing Face of Beauty* (St. Louis MT: Mosby Year Book, 1992)
- **Sartore, Richard** *Body Shaping: Trends, Fashions, and Rebellions* (Commack NY: Nova Science Publishers, 1996)
- **Waldfogel, Sabra** *The Body Beautiful, The Body Hateful: Feminine Body Image and the Culture of Consumption in 20th-Century America* (Diss.; University of Minnesota, 1986)
- **Wolf, Naomi** *The Beauty Myth: How Images of Female Beauty are used against Women* (New York NY: W. Morrow, 1991); *El mito de la belleza* (Barcelona: Publicaciones y Ediciones Salamandra, 1992)
- **Yalom, Marilyn** *History of the Breast* (New York NY: Random House, 1998); *Historia del pecho* (Barcelona: Tusquets Editores, 1997)

Advisory Books on Aesthetic Surgery

- **Antonic, Magda; Hollos, Peter** *Schönheitsoperationen: Methoden, Erfolge, Risiken, Kosten, Adressen* (Berlin: Urania, 1998)

- **Arion, Ingrid** *Changer ou s'accepter : Du bon usage de la chirurgie esthétique* (Paris : Albin Michel, 2002)
- **Banic, A.; Biemer J.; Exner, K.; Frey; M. E., Mühlbauer, W.; Olbrisch, R. (ed.)** *Medführer Plastische und Ästhetische Chirurgie Deutschland, Österreich, Schweiz 2005* (Düsseldorf: medführer, 2004)
- **Bassot, Jacques** *Bien-être et la beauté : chirurgie esthétique* (Meolans-Revel: Désiris, 1998)
- **Beauty Colosseum production staff (ed.)** *Beauty Colosseum* (Tokyo: Gentosha, 2002)
- **Biegi, Ditta** *Makellose Schönheit durch kosmetische Eingriffe: Was Sie wissen müssen über Erfolge und Risiken, Dauer und Kosten der Behandlung, Praxen und Kliniken* (München: Heyne, 1999)
- **Cariel, Laura** *La chirurgie esthétique* (Paris: Flammarion, 2005)
- **Casbas Cancer, María Pilar** *Estírame: locos por la cirugía estética* (Barcelona: Plaza & Janés, 2002)
- **Cimorra, Gustavo A.; Sánchez-Ocaña Serrano, Ramón** *Cirugía estética: todas las respuestas* (Madrid: Meditor, 1992)
- **Colinon, Marie-Christine et Lemoult, Sandrine** *Modifier son corps : Chirurgie, tatouage, piercing* (Paris: Edition de la Martinière Jeunesse, 2003)
- **Dallée, Marie** *To lift or not to lift: Mes déboires au pays de la chirurgie esthétique* (Paris: Albin Michel, 2003)
- **Dardour, Jean-Claude; Charpentier, Laure** *Les tabous du corps* (Paris: Grancher, 1999)
- **de Laval, Rose** *La chirurgie esthétique* (Paris: Milan, 2000)
- **Engler, Alan M.** *The Slim Book of Liposuction* (New York, NY: Vantage Press, 1993)
- **Fatemi, Afschin; Brück, Sebastian** *Die gefragtesten Schönheitsoperationen* (München: Goldmann, 2004)
- **Ganny, Charlee; Collini, Susan J.** *Two Girlfriends get real about Cosmetic Surgery: A Woman-to-Woman Guide to today's most Popular Cosmetic Procedures* (Los Angeles CA: Renaissance, 2000)
- **Gaynor, Alan** *Todo lo que usted siempre quiso saber sobre la cirugía estética y nunca se atrevió a preguntar: una guía completa sobre los últimos avances que han revolucionado la cirugía estética por uno de los más prestigiosos especialistas* (Barcelona, Editorial Gedisa, 1999)
- **Haddad, Guy** *La chirurgie esthétique* (Lyon: Josette Lyon, 2004)
- **Haddad, Guy; Saurat, Marie-France** *Jeunesse pour tous* (Paris: Livre de Poche, 1995)
- **Ishii, Mieko** *Biyou Seikei Catalog – Plastic Surgery Catalog* (Tokyo: Magazine House, 2003)
- **Koncilia, Heimo; Graf, Edda** *Operation Schönheit* (Wien: Ueberreuter, 2002)
- **Kyo, Kongen** *Shippai Shinai Biyou seikei No Hon – Plastic surgery you never fail* (Tokyo: Waseda Shuppan, 2004)
- **Latouche, Xavier; Krotenberg, Alain** *Mon corps et moi : chirurgie esthétique et désir de changement* (Paris: Payot, 2002)
- **Le Gouès, Gérard** *Un désir dans la peau : La Chirurgie plastique sur le divan* (Paris: Hachette Littératures, 2004)
- **Lewis, Wendy** *The Lowdown on Facelifts and other Wrinkle Remedies* (London: Quadrille, 2001)
- **Mang, Werner L. et al.** *Schönheitsoperationen* (Stuttgart: Hippokrates, 2001)
- **Mang, Werner L.; Wülker, Andrea** *Ratgeber Schönheits-Operation* (Stuttgart: Trias, 2005)
- **Martínez-Pereda Rodríguez, José Manuel** *La cirugía estética y su responsabilidad* (Granada: Editorial Comares, 1997)
- **Mitrofanoff, Marc** *La chirurgie esthétique* (Paris: Flammarion, 2005)
- **Mitz, Vladimir** *Le vademecum de chirurgie esthétique* (Paris: Masson, 2002)
- **Nahon, Pierre** *La vérité en chirurgie esthétique* (Paris: LCCI, 2001)
- **Nakamura, Usagi** *Bijin Ni Naritai - I want to be a beauty* (Tokyo: Shogakukan, 2003)
- **Ohana, Jacques** *Esthétiquement votre. Entretiens avec Minou Azoulai* (Paris: J.-C. Lattès, 1996)
- **Rehra, Sabine; Exner, Klaus** *Die weibliche Brust: Der kritische Ratgeber bei medizinischen Eingriffen* (Berlin, München: Gesundheit / Econ-Ullstein-List, 2000)
- **Sánchez-Ocaña Serrano, Ramón** *El libro de la cirugía estética* (Barcelona: Alba Editorial, 1996)
- **Serena, Rafael** *El arte de rejuvenecer: el Botox, nuestro aliado* (Barcelona: Amat Editorial, 2004)
- **Tapia, Antonio** *Tú decides : todo sobre la cirugía estética* (Barcelona: Editorial Planeta, 2003)
- **Vilain, Raymond** *Jeux de mains* (Paris: Arthaud, 2001)
- **Willen, Karin** *Schönheitsoperationen* (Reinbek: Rowohlt, 2003)
- **Zelicovich, Roberto Héctor** *Cirugía estética: todo lo que debe saber* (Madrid: Ediciones Librería Argentina, 2003)

XI.2

Websites for Plastic Surgery

compiled by NANNETTE BUEHL, Paris

XI.2.1

International and National Societies and Associations for Plastic Surgery

International Societies:
IPRAS
IPRAF
FILACP
ISAPS
EURAPS

National Societies in:
USA and Canada
Latin America
European Union / Switzerland / Iceland
Mid-Eastern Europe
South Eastern Europe
Baltic States
Russian Federation
Northern Africa and South Africa
Near East
Middle East
Asia
Australia
New Zealand

XI.2.2

Plastic Surgery on the Web

XI.2.2.1

General information – from liposuction and breast augmentation to rhinoplasty and facelifts to hair transplants and Botox injections...

XI.2.2.2

Teenagers: What's first, the nose or the driver's licence?

XI.2.2.3

Transgender

XI.2.2.4

Computer-generated Beauty

XI.2.2.5

Online Surgeon Search

XI.2.2.6

International Medical Journals, Online Journals and Magazines

International and National Societies and Associations for Plastic Surgery

compiled by NANNETTE BUEHL, Paris

IPRAS – The International Confederation for Plastic Reconstructive and Aesthetic Surgery

This international governing body, founded in 1955, incorporates the world's leading national societies and associations for plastic surgery. The prime objective of IPRAS is to foster both scientific and practice-related research in the field of plastic surgery, as well as facilitating professional exchange between the national organisations it hosts.
Website: http://www.ipras.org

IPRAF – The International Plastic, Reconstructive and Aesthetic Surgery Foundation

This IPRAS offshoot was founded in 1993. IPRAF is dedicated to research, teaching programmes and humanitarian projects.
Website: http://www.ipraf.org

FILACP – Federación Ibero Latinoamericana de Cirugía Plástica y Reconstructiva

Founded in 1974, FILACP is an international association incorporating national societies from Latin America as well as Spain and Portugal. The Federación is the Ibero-Latin American branch of IPRAS.
Website: http://www.filacp.org *(in Spanish)*

ISAPS – International Society of Aesthetic Plastic Surgery

This international society was founded in 1970 and has been part of IPRAS since 1975, representing the branch of aesthetic surgery. It has individual members from all over the world.
Website: http://www.isaps.org
An online global surgeon search is also available from this website, providing contact details for all of the society's members.

EURAPS – European Association of Plastic Surgeons

This international association was founded in 1989, bringing together members from 18 European countries with the objective of setting and fostering an excellent standard of quality for plastic surgery throughout Europe. EURAPS also organises international conferences that are hosted in a different European country each year.
Website: http://www.euraps.org

National Societies and Associations for Plastic Surgery

The prime objective of the national societies is to ensure a high standard of quality in the fields of plastic, aesthetic and reconstructive surgery by fostering medical research and technical development. Their members have to meet scrupulously chosen selection criteria before being accepted. National associations and societies also act as representative bodies for their members, providing training opportunities and facilitating professional exchange on an international level. For prospective patients and the public, the national societies and associations are a first point of contact when searching for appropriately qualified surgeons. They also provide a comprehensive information base for all matters pertaining to plastic surgery.

Most of the national societies and associations for plastic surgery listed below are members of IPRAS or one of the IPRAS branches.

USA and Canada

American Society of Plastic Surgeons (ASPS)

444 E. Algonquin Rd.
Arlington Heights, IL 60 005
USA
Plastic Surgeon Referral Service
+1-888-4-PLASTIC (475-2784)
Public Relations

Tel: +1-847-228-9900
E-mail: media@plasticsurgery.org
http://www.plasticsurgery.org *(English)*

The aim of the *American Society of Plastic Surgeons (ASPS)* is to promote quality and research in the field of plastic surgery and to provide thc general public with comprehensive, up-to-date information in this field.
Founded: 1931
Members: 4466 active members worldwide
Member qualifications: Members must be certified by the *American Board of Plastic Surgery (ABPS)* as specialists in plastic surgery, prove that they have completed comprehensive training in all fields of plastic surgery and must attend further education measures on a continuous basis (at least 150 hours of medical further education within three years).
Online search for surgeons: Via the website, listed according to name, US state or country.

American Society for Aesthetic Plastic Surgery (ASAPS)

Media contact:
ASAPS Communications Office
36 West 44th Street, Suite 630
New York, New York 10 036
Tel: +1-212-921-0500
Fax: +1-212-921-0011
E-mail: media@surgery.org
Medical Professionals:
ASAPS Central Office
11 081 Winners Circle
Los Alamitos, California 90 720
USA
Tel:+1-800-364-2147 / +1-562-799-2356
Fax: +1-562-799-1098
E-mail: asaps@surgery.org
Public contact:
ASAPS Find-a-Surgeon Referral Service
+1-888-ASAPS-11 (272-7711)
http://www.surgery.org *(English)*

The *American Society for Aesthetic Plastic Surgery (ASAPS)* is a teaching and research organisation which supports scientific meetings and studies, and annually publishes statistics on developments in the field of cosmetic surgery. It also aims to supply the general public with detailed information on all fields of plastic surgery.
Founded: 1967
Members: 2100 members worldwide
Member qualifications: Full members must be certified as plastic surgeons by the *American Board of Plastic Surgery (ABPS)* in the USA or, in Canada, by the *Royal College of Physicians and Surgeons of Canada*. They must be at least in their third year of practice since certification and prove that they are fully up-to-date with developments in the field. Membership applications must be recommended by two members of the Society.
Online search for surgeons: Via the website, listed according to name, US state or country.

Canadian Society of Plastic Surgeons (CSPS)

Secretary
Karyn Wagner
1469 St. Joseph Blvd. E. #4
Montreal, QC H2J 1M6
CANADA
Tel: +1-514-843-5415
Fax: +1-514-843-7005
E-mail: csps_sccp@bellnet.ca
http://www.plasticsurgery.ca *(English and French)*

Teaching and educating the general public as well as the membership is an important activity of the *Canadian Society of Plastic Surgeons (CSPS)*, which documents its research and studies in annual meetings.
Founded: 1947
Member qualifications: Members must be certified by the *Royal College of Physicians and Surgeons of Canada* or the *Collège des Médecins du Québec*. Conditions of certification are training in general surgery followed by specialisation in all aspects of plastic surgery, as well as passing the examination of the *Royal College of Physicians and Surgeon of Canada*.

Online search for surgeons: Via the website, structured according to name and country (USA /Canada/international).

Canadian Society for Aesthetic (Cosmetic) Plastic Surgery (CSAPS)

2334 Heska Rd.
Pickering, ON CA L1V 2P9
CANADA
Tel: +1-905-831-7750
Fax: +1-905-831-7248
E-mail: information@csaps.ca
http://www.csaps.ca *(English and French)*

The *Canadian Society for Aesthetic (Cosmetic) Plastic Surgery (CSAPS)* is an association specialising in cosmetic surgery (many doctors of the CSAPS are also members of the *Canadian Society of Plastic Surgeons – CSPS*). It aims to develop and disseminate modern surgical techniques, to promote the exchange of ideas between qualified plastic surgeons and to guarantee a high standard of practice.
Founded: 1972
Member qualifications: All members must be certified by the *Royal College of Physicians and Surgeons of Canada*. Having obtained a qualification in general medicine they must further have completed a minimum of five years of specialist training and then have specialised in all aspects of cosmetic surgery.
Online search for surgeons: Via the website, structured according to name and country (USA /Canada/international)

Latin America

Sociedad Argentina de Cirugía Plástica, Estética y Reparadora (SACPER)

Av. Santa Fe 16 11 3° (1060)
Buenos Aires
ARGENTINA
Tel: +54-11-4 816 3757
Fax: +54-11-4 816 0346
E-mail: sacper@cirplastica.org.ar
http://www.sacper.org.ar *(Spanish)*

The *Sociedad Argentina de Cirugía Plástica, Estética y Reparadora (SACPER)* is a branch of the *Asociación Médica Argentina (AMA)* and is composed of members of regional Argentinean associations.
Founded: 1952
Members: approx. 200
Member qualifications: Plastic surgeons are required to be members of their regional association and have proven, comprehensive training in the field of plastic surgery.

Online search for surgeons: Via the website. An alphabetical list is provided, but contact addresses are not. These can be supplied by the regional associations, such as the *Sociedad de Cirugía Plástica de Buenos Aires (SCPBA)* – see below.

Sociedad de Cirugía Plástica de Buenos Aires (SCPBA)

Avenida Santa Fe 1611, 3° Piso
Capital Federal, Buenos Aires
CP: A1060BCD
ARGENTINA
Tel: +54-11-4816-3757/+54-11-4816-3758
Fax: +54-11-4816-0342
E-mail: scpba@intramed.net.ar
Office hours: Monday to Friday 1 p. m. – 8 p. m.
http://www.scpba.com.ar *(Spanish and English)*

The members of the *Sociedad de Cirugía Plástica de Buenos Aires (SCPBA)* practise as surgeons in Buenos Aires and the surrounding area. The Society is a branch of the *Sociedad Argentina de Cirugía Plástica, Estética y Reparadora (SACPER)*.
Founded: 1978
Member qualifications: Full members have to prove that they have practised as general surgeons, orthopaedists or plastic surgeons for an appropriate period of time, have been associate members for at least two years and are also members of the Argentinean Medical Association *Asociación Médica Argentina (AMA)*.
Online search for surgeons: Via the website, alphabetical listings.

Sociedad Boliviana de Cirugía Plástica

Cajou Postal 228
C. Padilla 74
Sucre
BOLIVIA
Tel: +591-4-645 5259/+591-4-644 0305
Fax: +591-4-645 5559
E-mail: ferurriola@hotmail.com
http://www.bago.com.bo/sbcp/index.html *(Spanish)*

Sociedade Brasileira de Cirurgia Plástica (SBCP)

Av. Pacaembú, 746 –
11° andar – Perdizes
CEP: 01 234 – 000
São Paulo – SP
BRAZIL
Tel: +55-11-3 826 1499
Fax: +55-11-3 826 1710
E-mail: sbcp@cirurgiaplastica.org.br
http://www.cirurgiaplastica.org.br *(Portuguese)*

The *Sociedade Brasileira de Cirurgia Plástica (SBCP)* aims to train excellent surgeons and to promote the dissemination of the latest scientific developments and techniques in the field of plastic surgery.
Founded: 1948
Member qualifications: Members are required to have worked as assistant doctors (residência) in general surgery, to have worked in the field of plastic surgery for at least three years and to have passed the examination for the official title as a specialist, which can only be awarded by the SBCP in agreement with the Brazilian Medical Association *Associação Médica Brasileira* and the Federal Medical Council *Conselho Federal de Medicina*. The examination for full membership of the Society can be taken two years later at the earliest.
Online search for surgeons: Via the website, listed alphabetically or according to regions.

Sociedad Chilena de Cirugía Plástica Reconstructiva y Estética

Esmeralda 678 – 2° Piso interior
Santiago
CHILE
Tel: +56-2-632 0714 / +56-2-632 8731
Fax: +56-2-639 1085
E-mail: cirplastica@terra.cl
http://www.cirplastica.cl *(Spanish)*

The aim of the *Sociedad Chilena de Cirugía Plástica, Reconstructiva y Estética* is to advance scientific and ethical quality in plastic surgery, to perfect existing techniques and train new generations of plastic surgeons.
Founded: 1941
Members: approx. 80
Member qualifications: To become a licensed specialist for plastic surgery, one has to be a certified surgeon, be recognised as a specialist for general surgery by the *Corporación Nacional Autónoma de Certificaciones Médicas (CONACEM)* and then have completed an additional special training course in plastic, reconstructive and aesthetic surgery which is in keeping with the guidelines of the Society.
Online search for surgeons: Alphabetical list of members via website. Contact addresses are not included.

Sociedad Colombiana de Cirugía Plástica-Estética, Maxilofacial y de la Mano (SCCP)

Edificio Los Hexágonos
Avenida 15 No. 119 A-43 Oficina 406
Santa Fe De Bogotá
COLUMBIA
Tel: +57-1-214 0462/+57-1-213 9028/+57-1-612 7774
E-mail: cirugiaplastica@sky.net.co
http://www.cirugiaplastica.org.co *(Spanish)*

The *Sociedad Colombiana de Cirugía Plástica-Estética, Maxilofacial y de la Mano (SCCP)* promotes the art and science of plastic, reconstructive and aesthetic surgery through qualified surgeons and public access to information.
Founded: 1956
Member qualifications: Members must have completed a specialist training in plastic surgery (one year assistant doctor in general surgery, three years in the area of plastic surgery), and be active in the field of research.
Online search for surgeons: Via the website, listed according to cities.

Asociación de Costa Rica de Cirugía Plástica, Reconstructiva y Estética

Apartado Postal 767–3000
Heredia
COSTA RICA
Tel / Fax: +506-261 1914
E-mail: saraya@racsa.co.cr

Sociedad Dominicana de Cirugía Plástica y Reconstructiva

Plaza Gascue, Of. N° 308
Av. Máximo Gómez N° 29 esq. Calle José Contreras
Santo Domingo
DOMINICAN REPUBLIC
Tel:+1-809-688 8451/+1-809-682 5229
Fax: +1-809-688 8451/+1-809-682 8560
E-mail: julio.pena@codetel.net.do

Sociedad Ecuatoriana de Cirugía Plástica, Reconstructiva y Estética

Av. Villalengua, OE4 - 319 (1511)
Urb. Granda Centeno
Quito
ECUADOR
Tel: +593-2-243 5293 / +593-2-2 921 184
Fax: +593-2-2 921 178
E-mail: pablo_davalos@hotmail.com

Sociedad de Cirugía Plástica de El Salvador

Paseo General Escalón
Apartado Postal 2894
Edif. Villavicencio Plaza, 3er Piso, Local 3 – 13
San Salvador
EL SALVADOR
Tel: +503-263 8188
E-mail: eduardorevelojiron@hotmail.com

Sociedad Guatemalteca de Cirugía Plástica, Reconstructiva y Estética

17 calle 1–61 Zona 1
Colegio de Médicos y Cirujanos de Guatemala

Ciudad de Guatemala
GUATEMALA
Tel: +502-238 1121
Fax: +502-238 1121
E-mail: arruga@intelnet.net.gt

Founded: 1964
Members: 23
Member qualifications: Members are required to be certified doctors and to have completed a three-year training course in general surgery, as well as two to three years of further training in plastic surgery at a recognised university.

Sociedad Hondureña de Cirugía Plástica, Estética y Reparadora

Colonia Florencia Sur, 1ª Calle, Nº 4076
Tegucigalpa
HONDURAS
Tel: +504-235 3328
Fax: +504-235 3329
E-mail: osarmiento@cablecolor.hn

Founded: 1989
Members: 16
Member qualifications: Members must prove that they have completed training in general surgery followed by specialist training at an internationally recognised institution; three years as an assistant doctor (resident) in general surgery, three years plastic surgery.

Asociación Mexicana de Cirugía Plástica, Estética y Reconstructiva

Flamencos Nº 74, Col. San José Insurgentes, México, D. F.
C. P. 03 900
MEXICO
Tel: +52-55-5 615 4911/52-55-800 711 8732
Fax: +52-55-5615-4923
E-mail: amcper@cirugiaplastica.org.mx
asociacion@cirugiaplastica.org.mx
http://www.cirugiaplastica.org.mx *(Spanish and English)*

Founded: 1948
Member qualifications: Doctors who have a university degree in general surgery and are licensed by the *Dirección General de Profesiones* and the *Secretaría de Salud*, have completed three year's training in general surgery, plus three years' experience in plastic surgery and have passed the examination of the *Consejo Mexicano de Cirugía Plástica, Estética y Reconstructiva*.
Online search for surgeons: Via the website, listed according to regions.

Sociedad Nicaragüense de Cirugía Plástica, Estética y Reparadora

Clínica López Galo, Hotel Princess 200 mts abajo-Colonial Los Robles
Managua
NICARAGUA
Tel: +50-5-278 0054
Fax: +50-5-278 0657
E-mail: osnsiu@ibw.com.ni

Sociedad Paraguaya de Cirugía Plástica

Mayor Bullo 541 casi Cerro Corá
Asunción
PARAGUAY
Tel: +595-21-205 323
Fax: +595-21-505 323
E-mail: elvio@webmail.com.py

Sociedad de Cirugía Plástica, Reconstructiva y Estética del Perú

Calle Ramón Ribeyro, Nº 672, Of. 102
San Antonio, Miraflores
Lima 18
PERU
Tel.: +51-1-241 1883
Fax: +51-1-225 6812
E-mail: info@sociprep.org
http://www.sociprep.org *(Spanish)*

Founded: 1950
Members: 110
Member qualifications: Doctors are required to hold a university degree in plastic surgery and have two years' practical experience in this field. They require a letter of recommendation from three other members and must submit a scientific paper.

Sociedad Puertoriqueña de Cirugía Plástica

División de Cirugía Plástica
Recinto de Ciencias Médicas
UPR – P. O. Box 365 067
San Juan
Puerto Rico 00 936–5067
PUERTO RICO
Tel: +1-787-758 2525 Ext 1050
Fax: +1-787-758 119
E-mail: normacruz@sanjuanstar.net

Members: 18
Member qualifications: Membership is open to all plastic surgeons resident in Puerto Rico who have a certificate proving they have completed training as a plastic surgeon in the USA or its territories and have passed the examination of the *American Board of Plastic Surgery (ABPS)*.

Sociedad de Cirugía Plástica, Reparadora y Estética del Uruguay
Laboratorio Galien S. A.
Zelmar Michelini 1230 – CP 11 100
Montevideo
URUGUAY
Tel/Fax: +598-2-336 6646
E-mail: secre@scpu.org
http://www.scpu.org *(Spanish)*

The aim of the *Sociedad de Cirugía Plástica Reparadora y Estética del Uruguay* is to promote progress in the field of plastic surgery, guarantee the high quality work of its members and to support scientific communication.
Founded: 1957
Members: approx. 80
Member qualifications: Full membership is open to doctors who have a specialist qualification in plastic surgery, are licensed to work in this field, have been an "active member" for five years and also work in the field of research.
Online search for surgeons: List of members via website. Contact addresses are not supplied.

Sociedad Venezolana de Cirugía Plástica, Reconstructiva, Estética y Maxilofacial (SVCPREM)
Santa Fé Norte
Av. José María Vargas
Torre del Colegio, Piso 2, Oficina F-2.
Caracas 1060
VENEZUELA
Tel/Fax: +58-212-979 7380
E-mail: svcprem@cantv.net
http://www.sociedadcirugiaplasticavenezolana.org *(Spanish)*

The aim of the *Sociedad Venezolana de Cirugía Plástica, Reconstructiva, Estética y Maxilofacial (SVCPREM)* is to keep its members and the general public updated on developments in the field of plastic and reconstructive surgery and to facilitate contact between members (95 % of plastic surgeons in Venezuela) and patients.
Founded: 1956
Members: 95 % of Venezuelan plastic surgeons
Member qualifications: Members are doctors who have completed an additional training in general surgery for a minimum of three years, and have been assistant doctors (residencia) in plastic surgery for at least three years at an institution recognised by the Society.
Online search for surgeons: Via the website, listed according to regions.

European Union / Switzerland / Iceland

Österreichische Gesellschaft für Plastische, Ästhetische und Rekonstruktive Chirurgie
Secretariat
Frau Eva Klausner
Institut für Biomedizinische Forschung
Währinger Gürtel 18–20
1090 Vienna
AUSTRIA
Tel: +43-1-40 400-5221
Fax: +43-1-40 400-5229
E-mail: office@plastischechirurgie.org
http://www.plastischechirurgie.org *(German)*

The *Österreichische Gesellschaft für Plastische, Ästhetische und Rekonstruktive Chirurgie* is the national representative body for specialists in plastic surgery in Austria. It aims to promote and monitor training and further education of both the practice of and research in plastic surgery, and to represent the professional interests of its members.
Members: approx. 146 full members
Member qualifications: Members must be specialists in plastic surgery, i. e. they must have completed a six-year training at an educational institute that is recognised by the Austrian Ministry of Health.
Online search for surgeons: Via the website, listed according to name or federal state.

Belgian Society for Plastic, Reconstructive & Aesthetic Surgery (BSPRAS)
Société Belge de Chirurgie Plastique, Reconstructrice et Esthétique /
Belgische Vereniging voor Plastische, Reconstructieve en Esthetische Chirurgie
Secretariat
Prof. Dr. P. Wylock
Academic Hospital VUB
Department of Plastic Surgery
Laarbeeklaan 101
1090 Brussels
BELGIUM
Tel: +32-2-477 65 33
Fax: +32-2-477 65 63
E-mail: plhwkp@az.vub.ac.be
http://www.bspras.org *(Dutch, French and soon also English)*

The aim of the *Belgian Society for Plastic, Reconstructive and Aesthetic Surgery (BSPRAS)* is to promote the scientific development of plastic surgery and its related disciplines, and to organise congresses to disseminate new developments in the field.

Founded: 1955
Members: 145 active members
Member qualifications: All active members are Belgian or Luxembourgian doctors recognised by the Belgian Ministry of Health as specialists in plastic, reconstructive and aesthetic surgery who practise only in this field.
Online search for surgeons: Alphabetical list of members. Contact addresses are not included.

Dansk Selskab for Plastik- og Rekonstruktionskirugi

(Danish Society of Plastic and Reconstructive Surgery)
Rigshospitalet Univ. of Copenhagen
Clinic for Plastic Surgery and Burns
Blegdamsvej 9
Copenhagen DK-2100
DENMARK
Tel: +45-3545-3339
Fax: +45-3545-3032
E-mail: jl.z@dadlnet.dk
http://www.dspr.dk *(Danish)*

Members: 105
Member qualifications: Membership is open to Danish specialists in plastic surgery or to doctors who have completed at least one year of training in the field of plastic surgery.

Chirurgi Plastici Fenniae

Finnish Society of Plastic Surgeons
Helsinki Univ. Central Hosp.
Dpt. Plastic Surgery
Topeliuksenkatu, 5
Helsinki SF-00 260
FINLAND
Tel: +358-0-471 7443
Fax: +358-0-471 7570
E-mail: erkki.suominen@huch.fi
http://www.chirurgiplasticifenniae.fi *(Finnish)*

Founded: 1957
Members: 63 members
Member qualifications: Members must be qualified specialists in plastic surgery.
Online search for surgeons: Alphabetical list of members. Contact addresses are not included.

Société Française de Chirurgie Plastique Reconstructrice et Esthétique (SOFCPRE)

SOFCPRE/SNCPRE/CFCPRE
26 rue de Belfort
92 400 Courbevoie
FRANCE
Tel: +33-1-466 774 85
Fax: +33-1-466 774 89
E-mail SOFCPRE: sofcpre@wanadoo.fr
E-mail SNCPRE: contacts@esthetique-chirurgie.org
Business hours: Monday to Friday 10 a. m.–12 p. m. and 2 p. m.–7 p. m.
http://www.plasticiens.org *(French)*

The aim of the *Société Française de Chirurgie Plastique Reconstructrice et Esthétique (SOFCPRE)* is to promote the further development of plastic surgery by coordinating and disseminating the work achieved by specialists in the field.
Founded: 1953
Members: ca. 550
Member qualifications: Active membership is open to doctors who have a specialist qualification in plastic, reconstructive and aesthetic surgery. Since 1988 this has meant: full medical training, followed by a five-year specialisation as a plastic surgeon, as well as a minimum of two further years as an assistant doctor. One can then be registered as a specialist in the *Ordre National des Médecins.*
Online search for surgeons: Via the website, listed according to name, region or city.
Beside the scientific society SOFCPRE, which is responsible for congresses and publications, there are two further branches: the *Collège Français de Chirurgie Plastique Reconstructrice et Esthétique (CFCPRE)* which is responsible for teaching and further education and the *Syndicat National de Chirurgie Plastique Reconstructrice et Esthétique (SNCPRE)*, responsible for public relations. All three associations can be contacted via the website given above.

Vereinigung der Deutschen Plastischen Chirurgen (VDPC)

Geschäftsstelle der Vereinigung der
Deutschen Plastischen Chirurgen
Bleibtreustrasse 12 a
10 623 Berlin
GERMANY
Tel: +49-30-885 1063
Fax: +49-30-885 1067
E-mail: info@plastische-chirurgie.de
http://www.plastische-chirurgie.de *(German)*

Business hours: Monday to Friday 10 a. m. to 2 p. m.
The *Vereinigung der Deutschen Plastischen Chirurgen (VDPC)* is the professional representative body of plastic surgeons in Germany and aims to develop and preserve plastic surgery as an independent monospeciality in Germany, as well as monitor the quality of both the theory and practice of further education in plastic surgery.
Founded: 1968
Members: approx. 460
Member qualifications: Ordinary membership is open to doctors who have completed an additional training in plastic surgery at an institute of higher education officially

recognised in this field. Members must be continually and exclusively practicing plastic surgeons.
Online search for surgeons: Via the website, listed according to name or postal code.

British Association of Plastic Surgeons (BAPS)

The Royal College of Surgeons
35–43 Lincoln's Inn Fields
London, WC2A 3PE
GREAT BRITAIN
Tel: +44-207-831-5161
Fax: +44-207-831-4041
E-mail: secretariat@baps.co.uk
http://www.baps.co.uk *(English)*

The *British Association of Plastic Surgeons (BAPS)* is the professional representative body of plastic and reconstructive surgeons in the United Kingdom, based at the *Royal College of Surgeons*.
The aim of the Association is to protect public health through progress and development in the field of plastic surgery.
Founded: 1946
Members: 300 full members and 300 further members from 54 countries
Member qualifications: Full members must be listed in the Specialist Register of Plastic Surgery of the *General Medical Council* and hold or have held a consultant appointment in plastic surgery in the National Health Service in the United Kingdom or in the Republic of Ireland. They must also be recommended by two full members of the society and be elected by the remaining members.
Online search for surgeons: Unfortunately not possible via the website, but there is a link to the *General Medical Council* (**http://www.gmc-uk.org**) where the qualifications and registration of individual doctors (via name search) can be checked.

Hellenic Society of Plastic Reconstructive & Aesthetic Surgery

32, Xenias street
Zografou
15 771 Athens
GREECE
Tel/Fax: +30-210-77 10 116
E-mail: plastiki@otenet.gr
http://www.hespras.gr *(Greek and English)*

Founded: 1963
Members: approx. 165 full members
Online search for surgeons: Via the website, listed alphabetically.

Félag íslenskra lýtalækna

Icelandic Society of Plastic Surgeons
Landspítalinn Univ. Hospital
P. O.Box 10
Reykjavík – 121
ICELAND
Tel: +354-560 1000
Fax: +354-560 1329
E-mail: rafna@rsp.is

Founded: 1987
Member qualifications: All members are fully qualified plastic surgeons as required by Icelandic law.

Società Italiana di Chirurgia Plastica Ricostruttiva ed Estetica (SICPRE)

Secretariat
Via Campiglione, 18
80 122 Naples
ITALY
Tel: +39-081-7 612 063
Fax: +39-081-2 470 389
E-mail: info@sicpre.org
http://www.sicpre.org *(Italian)*
Business hours: Monday to Thursday 2 p. m. to 6 p. m.

The *Società Italiana di Chirurgia Plastica Ricostruttiva ed Estetica (SICPRE)* aims to promote the scientific and technical development of all aspects of plastic surgery, to protect the reputation of the field and to guarantee a high quality of practice.
Founded: 1934
Members: approx. 800, of which 400 are full members
Member qualifications: Full membership is open to doctors who are specialists in plastic surgery, can provide proof of their qualification and are full-time practicing plastic surgeons.
Online search for surgeons: Via the website, structured according to region.

Nederlandse Vereniging voor Plastische Chirurgie

Netherlands Society for Plastic Surgery
Centraal secretariaat
Pottenbakkerij 12
2993 CN Barendrecht
THE NETHERLANDS
Tel: +31-180-690 996
Fax: +31-180-690 995
E-mail: secretariaat@nvpc.nl
http://www.nvpc.nl *(Dutch)*

Founded: 1950
Members: 302 in total (164 plastic surgeons)
Member qualifications: Full membership is open to doc-

tors who are registered as plastic surgeons in the Netherlands and are recommended by other members (plastic surgeons).
Online search for surgeons: Not possible.

Sociedade Portuguesa de Cirurgia Plástica Reconstrutiva e Estética (SPCPRE)

Av^a^ da República, 34 – 1°
1050–193 Lisbon
PORTUGAL
Tel/Fax: +351-21-793 74 12
E-mail: spcpre@mail.telepac.pt
http://www.spcpre.org *(Portuguese)*

The *Sociedade Portuguesa de Cirurgia Plástica Reconstrutiva e Estética (SPCPRE)* has the aim of promoting communication between plastic surgeons as well as providing programmes to support teaching in this field and to facilitate international contacts with other scientific societies.
Founded: 1961
Members: approx. 126
Member qualifications: Membership is open to doctors who, having gained a qualification in general medicine, have completed a comprehensive, six-year specialist training in all fields of plastic surgery and are recognised by a national jury, some of whom are members of the national medical council. Continuous further training through participation at congresses and courses is also mandatory.
Online search for surgeons: Via the website, listed according to name and hospital/region.

Svensk Plastikkirurgisk Förening

Swedish Association of Plastic Surgeons
http://www.svls.se/sektioner/pk *(Swedish, only first page in English)* Affilated to:

Sociedad Española de Cirugía Plástica Reparadora y Estética (SECPRE)

Villanueva 11 – 3ª Planta
28 001 Madrid
SPAIN
Tel: +34-91-576 5995
Fax: +34-91-431 5153
E-mail: info@secpre.org
http://www.secpre.org *(Spanish)*

The aim of the *Sociedad Española de Cirugía Plástica Reparadora y Estética (SECPRE)*, which includes the majority of Spanish plastic surgeons, is to promote the reputation of the field of plastic surgery, to cooperate with public and private organisations, to guarantee high quality standards and to promote scientific research and teaching.
Founded: 1956
Members: approx. 650
Member qualifications: Members must have gained a qualification in general medicine, followed by five year's specialist training at an accredited hospital, at least three of which must have been devoted to the field of plastic, reconstructive and aesthetic surgery.
Online search for surgeons: Via the website, listed according to region.

The Swedish Society of Medicine

(Svenska Läkaresällskapet)
Klara Östra Kyrkogata 10
P. O. Box 738
SE-101 35 Stockholm
SWEDEN
Tel: +46-8-440 88 60
Fax: +46-8-440 88 99
E-mail: sls@svls.se
http://www.svls.se *(Swedish and English)*

Schweizerische Gesellschaft für Plastische, Rekonstruktive und Ästhetische Chirurgie (SGPRAC)

Société Suisse de Chirurgie Plastique, Reconstructive et Esthétique (SSCPRE)
SGPRAC-SSCPRE Office
15, avenue des Planches
1820 Montreux
SWITZERLAND
Tel: +41-21-963 21 39
Fax: +41-21-963 21 49
Mobil: +41-79-300 30 33
E-mail: info@plastic-surgery.ch
http://www.plastic-surgery.ch *(German, French and English)*

The *Schweizerische Gesellschaft für Plastische, Rekonstruktive und Ästhetische Chirurgie (SGPRAC)* aims to promote research and teaching in the field of plastic surgery, maintain contact to related societies and organisations at home and abroad and promote the professional interests and the ethical principles in the medical practice of its members.
Founded: 1965
Members: 111 ordinary members
Member qualifications: Ordinary membership is open to specialists in plastic surgery who practice mainly in Switzerland, can provide proof of a confederate specialist qualification or the EU equivalent and who have passed the EBOPRAS examination.
Online search for surgeons: Via the website, listed according to region.

Mid-Eastern Europe

Czech Society of Plastic Surgery

Univerzita Karlova
Teaching Hospital
500 36 Hradec Králové
CZECH REPUBLIC
Tel: +420-49-23 641
Fax: +420-49-27 758
E-mail: ldrazan@med.muni.cz

Hungarian Society of Plastic, Reconstructive and Aesthetic Surgeons (HSPRAS)

Magyar Plasztikai Helyreállító és Esztétikai Sebész Társaság
Tátra Street 43
1136 Budapest
HUNGARY
Tel/Fax: +36-1-3 291 425
E-mail: esorba@sage.hu
Website: http://www.plasztika.org.hu *(Hungarian)*

Slovak Society of Plastic and Aesthetic Surgery

Slovenská spolocnost plastickej a estetickej chirurgie
NsP Ruzinov – Ruzinovská 6
Bratislava 82 606
SLOVAKIA
Tel/Fax: +421-2-4 333 6741
E-mail: koller@nspr.sk

Founded: 1962
Members: 124
Member qualifications: Members are plastic surgeons, although general surgeons and specialists from related fields are also admitted.

Croatian Society of Plastic, Reconstructive and Aesthetic Surgery (CSPRAS)

Hrvatsko društvo za plastičnu, rekonstrukcijsku i estetsku kirurgiju (HDPREK)
University Hospital Dubrava Zagreb
Department of Plastic Surgery
Av. Gojka Šuška 6
10 000 Zagreb
CROATIA
Tel: +385-1-28 63 695
Fax: +385-1-290 2451
E-mail: plkir@kbd.hr
http://www.kbd.hr/plastkir *(Croatian and English)*

Founded: 1997
Members: approx. 40
Member qualifications: Plastic surgeons who qualified before 1994 (three to five years of training) and are recognised by the Ministry of Health, and plastic surgeons who qualified after 1994 (seven years' training). Also admitted are general surgeons who have worked in the field of plastic and reconstructive surgery for over ten years and are recognised by the Croatian Ministry of Health.

Romanian Society of Plastic and Reconstructive Surgery

Emergency Hospital Bagdasar
Sos. Berceni nr. 10
Bucharest
ROMANIA
Tel: +40-21-4 610 502
Fax: +40-232-216 588
E-mail: noela@pcnet.ro
tstamate@mail.dntis.ro

Founded: 1990

Yugoslav Society of Plastic, Reconstructive and Aesthetic Surgery

Jugoslovensko udruženje za plastičnu, rekonstruktivnu i estetsku hirurgiju
Bulevar Kralja Aleksandra 280
11 000 Belgrade
SERBIA and MONTENEGRO
Tel: +381-11-380 8309
Fax: +381-11-380 6434
E-mail: office@yupras.co.yu
Members of the Association are plastic surgeons in Serbia and Montenegro.
http://www.yupras.co.yu *(English)*

Founded: 1996
Members: ca. 42
Online search for surgeons: Via the website, alphabetical listing.

South Eastern Europe

Bulgarian National Society of Plastic Surgery and Burns

Medical Institut Pirogov
21 Bul. Macedonia
Sofia 1606
BULGARIA
Tel: +359-2-546 108
www.bapras.gr

Founded: 1962

Turkish Society of Plastic Reconstructive and Aesthetic Surgeons
Türk Plastik, Rekonstrüktif ve Estetik Cerrahi Derneği
Billur Sokak No: 35/3
Kavaklıdere
06 700 Ankara
TURKEY
Tel: +90-312-427 22 23,
Fax: +90-312-427 52 73
E-mail: tprec@tpcd.org.tr
http://www.tpcd.org.tr. *(Turkish and English)*

The aim of the *Turkish Society of Plastic Reconstructive and Aesthetic Surgeons* is to promote the development of plastic surgery in Turkey, to guarantee international standards of quality, to support scientific studies and to make and maintain international contacts with other societies and leading foreign hospitals.

Founded: 1961
Members: approx. 335 active members
Member qualifications: Active membership is open to specialists in plastic, reconstructive and aesthetic surgery who are recommended for membership by two other active members.
Online search for surgeons: Via the website, alphabetical listing.

Baltic States

Latvian Association of Plastic Surgeons
Latvijas Plastisko ķirurgu asociācijas
Hipokrāta iela 2
1038 Rīga
LATVIA
Tel: +371-7 042 641
Fax: +371-2 539 524
http://www.pka.lv *(Latvian)*

Founded: 1992
Members: 21
Member qualifications: Members must be recognised specialists for plastic surgery.

Lithuanian Plastic and Reconstructive Surgery Society
Lietuvos Plastines & Rekonstrukcines Chirurgijos Draugija
Clinic for Plastic and Reconstructive Surgery
Tilto str. 11
Vilnius 01 101
LITHUANIA
Tel: +370-5-262 94 90
Fax: +370-5-212 51 36
E-mail: vitkus@takas.lt

Founded: 1990
Members: 23
Member qualifications: Following the successful completion of a three-year course in general surgery at the University of Vilnius, members must complete an additional two-years' training in plastic surgery. An application for membership must be supported by at least two other members of the Society.

Russian Federation

Russian Society of Plastic Reconstructive and Aesthetic Surgeons
SPRAS
Abricosovski Pereulok 2
Moscow GSP-2 199 921
RUSSIAN FEDERATION
Tel: +7-095-248-12-66
Fax: +7-095-248-60-77
E-mail: radamian@mail.med.ru
http://www.spras.ru *(Russian)*

Founded: 1994
Members: 560
Member qualifications: Doctors wishing to join are required to have at least five years' practical experience in the field of plastic surgery. They must be recommended by two other members of the Society.

Northern and South Africa

Egyptian Society of Plastic and Reconstructive Surgeons (ESPRS)
2 El-Thawra Street
Dokki
Cairo 12 311
EGYPT
Tel: +20-2-748 8728
Fax: +20-2-337 9110
E-mail: ESPRS@hotmail.com
http://www.geocities.com/esprs *(Arabic and English)*

The *Egyptian Society of Plastic and Reconstructive Surgeons (ESPRS)* is the official representative body of plastic surgeons in Egypt.
Founded: 1962
Members: approx. 170
Online search for surgeons: Via the website, listed in alphabetical order.

Société Marocaine de Chirurgie Plastique, Reconstruction et Esthétique

Clinique de La Nichée
34, rue Zerhoun
Mers Sultan
21 000 Casablanca
MOROCCO
Tel: +212-22- 26 47 55

Association of Plastic and Reconstructive Surgeons of Southern Africa (APRSSA)

P.O. Box 130 891
Bryanston
Johannesburg 2021
SOUTH AFRICA
Tel: +27-11-463 1210
Fax: +27-11-463 2485
E-mail: tomford@pixie.co.za
www.plasticsurgeons.co.za *(English)*

The *Association of Plastic and Reconstructive Surgeons of Southern Africa (APRSSA)* aims to support its members in their efforts to achieve highest quality patient care and attain and maintain professional and ethical standards.
Founded: 1956
Members: over 120
Member qualifications: Full members must be registered at the *Health Professions Council of South Africa (HPCSA)*, and should also be full members of the *South African Medical Association (SAMA)*. To be admitted, candidates require the support of a voting member of the Association and be elected by the other members.
Online search for surgeons: Via the website, listed according to regions. Includes tips for overseas patients.

Société Tunisienne de Chirurgie Plastique Reconstructrive, Maxillo-Faciale et Esthétique

Hôpital Sahloul
4011 Hammam Sousse
TUNISIA
Tel: +216-71-367 447 / +216-73-367 451

Near East

Israel Society of Plastic Surgeons

The Chaim Sheba Medical Center, Advanced Technology Center
Tel Hashomer 52 621
ISRAEL
Tel: +972-3-530 3114
Fax: +972-3-530 314

Jordanian Society for Plastic and Reconstructive Surgery

Jordan Medical Association
P. O. Box 921 919
Amman
JORDAN
Tel: +962-6-665 620
Fax: +962-6-644 700

Lebanese Society of Plastic, Reconstructive and Aesthetic Surgery (LSPRAS)

E-mail: Info@estheticlebanon.com
http://www.estheticlebanon.com *(English)*

The aim of the *Lebanese Society of Plastic, Reconstructive and Aesthetic Surgery* (LSPRAS) is to supply the general public with up-to-date information on the latest techniques in the field of plastic surgery and to facilitate contact with qualified doctors.
Founded: 1966
Members: ca. 52
Member qualifications: Members must be recognised by the *Lebanese Order of Physicians* and the Lebanese Ministry of Health. They must also prove that they have intensively studied the latest developments and techniques in this field.
Online search for surgeons: Via the website, alphabetical listing.

Middle East

Iranian Society of Plastic and Reconstructive Surgery

P. O. Box 14 335
Teheran 1313
IRAN
Tel: +98-21-655 573
Fax: +98-21-7 155 198

Kuwait Society of Plastic Surgeons

P. O. Box 31 420
Al-Sulaibikhat 90 805
KUWAIT
Tel: +965-483 4785
Fax: +965-481 1784
E-mail: abrelari@ipras.org

Plastic Surgery Society – Emirates Medical Association
P. O. Box 6600
Dubai
UNITED ARAB EMIRATES (UAE)
Tel: +971-4-377 377
Fax: +971-4-344 082
E-mail: numairy@emirates.net.ae

Founded: 1993
Members: 25
Member qualifications: Full membership is open to doctors who live in the United Arab Emirates, hold a degree in plastic surgery (not aesthetic or cosmetic surgery) from a reputable university and are licensed as specialists in this field.

Asia

Chinese Plastic Surgery Society
Institute Plastic Surgery
Chinese Academy of Medical Sciences
Ba-da-chu
Beijing 100 041
PEOPLE'S REPUBLIC OF CHINA
Tel: +86-1-886 4812
Fax: +86-1-886 4137
E-mail: yeguang@126.com

Hong Kong Society of Plastic and Reconstructive Surgeons
Room 2210, Bank of America Tower
12 Harcourt Road Central
HONG KONG
Tel: +852-2 523 7690
Fax: +852-2 523 7363
E-mail: info@plasticsurgery.org.hk
http://www.plasticsurgery.org.hk *(English)*

Founded: 1967
Members: 36
Member qualifications: Members must be recognised as plastic surgeons by the *Hong Kong College of Surgeons*.

Association of Plastic Surgeons of India (APSI)
Dr. Rajeev B. Ahuja
B-18, Swasthya Vihar
Vikas Marg, Delhi 110 092
INDIA
Tel: +91-11-2 251 6733 /+91-11-2 323 1871
Fax: +91-11-243 2275
E-mail: rbahuja@vsnl.com

Founded: 1957
Members: 826
Member qualifications: Members must be trained plastic surgeons or trained general surgeons with proven experience in plastic surgery.

Japan Society of Plastic and Reconstructive Surgery
Nihon keiseigeka gakkai
Rakuyô Bldg. 3 F
Tsurumaki 519
Waseda, Shinjuku-ku
Tokyo-to 162-0041
JAPAN
Tel: +81-3-5287-6773
http://www.jsprs.or.jp *(Japanese)*

Founded: 1958
Members: 4100
Member qualifications: Plastic surgeons wishing to apply for membership require a letter of recommendation from two members of the council.

Philippine Association of Plastic Reconstructive and Aesthetic Surgeons (PAPRAS)
2nd floor, Bldg. A
SM Megamall
Ortigas Center
Mandaluyong Metro
Manila
PHILIPPINES
Tel: +63-2-638 69 34/+63-2-638 69 35
E-mail: laserpsg@skyinet.net
http://www.plasticsurgery-phil.org *(English)*

Members: approx. 40

Society of Plastic and Reconstructive Surgeons of Thailand (TSPRS)
Royal Golden Jubilee Building (9th floor)
2 soi Soonvijai, New Petchaburi Road
Bangkok 10 320
THAILAND
Tel: +66-2-716 6214
Fax: +66-2-716 6966
E-mail: kamol@plasticsurgery.or.th
http://www.plasticsurgery.or.th *(Thai)*

Online search for surgeons: Currently under construction.

Australia / New Zealand

The Australian Society of Plastic Surgeons (ASPS)

Suite 503, Level 5
69 Christie Street
St Leonards NSW 2065
AUSTRALIA
Toll Free: 1 300 367 446
Tel: +61-2-94 379 200
Fax: +61-2-94 379 210
E-mail: info@plasticsurgery.org.au
http://www.plasticsurgery.org.au *(English)*

The *Australian Society of Plastic Surgeons (ASPS)* is devoted to the maintenance of a high professional and ethical standard in the field of plastic surgery and to the provision of information to all interested parties.
Founded: In 1971 as the Australian branch of the *Division of Plastic and Reconstructive Surgery*, which is part of the *Royal Australasian College of Surgeons (RACS)* responsible for Australia and New Zealand.
Members: 224
Member qualifications: All members must be members of the RACS or apply for membership thereof, must be recommended by other plastic surgeon members and elected by the remaining members. All members are fully qualified specialists in the field of plastic surgery. They are only accepted once they have completed the RACS-required training and if they are full-time practicing plastic surgeons.
Online search for surgeons: Via the website, listed according to name. A geographical list is available from the Society office upon request.

New Zealand Association of Plastic Reconstructive and Aesthetic Surgeons

243 Remuera Road
Remuera
Auckland
NEW ZEALAND
Tel: +64-9-5 295 002
Fax: +64-9-5 246 043
E-mail: jsj@plasticsurgeons.co.nz

Founded: 1976
Members: 34
Member qualifications: All members are also members of the *Royal Australasian College of Surgeons* (or an equivalent organisation) and are registered at the *New Zealand Medical Council* as specialists in plastic and reconstructive surgery.

Plastic Surgery on the Web

compiled by NANNETTE BÜHL, Paris

XI.2.2.1 General information – from liposuction and breast augmentation to rhinoplasty and facelifts to hair transplants and Botox injections...

Websites and local information, e. g. websites for surgeons, private clinics etc. can be found at:

United States: **http://google.com** > search term "plastic surgery"
Canada: **http://google.ca** > search term "plastic surgery"
Great Britain: **http://www.google.co.uk** > search term "plastic surgery"

http://www.plasticsurgery.org *(English)*
Well designed and highly accessible website by the *American Society of Plastic Surgeons (ASPS)* and the *Plastic Surgery Educational Foundation (PSEF).*

As well as a detailed history of plastic surgery, this website presents a Procedures section with detailed explanations of all the surgical procedures available (also in Spanish), a Photo Gallery with before/after photos, and statistics for individual procedures (collected in the US).
For visitors with a special interest in this latter subject, the areas Statistics and Costs have plenty of detail to offer – all relevant figures after 1992, visual overviews and charts etc.
Patient Advocacy is dedicated to providing legal information to patients (US law) and offers links to organisations and self-help groups e. g. for women suffering from breast cancer.
The Newsroom is designed for media use, providing additional background information, press releases etc.
The surgeon search engine, Find a Plastic Surgeon, accesses an extensive directory. Users can search by name or state, or enter their own address to find a local surgeon.
ASPS members, i. e. the society's plastic surgeons, have access to a restricted Members section (login / password-protected); non-member practitioners can access the Medical Professionals section to inform themselves about conferences and international programmes or to search for work offers.
The site also provides links to related organisations and associations, as well as to the electronic magazine Plastic Surgery Today and the *ASPS* Newsletter, an online version of the weekly *ASPS* supplement to the popular American newspaper *USA Today*.
For English-speaking persons (also outside the US) interested in gaining a detailed overview of plastic surgery or looking for a qualified practitioner; for journalists requiring background information, statistics and diagrams; for practitioners seeking information about events etc.

http://www.surgery.org *(English)*
The website of the *American Society for Aesthetic Plastic Surgery (ASAPS)* has a similar structure to the one described above, offering the same amount of extensive information in a different format.

In Procedures, the different types of surgical procedures are explained in great detail (partially also in Spanish). As well as techniques, non-surgical aspects are addressed: "Will my insurance cover the procedure?", "What will happen on the day of my operation?", "How long will the changes last?" etc. The text explanations often contain links to the Photo Gallery, a before/after collection of photos that can also be searched directly for specific procedures.
The Public Site presents current studies and news from all areas related to plastic surgery.

Visitors who want to communicate directly with a surgeon may do so via email in the section Ask a Surgeon. A selection of professional replies to visitors' questions, e. g. in regard to Botox, facial implants, surgery for teenagers etc., is posted here (updated weekly).
The website also features online searching for practitioners; the Find a Surgeon directory lists contact details for professional members based in the US and many other countries.
The Press Center provides journalists with press releases and detailed statistics, and also lists contact details for practitioners acting as official media representatives for ASAPS. These designated practitioners are also available for interviews. For visitors requiring further visual information, the Press Center additionally provides online ordering for videos of surgical procedures.
Members and other interested practitioners can access the Medical Professionals section for details about conferences and international events. A link to the ASAPS Aesthetic Surgery Journal leads to a section where visitors can read summaries of the articles free of charge (some of the articles are also available in Portuguese), or download full-length versions for a fee.
For English-speaking persons interested in gaining a detailed overview of plastic surgery or looking for a qualified practitioner; for journalists requiring background information, news and contact persons; for practitioners seeking information about international events etc.

http://www.facial-plastic-surgery.org *(English)*
The website of the *American Academy of Facial Plastic and Reconstructive Surgery (AAFPRS)* is structured like a consultation session.
First, the virtual patient enters a Virtual Exam Room, located in the Procedures section. Here, the medical terms for different parts of the face are explained. Thus informed and knowing which procedure to pursue, the patient can then read up on the before, during and after details of the operation in Procedure Types. If there is still confusion despite all these medical details, he or she can browse the FAQ's – Frequently Asked Questions or look at the before/after photos. There is also a Glossary of Terms for those who want to learn even more about the different surgical aspects, and an archive of the online magazine Facial Plastic Surgery Today for further perusal. Prospective patients who were sufficiently impressed by this virtual consultation can use the Physician Finder to obtain contact details for AAFPRS surgeons.
Journalists are provided with press releases and statistics in the Media &Exhibitors area, and practitioners can find out about international conferences and humanitarian projects in the Physicians section.
For English-speaking prospective patients looking for a detailed introduction to facial plastic surgery.

http://www.cosmeticplasticsurgerystatistics.com
(English)
This in-depth reference site on cosmetic surgery presents detailed information about the costs of operations and the eligibility of prospective patients for specific procedures, extremely detailed descriptions of all procedures, an exhaustive list of risks and complications, and guidelines for the time before and after the operation.
The section Find a Surgeon can be used to search for registered specialists and verify their qualifications, and specific questions can be posted at Ask a Surgeon. An interesting additional feature is provided by the Financing section, which is linked to a separate website for financing cosmetic surgical procedures (US citizens only). The terms of payment, i. e. the loan, can be arranged online!
For English-speaking persons seeking reliable in-depth information on the surgical procedures available and the risks associated with them, and for US citizens investigating financing options for their operation.

http://www.abplsurg.org *(English)*
The website of the *American Board of Plastic Surgery (ABPS)*, one of the 24 sections of the *American Board of Medical Specialties (ABMS)*, is formatted for professional medical use. It provides details about the qualifications required by

different specialists, the training programmes available, practical training, diplomas etc.
For English-speaking medical professionals looking for information about the qualification requirements of the ABPS, and for prospective patients who want to know exactly which qualifications their plastic surgeon should have.

Further **French-language** websites containing general and local information, e. g. websites for surgeons, private clinics etc. can be found at:

http://www.google.fr > Search term "chirurgie plastique"

http://plasticiens.org *(French)*
Website for the *Société Française de Chirurgie Plastique Reconstructrice et Esthétique (SOFCPRE)*. These internet pages, presented as the web portal to plastic surgery in France (Portail Français de la Chirurgie Plastique Reconstructice et Esthétique), offer French-only overviews of surgical procedures similar to those provided by the US websites described above. However, this portal offers much less detailed information than its American counterparts.
As well as describing details of operations (Interventions) in the area of aesthetic surgery, the sections of the website also explain procedures of general plastic surgery, microsurgery, burns surgery and humanitarian plastic surgery," and provides links to relevant articles.
The surgeon address book (Annuaire des plasticiens) is also very useful. Sorted by name and city, it lists all SOFCPRE members complete with contact details.
Of course, the society itself and its training programmes are also represented with extensive sections. Cyberstaff is a members-only forum, and surgeons looking for employment can search the classifieds (Petites annonces).
For French-speaking persons interested in an overview of the procedures available or looking for a surgeon in France.

http://www.sofcep.org *(French)*
Website of the *Société Française des Chirurgiens Esthétiques Plasticiens (SOFCEP)*, a French society of plastic surgeons. The site presents details about plastic surgical procedures similar to the SOFCPRE pages, as well as additional information. The different types of operations are described extensively in the section Les opérations en Chirurgie Esthétique.
There are also hints and tips – Comment choisir son Chirurgien (How to choose a surgeon) – and useful French legal information, for example that French surgeons are obligated to supply prospective patients with a quotation (Le devis obligatoire). As well as the operative costs, this quotation lists the practitioner's registration number. An article about aesthetic surgery in France (La Chirurgie Esthétique en France) is of similar interest – it discusses the medical qualifications required by surgeons and different categories of specialisation.
Again, visitors can search for surgeons online (all SOFCEP members are also SOFCPRE members), listed by name and by region in the Liste des membres. Members of the society have an additional area, which can only be accessed with a login and password. Links to several other international societies are also supplied.
For French-speaking persons interested in an overview of plastic surgery in France or looking for a qualified surgeon in France.

http://doc.esthetique.free.fr *(French and English)*
This French website, which is also available in English, is designed without any photos or diagrams but as a question/answer game:
There are six sections – Chirurgie du visage (face), Traitement des rides (folds/wrinkles), Calvitié (baldness), Chirurgie des seins (breasts), Chirurgie de l'abdomen (tummy), Lipoaspiration (liposuction) and Chirurgie du sexe feminin (female genitalia) – each of which is subdivided into specific categories (lifting, nose, etc). Each of the categories has approx. 15 questions and answers: "What exactly is...?", "Who is this suitable for?", "How long does the change last for?", "What will the operation cost?", etc.
Nouveautés (news) presents surgical techniques that are currently popular (e. g. Botox injections, hair transplants). Liens utiles provides a modest collection of links.
For French or English speaking persons seeking clear, detailed answers to specific questions regarding different areas of plastic surgery.

http://www.infoesth.com *(French)*
Website of the French association *AIME (Association pour l'Information Médicale en Esthétique)* – medical information about aesthetic surgery.
To gain access to the independent data provided by this non-commercial association, visitors needs to pay a subscription fee (EUR 40 per annum). This unlocks the INFOESTH database run by *AIME*, who are fully focused on the advocacy of consumers, i. e. prospective patients. The database contains detailed independent information on all available techniques, realistic assessments of the associated risks, studies, photos, legal aid for botched operations etc. Before subscribing, visitors can get a taste of the site by browsing the archived editorials (Archives des éditoriaux). These frequently question the qualifications of experts in the field and critically examine new techniques and products.
For French-speaking persons interested in general information as well as critical assessments of plastic surgery and the possibilities and risks it entails, and who are willing to pay EUR 40 per year for site access.

Further **German-language** websites containing general and local information, e. g. websites for surgeons, private clinics etc. can be found at:

http://www.google.de > Search term "Plastische Chirurgie"

http://www.plastische-chirurgie.de *(German)*
Website for the *Vereinigung der Deutschen Plastischen Chirurgen (VDPC)*.
This transparently structured website is free of confusing visual design elements and focuses on the four tiers of plastic surgery: Rekonstruktive Chirurgie (reconstructive surgery), Handchirurgie (hand surgery), Ästhetische Chirurgie (aesthetic surgery) and Verbrennungschirurgie (burns surgery). As well as the specific details of the procedures, the potential success and limitations of each area are described. Questions such as "How do I prepare for the operation?" or "What happens after the operation?" are also addressed.
Like most of the websites described, this site contains an online directory of the association's members, available in the section Wie Sie Ihren Arzt finden and searchable by post code or name. A small selection of surgeons in other European countries is also included.
Für Ärzte und Mitglieder provides practitioners and members with details about conferences and symposiums, training programme details and an employment notice board. Members additionally have password-protected access to a restricted section, the Interner Bereich.
For German-speaking persons interested in a well-structured overview of the different surgical procedures available or looking for a qualified surgeon in Germany.

http://www.lifeline.de/ilchirurg *(German)*
These German-language web pages are part of the larger health website *Lifeline*, whose authors are scientific and medical journalists, medical professionals and other health experts. Different surgical techniques are reviewed by individual studies, essays and articles, e. g. "The dangers of treating wrinkles with silicone oil", "How to find a good cosmetic surgeon", "The essential aspects of an operation", etc. Although the titles frequently read like they're out of a women's magazine, the articles associated with them offer a good, accurate introduction to the themes described. When browsing these pages, visitors can also quickly cross-reference to the other health topics presented by Lifeline.
For German-speaking persons interested in gaining an introduction to plastic surgery and its procedures.

XI.2.2.2 Teenagers – what's first, the new nose or the driver's licence?

Parent advice *(English)*
http://www.entdr.com/teenplastice.html
The web pages of this site, hosted by the *Associates in Otolaryngology, Head & Neck Surgery*, provide a Parents Guide on Facial Plastic Surgery for Teens. The guidelines presented here are supplied by the *American Academy of Facial Plastic and Reconstructive Surgery (AAFPRS)* and answer questions such as "Should teenagers have cosmetic surgery?", "Which operations are suitable?" etc. The guide emphasises the importance of communication between parents and children, outlines what to expect from the first consultation with the surgeon, and addresses the possible operative results, associated risks and costs.

Patients like any other? *(English)*
http://www.facial-plastic-surgery.org/patient/fps_today/vol15_3/vol15_3pg1.html
This article, taken from the online journal of the *American Academy of Facial Plastic and Reconstructive Surgery (AAFPRS)*, presents a brief overview of issues specifically related to plastic surgery for teenagers.

Briefing *(English)*
http://www.plasticsurgery.org/news_room/Briefing-Papers-Index.cfm
These "briefing papers" on plastic surgery for teenagers, to be found on the website of the *American Society of Plastic Surgeons (ASPS)*, review the surgical procedures relevant to teenage patients, outline the legal situation (US law) and urge parents to closely examine their children's level of maturity and self-understanding.
All three of the websites described are targeted at English-speaking parents of teenagers that wish to undergo plastic surgery. The sites focus on providing answers to essential questions and issues.

TeensHealth *(English)*
http://kidshealth.org/teen/your_mind/body_image/plastic_surgery.html or **www.kidshealth.org** > Teens > Your Body > Getting Medical Care > Plastic Surgery
TeensHealth comprises the teenager-oriented pages of the child health website "KidsHealth," created by the US-based *Nemours Foundation*.
The "Plastic Surgery" page is aimed at teenagers who are unhappy with their bodies and are considering plastic surgery as a solution to their issues. The article describes

plastic surgery and the results it can produce from an educational perspective, and suggests ways of how teenagers can communicate the subject to their parents.
For English-speaking teenagers who are considering plastic surgery as a solution to their problems.

XI.2.2.3 Transgender

http://www.transgender-net.de *(German with English-language links)*
This website is presented as the main portal for German-language transgender sites on the internet. It provides links for areas such as people, books, films, music, life, celebrities, beauty, law/politics, and Medizin. This "Medicine" section is subdivided into Allgemeine Übersichtsseiten (general overview pages), describing everything men and women should know about the medical treatment of transsexuality, Definitionen (definitions) of concepts such as transgender, transsexuality and transvestism, and Geschlechtsangleichende Operationen (sex change operations), outlining surgical techniques, surgeons, experiences etc. Further sections include Psyche, Stimme und Hormone (psychology, voice and hormones) and lastly Plastische Chirurgie (plastic surgery) – the Pamela Anderson dream and its limitations. This section provides numerous links to personal accounts, surgical reports and impressive before/after photos (mostly of men being transformed into women). Many of the links lead to English-language sites.
For German-speaking men and women with a general interest in the transgender phenomenon or seeking specific information about the possibilities of transgender plastic surgery.

http://www.transhistory.org *(English)*
This website focuses on transgender history. The main historical developments are outlined in TransHistory; Organizations provides links to US-based transgender organisations; Medical describes the first transsexual operations at the beginning of the 20th century and traces the developments of this specific branch of medicine through the biographies of the pioneering surgeons involved (Magnus Hirschfeld, Felix Abraham, Harry Benjamin etc.).
For English-speaking men and women looking for an overview of transgender history.

http://www.tsroadmap.com *(English)*
The most interesting sections of this largely text-based website are Info Sources, listing details of US-based and international transgender organisations, and Transition's Real World Issues, which provides information about legal aspects, deed poll changes and insurance. An interesting description of surgical details can be found in Facial Feminization Surgery (FFS), a subsection of Your physical well-being and appearance. "FFS" provides in-depth details about all the possible surgical techniques of feminisation after a sex change, e. g. for the brow, nose, ears or chin, as well as implants, risks etc.
If you would like some visual illustrations to complement the detailed descriptions found on sites such as the TS Road Map, make sure to also visit the pages of the *Transsexual Women's Resources* described below.
For English-speaking men and women interested in the specific aspects of a sex change and the associated follow-up operations or in other aspects of transgender existence.

http://www.annelawrence.com/twr *(English)*
This website, designed predominantly in the colours pink and light blue, addresses all the medical topics of the male to female sex change: Sex Reassignment Surgery, Hormone Therapy, Breast Augmentation Surgery and Facial Feminization Surgery, but also Voice Feminization Techniques, Psychological Resources, Sexuality and many more. All of the sections contain numerous links to medical studies, international organisations, personal accounts of surgery etc. The before/after photos some links lead to are often surprising and impressive, particularly the photos of the Facial Feminization Surgery and Sex Reassignment Surgery sections (the latter of which is very graphic, so be warned!). For Medical Professionals is aimed at practitioners who are looking for peer discussion groups or simply want to inform themselves about the topic.
The most comprehensive site for transsexual women planning to have genital surgery or plastic surgery for further feminisation and seeking detailed information.

XI.2.2.4 Computer-generated beauty

Let's be honest: who hasn't ever stood in front of the mirror and stretched their face towards their ears or their hairline, imagining what a facelift would look like – or pretending that ever-growing double chin was eliminated? Or taken it a step further and retouched their portrait photos in an image-editing program like Photoshop?
In fact there are specifically developed computer techniques for this very purpose, used by many surgeons to give their patients a mock preview of the operative result – virtual before/after photos. Prospective patients who haven't dared make an appointment for a consultation but would still like to get some idea of what's possible should visit one of the two websites described below – just send in your photo, and for a fee, it will be beautified using the latest in photo manipulation technology!
For anyone who would like a virtual "after" photo without ever committing to an operation.

http://www.aprille.com *(English)*
Even virtual beauty has its price: A computer-corrected photo costs US $ 35 at *Aprille.com*. First, you "purchase" the desired modification by clicking on a technique (facelift, rhinoplasty, breast augmentation etc.) – it's almost like online book shopping ("You have added a Facelift to your basket"), then you take this "basket" to the "till." After the obligatory question if you'd like any other procedures with that facelift, you get to enter your credit card number. Only then can you email your photo to *Aprille* – if you don't own a digital camera, you'll need to have the photo scanned yourself. The "after" photo is also returned as an email.

http://www.angelslab.com *(English)*
Beautification at *Angels LAB* is a similar process – as a bonus, this company also offers to fix your teeth! Again, you first need to select a technique, then pay for the service (significantly more expensive at US$90), and then send off the photo. As well emailing it, however, you can also upload your digital photo to the website – or even send your physical photograph by snail mail.

XI.2.2.5 Online surgeon search

The most reliable method of finding a qualified surgeon via the internet is to use the search functions offered by official websites for plastic surgery associations and societies. These directories readily provide contact details for member surgeons, usually sorted by name or region.

International

International Society of Aesthetic Plastic Surgery (ISAPS) – Branch of the *International Confederation for Plastic Reconstructive and Aesthetic Surgery (IPRAS)*
http://www.isaps.org *(English)*
Members worldwide

USA / Canada / International

American Board of Medical Specialties (ABMS)
http://www.abms.org *(English)*
This website provides a quick and efficient method of verifying the surgeon envisioned for a prospective operation. Visitors simply register online and receive a password, which is required to access the search page. After the name of the surgeon and the country/state is entered (the surgeons registered with this service are predominantly American), the qualifications are checked. This is an easy way of establishing whether the practitioner in question has had sufficient specialist training to successfully perform the desired operation. The search function also works for the other 23 areas of medical specialisation encompassed by the ABMS. Only five searches may be performed per day; if this isn't enough, one of the following services can be used in addition:
ChoicePoint www.choicepoint.net
Certifacts Online www.certifacts.org
Reed Elsevier, Inc. www.boardcertifieddocs.com
GeoAccess www.primesourceweb.com

American Society for Aesthetic Plastic Surgery (ASAPS)
http://www.surgery.org *(English)*

American Society of Plastic Surgeons (ASPS)
http://www.plasticsurgery.org *(English)*

Canadian Society of Plastic Surgeons (CSPS)
http://www.plasticsurgery.ca *(English, French)*

Latin America

ARGENTINA
Sociedad Argentina de Cirugía Plástica, Estética y Reparadora (SACPER)
http://www.sacper.org.ar *(Spanish)*

BRAZIL
Sociedade Brasileira de Cirurgia Plástica (SBCP)
http://www.cirurgiaplastica.org.br *(Portuguese)*

COLUMBIA
Sociedad Colombiana de Cirugía Plástica-Estética, Maxilofacial y de la Mano (SCCP)
http://www.cirugiaplastica.org.co *(Spanish)*

MEXICO
Asociación Mexicana de Cirugía Plástica, Estética y Reconstructiva
http://www.cirugiaplastica.org.mx *(Spanish, English)*

VENEZUELA
Sociedad Venezolana de Cirugía Plástica, Reconstructiva, Estética y Máxilofacial (SVCPREM)
http://www.svcprem.org *(Spanish)*

Europe

AUSTRIA
Österreichische Gesellschaft für Plastische, Ästhetische und Rekonstruktive Chirurgie
http://www.plastischechirurgie.org *(German)*

BELGIUM
Belgian Society for Plastic, Reconstructive & Aesthetic Surgery (BSPRAS)
http://www.bspras.org *(Dutch, French; English to be added soon)*

FRANCE
Société Française de Chirurgie Plastique Reconstructrice et Esthétique (SOFCPRE)
http://plasticiens.org *(French)*

Société Française des Chirurgiens Esthétiques Plasticiens (SOFCEP)
http://www.sofcep.org *(French)*

Ordre National des Médecins
http://www.conseil-national.medecin.fr *(French)*
This website is used to check if the practitioner in question has been admitted by the French Medical Association, and if so, for which area of specialisation. Simply enter the doctor's name (and area of specialisation, if required) into the search boxes of the address book (Annuaire). If the practitioner is registered, his or her title, address and area of specialisation will be displayed.

GERMANY
Vereinigung der Deutschen Plastischen Chirurgen (VDPC)
http://www.plastische-chirurgie.de *(German)*

GREAT BRITAIN
General Medical Council
http://www.gmc-uk.org *(English)*
Although this site doesn't specifically include a directory of plastic surgeons, it can be used to verify the registrations and qualifications of medical practitioners recorded by the UK General Medical Council (searching by name only).

GREECE
Hellenic Society of Plastic Reconstructive & Aesthetic Surgery
http://www.hespras.gr *(Greek, English)*

ITALY
Società Italiana di Chirurgia Plastica Ricostruttiva ed Estetica (SICPRE)
http://www.sicpre.org *(Italian)*

PORTUGAL
Sociedade Portuguesa de Cirurgia Plástica Reconstrutiva e Estética (SPCPRE)
http://www.spcpre.org *(Portuguese)*

SPAIN
Sociedad Española de Cirugía Plástica, Reparadora y Estética (SECPRE)
http://www.secpre.org *(Spanish)*

South Eastern Europe

CROATIA
Croatian Society of Plastic, Reconstructive and Aesthetic Surgery (CSPRAS)
http://www.kbd.hr/plastkir *(Croatian, English)*

TURKEY
Turkish Society of Plastic Reconstructive and Aesthetic Surgeons
http://www.tpcd.org.tr. *(Turkish, English)*

Near East

LEBANON
Lebanese Society of Plastic Reconstructive and Aesthetic Surgery
http://www.estheticlebanon.com *(English, French)*

Asia

PHILIPPINES
Philippine Association of Plastic Reconstructive and Aesthetic Surgeons (PAPRAS)
http://www.plasticsurgery-phil.org *(English)*

THAILAND
Society of Plastic and Reconstructive Surgeons of Thailand (TSPRS)
http://www.plasticsurgery.or.th *(Thai, English)*
A surgeons' directory is under construction.

Africa

EGYPT

Egyptian Society of Plastic & Reconstructive Surgeons (ESPRS)
http://www.geocities.com/esprs *(Arabic, English)*

SOUTH AFRICA

Association of Plastic and Reconstructive Surgeons of Southern Africa (APRSSA)
http://www.plasticsurgeons.co.za *(English)*

Australia

Australian Society of Plastic Surgeons (ASPS)
http://www.plasticsurgery.org.au *(English)*

XI.2.2.6 International medical journals, Online journals and magazines

All medical journals are in English.

- **European Journal of Plastic Surgery**
  http://link.springer.de/link/service/journals/00238/
  Journal of the *European Association of Plastic Surgeons (EURAPS)* and the *European Burns Association.*
  - Summaries of print articles may be read free of charge. Subscribers can download full-length texts.

- **Plastic and Reconstructive Surgery**
  http://plasreconsurg.org
  Journal of the *American Society of Plastic Surgeons (ASPS).*
  - Summaries of print articles may be read free of charge. Registered users can download full-length texts for a fee. Online subscription is possible.

- **Aesthetic Surgery Journal**
  http://www2.us.elsevierhealth.com/scripts/om.dll/serve?action=searchDB&searchDBfor=home&id=AQ
  Journal of the *American Society for Aesthetic Plastic Surgery (ASAPS).*
  - Summaries of print articles may be read free of charge. Subscribers can download full-length texts. Online subscription is possible.

- **Scandinavian Journal of Plastic and Reconstructive Surgery and Hand Surgery**
  http://www.tandf.co.uk/journals/titles/02844311.html
  International journal on plastic and reconstructive surgery.
  - After registering free of charge, users can access a collection of summarised print articles ("Online sample copy"). Online subscription is possible.

- **The Canadian Journal of Plastic Surgery**
  http://www.pulsus.com/plastics/home2.htm
  Journal of the *Canadian Society of Plastic Surgeons (CSPS).*
  - Summaries of print articles may be read free of charge. Individual articles may be ordered for a small fee. Registered users can download all of the articles for a fee.

- **BJPS: British Journal of Plastic Surgery**
  http://www.harcourt-international.com/journals/bjps
  Journal of the *British Association of Plastic Surgeons (BAPS).*
  - Online subscription is possible. Summaries of articles are not available.

- **FACE – Facial Aesthetic Communications in Europe**
  http://www.sfcpefc.org/1/revue/index.html
  International specialist journal on facial plastic surgery.
  - Each issue's table of contents is online, but no summaries of print articles are available. Online subscription is possible.

- **Aesthetic Plastic Surgery**
  http://link.springer.de/link/service/journals/00266/index.htm
  US journal for the latest developments in the field of aesthetic plastic surgery.
  - Summaries of articles may be read free of charge. Subscribed users can download full-length articles. Subscription is possible via email.

- **International Journal of Plastic & Aesthetic Surgery (IJPAS)** (Formerly: *Brazilian Journal of Plastic Surgery*)
- **http://www.imedical.com/ijpas/**
  Extensive articles and medical studies of all areas of plastic surgery by international specialists – online. Also of interest to untrained readers.

- **Cosmetic Surgery Times**
  http://www.cosmeticsurgerytimes.com
  Online version of the print magazine, featuring a wealth of detailed scientific articles, columns, reports and plastic surgery news. Partially of interest to non-specialists.

- **Plastic Surgery Today**
  http://www.plasticsurgery.org/news_room/PST-Index.cfm
  Online version of the weekly *American Society of Plastic Surgeons (ASPS)* supplement to the newspaper *USA Today*. Also contains many articles interesting to non-specialists.

Aesthetic Surgeons' Biographies and Addresses

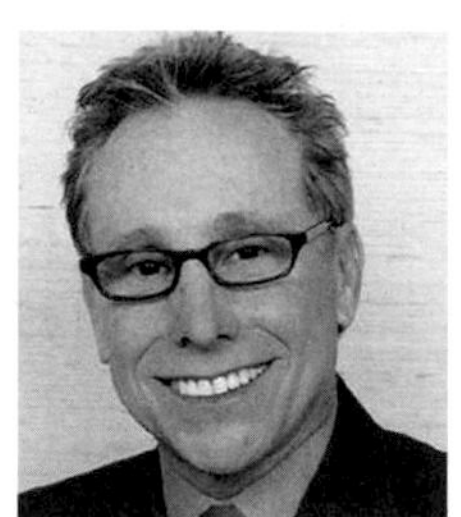

Dr. Gary J. Alter
416 North Bedford Drive, Suite 400
USA – Beverly Hills, CA 90 210
Tel: +1-310-275 5566
Fax: +1-310-271 0521
E-mail: altermd@earthlink.net
www.altermd.com
www.garyaltermd.com

Biography:
Born 2 July 1948. Single.
1966–1969 student at the University of California at Berkeley.
1969–1973 UCLA Medical School in Los Angeles, California.
1973–1975 General Surgery internship and residency at UCLA Medical School.
1975–1979 Urology residency at Baylor College of Medicine in Houston, Texas.
1979–1990 private practice in urology in Los Angeles, California.
1981 Board Certification of American Board of Urology.
1990–1992 Plastic Surgery residency at Mayo Clinic in Rochester, Minnesota.
1992 Plastic Surgery fellowship emphasising genital reconstruction at Eastern Virginia Graduate School of Medicine, Norfolk, Virginia.
1993–present: private practice in plastic surgery in Beverly Hills, California.
1997 Board Certification of American Board of Plastic Surgery.
Hospital affiliations: UCLA Center for the Health Sciences, Los Angeles; Cedars-Sinai Medical Center, Los Angeles; Midway Hospital, Los Angeles.

Societies:
— *American Society of Plastic Surgeons (ASPS)*
— *American Society for Aesthetic Surgery (ASAPS)*
— *American Urological Association*
— *Western Section of American Urological Association*
— *Society of Genitourinary Reconstructive Surgeons*

Publications:
Alter, Gary J. and Ehrlich, Richard M. eds. *Reconstructive and Plastic Surgery of the External Genitalia.* Philadelphia: W. B. Saunders and Co, 1999.
Numerous articles and contributions to books about urology, plastic surgery and genital surgery.

Key aspects of activity:
— Plastic aesthetic facial and body surgery
— Genital plastic and reconstructive surgery

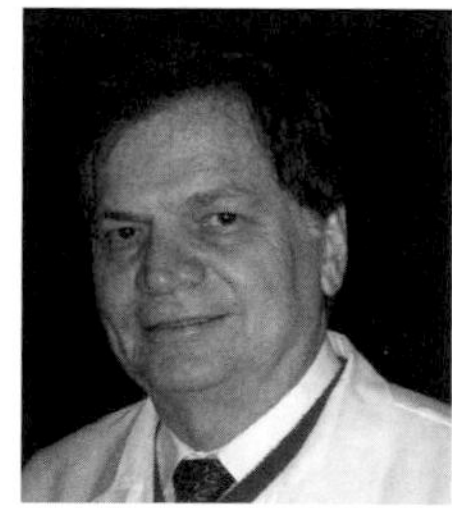

Prof. Juarez Avelar
620 Alameda Gabriel Monteiro da Silva
BR – SP 01 442–000 Jardim Europa, São Paulo
Tel: +55-11-3085 4211
Fax: +55-11-3088 1993
E-mail: juarezavelar@bol.com.br

Biography:
Born 23 July 1946. Married, one son.

1964–1968 medical student in
Rio de Janeiro, Brazil.
1968–1969 resident in General Surgery
in Rio de Janeiro.
1970–1972 resident in Plastic Surgery
at Pitanguy's Clinic in Rio de Janeiro.
1973 advanced professional training in Miami,
New York, London, Glasgow, Paris and Berlin.
1974 began working in São Paulo, at the
Albert Einstein Israeli Hospital.
1982–1983 president of the Plastic Surgery
Society of São Paulo.
1984–1985 general secretary of the Brazilian
Society of Plastic Surgery.
1986–1987 president of the Brazilian Society
of Plastic Surgery.
1990–1991 president of the Brazilian Society
of Plastic Surgery.
1992–1997 general secretary of the Brazilian
Medical Association.
Since 1987 member of the Brazilian
Academy of History.
Since 1988 plastic surgeon at the
Heart Hospital in São Paulo.
Since 1991 member of the Academy
of Medicine in São Paulo.
Since 1999 professor of courses of the *International Society of Aesthetic Plastic Surgery* (*ISAPS*).
Postgraduate Professor of the *International Society of Aesthetic plastic Surgery* (*ISAPS*).
Professor of Marilia Medical School, São Paulo.
Has lectured in Brazil and abroad

Publications:
13 books published about various fields of plastic surgery and other areas of medicine. 180 scientific articles in journals of medicine, together with chapters in books on medicine, published in Brazil and abroad

Key aspects of activity:
— Correction of negroid nose
— Creation of a new technique for umbilicoplasty during abdominoplasty
— Correction of blepharoptosis
— Ear reconstruction after traumatic amputation
— Ear reconstruction in congenial absence of the auricle
— Ear reconstruction after burn
— Abdominoplasty
— Liposuction
— Body contour surgery
— Breast surgery
— Facelift by tunnelization without subcutaneous undermining
— Abdominoplasty without panniculus undermining
— Plastic surgery of the axilla without panniculus undermining
— Torsoplasty without panniculus undermining
— Medial thigh lifting without panniculus undermining

Wishes for the future:
To work as if I will never die and
live as if I will die tomorrow.
To perform each operation with so much care and meticulous attention as if it were the first one in my life and to perform it with so much enthusiasm and delight as if it were the last one in my life (of course one day it will be the last one).
Medicine is like love—it is always starting and never finishes (love is the reason for living). Medicine is like a mother's heart—it is always capable of embracing one more child. Performing an operation is like being hurt in love—it always leaves a scar of happiness.
To be wise enough to live the glories of what one has accomplished in life and keep the flames of expectation burning in search of new accomplishments.
To have faith and hope
for every extra minute one breathes.
To believe in the love of the loved one

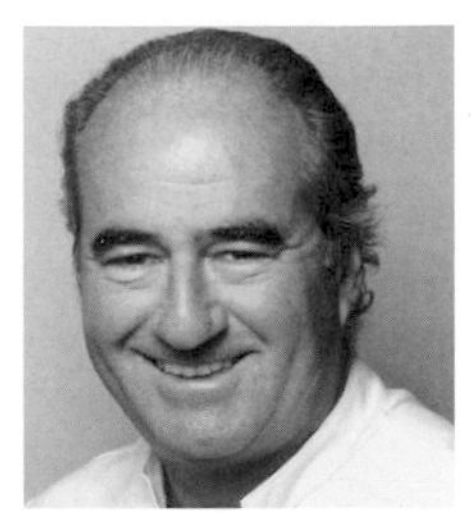

Dr. Javier de Benito

12, Marquesa de Vilallonga
E – 08 017 Barcelona
Tel: +34-93-253 0282
Fax: +34-93-253 0283
E-mail: debenitoworld@terra.es
www.institutodebenito.com

Biography:

Born 14 January1948. Married, one daughter.
1968–1973 University of Barcelona.
1973–1979 Clinica Planas de Cirugía Plástica y Estética.
1986–1997 director of Plastic Surgery department of Clínica Quirón.
1992–2003 expert on nonactive surgical implants in the European Committee.
Conferences and workshops.
1997–present: director of Instituto Javier de Benito at the Centro Médico Teknon, Barcelona.
Coordinator and director of the First, Second, Third, Fourth and Fifth International Courses Advances in Aesthetic and Plastic Surgery.
Conferences and workshops.

Societies:

– Vice-president of the *International Society of Aesthetic Plastic Surgery (ISAPS)*
– *The American Society for Aesthetic Plastic Surgery (ASAPS)*
– *The Royal Academy of Medicine of Zaragoza*

Publications:

El Gran Libro de la Cirugia Estética. Barcelona: Rba Editores 2002.
Estética y cirugía. Barcelona: Emeka Editores

Key aspects of activity:

— Endoscopy of foreheads
— Face and neck lift
— Upper and lower eyelids
— Breast augmentation: expert in breast anatomical implant development and research
— Breast mastopexy
— Body contouring, thigh lifting, abdominoplasty, liposuction

Wishes for the future:

To work on the development of a medicine and integral rejuvenation surgery that will treat from the gene to the epidermis. This will be achieved through anti-aging medication, plastic surgery, skin rejuvenation and research into stem cells for skin, hair and connective tissue.

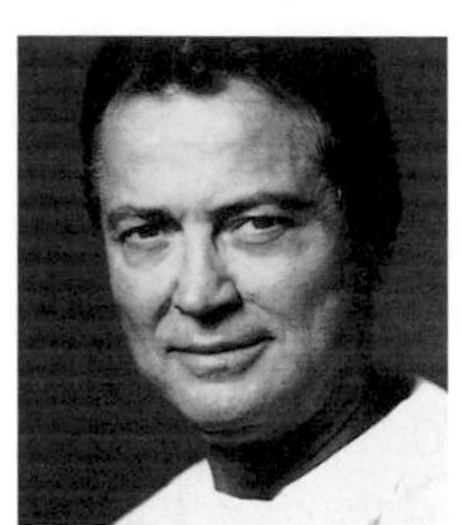

Dr. Bernard Cornette de Saint Cyr

15, Rue Spontini
F – 75 116 Paris
Tel: +33-1-47 04 25 02
Fax: +33-1-47 04 60 66
E-mail: bdesaintcyr@hotmail.com
www.cornettedesaintcyr.com

Biography:

Married, two children.
Faculté de Médecine de Paris.
Concours international des hôpitaux de Paris.
Qualified in general surgery.
Board of plastic reconstructive and aesthetic surgery.
Colleague and successor to Dr. Jean Paul Lintilhac.
Professor of postgraduate education in aesthetic plastic surgery

Societies:

— *Société Française de Chirurgie Plastique Reconstructrice et Esthétique (SOFCPRE)*
— Became president of *SOFCPRE* in 2003
— *International Society of Aesthetic Plastic Surgery (ISAPS)*

Key aspects of activity:

— Facial rejuvenation and embellishment
— Breast surgery
— Body sculpturing

Wishes for the future:

Always to keep the same enthusiasm and passion for this wonderful activity, which gives happiness to my patients. Always to try to achieve excellence and never stop learning. A professional must be an eternal student. Being able to practice sports and golf for a long time

— Teaching cosmetic surgery
— Surgical expert witness for Medical Defense Unions

Wishes for the future:
To improve the profile of cosmetic surgery.
To know my grandchildren for a long time.

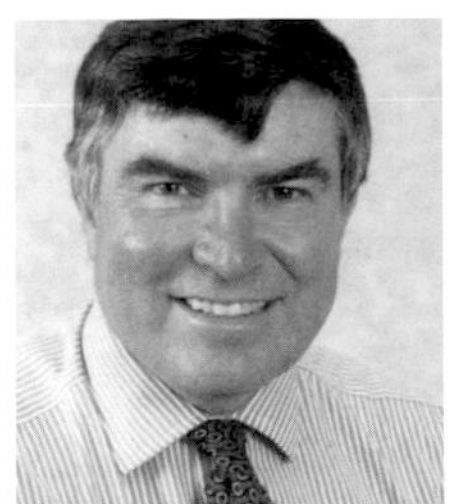

Dr. Dai M. Davies

55 Harley Street
GB – London W1G 8QR
and
Institute of Cosmetic and Reconstructive Surgery
West London Clinic, The Wakefield Centre,
Ravenscourt Gardens, Ravenscourt Park,
GB – London W6 0AE
Tel: +44-207-462 0030
E-mail: enquiries@renascence.co.uk
www.renascence.co.uk

Biography:
Born 10 July 1947. Married, three children.
1965–1970 student at the Barts (St. Bartholomews) Hospital, London.
1974 fellow of the Royal College of Surgeons (FRCS)
1981 certification of higher surgical training in plastic and reconstructive surgery.
1982 consultant plastic surgeon, Hammersmith Hospitals NHS Trust. Royal Postgraduate Medical School, Imperial College, London.
Since 2000 director of The Institute of Cosmetic and Reconstructive Surgery, West London Clinic

Societies:
— *British Association of Plastic Surgeons (BAPS)*
— *British Association of Aesthetic Plastic Surgeons (BAAPS)*
— *British Hand Society*
— *International Society of Aesthetic Plastic Surgery (ISAPS)*
— *Hellenic Society of Plastic Reconstructive & Aesthetic Surgery* (Life member)
— *Argentinean Society of Plastic Surgeons* (Honorary member)
— *American Society of Plastic Surgeons (ASPS)* (Corresponding member)

Publications:
Many publications and lectures worldwide

Key aspects of activity:
— Facial aesthetic surgery
— Breast aesthetic and reconstructive surgery
— Secondary corrective surgery (rhinoplasty and breast)
— Skin care

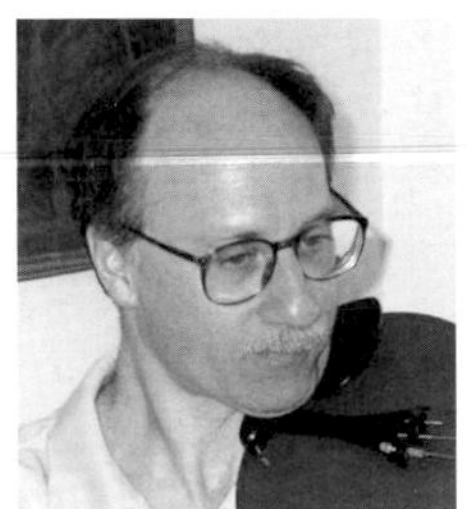

Dr. Alan M. Engler

122 East 64th Street
USA – New York, NY 10 021
Tel: +1-212-308 7000
Fax: +1-212-308 7094
E-mail: dralanengler@aol.com
www.bodysculpture.com

Biography:
Born 14 April 1954. Married, two children.
1972–1976 Yale University, New Haven, Connecticut. B. A., Russian Studies.
1976–1980 Columbia University, College of Physicians and Surgeons New York, M. D.
1974–1975 junior year in Paris (Université de Paris).
1980–1984 Montefiore Medical Center, New York, General Surgery.
1984–1986 Montefiore Medical Center, New York. Plastic and Reconstructive Surgery.
1986–present: assistant clinical professor of plastic surgery, Albert Einstein College of Medicine, New York.
1986–present: private practice in plastic surgery, New York.
1988 Board Certification of *American Board of Plastic Surgery*.
Office accredited by the American Association for the Accreditation of Ambulatory Surgical Facilities (AAAASF).
Inventor of a surgical instrument, (US Patent – 2002)

Societies:
— *American Society for Aesthetic Plastic Surgery (ASAPS)*
— *American Society of Plastic Surgeons (ASPS)*
— *American College of Surgeons (ACS)*

Publications:
Listed as "One of the Best Doctors in New York" by *New York Magazine*, and in *How to Find the Best New York Metro Area Doctors* (a guide published by Castle Connolly Medical Ltd, New York)
The Slim Book of Liposuction. New York: Vantage Press Inc., 1993.
BodySculpture. New York: Hudson Publishing, 1998 and 2000 (with Sonia Weiss).
Restylane. New York: Berkley Books, 2003.
Numerous Radio and Television Appearances (including *The Ricki Lake Show* – four times)

Key aspects of activity:
— Plastic surgery of the face and body
— Minimally invasive surgical techniques
— Breast surgery (enlargements, lifts, reductions)
— Liposuction and tummy tucks
— Facial aesthetic surgery including facelifts and eyelid surgery

Wishes for the Future:
Good health for my loved ones. Peaceful resolution to the awful inequities and conflicts around the world.
Unending beauty in all its forms.

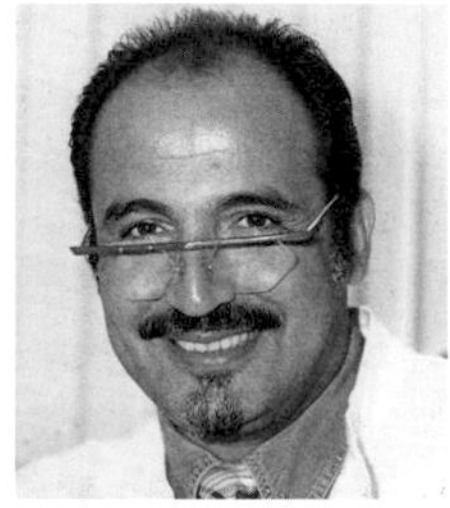

Dr. Serdar Eren

Im MediaPark 3
DE – 50 670 Cologne
Tel: +49-221-979 7888
Fax: +49-221-979 79880
E-mail: dr-eren@dr-eren.de
www.dr-eren.de

Biography:
Born 11 October 1954. Married, one child.
1971–1977 student of Medicine at the University of Istanbul, Turkey.
1977 assistant doctor at Istanbul University surgical clinic.
1978–1981 assistant doctor at the surgical clinic of St. Agatha's Hospital, Cologne.
1981–1984 assistant doctor to the II. surgical professorship at Cologne University, Cologne-Merheim.
1985 certification as a surgeon.
1984–1988 assistant doctor at the Clinic for Plastic Surgery and Severe Burns Center in Cologne-Merheim.
1987 certification as a specialist in plastic surgery.
1988 senior physician at the Clinic for Plastic Surgery and Severe Burns Center in Cologne-Merheim.
1988–1992 leading senior physician at the Clinic for Burns and Plastic Reconstructive Surgery at the Medical Faculty of the RWTH Aachen.
1993–2002 head physician of the Department of Plastic Surgery / Hand Surgery at St. Agatha's Hospital, Cologne.
2003–present head of the Center for Aesthetic Plastic Surgery/Hand Surgery at the MediaPark Clinic, Cologne

Key aspects of activity:
— Aesthetic facial surgery
— Facelifts and facial rejuvenation
— Eyelid correction/blepharoplasty
— Nose surgery/rhinoplasty
— Ear surgery/otoplasty
— Breast enlargement, reduction and lifting
— Breast reconstruction after tumors
— Tummy tucks
— Combined body shaping operations
— Liposuction
— Wrinkle treatment
— Aesthetic surgery for men
— Anti-aging, nutrition
— Obesity treatment
— Selective hand surgery
— Treatment of hand diseases and congenital malformations
— Peripheral nerve surgery
— Reconstructive hand surgery after accidents
— Reconstructive tumor surgery, skin flaps

Wishes for the future:
To stop operating by the end of my 50s, before my manual dexterity is reduced. I then intend to concentrate on teaching the philosophy of plastic surgery and plastic surgeons.

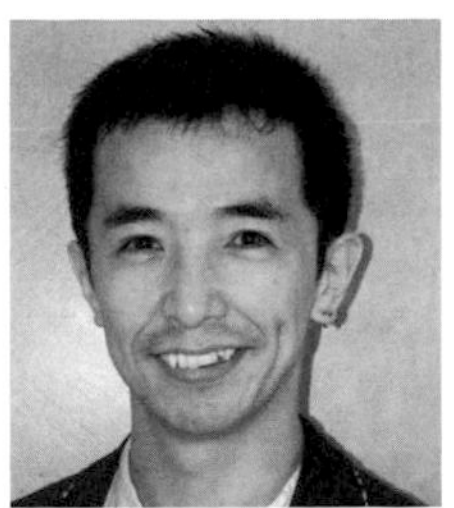

Dr. Keizo Fukuta
Verite Clinic
3F New Ginza Building, 5-5-7 Ginza Chuo-ku
J – 104-0061 Tokyo
Tel: +81-3-3573 0333
Fax: +81-3-6253 8588
E-mail: fukuta@veriteclinic.com
www.veriteclinic.com

Biography:
Born 12 August 1960. Married, no children.
1979–1985 student of medicine at Nagoya University School of Medicine, Nagoya, Japan.
1985–1994 advanced professional training in Nagoya, Japan and USA.
1987–1989 Mayo Clinic, Rochester, Minnesota.
1990–1991 Institute for Craniofacial Surgery, Southfield, Michigan.
1991–1992 Providence Hospital, Southfield, Michigan.
1995–2001 chief plastic surgeon at Komaki City Hospital, Komaki, Japan.
2001–2004 assistant professor of Aesthetic Plastic Surgery at Aichi Medical University, Aichi, Japan.
Since 2004 chief surgeon at Verite Clinic, Tokyo, Japan

Societies:
— *International Society of Aesthetic Plastic Surgery (ISAPS)*
— *International Society of Craniofacial Surgery*
— *Japanese Society of Plastic and Reconstructive Surgery*
— *Japanese Society of Aesthetic Plastic Surgery*
— *Board certificate of the Japanese Society of Plastic and Reconstructive Surgery*

Key aspects of activity:
— Rhinoplasty particularly for Oriental nose
— Upper blepharoplasty including Oriental double fold procedure
— Facelift technique with ligament suspension
— Facial bone contouring and osteotomy
— Treatment of skin pigmentation

Wishes for the future:
I have not yet reached the point where I am truly satisfied with my skill at aesthetic surgery. I am not afraid of hard work and intend to become a master aesthetic surgeon by the time I retire.

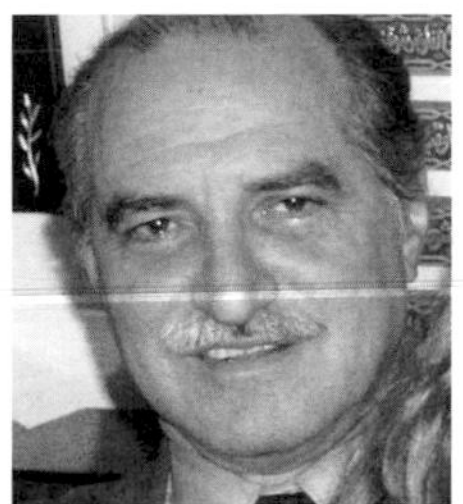

Prof. Alaa El Din Gheita
12, Hassan Sabry street, Zamalek
EG – 111 211 Cairo
Tel: +20-2-736 7734
Fax: +20-2-736 7734
E-mail: Gheita@link.net

Biography:
Born 16 March 1945. Divorced, two children.
1963–1969 student of medicine at Cairo University, Egypt.
1969–1979 resident and lecturer General Surgery Faculty of Medicine, Cairo University.
1979–1982 plastic surgery training in Paris at Hôpital St. Louis with Prof. Claude Dufourmentel, Roger Mouly, Pierre Banzet and others.
1982 trained with Tom Rees at Manhattan Eye, Ear and Throat Hospital, New York.
1983 Faculty of Medicine, Cairo University.
1983–present practice at the Kasr El Einy Hospital, Cairo University and (privately) at Assalam International Hospital, Meadi, Cairo.
1987 obtained Egypt's National Academic Award in Medical Sciences for his research and publications.
1992 named Professor of Plastic Surgery and Head of Department of Plastic & Reconstructive Surgery at the University Hospital.
Invited speaker at many international meetings around the world, mostly on the subjects facial rejuvenation, breasts, craniofacial correction of congenital anomalies

Societies:
— Previous President of *Egyptian Society of Plastic & Reconstructive Surgeons*
— Honorary member of *French Society of Plastic, Reconstructive & Aesthetic Surgery*
— Honorary member of the *South African Society of Plastic & Reconstructive Surgeons*

— Honorary life membership of *The Emirates Society of Plastic Surgery*
— 1998 Co founder of the *Pan African Society of Plastic & Reconstructive Surgery*
— 1995–2003 member of the Executive Committee of *International Confederation for Plastic Reconstructive & Aesthetic Surgery (IPRAS)*

Key aspects of activity:
— Facial rejuvenation (lids & lifting)
— Breast augmentation, reduction, elevation (mastopexy)
— Liposuction on various areas of the body
— Abdominoplasty
— Nose refinement either reduction or augmentation
— Craniofacial correction of various congenital anomalies

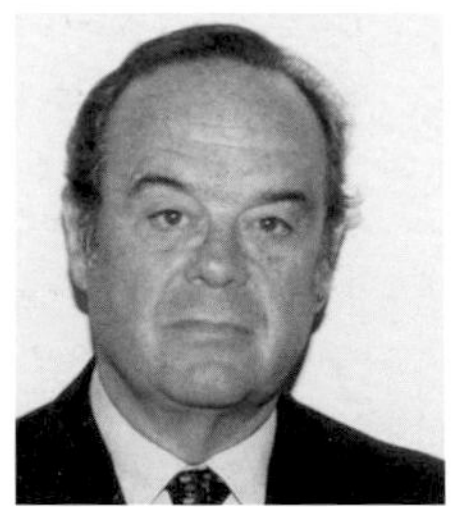

Dr. Jorge Herrera

1346 J. E.Uriburu
RA – Buenos Aires
Tel: +54-11-4822 2014/4 826 0178
Fax: +54-11-4804 0165
E-mail: jherrera@sminter.com.ar

Biography:
Born 26 September 1942. Married, three daughters.
1961–1967 student in the School of Medicine at Buenos Aires University.
1967–1970 resident in General Surgery in the Rawson Hospital in Buenos Aires.
1970–1978 advanced professional training in plastic surgery in Buenos Aires and USA with renowned professionals: J. M. Converse (in NYC), Ralph Millard (Miami, FL), John Owsley, Bruce Conell (California). In Europe with Jaime Planas (Barcelona, Spain), in Brazil with Ivo Pitangy and Liacyr Ribeiro (Rio de Janeiro).
Since 1980, professor of the Plastic Surgery Division at Salvador University in Buenos Aires (U. S. A. L.).
1980–present: numerous national and international lectures.
Certified Plastic Surgeon of the *Sociedad Argentina de Cirugia Plastica Estetica y Reparadora (SACPER)* full-time in Buenos Aires. Presently head professor in Aesthetic Plastic Surgery at U. S. A. L.

Societies:
— *The Argentine Plastic Surgery Society*
— *The Buenos Aires Plastic Surgery Society*
— *The International Society of Aesthetic Plastic Surgery (ISAPS)*
— *The Iberolatinamerican Federation of Plastic Surgery*
— Corresponding member of the *American Society of Plastic Surgerons, American Society of Aesthetic Plastic Surgery, Brazilian Society of Plastic Surgery, Uruguayan Society of Plastic Surgery*. Honorary member of *the Ecuatorian Society of Plastic Surgery, Cordoba Society of Plastic Surgery* and *Parana Society of Plastic Surgery*

Key aspects of activity:
— Facial rejuvenation surgery
— Aesthetic and reconstructive eyelid surgery
— Aesthetic and reconstructive breast surgery

Wishes for the future:
To keep developing professional skills and the ability to continue teaching and transmitting knowledge to upcoming generations of plastic surgeons, balanced with the needs of family and leisure time.

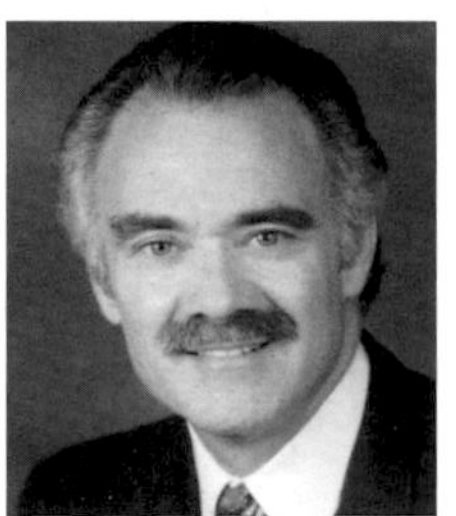

Dr. Steven M. Hoefflin

1530 Arizona Avenue
USA – Santa Monica, California 90 404
Tel: +1-310-451 4733
Fax: +1-310-451 5653
E-mail: steven@hoefflin.com
www.hoefflin.com

Biography:
Born 7 February 1946. Married, two sons.
1972 graduated first in his class at UCLA Medical School.
Completed his education in general surgery and completed a full plastic surgical residency training program at the UCLA Medical Center where

he received the coveted Surgical Medal Award.
1980–1985 Chief of Plastic Surgery at Brotman Medical Center.
1982–1989 Chief of Plastic Surgery at Santa Monica Hospital Medical Center. Board certified by the *American Board of Plastic Surgery*.
Fellow of the American College of Surgeons.
Past Associate Clinical Professor at UCLA Medical Center (where he received the Teacher of the Year Award, 1985–1986)

Societies:
— President of the *Los Angeles Society of Plastic Surgeons*

Key aspects of activity:
— Specialises in difficult revision surgeries of the face, breast and body

Wishes for the future:
To continue to participate in the health and happiness of family, friends and patients.
To contribute and assist in advancements and progress in the field of plastic surgery.

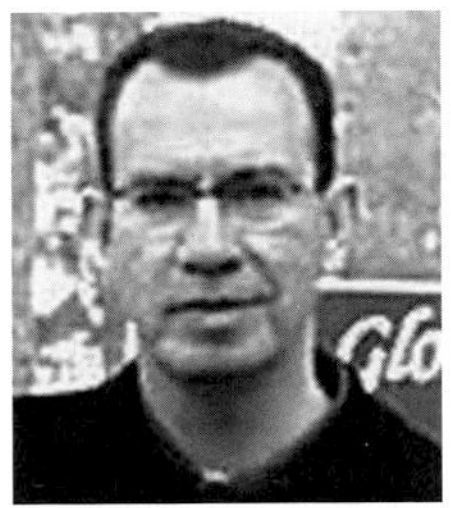

Associate Professor Ismail Kuran
Halaskargazi cad. 340/2 Şişli
TR – Istanbul
Tel: +90-532-322 0598
Fax: +90-212-224 2528
E-mail: ikuran@tnt.net
Web: www.kuranestetik.com

Biography:
Born 21 December 1960. Married, two children.
1978–1984 student at Istanbul Medical Faculty.
1984–1986 obligatory duty for Health Ministry in Kutahya, Turkey.
1986–2001 plastic surgery training in Şişli Etfal State Teaching Hospital, Istanbul.
1990 six months practice at Warwickshire Regional Plastic Surgery Unit, England.
1990 microsurgery training in Kantonspital Aarau, Switzerland.
1993 microsurgery training and clinical observation in Baylor College of Medicine, USA.
1991–1998 chief of residents at Şişli Etfal State Teaching Hospital Plastic Surgery Unit, Istanbul.
1998–2000 registrar in Şişli Etfal State Teaching Hospital Plastic Surgery Unit, Istanbul.
2000 awarded associate professorship.
2000–2004 chief of the Şişli Etfal State Teaching Hospital Plastic Surgery Unit, Istanbul.
Since 2004 chief of the Plastic Surgery Department of Maltepe University.
More than 80 presentations made at national and international congresses

Societies:
— *International Society of Plastic, Reconstructive and Aesthetic Surgery*
— *American Society for Facial Plastic and Aesthetic Surgery*
— Member of *Executive Committee of Turkish Society of Plastic Surgery*
— General Secretary of *Turkish Plastic Surgery Board*
— Turkish Representative to *European Board of Plastic Surgery*

Publications:
More than 60 national and international articles published in scientific journals

Key aspects of activity:
— Facial aesthetic surgery
— Forehead, eyebrow, mid-face, lower face and neck
— Prominent ear correction
— Soft tissue augmentation
— Lip augmentation or reduction
— Laser resurfacing
— Rhinoplasty
— Liposuction
— Breast reduction and augmentation
— Breast reconstruction
— Reconstructive surgery
— Congenital deformities
— Post-traumatic reconstructions
— Reconstruction after oncological resections

Wishes for the future:
Publishing a book on plastic surgery based on personal experiences. Trying to find new techniques with better results and less invasive procedures. Peace in the world.

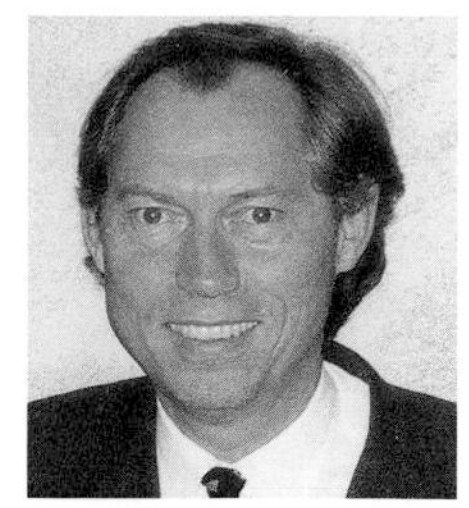

Prof. Dr. Dr. Werner L. Mang
Bodenseeklinik Lindau
Clinic for Plastic and Aesthetic Surgery
Unterer Schrannenplatz 1
DE – 88 131 Lindau
Tel: +49-8382-5094
Fax: +49-8382-28 932
E-mail: info@bodenseeklinik.de
www.bodenseeklinik.de

Biography:
Born 4 September 1949. Married, two children. Studied medicine at the Ludwig-Maximilian University in Munich including two spells of study abroad in London and San Francisco. Took state examination at the age of 23 then spent some time as an assistant surgeon before training as a specialist in ENT (completed at the age of 30) and plastic surgery (completed at the age of 32) at the Großhadern Clinic in Munich.
1980 appointed senior physician at the Rechts der Isar Clinic at the Technical University of Munich.
1983 awarded habilitation degree.
1989 awarded professorship, then became Medical Director of the Bodenseeklinik in Lindau. Has been a pioneer of plastic and aesthetic surgery in Germany ever since.
2003 opens "the most modern and exclusive beauty clinic in Europe."
Honorary professor at St. Petersburg University.
Internationally acclaimed surgeon and guest speaker.
Has so far performed more than 30,000 operations himself (approx. 2000 per year, which ranks him among the world's top ten).
Founder of the Prof. Mang Foundation to help children in need. The foundation also supports young surgeons who have shown particular promise in the field of aesthetic surgery.

Societies:
— Honorary president of the *German Society for Aesthetic Surgery (DGÄC)*
— President of the *International Society for Aesthetic Surgery*
— Member or honorary member of numerous national and international societies, e. g. the *American Academy of Facial Plastic and Reconstructive Surgery*, *Colégio Brasileiro de Cirurgia & Traumatologia*, *Canadian Institute of Facial Plastic Surgery*

Publications:
Several books, including *The Manual of Aesthetic Surgery*. 2 Vol., Berlin: Springer, 2001 and 2004. Many printed articles and contributions to TV programs and reports

Key aspects of activity:
— Specialist in ENT and plastic surgery
— Nose corrections
— Face lifts
— Breast enlargement
— Liposuction
— Lifting of all parts of body (body contouring)

Wishes for the future:
A training centre for doctors. Worldwide increase and maintenance of quality standards in aesthetic surgery via specialist text books, TV and the Internet. Factual reports on aesthetic surgery. Biological anti-aging.Research in the field of nutritional supplements and cosmetics (intensive medical cosmetics).

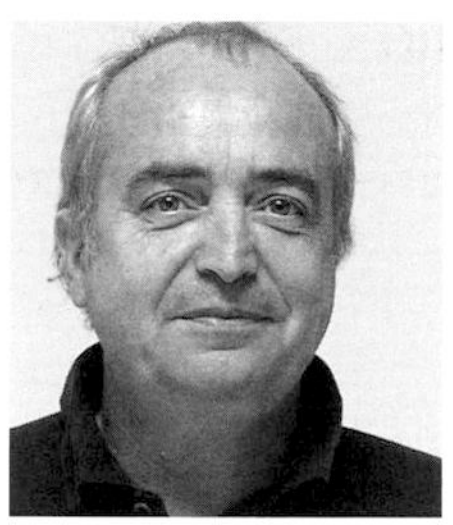

Dr. Hans-Leo Nathrath
Arabella Str. 5
DE – 81 925 Munich
Tel: +49-89-91 91 10
Fax: +49-89-91 91 12
E-mail: nathrath@plast-arabella.com
www.plastische-chirurgie-muenchen.de
www.dr-nathrath.de

Biography:
Born 23 December 1949. Married, three daughters.
1969–1974 studied languages, German literature, and photography.
1974–1980 studied medicine.
1980–1982 freelance work as a photographer, e. g.

for magazines in Southern Europe, Nepal, Australia and also in Germany.
1982–1991 trained as a surgeon and specialist in plastic and aesthetic surgery at the Clinic Munich Bogenhausen, Rechts der Isar Clinic.
1991–1994 aesthetic surgery at the Arabella Clinic, Munich.
1994 permanent position at the Arabella Clinic, Munich.
2000 head physician at the Department of Plastic Surgery at the Arabella Clinic, Munich

Societies:
— *German Society of Surgery (DGCH)*
— *Association of German Plastic Surgeons (VDPC)*
— *Association of German Aesthetic Plastic Surgeons (VDÄPC)*
— *International Consortium of Aesthetic Plastic Surgeons (ICAPS)*
— *International Society of Aesthetic Plastic Surgery (ISAPS)*

Key aspects of activity:
— Aesthetic facial surgery (including neck, eyelid, forehead, chin and lip corrections)
— Surgery on fatty tissues (liposuction, volume reduction and volume displacement)
— Aesthetic female breast surgery (reduction and enlargement)

Wishes for the future:
To devote much more time to my family—and everything listed above. If only surgery and working with the people who come into the practice every day weren't so enjoyable!

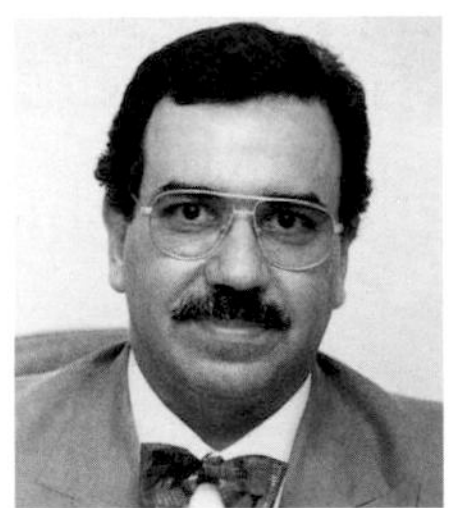

Dr. Ali Al-Numairy
Medical Director
Gulf Plastic Surgery Hospital
P.O. Box: 111 178
AE – Dubai
Tel: +971-4-269 9717
Fax: +971-4-268 1771
E-mail: numairy@emirates.net.ae
www.gulfplasticsurgery.com

Biography:
Born 18 May 1956. Married, five children.
1979 MBBCh from the Faculty of Medicine, University of Cairo, Egypt.
1980–1987 worked as intern house officer at surgical and medical departments, general duty medical officer at the Department of Surgery, General and Emergency Surgery Unit, Rashid Hospital, Dubai.
1987–1989 resident in plastic surgery at the unit of Dr. Ch. L. Masson, Saint Luc Hospital, Lyon, France; resident in hand, upper limb and microsurgery at the unit of Prof. J. J. Comtet, Edouard Herriot Hospital and the Faculty of Medicine, University of Lyon, France; assistant at the University of Lyon, Faculty of Medicine, Department of Stomatology, Maxillo-Facial and Plastic Surgery of the Face at Centre Hospitalier Lyon-Sud, France; visiting plastic surgeon at the unit of Dr. Ch. Masson, Lyon, France; visiting plastic surgeon with Dr. B. Dessapt, Plastic Surgery Centre, Lyon, France.
1990–2004 registrar (plastic surgery), department of surgery, Rashid Hospital, Dubai, United Arab Emirates, promoted to senior registrar, specialist and consultant (plastic surgery) and head of Plastic Surgery and Burns Unit, Rashid Hospital.
1990–2004 tutor and lecturer, Academic Dept. of Surgery, senior lecturer and head of Academic Division of Plastic Surgery, Dubai Medical College.
1996–present medical director, Gulf Plastic Surgery Hospital, Dubai, United Arab Emirates.
1997 lecturer on the postgraduate full course of Dermatological Surgery at the Arab Board of Dermatology.
1998–present Dubai Medical College. Chairman of the Scientific Committee, The Arab Board of Plastic Surgery.
From 2004 Chairman, Ethics Committee of IPRAS (International Confederation for Plastic, Reconstructive and Aesthetic Surgery).
2004 international visiting professor at the Albany Medical College and Albany Plastic Surgery Center, Albany, New York.
Diploma, Lipoplasty University, U. S. A.
Keen interest in teaching and research.
Research, lectures and presentation of scientific papers at various international conferences

Societies:
— Fellow of the *Royal Society of Medicine* in England
— *International Society for Burn Injuries* – National Representative of the U. A. E.
— *International Microsurgical Society*
— Fellow of the *American Academy of Cosmetic Surgery*

— *European Association of Plastic and Aesthetic Surgeons*
— *American Academy of Aesthetic and Restorative Surgery*
— Member of the Council and the Board of Directors, *Pan-Arab Association of Burns and Plastic Surgeons* (chairman of Arab Board of Plastic Surgery Committee 1997, president of the Association 2000–2001)
— *International Society of Cosmetic Laser Surgeon*
— Founding member and president, *Plastic Surgery Society, Emirates Medical Association*
— Founding member and first president, *G. C. C. Association of Plastic Surgeons* (chairman of Standing Committee for Ethics in Plastic Surgery 1995)
— *International Confederation for Plastic, Reconstructive and Aesthetic Surgery (IPRAS)*
— *North American Academy of Cosmetic and Restorative Surgery*
— National secretary of *International Society of Aesthetic Plastic Surgery (ISAPS)*
— *American Society of Plastic Surgeons (ASPS)*
— *International Academy of Cosmetic Surgery (IACS)*

Key aspects of activity:
— Abdominoplasty
— Liposuction
— Rhinoplasty
— Breast surgeries
— Eyelid surgery
— Filling procedures
— Laser resurfacing
— Chemical peeling
Interests include application of computers in medicine and photography, mainly medical

Wishes for the future:
To aim for perfection in every field of this profession and to impart the knowledge gained from my experiences to colleagues.

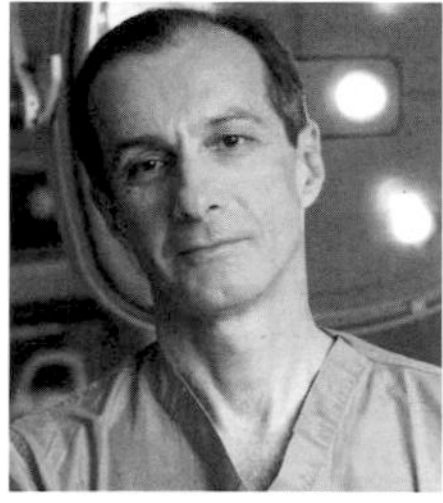

Dr. Gerald H. Pitman

170 East 73rd Street
USA – New York, NY 10 021
Tel: +1-212-517 2600
Fax: +1-212-628 0774
E-mail: drpitman@drpitman.com
www.drpitman.com

Biography:
Married, four children.
Bachelor of Arts in American History, Williams College, Williamstown, Massachusetts, USA.
Doctor of Medicine, University of Pennsylvania, Philadelphia, Pennsylvania, USA.
Resident in General Surgery, Columbia-Presbyterian Medical Center, New York, NY.
Resident in Plastic Surgery and fellow in Microsurgery Institute for Reconstructive Plastic Surgery, New York University Medical Center, New York.
Certified by the American Board of Plastic Surgery.
Certified by the American Board of Surgery.
Clinical associate professor of surgery (plastic), Institute for Reconstructive Plastic Surgery New York University School of Medicine, New York.
Hospital Affiliations (all in New York): Bellevue Hospital Center, Lenox Hill Hospital, Manhattan Eye, Ear and Throat Hospital, New York Eye and Ear Infirmary, Tisch Hospital of New York University Medical Center.
International lecturer to plastic surgeons

Societies:
— *American Society of Plastic Surgeons (ASPS)*
— *American Society for Aesthetic Plastic Surgery (ASAPS)*
— *New York Regional Society of Plastic and Reconstructive Surgeons*
— *New York State and County Medical Societies*

Publications:
Liposuction and Aesthetic Surgery. St. Louis: Quality Medical Publishing, 1993.
Many professional papers, chapters and videos on aesthetic surgery.
"Foundation face lift", in Nahai, F., ed., *Aesthetic Plastic Surgery*. St. Louis: Quality Medical Publishing, 2005.
(With Giese, S. Y.) "Liposuction", in Mathes, S. ed., *Plastic Surgery*. Philadelphia: Elsevier, 2005.
(With Stoker, D., Stevens, G.) "Liposuction and body-contouring", in McCarthy, Galiano, Boutros, *Current Therapy in Plastic Surgery*. Philadelphia: Elsevier, 2005

Key Aspects of Activity:
— Aesthetic facial rejuvenation: face lifts, neck lifts, brow lifts and eyelid surgery
— Liposuction and body lifts: tummy tucks, thigh lifts and buttocks lifts

Wishes for the future:
To remain enthusiastic about my work. To learn something new every day.
To remember that "doctor" means "teacher" and to educate my patients, my students, my fellow surgeons and, most importantly, myself. To take adequate time for family and leisure.

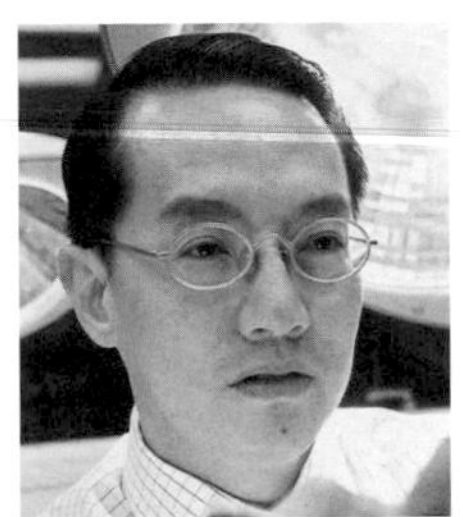

Dr. Woffles Wu

Woffles Wu Aesthetic Surgery and Laser Centre
Suite 09–02 Camden Medical Centre,
1 Orchard Boulevard,
SGP – Singapore 249 615
Tel: +65-6733-9771 / +65-9630-3686
Fax: +65-6733-2820
E-mail: woffles@woffleswu.com
www.woffleswu.com

Biography:
Born 2 February 1960. Married, two children.
1984 graduated with MBBS from Singapore University
1987 Medical officer in plastic surgery.
1989 FRCS (Edinburgh).
1992 Finished plastic surgery training in Singapore under Prof. S. T. Lee. Cleft and aesthetic fellowships to Bangkok (Siriraj, Chulalongkorn, Ramathibodi and Bumrungrad Hospitals) and Tokyo (in 1991).
1992–1993 Craniofacial fellow at Royal Children's Hospital, Melbourne under Anthony D. Holmes.
Numerous visits to clinics in the USA.
1994–1999 Craniofacial surgeon & head of Aesthetic Surgery Division, Department of Plastic Surgery, Singapore General Hospital.
Since 2000 aesthetic private practice.
Advanced Trainer for Botox and pioneer of Botox facial sculpting, masseteric reduction, brow lifting and Mesobotox (microBotox) for skin tightening and lifting.
Pioneer of the Woffles Lift non-surgical face lifting system using patented Woffles Threads, allowing for rapid recovery and natural results.
Young Surgeon's Award 1991 presented at the 25th Annual Combined Surgical Meeting (Silver Jubilee), Singapore, Nov 1991, for the Best Research Paper entitled: "The Oriental Nose: An Anatomical Basis for Surgery".
SEAMIC/IMFJ Travel Research Award 1991—travel scholarship awarded for the best proposal for a basic research/epidemiological study on cleft lip repair in ASEAN—Nov/Dec 1991

Publications:
"Barbed Sutures in Facial Rejuvenation" *Aesthetic Surgery Journal* 2004; 24: pp. 582–587.
"The Oriental Nose: An Anatomical Basis for Surgery" *Annals Academy of Medicine*, 1992; 21: pp. 176–189
Many appearances in over 250 magazines, journals and newspaper articles and television interviews

Societies:
— *International Society of Aesthetic Plastic Surgery (ISAPS)*
— *Singapore Association of Plastic Surgeons (SAPS)*
— *Cosmetic Surgery Society of Singapore (CSSS)*
— Associate member of *American Society of Plastic Surgeons (ASPS)*

Key aspects of activity:
— Aesthetic facial surgery, skin care and body contouring surgery
— Non-surgical facial rejuvenation using the 4R principle: Botox to relax facial muscles, contour jawline, create brow lift effect and refine pore size and skin texture; Fillers for volume restoration; IPL / Thermage for skin quality; Woffles Lift and Aptos for skin redraping
— Scarless upper (suture technique) and lower transconjunctival lid surgery with fat repositioning
— Facial contouring with implants, autogenous fat grafts and synthetic fillers
— Composite rhinoplasties using silastic dorsal implants and cartilage graft tips
— MACS, Minimal Access Cranial Suspension facelifts and multiplane facelifts
— The 20-minute facelift and neck lift: The Woffles Lift with Woffles Barbed Sutures
— The WW Stealth – Invisible Scar Breast Augmentation Refinement
— High-volume liposuction HVL using the STARS rotary power assisted system

Wishes for the future:
To push the envelope of Non-Surgical Facial Rejuvenation and the creation of the beautiful face, never to stop in the pursuit of Beauty and Youth, to see more of the world and understand more about human nature, to start a Modern Art Museum, to play more squash, to raise a decent family

whose members can contribute to the world and to find the elixir of youth so that I can remain vibrant and vital till well over 100 years old!

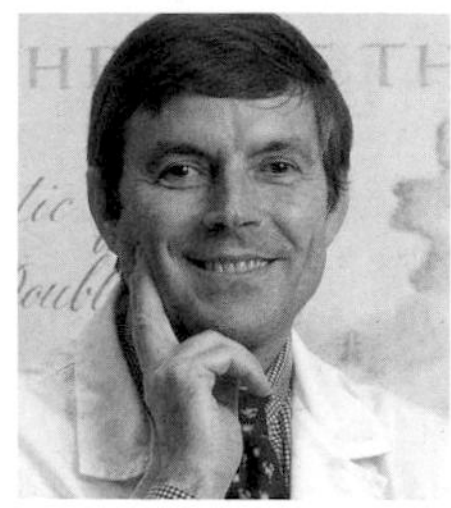

Dr. Christoph Wolfensberger
Bodmerstrasse 2
CH – 8002 Zurich
Tel: +41-1-202 72 32
Fax: +41-1-202 43 53
E-mail: christoph.wolfensberger@bluewin.ch
www.facelifting.ch

Biography:
Born 19 January 1946. Married.
1964 student of medicine at Neuchâtel University and in Zurich.
1972 doctor at Zurich Medical Faculty. Assistant doctor at the Altein lung sanatorium in Arosa.
1972–1978 trains as a surgeon at the Clinic of Orthopaedics and Traumatology at the St. Gallen Canton Hospital and at the surgical clinic of the Lucerne Canton Hospital. Appointed senior physician.
1979–1987 trains as a specialist in plastic, reconstructive and aesthetic surgery including hand surgery, microsurgery, replant surgery and free tissue transplantation at Berufsgenossenschaftliches Unfallkrankenhaus Hamburg, Department of Plastic, Reconstructive and Hand Surgery; Aarau Canton Hospital (Switzerland), Plastic and Reconstructive Surgery Clinic, where he is appointed senior physician; Bellevue Clinic for Aesthetic Surgery, Zurich; and the Plastic and Reconstructive Surgery Clinic at the Technical University of Munich.
Study visits to the USA, including the Jewish Hospital Louisville, Kentucky, Hand and Reconstructive Surgery Clinic and the Plastic Surgery Clinics of the Manhattan Eye, Ear & Throat Hospital, New York.
1984 receives Spezialarztdiplom FMH (Swiss specialist certificate) for Plastic, Reconstructive and Aesthetic Surgery.
1988–present private practice in Zurich and visiting physician at the Clinic im Park and at the Swissana Clinic, Zurich-Schwerzenbach.
With his increasing focus on aesthetic plastic surgery, he has been a frequent guest speaker at international congresses, and has had regular further training in the USA, South America and Europe

Societies:
— *Society for Plastic, Reconstructive and Aesthetic Surgery* (Switzerland)
— *International Society of Aesthetic Plastic Surgery (ISAPS)*
— *International Consortium of Aesthetic Plastic Surgeons (ICAPS)*
— *American Society of Plastic Surgeons (ASPS)* (Corresponding Member)
— *Société Française des Chirurgiens Esthétiques Plasticiens)* (Foreign Member)
— *German Society of Anti-Aging Medicine (GSAAM)*

Publications:
Regular publications in specialist literature, most recently: "Die Prehairline Incision in der zervikofazialen Rhytidektomie" ("The pre-hairline incision in a cervicofacial rhytidectomy") in G. Lemperle, *Handbuch für Ästhetische Chirurgie*. Landsburg: Ecomed, 2004
Currently working on: "Das volumetrische Facelifting" ("Volumetric Face Lifting") a textbook chapter commissioned by Springer Publishers in 2005

Key aspects of activity:
— Aesthetic plastic facial surgery with all modern facelifting techniques, including endoscopy, rhinoplasty, laser resurfacing, various peeling methods, dermabrasion, fat grafting and Botox injections, as well as body-shaping aesthetic surgery (body contouring, breast surgery, liposuction, body-lifting surgery)
— His practice has its own Day Spa for medical skin care and endermology, IPL skin rejuvenation and high-frequency radiosurgery as well as anti-aging medicine
— The practice also has an information center about aesthetic surgery with video/DVD-assisted patient counseling

Addresses of the interviewed surgeons – Europe

Norway

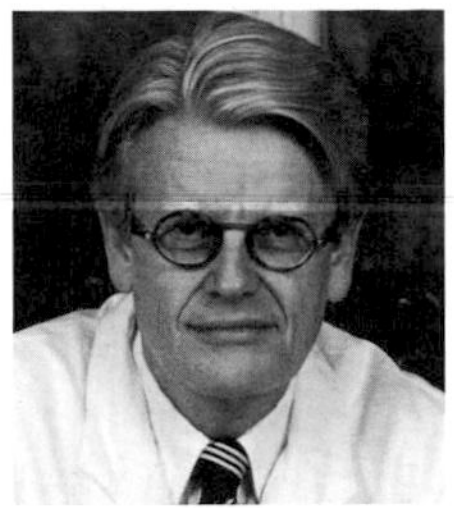

Dr. Morten H. Rynning Kveim
Smestadyn 1
N – Oslo, 0376
Tel: +47-22-139 520
Fax: +47-22-139 529
E-mail: kveim@online.no

Great Britain

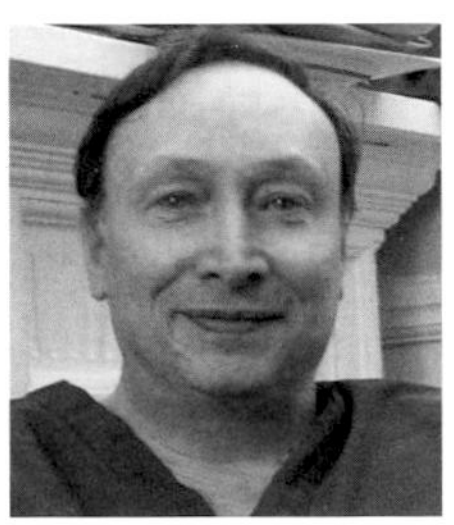

Prof. Dr. John F. Celin
Clinical Associated Professor of Surgery
University of Virginia School of Medicine
19 Wimpole Street
GB – London W1G 8GE
Tel: +44-207-636 6161
Fax: +44-207-636 8181
E-Mail: celinjohn@aol.com

Dr. Dai M. Davies
55 Harley Street
GB – London W1G 8QR
and
Institute of Cosmetic and Reconstructive Surgery
West London Clinic, The Wakefield Centre,
Ravenscourt Gardens, Ravenscourt Park,
GB – London W6 0AE
Tel: +44-207-462 0030
E-mail: enquiries@renascence.co.uk
www.renascence.co.uk

Dr. Barry M. Jones
14a Upper Wimpole Street
GB – London W1G 6LR
Tel: + 44-207-935 1938
Fax: + 44-207-935 6607
E-mail: bmj@barrymjones.co.uk

Dr. Jean-Louis Sebagh
French Cosmetic Clinic
25 Wimpole Street
GB – London W1
Tel: + 44-207-637 0548
Fax: + 44-207-637 5110
E-Mail: doctor@frenchcosmetic.com

Germany

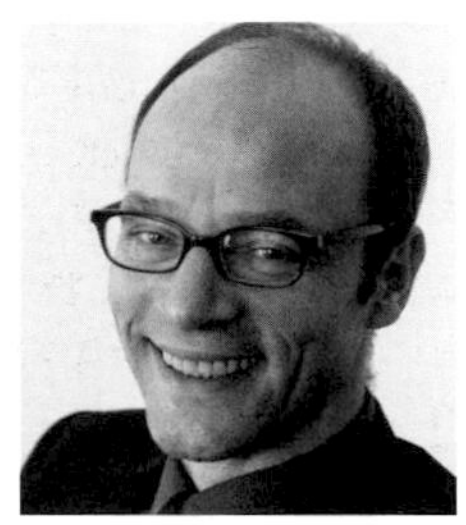

Dr. Bernhard Brinkmann
Mund-Kiefer-Gesichtschirurgie
Kollaustr. 239
DE – 22 453 Hamburg Fuhlsbüttel
Tel: +49-40-589 7789 0

Dr. Dr. Johannes C. Bruck
Martin-Luther-Krankenhaus
Abt. f. Plastische Chirurgie
Caspar-Theyß-Str. 27–31
DE – 14 193 Berlin
Tel: +49-30-895 525 11
Fax: + 49-30-895 525 15
E-mail: bruck.pc@t-online.de

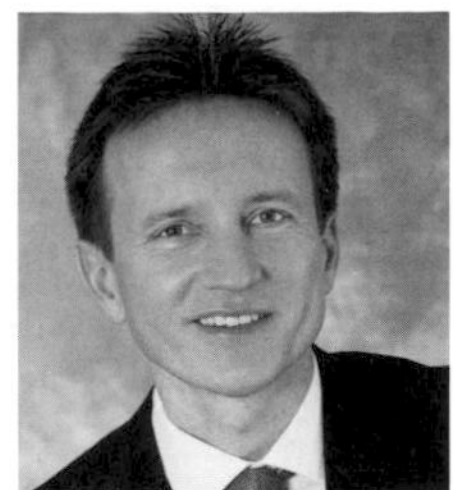

Dr. Stefan Duve
Perusastr. 5
DE – 80 333 Munich
Tel: +49-89-260 224 42
Fax: +49-89-268 792
E-mail: praxis@laser-haut-center.de
www.laser-haut-center.de

Dr. Serdar Eren
Im MediaPark 3
DE – 50 670 Cologne
Tel: +49-221-979 7888
Fax: +49-221-979 79880
E-mail: dr-eren@dr-eren.de
www.dr-eren.de

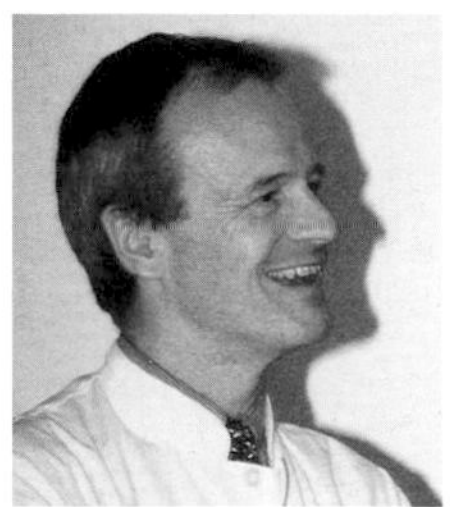

Prof. Dr. Dr. Axel-Mario Feller
Maximilianstr. 38–40
DE – 80 539 Munich
Tel: +49-89-211 130 0
Fax: +49-89-211 130 29
E-mail: a. m.feller@professor-feller.de
www.professor-feller.de

Dr. Thomas Klosterhalfen
Viamedic
Maximilianstr. 36
DE – 80539 Munich
Tel: +49-89-24 44 2000
Fax: +49-89-24 44 2001
E-Mail: doc@viamedic.de

Prof. Dr. Werner L. Mang
Bodenseeklinik Lindau
Clinic for Plastic and Aesthetic Surgery
Unterer Schrannenplatz 1
DE – 88 131 Lindau
Tel: +49-8382-5094
Fax: +49-8382-28 932
E-mail: info@bodenseeklinik.de
www.bodenseeklinik.de

Dr. Hans-Leo Nathrath
Arabella Str. 5
DE – 81 925 Munich
Tel: +49-89-919 110
Fax: +49-89-919 112
E-mail: nathrath@plast-arabella.com
www.plastische-chirurgie-muenchen.de
www.dr-nathrath.de

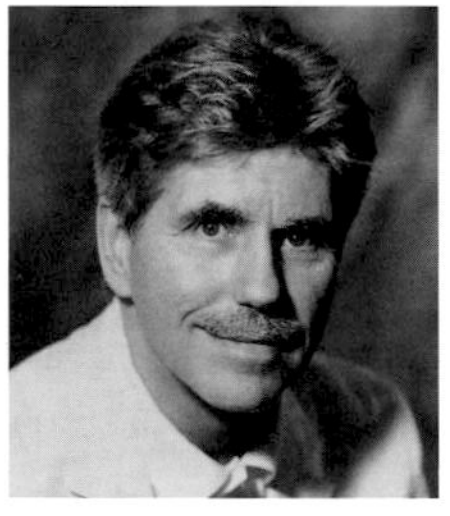

Dr. Axel Neuroth
Schönheitschirurgie
Kaiserswerther Str. 140–144
DE – 40 474 Düsseldorf
Tel: +49-211-453 525
Fax: +49-211-452 000
E-mail: info@vip-klinik.de
www.vip-klinik.de

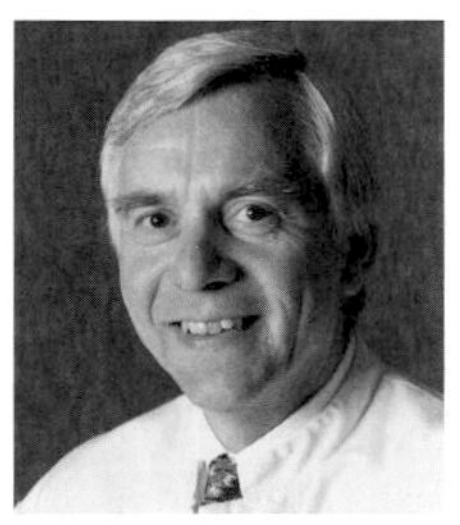

Prof. Dr. Rolf-Rüdiger Olbrisch
Klinik für Plastische und Ästethische Chirurgie
Kreuzbergstr. 79
DE – 40489 Düsseldorf
Tel: +49-211-409 25 22
Fax: +49-211-409 26 22
E-mail: olbrisch@fuk.de

Austria

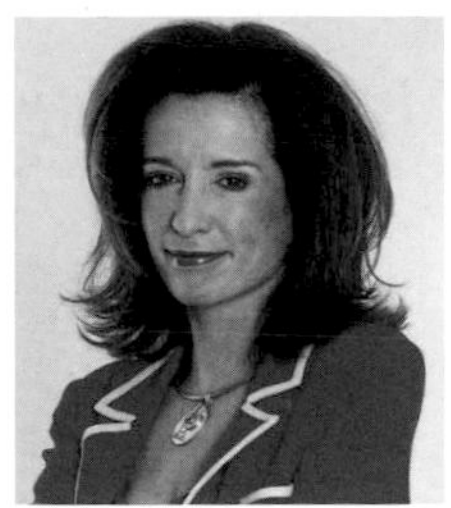

Dr. Dagmar Millesi
Naglergasse 9
A – 1010 Wien
Tel: +43-1-533 26 70
E-mail: dagmar@millesi.com
www.millesi.com

Switzerland

Dr. Carlo Gasperoni
Ars Medica Clinic
Via Cantonale
CH – 6929 Lugano-Gravesano
Tel: +41-91-6116211
Fax: +41-91-6051559
Dir: +41-91-6116161
E-mail: info@carlogasperoni.ch
www.carlogasperoni.ch

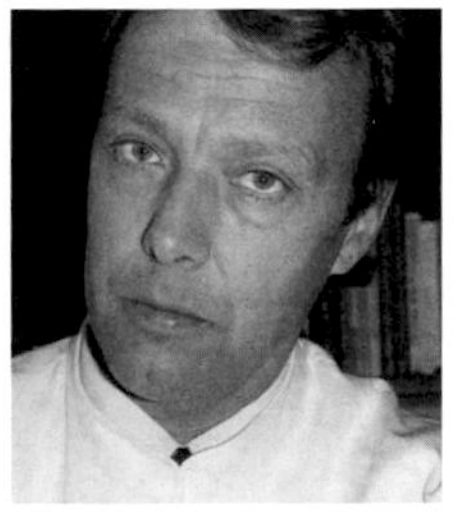

Dr. Ulrich K. Kesselring
Avenue Marc-Dufour 4
CH – 1007 Lausanne
Tel: +41-21-311 23 76
Fax: +41-21-311 16 08
E-mail: plaesthethics@bluewin.ch

Dr. Christoph Wolfensberger
Bodmerstr. 2
CH – 8002 Zurich
Tel: + 41-1-202 72 32
Fax: +41-1-202 43 53
E-mail: christoph.wolfensberger@bluewin.ch
www.facelifting.ch

France

Dr. Bernard Cornette de Saint Cyr
15, Rue Spontini
F – 75 116 Paris
Tel: +33-1-470 425 02
Fax: +33-1-470 460 66
E-mail: bdesaintcyr@hotmail.com
www.cornettedesaintcyr.com

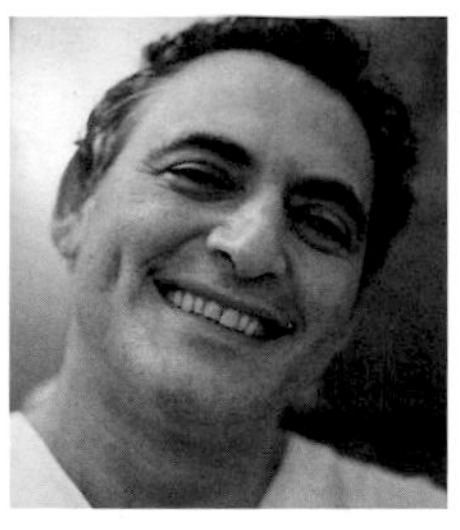

Dr. Jean-Louis Sebagh
64, Rue de Longchamp
F – 75 116 Paris
Tel: + 33-1-470 465 75
Fax: +33-1-455 345 18
E-Mail: doctor@frenchcosmetic.com

Spain

Dr. Javier de Benito
12, Marquesa de Vilallonga
E – 08 017 Barcelona
Tel: +34-93-253 0282
Fax: +34-93-253 0283
E-mail: debenitoworld@terra.es
www.institutodebenito.com

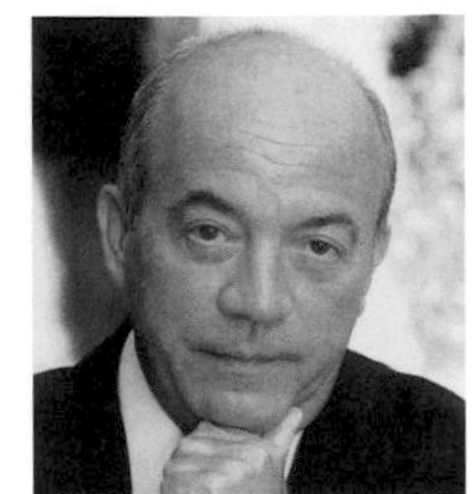

Dr. Antonio Tapia
Balmes, 203, 4°
E – 08 006 Barcelona
Tel: +34-932-376 643
Fax: +34-934-151 262
E-mail: info@drtapia.com
www.drtapia.com

Italy

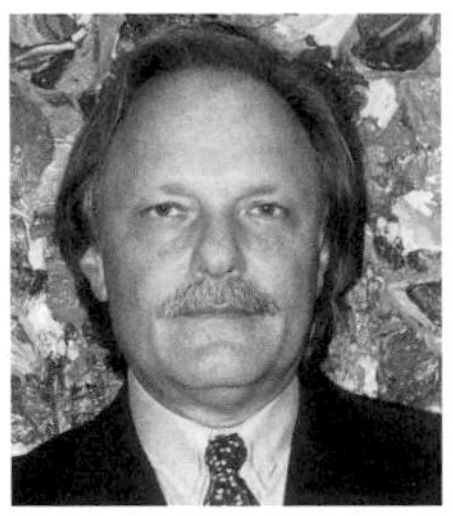

Dr. Carlo Gasperoni
Clinica Quisisana
Via Gian Giacomo Porro 5
I – 00197 Rome
Tel: +39-06-8088513
Fax: +39-06-8073348
E-mail: cgasperoni@hotmail.com

Dr. Egle Muti
Piazza Maria Teresa2
I – 10 123 Turin
Tel: +39-011-883 619
Fax: +39-011-883 619
E-mail: eglemu@tin.it

Turkey

Associate Professor Ismail Kuran
Halaskargazi cad. 340/2 Şişli
TR – Istanbul
Tel: +90-53-2322 0598
Fax: +90-21-2224 2528
E-mail: ikuran@tnt.net
www.kuranestetik.com

Middle East

Prof. Alaa El Din Gheita
12, Hassan Sabry street, Zamalek
EG – 111 211 Cairo
Tel: +20-2-7367 734
Tel: +20-2-7367 734
E-mail: Gheita@link.net

Dr. Ali Al-Numairy
Medical Director
Gulf Plastic Surgery Hospital
P.O. Box: 111 178
AE – Dubai
Tel: +971-4-269 9717
Fax: +971-4-268 1771
E-mail: numairy@emirates.net.ae
www.gulfplasticsurgery.com

USA

Dr. Gary J. Alter
416 North Bedford Drive, Suite 400
USA – Beverly Hills, CA 90 210
Tel: +1-310-275 5566
Fax: +1-310-271 0521
E-mail: altermd@earthlink.net
www.altermd.com
www.garyaltermd.com

Dr. Sherrell J. Aston
728 Park Avenue
USA – New York, NY 10 021
Tel: +1-212-249 600 0
Fax: +1-212-249 600 2
E-mail: sjaston@sjaston.com

Dr. Sydney R. Coleman
44 Hudson Street
US A – New York, NY 10 021
Tel: +1-212-571 5200
Fax: +1-212-571 5255
E-mail: lipostructure@yahoo.com

Dr. Alan M. Engler
122 East 64th Street
USA – New York, NY 10 021
Tel: +1-212-308 7000
Fax: +1-212-308 7094
E-mail: dralanengler@aol.com
www.bodysculpture.com

Dr. Steven M. Hoefflin
1530 Arizona Avenue
USA – Santa Monica, CA 90 404
Tel: +1-310-451 4733
Fax: +1-310-451 5653
E-mail: steven@hoefflin.com
www.hoefflin.com

Dr. Norman Orentreich
Orentreich Medical Group, LLP
909 Fifth Avenue
USA – New York, NY 10 021
Tel: +1-212-794 0800
Fax: +1-212-794 62 63
E-mail: info@orentreich.com
www.orentreich.com

Dr. Gerald H. Pitman
170 East 73rd Street
USA – New York, NY 10 021
Tel: +1-212-517 2600
Fax: +1-212-628 0774
E-mail: drpitman@drpitman.com
www.drpitman.com

Latin America

Prof. Juarez Avelar
620 Alameda Gabriel Monteiro da Silva
BR – SP 01 442–000 Jardim Europa, São Paulo
Tel: +55-11-3085 4211
Fax: +55-11-3088 1993
E-mail: juarezavelar@bol.com.br

Dr. Jorge Herrera
1346 J. E.Uriburu
RA – Buenos Aires
Tel: +54-11-4822 2014
Fax: +54-11-4804 0165
E-mail: jherrera@sminter.com.ar

Dr. Ivo Pitanguy
Ivo Pitanguy Clinic
65, Rua Dona Mariana
BR – 22280-02 Botafogo/ Rio de Janeiro
Tel: +55-21-253 75 812
Fax: +55-21-253 90 314
E-mail: pitanguy@visualnet.com.br
www.pitanguy.com.br

Asia

Dr. Keizo Fukuta
Verite Clinic
3F New Ginza Building, 5-5-7 Ginza Chuo-ku
J – Tokyo 104–0061
Tel: +81-3-3 573 0333
Fax: +81-3-6 253 8588
E-mail: fukuta@veriteclinic.com
www.veriteclinic.com

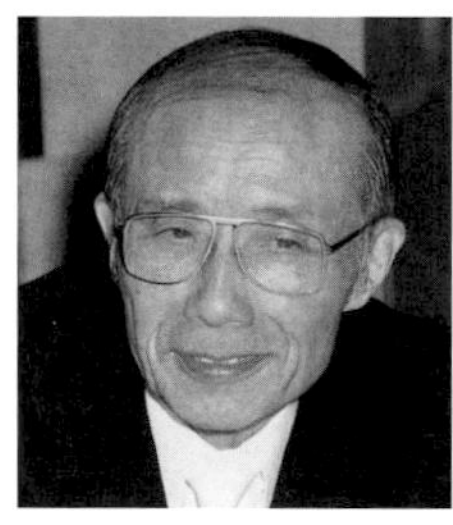

Dr. Kiyotaka Watanabe
Tokyo Seven Bell Clinic
9F Watanabe Building
1-1-18 Higashi Shinbashi Minato-ku
J – Tokyo 105–0021
Tel: +81-3-3 572 3719
Fax: +81-3-3 289 2577
E-mail: sevenbell@e-mail.ne.jp

Dr. Woffles Wu
Woffles Wu Aesthetic Surgery and Laser Centre
Suite 09–02 Camden Medical Centre,
1 Orchard Boulevard,
SGP – Singapore 249 615
Tel: +65-6733 9771
Fax: +65-6733 2820
E-mail: woffles@woffleswu.com
www.woffleswu.com

The editor:
Angelika Taschen studied art history and German literature in Heidelberg, gaining her doctorate in 1986. Working for TASCHEN since 1987, she has published numerous titles on the themes of architecture, photography, design, and contemporary art.

The authors:
Sander L. Gilman is distinguished professor of the Liberal Arts and Sciences at Emory University, Atlanta. A cultural and literary historian, he is the author or editor of over 70 books. His widely reviewed monograph *Fat Boys: A Slim Book* appeared in 2004, as well as his most recent edited volume, *Smoke: A Global History of Smoking* (with Zhou Xun). He is also the author of *Creating Beauty to Cure the Soul: Race and Psychology in the Shaping of Aesthetic Surgery* (1998) and *Making the Body Beautiful: A Cultural History of Aesthetic Surgery* (1999). **Eva Karcher** has been working in journalism for the past 15 years, specialising in contemporary arts. She lives in Munich and regularly writes for magazines and newspapers including *Vogue*, *Focus*, *Bunte*, *AD*, *SZ*, *Die Zeit*, and *Der Tagesspiegel*. She has published several books, and developed new magazine concepts for *artinvestor* and *sleek*, for example. She also curates exhibitions and is an art consultant for galleries, companies and private collectors. **Jürgen Müller** studied art history in Bochum, Paris, Pisa, and Amsterdam. He has worked as an art critic, a curator of numerous exhibitions, a visiting professor at various universities, and has published books and numerous articles on cinema and art history. Currently he holds the chair of Art History at the University of Dresden, where he lives. Müller is also the series editor of TASCHEN's *Movies* decade titles. **Richard Rushfield** is a native Los Angeles journalist. He is founder and co-editor of the satirical review *The LA Innuendo*, a contributing editor of *Vanity Fair* and author of the novel *On Spec*. His is currently working on a history of the Grunge Era.

Keep abreast of upcoming TASCHEN titles and request our magazine at www.taschen.com, or write to TASCHEN America, 6671 Sunset Boulevard, Suite 1508, USA–Los Angeles, CA 90028, Fax: +1-323-463.4442. We're happy to send you a free copy of our magazine packed with information about all our books.

Hohenzollernring 53, D–50672 Köln
www.taschen.com

Idea, Concept and Editing: Angelika Taschen, Berlin
Design: Sense/Net, Andy Disl and Birgit Reber, Cologne
General Project Management:
Stephanie Bischoff, Cologne
Captions for all chapters, excluding chapter V.:
Christiane Reiter, Berlin
English Translation:
Johannes Contag for English Express, Berlin
Coordination for typesetting:
Kirsten E. Lehmann, Cologne
Lithography: Horst Neuzner, Cologne

Cover:
David LaChapelle: *Makeover – The Plastic Surgery Story*, 1997.

Printed in Italy
ISBN 3-8228-3003-8